Macrocycles in Drug Discovery

RSC Drug Discovery Series

Editor-in-Chief:
Professor David Thurston, *King's College, London, UK*

Series Editors:
Professor David Rotella, *Montclair State University, USA*
Professor Ana Martinez, *Medicinal Chemistry Institute-CSIC, Madrid, Spain*
Dr David Fox, *Vulpine Science and Learning, UK*

Advisor to the Board:
Professor Robin Ganellin, *University College London, UK*

Titles in the Series:
1: Metabolism, Pharmacokinetics and Toxicity of Functional Groups
2: Emerging Drugs and Targets for Alzheimer's Disease; Volume 1
3: Emerging Drugs and Targets for Alzheimer's Disease; Volume 2
4: Accounts in Drug Discovery
5: New Frontiers in Chemical Biology
6: Animal Models for Neurodegenerative Disease
7: Neurodegeneration
8: G Protein-Coupled Receptors
9: Pharmaceutical Process Development
10: Extracellular and Intracellular Signaling
11: New Synthetic Technologies in Medicinal Chemistry
12: New Horizons in Predictive Toxicology
13: Drug Design Strategies: Quantitative Approaches
14: Neglected Diseases and Drug Discovery
15: Biomedical Imaging
16: Pharmaceutical Salts and Cocrystals
17: Polyamine Drug Discovery
18: Proteinases as Drug Targets
19: Kinase Drug Discovery
20: Drug Design Strategies: Computational Techniques and Applications
21: Designing Multi-Target Drugs
22: Nanostructured Biomaterials for Overcoming Biological Barriers
23: Physico-Chemical and Computational Approaches to Drug Discovery
24: Biomarkers for Traumatic Brain Injury
25: Drug Discovery from Natural Products
26: Anti-Inflammatory Drug Discovery
27: New Therapeutic Strategies for Type 2 Diabetes: Small Molecules
28: Drug Discovery for Psychiatric Disorders
29: Organic Chemistry of Drug Degradation
30: Computational Approaches to Nuclear Receptors
31: Traditional Chinese Medicine

How to obtain future titles on publication:
A standing order plan is available for this series. A standing order will bring delivery of each new volume immediately on publication.

For further information please contact:
Book Sales Department, Royal Society of Chemistry, Thomas Graham House, Science Park, Milton Road, Cambridge, CB4 0WF, UK
Telephone: +44 (0)1223 420066, Fax: +44 (0)1223 420247,
Email: booksales@rsc.org
Visit our website at www.rsc.org/books

Macrocycles in Drug Discovery

Edited by

Jeremy Levin
Email: Jeremy.Levin@boehringer-ingelheim.com
Boehringer Ingelheim, Connecticut, USA

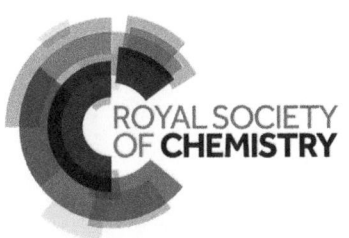

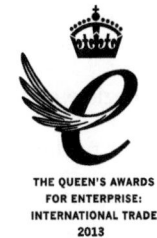

RSC Drug Discovery Series No. 40

Print ISBN: 978-1-84973-701-2
PDF eISBN: 978-1-78262-311-3
ISSN: 2041-3203

A catalogue record for this book is available from the British Library

Published by The Royal Society of Chemistry,
Thomas Graham House, Science Park, Milton Road,
Cambridge CB4 0WF, UK

Registered Charity Number 207890

For further information see our web site at www.rsc.org

Preface

Macrocycles are an exceptionally interesting structural class of small molecules with proven therapeutic value that have been the subject of medicinal chemistry research for many years. The increasing effort devoted to the design and synthesis of macrocyclic molecules in both academic and industrial drug discovery programmes, with exciting developments in understanding the determinants of properties such as potency, selectivity, permeability and bioavailability for these molecules, as well as advances in the synthetic methodologies that provide access to them, has provided the impetus for the construction of this volume.

It is the goal of this book to bring together scientific experts, who have been directly involved in research to discover and develop drugs based on macrocyclic scaffolds, and afford them a forum to present the state of the art in their field including, in some cases, drugs with exciting potential that have advanced to clinical trials or to the market. It is my hope that the topics covered herein will provide essential background information on the genesis and evolution of macrocyclic compounds in drug discovery, as well as offering a sense of the promise of what this field may deliver in the future.

I would like to express my great appreciation to each of the chapter authors for the time and effort spent to write informative reviews on their respective areas of research. I would also like to express my appreciation to Professor David Rotella (Montclair State University), and Rosalind Searle, Helen Prasad and Rowan Frame at the Royal Society of Chemistry for their help, support and patience in the course of putting together this book.

Jeremy I. Levin

RSC Drug Discovery Series No. 40
Macrocycles in Drug Discovery
Edited by Jeremy Levin
© The Royal Society of Chemistry 2015
Published by the Royal Society of Chemistry, www.rsc.org

Acknowledgements

The editor would like to thank Anthony Slavin, John Proudfoot, Craig Miller, Ingo Mugge, Gene Hickey, Lee Fader, Philipp Emert, Edmund Graziani, Montse Llinas-Brunet, Maurizio Botta, Yongxin Han, Nathan Yee, Didier Picard, Tai Wang, Novak Predrag, Klaus Zangger, Ian Sayers, Manfred Jung, Jason Gestwicki, John Robinson, Ash Jogalekar and David Rotella for their prompt, thorough and thoughtful review of chapters in this volume. Thanks are also due to his family, Leslie Feiner, Hannah Levin and Lucy Levin, for their patience and support during the compilation of this volume.

RSC Drug Discovery Series No. 40
Macrocycles in Drug Discovery
Edited by Jeremy Levin
© The Royal Society of Chemistry 2015
Published by the Royal Society of Chemistry, www.rsc.org

Biography

Jeremy I. Levin has been a Director of Medicinal Chemistry for Boehringer-Ingelheim in Ridgefield, Connecticut, since 2010. He received his BA from Johns Hopkins University in 1978 and a PhD in organic chemistry with Professor Steven Weinreb at the Pennsylvania State University in 1983. Following a post-doctoral fellowship at the University of California at Irvine with Professor Larry Overman, he spent 25 years in the pharmaceutical industry at American Cyanamid (Lederle laboratories) and Wyeth Research.

Dr Levin has worked in a variety of therapeutic areas including CNS, inflammation and immunology, and oncology. He is the author/co-author of more than 75 papers and an inventor on more than 60 US Patents.

RSC Drug Discovery Series No. 40
Macrocycles in Drug Discovery
Edited by Jeremy Levin
© The Royal Society of Chemistry 2015
Published by the Royal Society of Chemistry, www.rsc.org

Contents

RSC Drug Discovery Series No. 40
Macrocycles in Drug Discovery
Edited by Jeremy Levin
© The Royal Society of Chemistry 2015
Published by the Royal Society of Chemistry, www.rsc.org

Macrocycles in Drug Discovery: Introduction

It is the aim of this volume to explore the study of macrocycles in drug discovery, both those of natural origin and semi-synthetic derivatives of natural products, and those designed and synthesized based on principles of medicinal chemistry. Macrocyclic molecules, herein defined as molecules with rings of 12-members or larger, have figured prominently in the history of medicinal chemistry, with the most common source of these compounds being from natural products. In fact, numerous macrocycles have become important drugs or have been identified as leads to marketed drugs.

Of late, interest in macrocycles and their novel architectures has increased significantly as their potential for interacting with a variety of targets including kinases, ATPases, proteases, GPCRs and others has been recognized. Furthermore, as more non-classical drug targets, such as protein–protein interactions (PPIs), are pursued in the pharmaceutical industry, macrocyclic molecules have attracted significant attention since they offer the potential to provide drug–protein interactions that cover a larger surface area than traditional small molecules. This text will discuss the identification, optimization, pharmacology and synthesis of biologically active macrocyclic compounds in the context of their broad chemotype as compounds composed of large rings.

In the first chapter of this volume the wide variety of bioactive macrocyclic natural products is explored, including examples of those with clinically validated anti-infective and anti-tumor activity. Many of these natural products have been the subject of drug discovery efforts that have leveraged semi-synthesis, biosynthesis and total synthesis in order to investigate or optimize their pharmacological effects and viability as drugs. The medicinal

RSC Drug Discovery Series No. 40
Macrocycles in Drug Discovery
Edited by Jeremy Levin
© The Royal Society of Chemistry 2015
Published by the Royal Society of Chemistry, www.rsc.org

chemistry of these macrocyclic natural products is interesting in itself, but lessons learned from these compounds, particularly in terms of the relationship between structure and desirable physicochemical properties, are now informing and driving the design of fully synthetic macrocyclic drug candidates.

Macrocyclic inhibitors of the chaperone protein Hsp90 are the subject of the second chapter. This ATPase is an important oncology target against which a variety of macrocyclic scaffolds have demonstrated activity, including the natural products geldanamycin and radicicol, and their derivatives, as well as fully synthetic, designed macrocyclic aminobenzamide derivatives, all of which bind to the *N*-terminal ATP binding domain. In this case structural information gathered on the binding of the natural products to Hsp90 was important for guiding the design of the fully synthetic macrocyclic inhibitors. Macrocyclic inhibitors of the Hsp90 *N*-middle domain related to the penta-depsipeptide sansalvamide A are also known and discussed in this section.

The third chapter of the volume describes the *in vitro* and *in vivo* activity of the natural occurring microtubule stabilizer epothilone B and its analogs. This macrocyclic natural product has been the subject of extensive medicinal chemistry research and numerous derivatives have been studied preclinically and clinically for oncology indications. One such compound, ixabepilone (BMS-247550; Ixempra®) was approved by the FDA in 2007 for the treatment of breast cancer.

Chapters 4 and 5 are also focused on macrocycles with potential utility as anti-cancer therapeutics. Thus, Chapter 4 describes drug discovery efforts directed at the identification of inhibitors of a family of zinc-dependent enzymes known as histone deacetylases (HDACs). Interestingly, a variety of macrocyclic natural product HDAC inhibitors are known, including cyclic peptides and depsipeptides with a diverse set of zinc-binding warheads, as well as fully synthetic inhibitors. This epigenetic target has afforded two FDA approved inhibitors as oncology therapeutics, one an acyclic hydroxamic acid derivative and the second a macrocyclic disulfide natural product, FK228, that undergoes reductive ring cleavage to reveal the active species bearing a thiol zinc chelator.

The search for macrocyclic kinase inhibitors is detailed in Chapter 5, starting from macrocyclic bisindolylmaleimide analogs of staurosporine, the initial foray into this area thirty years ago by chemists at Lilly in search of novel protein kinase C inhibitors, to more recent drug discovery efforts into potent inhibitors of CDKs, JAK2 and FLT3, among other kinases, driven by structure-based design. The rational design of macrocyclic kinase inhibitors with desirable, indication-specific, kinase selectivity profiles and oral bioavailability has been particularly exciting and has yielded several molecules now in clinical trials for the treatment of cancer and rheumatoid arthritis.

The sixth chapter of this volume explores the use of macrolides, macrocyclic lactone polyketide natural products best known for their antibacterial activity, for their anti-inflammatory activity. The propensity for these molecules, exemplified by azithromycin, to accumulate in inflamed tissue and polarize macrophages is discussed in detail. In addition, a creative and exciting drug discovery approach has been taken that investigates the ability of macrolides to act as carriers of small molecule payloads in order to transport them into immune cells. Thus, small molecule inhibitors with diverse biochemical targets including p38 kinase and lipoxygenase, as well as steroidal and non-steroidal anti-inflammatories, have been conjugated to macrolides and have demonstrated activity in *in vitro* assays and *in vivo* animal models of inflammatory disease and cancer.

The identification and optimization of macrocyclic molecules that inhibit a broad array of target classes such as proteases, G protein-coupled receptors (GPCRs), integrins and PPIs, is thoroughly reviewed in Chapters 7, 8 and 9. Chapter 7 focuses on providing background on the hugely important and competitive area of research surrounding the discovery and development of macrocyclic HCV protease inhibitors with multiple agents in clinical trials and progressing to the market. The concept of macrocyclization as applied to HCV protease inhibitors was driven by the seminal work from researchers at Boehringer-Ingelheim, and its translation into the optimization of boron-containing irreversible inhibitors of this enzyme is presented. This is followed by an extensive review in Chapter 8 of macrocycles that target GPCRs, both agonists and antagonists, integrin inhibitors and the rapidly expanding field of macrocyclic modulators of protein-protein interactions. That theme is further extended in Chapter 9 with a discussion of stapled peptides. These fascinating macrocyclic molecules are constructed to lock peptidic ligand molecules in an α-helical conformation, most often through the use of a hydrocarbon linker, for recognition by their targets. An extraordinary effort combining computational chemistry, structural biology, chemical biology and organic synthesis has enabled the evolution of this chemotype into one that can deliver stapled peptides with sufficient cell penetration and *in vivo* exposure to advance into the clinic, as is the case for the MDM2/MDMX antagonist ALRN-6924, being studied for the treatment of p53-dependent cancers.

This volume concludes with two chapters that describe efforts that will truly enable the expansion of the field of macrocyclic molecules for drug discovery and the treatment of disease. Chapter 10 covers ongoing efforts to understand the factors that affect the permeability and bioavailability of macrocyclic compounds and comes full circle with some of the natural products described in Chapter 1. Thus, the field of medicinal chemistry has, over the last 15 years in particular, focused on deciphering the relationship between the physical properties of a molecule and its oral bioavailability, since there is a great preference for small molecule drugs to have the convenience of oral dosing. With this in mind, the natural products that do not adhere to standard Rule of Five guidelines yet do display reasonable oral bioavailability have become the subject of intense scrutiny in an attempt to understand how and why they are able to be orally absorbed so that those principles can be applied to additional molecules outside of the Rule of Five space.

Finally, Chapter 11 provides the last piece in the puzzle for delivering macrocyclic molecules for drug discovery programs and advancing them into clinical trials and ultimately to the market for the benefit of patients. Therefore, in order to optimize macrocycles for potency against a target and pharmacokinetics, to make sufficient quantities to test in animal models of efficacy and toxicity, and to manufacture these materials on large scale for commercial use, one needs to be able to devise and execute practical, scalable routes for their synthesis. Chapter 11 provides an exhaustive survey of the methodologies that have been used to generate these molecules.

In summary, this volume covers a selection of the most active and promising areas of research ongoing in the discovery of macrocycles for therapeutic use and we hope it provides valuable insight into the challenges encountered and solved for this diverse class of molecules.

CHAPTER 1

Bioactive Macrocycles from Nature[†]

DAVID J. NEWMAN* AND GORDON M. CRAGG

Natural Products Branch, Developmental Therapeutics Program,
DCTD, NCI, Frederick National Laboratory, P. O. Box B, Frederick,
MD 21702, USA
*Email: dn22a@nih.gov

1.1   Introduction

Natural products have been an important source of pharmacologically active
molecules throughout the history of medicinal chemistry and a selection of
these molecules has advanced to provide clinically validated, marketed
therapeutics for numerous indications, most notably as antibiotics, im-
munosuppressives and anti-tumor agents. Among these, structurally diverse
and complex naturally derived macrocycles have demonstrated an impressive record of efficacy as pharmaceutical agents, and are playing an
increasingly important role in the treatment of a range of serious diseases.
These macrocycles have received intense recent interest from the medicinal
chemistry community driven in part by their activity in biological systems,
such as those mediated by protein–protein interactions, that are difficult to
prosecute with more typically drug-like small molecules. In addition, the
selectivity afforded by their complexity and the remarkable ability of some of
these macrocyclic natural products to provide significant systemic exposures

---

[†]The opinions expressed in this article are those of the authors, not necessarily those of the US
  Government.

RSC Drug Discovery Series No. 40
Macrocycles in Drug Discovery
Edited by Jeremy Levin
© The Royal Society of Chemistry 2015
Published by the Royal Society of Chemistry, www.rsc.org

on oral dosing despite physical properties that lie substantially outside of normal parameters for achieving oral bioavailability, make them an attractive chemical class. Thus, these macrocyclic natural products and related biosynthetically and semi-synthetically derived macrocycles are of great value not only for their own intrinsic pharmacological activity but also for their potential as tools used to understand how to design molecules with the properties necessary to produce highly effective therapeutics for the treatment of human disease.

Further testaments to the current level of focus on macrocycles in drug discovery are the excellent reviews published over the last five years on key aspects of the medicinal chemistry of this chemotype.[1–4] The most recent of these reviews, by Giordanetto and Kihlberg,[1] provides an analysis of the physical properties of macrocyclic drug molecules, including cLogP, polar surface area, hydrogen bond donor count and molecular weight, in relationship to their ability to be orally efficacious. In addition, in 2008, Driggers *et al.*[2] provided an excellent overview of macrocycles as drug leads and candidates at that time. This was followed by a review in 2011 by Marsault and Peterson[3] showing the use of macrocycles over a wide area of medicinal chemistry and, in 2012, a review from Mallinson and Collins focusing primarily on potential anticancer agents.[4]

In their 2014 review[1] Giordanetto and Kihlberg reported 68 registered macrocyclic drugs approved for human use (identified through mining of the GVK BIO online structure-activity relationship database (GOSTAR)), along with a set of 35 macrocyclic drug candidates in clinical development (identified using the Adis R&D Insight database). The latter set did not include compounds in early clinical trials whose structures were not in the public domain.[1] Most of these drugs, which have macrocyclic rings comprised of 12 or more atoms, fall into three chemical classes, namely macrolidic antibiotics, macrolides that have antitumor or immunological effects, and cyclic peptides that may or may not contain lactone (depsipeptide) linkages.

Of the 68 identified macrocyclic registered drugs,[1] 34 are used for the treatment of infections, mainly of bacterial origin, while 10 are used for the treatment of a variety of cancers; the remaining 28 are applied in cardio-vascular, gynecological and immunological therapeutic areas, as well as in a range of indications, including anesthesiology and pain (these numbers do not total 68 since some agents have two or more activities). The majority of these molecules are natural products or directly derived from natural products (48 and 18, respectively), while eribulin (*vide infra*) is totally synthetic but modeled on the marine natural product, halichondrin B, and Sugammadex is a modified γ-cyclodextrin. Nineteen of the 68 drugs are administered orally, with 15 of these belonging to the macrolide classes. The parenterally administered macrocyclic drugs include all of the cyclic peptides, with the exception of cyclosporin A which is orally delivered.

As with the registered drugs briefly discussed above, of the 35 macrocycles identified as agents in clinical development 14 are under investigation for the treatment of various cancers, 10 are in infectious disease trials, and the remaining 11 are under investigation for indications ranging from endocrinology to ophthalmology.[1] While these agents are also predominantly natural products (17) or natural product-derived molecules (8), with the largest chemical class being cyclic peptides (11), 10 of the clinical candidates are of *de novo* design. A total of 43% of these clinical candidates are administered orally, a significant increase over the 28% of all registered macrocyclic drugs that are orally administered, and nine of the 10 *de novo* designed macrocycles in trials are orally bioavailable. The increasing numbers of orally active macrocyclic drug candidates indicates that organic and medicinal chemists are learning to apply the lessons provided by bioactive natural macrocyclic agents, such as those presented in this chapter, for the design of fully synthetic molecules having desirable pharmacological properties, including oral bioavailability.

In strongly endorsing the impressive therapeutic record of natural product-derived macrocycles reported in earlier reviews and commentaries, the following sections will expand on the discussion of the macrocyclic chemical classes mentioned above, while adding a number of other chemical compounds that fall under the general description of "macrocycles" that have originated from plant and marine sources. Some of these compounds have arisen from the assessment of biosynthetic clusters that has led to the identification of novel agents, frequently not associated with the "expected" macro-organism source.

Also included are two short sections covering natural product macrocycles, which are described in detail in two later chapters of this volume. In the case of the ansamycin Hsp90 inhibitors, some of the very early work has been referenced, as the authors of this chapter were involved in the initial production of geldanamycin for the NCI's work with 17-AAG and 17-DMAG. This is followed by some current examples, where the manipulation of biosynthetic clusters in the producing bacteria has led to ansamycin structures that are completely novel and Hsp90 active. Similarly, with the epothilones, which are covered extensively in Chapter 3, particularly from a synthetic chemistry aspect, it is shown how genetic manipulation of the base-producing cluster and expressing it in heterologous hosts permitted the production of quantities of the four basic epothilones, and also materially aided in the utilization of myxobacteria as sources of novel agents, mainly *via* genomic techniques.

1.2 Macrolides and Peptide-based Bioactive Compounds

1.2.1 Non-Ansamycin Antibiotics (Anti-infective and Anti-tumor)

1.2.1.1 Actinomycins

It can be successfully argued that the discovery of the actinomycins by Waksman and Woodruff in 1940[5] led to at least two firsts: the first crystalline antibiotic and the first demonstration of anti-tumor activity (actinomycin C) *in vitro.*[6] This was followed by a report later in 1952 by Schulte demonstrating the first clinical studies with these agents.[7] Over the last 60 plus years, actinomycins, usually as actinomycin D (Figure 1.1, **1**), have been used as treatments for a variety of tumor types. Currently actinomycin D is used primarily for the treatment of rhabdomyosarcoma and Wilms' tumor in children and young adults, with a very recent example being its reported use in the treatment of a patient with uterine embryonal rhabdomyosarcoma,[8] 50 years after its formal launch in 1963.

Two major mechanisms of action, involving intercalation of DNA and stabilization of cleavable complexes of topoisomerases I and II with DNA, have been discussed in a review by Mauger and Lackner.[9] In 2003,

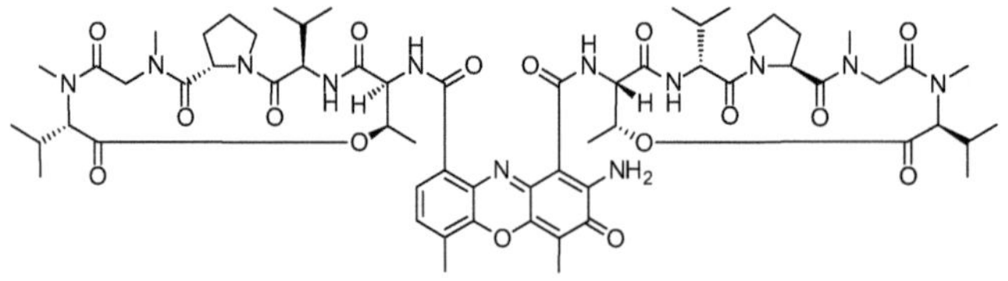

1. Actinomycin D

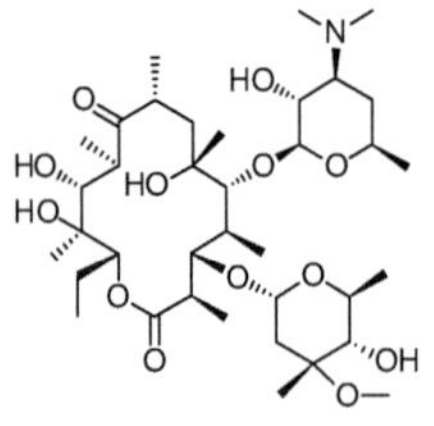

2. Erythromycin 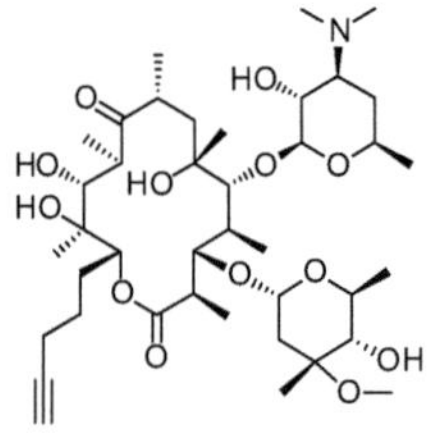   **3.** Propargyl-Derivative of 2 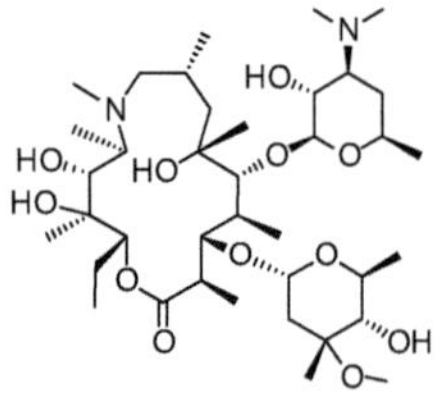   **4.** Azithromycin

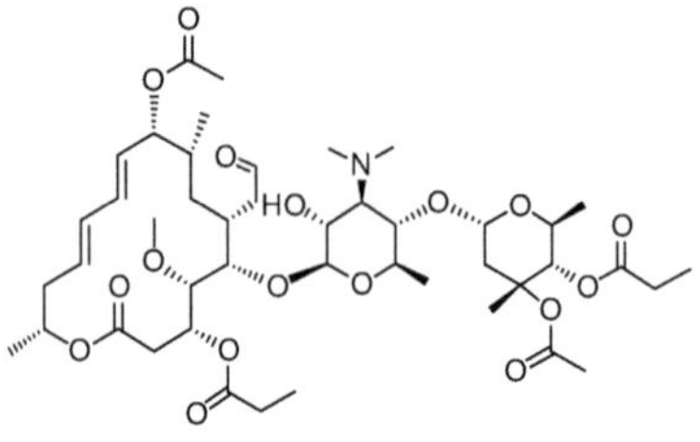

5. Midecamycin acetate 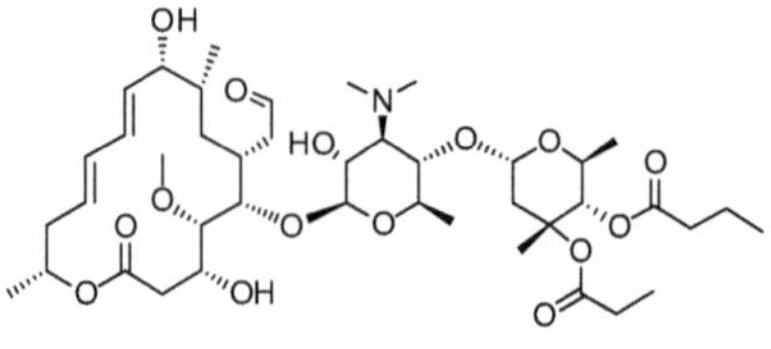   **6.** Rokitamycin

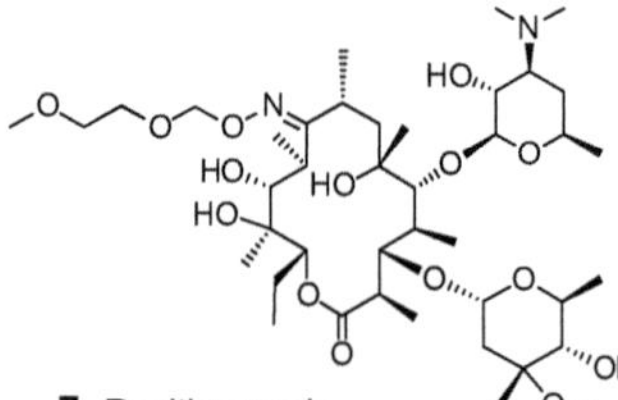

7. Roxithromycin 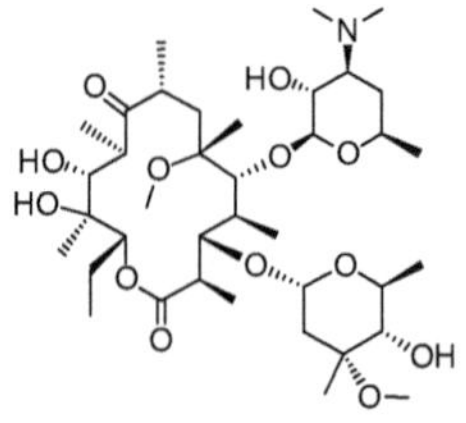   **8.** Clarithromycin

Figure 1.1 Structures **1** to **8**; Actinomycin D; Erythromycin and Early Derivatives.

Gniazdowski *et al.* reported that actinomycin D interacted with downstream proteins associated with transcription, and this activity appeared related to its DNA-intercalating ability, but at levels well below those demonstrating anti-tumor activity.[10] In contrast, in a recent review, Leung *et al.* did not confirm this earlier report but did show that another complex depsipetide, echinomycin demonstrated such activity at the transcription factor level (*vide infra*).[11] Studies reported in 2009 by Kang and Park showed that actinomycin D binds to oncogenic promoter G-quadruplex DNA repressing gene expression.[12] Formally, actinomycins can be considered as two separate depsipeptides (the macrocycles) linked *via* a phenoxazine nucleus with differing amino acids in the depsipeptides, depending upon the actinomycin variant in question. For a much fuller description of the history of actino-mycins, the significant chemical synthetic and semi-synthetic programs since its introduction and their activities, the 2012 review by Mauger and Lackner should be consulted.[9]

1.2.1.2 Erythromycin and Related Macrolides

Although not the first antibiotic to go into general clinical use, erythromycin (Figure 1.1, 2), which was introduced in 1952, was certainly the first of the bioactive macrolidic agents to become an anti-infective drug. Even today, 60 years later, variations, usually with a change in the salt form, are still in clinical trials, and the parent molecule has been almost a "poster child" for what could be done to follow the biosynthesis, initially by using radio-labeled production of the base aglycone, the macrolide erythronolide B[13] and then the work over many years by Abbott scientists and their successors in the production of variations of the base macrolide. These derivatives were prepared by biosynthetic manipulations as recombinant DNA technologies advanced, coupled to fundamental knowledge of how to manipulate gene clusters in antibiotic producing microbes. A large amount of the work using these techniques was performed by the now defunct Kosan, Inc., and modifications of the base structure using biosynthetic techniques to pro-duce what might best be called, un-natural natural products are still being published,[14] with the alkynyl substituted erythromycin (Figure 1.1, 3) being an excellent example.

Over the last 25 years, in addition to this type of biosynthetic process which has not yet led to an approved agent, a number of macrolide anti-biotics have been launched based upon the erythromycin core structure. In each case, the compounds were optimized to overcome problems with the parent molecule from an antibiotic perspective. These approved agents in-cluded the first azalide azithromycin (Figure 1.1, 4) launched in 1988, a long-acting agent that is now generic in the USA. Other approved drugs with the base erythronolide structure include midecamycin (Figure 1.1, 5) launched in 1985, rokitamycin (Figure 1.1, 6) in 1986, roxithromycin (Figure 1.1, 7) in 1987, clarithromycin (Figure 1.1, 8) in 1990, flurithromycin (Figure 1.2, 9) in 1997, dirithromycin (Figure 1.2, 10) in 1993, telithromycin, the first ketolide, (Figure 1.2, 11) in 2001, and fidaxomycin (Figure 1.2, 12) in 2011. In addition

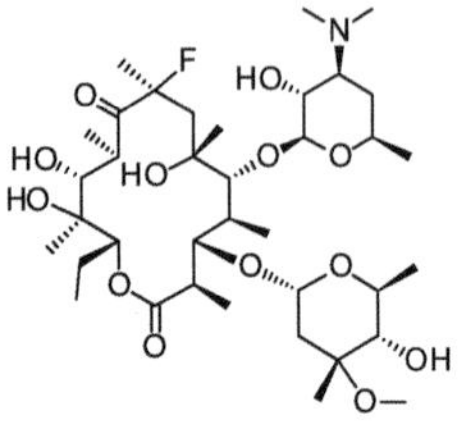

9. Flurithromycin 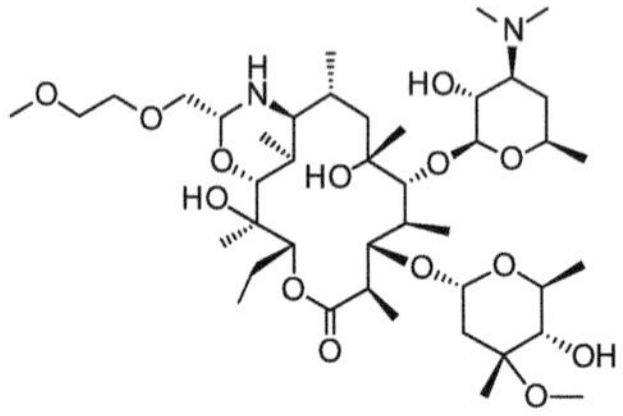   **10.** Dirithromycin

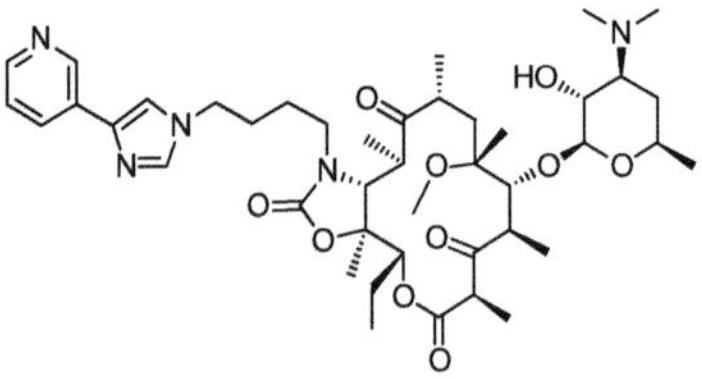

11. Telithromycin 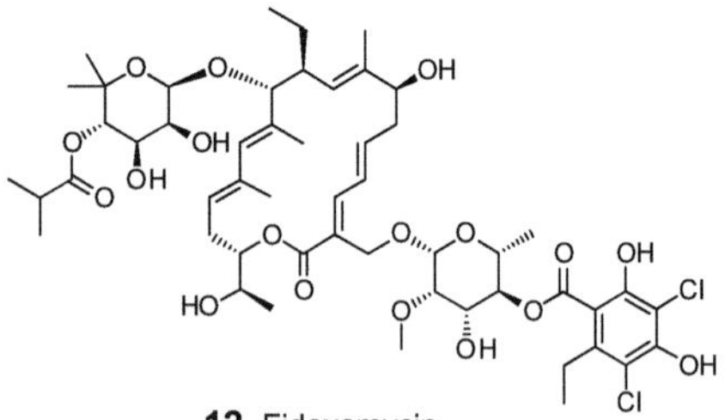   **12.** Fidaxomycin

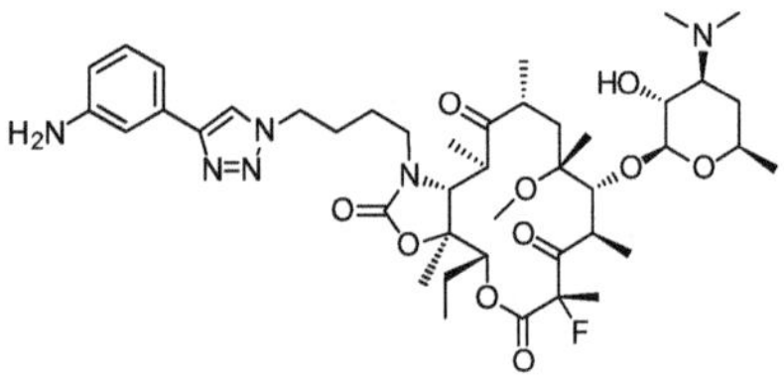

13. Solithromycin

Figure 1.2   Structures **9** to **13**; Later Erythromycin-based Derivatives.

to these, solithromycin (Figure 1.2, **13**) is now in Phase III clinical trials for the treatment of Community-acquired Bacterial Pneumonia (CaBP).

1.2.1.3   Synergistic Antibiotic Mixtures

In the 1960s and later, synergistic antibiotics that were mixtures of two macrolides, known collectively as streptogramins, were in use as agents to alter food uptake and metabolism, predominantly in ruminants. Following the advent of Gram positive resistant organisms, in particular methicillin resistant *Staphylococcus aureus* (MRSA), and the lack of suitable treatments for these and other more resistant Gram positive microbes in humans, these old compounds were used as templates for chemical modification, leading to the approval and subsequent launch in 1999 of the quinuprisitin (Figure 1.3, **14**)/dalfoprisitin (Figure 1.3, **15**) 1 : 1 mole ratio defined mixture under the name Synercid® in the USA. At this moment, another similar mixture of related compounds is in Phase II clinical trials with Novexel, using linopristine (Figure 1.3, **16**) and flopristine (Figure 1.3, **17**) as the components of the mixture.

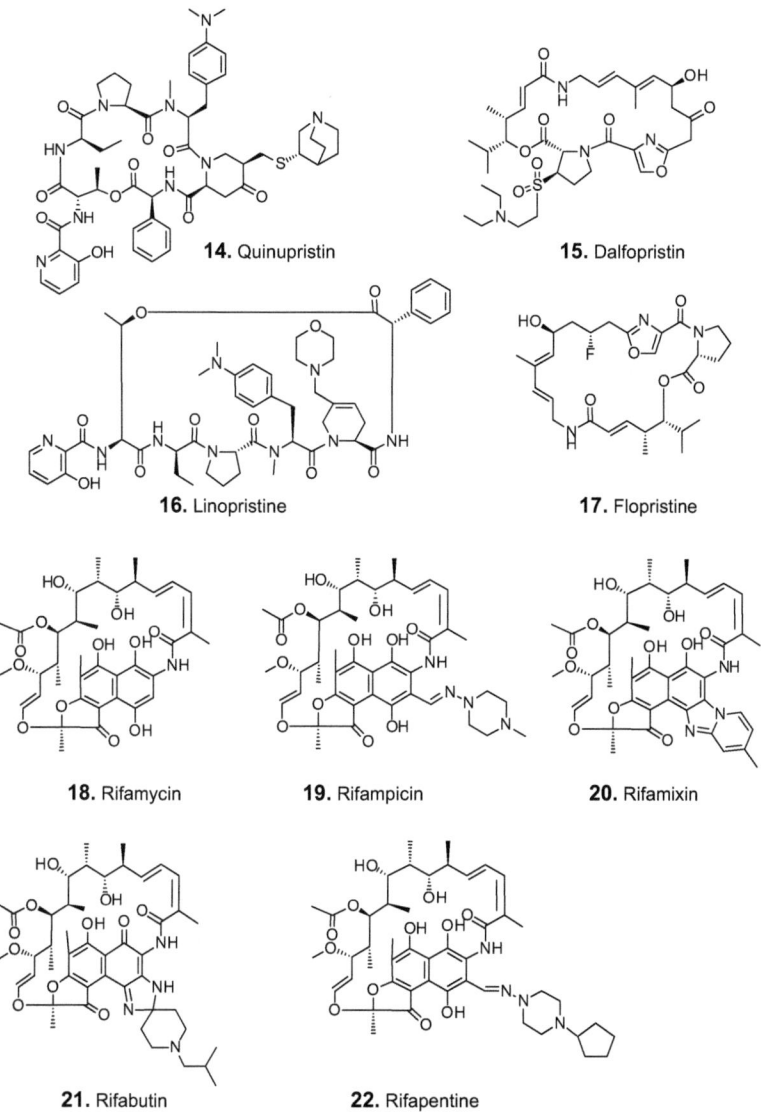

Figure 1.3 Structures **14** to **22**; Synergistic Antibiotic Pairs & Rifamycin-based Molecules.

1.3 Ansamycins (Antimycobacterial and Antibacterial)

1.3.1 Rifamycins

The base structure of the rifamycin class of macrocyclic antibiotics can be best thought of as a single or fused ring (usually two) linked within a larger macrolidic ring (Figure 1.3, **18**). The base molecule in this series was launched in the middle 1960s as an antimycobacterial (tuberculosis) agent, and in the intervening five decades, well over 300 variations on the structure have been reported as being in biological assessments ranging from *in vitro* testing, through clinical trials, to becoming approved drugs. A search of the Thomson–Reuters Integrity™ database in December 2013 showed 177 different compounds listed of similar structure, with 7 being shown as launched.

A relatively recent paper by Mariani and Maffioli[15] gives an excellent comparison of the various rifamycins and also leads into discussions of other ansamycin molecules including the geldanamycins and ansamitocins, both of which will be mentioned later.

In addition to rifamycin, four other variations have been marketed since that approval: rifampicin in 1967 (Figure 1.3, **19**), rifamixin in 1988 (Figure 1.3, **20**), rifabutin (Figure 1.3, **21**) in 1992 and rifapentine (Figure 1.3, **22**) in 1998. As of December, 2013, there appear to be no rifamycin-like molecules in clinical trials for mycobacterial infections, though a recent publication in the infectious disease literature does imply that increased doses of these agents in conjunction with other anti-tuberculosis drugs are still viable treatments.[16]

Of additional interest is the report in August 2012, that three rifamycins, rifampicin, rifamixin and rifabutin, have been found to be effective in preventing the growth and cellular respiration of multidrug resistant (MDR) *Acinetobacter baumanii* (MDRAb), which is an important pathogen associated with wound infections afflicting US military personnel.[17]

1.3.2 Anthracimycin

Although not an erythromycin-based molecule, nor an ansamycin of the normal basic structure for these agents due to the linkages of the macrolide ring, a very recent paper from the Fenical group at the Scripps Institute of Oceanography reported the isolation and identification of the 14-ring macrolide known as anthracimycin (Figure 1.4, **23**) from a streptomycete isolated from marine sediments.[18] The name chosen was due to its activity against both *Bacillus anthracis* and methicillin-resistant *Staphylococcus aureus* and according to the authors only one other structure similar to this has been reported to date and that was from a myxobacterium in 2008.[18] Thus, even today novel bioactive macrocyclic agents are still being found.

1.3.3 Ansamitocins (Tubulin Interactive Agents)

Very recently, one of the first "plant-derived" tubulin interactive compounds that can be considered a bioactive macrocycle to enter clinical trials, maytansine from the Ethiopian tree *Maytenus serrata*, was effectively granted a new lease of life as a slightly modified "warhead" that could be conjugated to a monoclonal antibody to provide potent and selective anti-tumor agents.

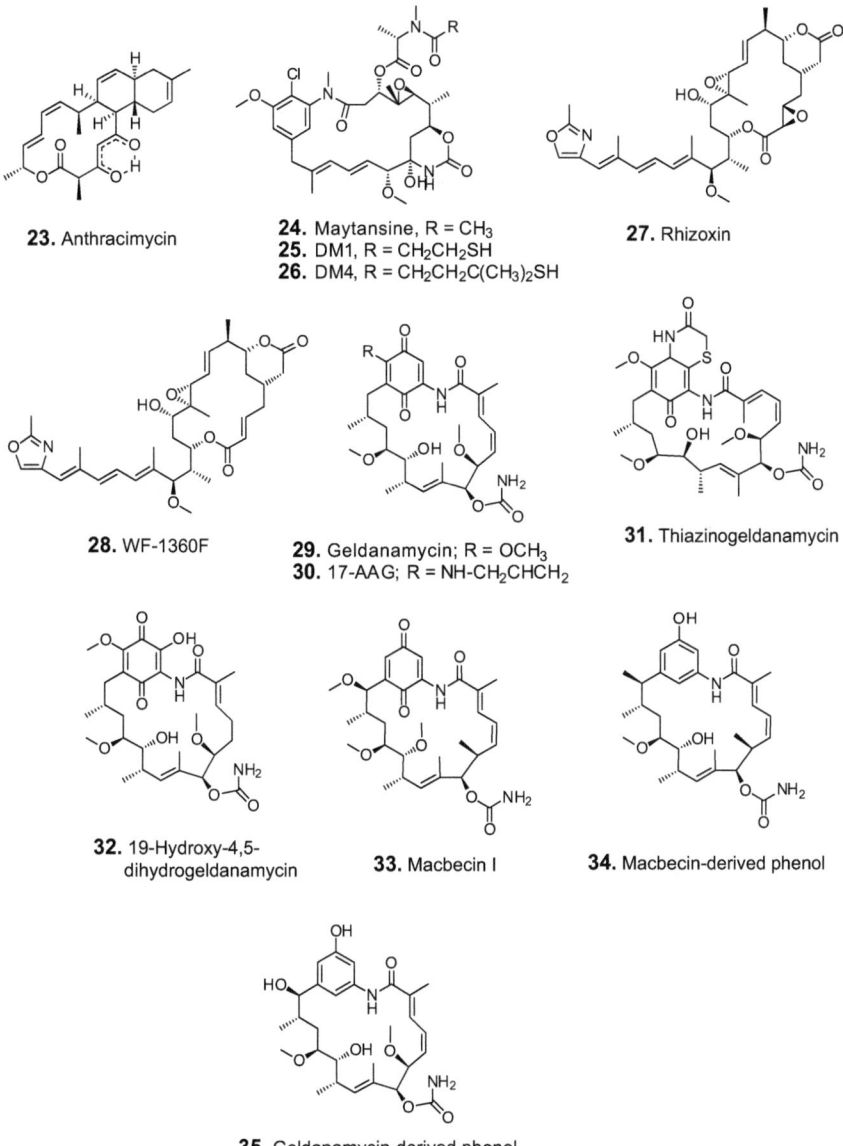

23. Anthracimycin

24. Maytansine, R = CH$_3$
25. DM1, R = CH$_2$CH$_2$SH
26. DM4, R = CH$_2$CH$_2$C(CH$_3$)$_2$SH

27. Rhizoxin

28. WF-1360F

29. Geldanamycin; R = OCH$_3$
30. 17-AAG; R = NH-CH$_2$CHCH$_2$

31. Thiazinogeldanamycin

32. 19-Hydroxy-4,5-dihydrogeldanamycin

33. Macbecin I

34. Macbecin-derived phenol

35. Geldanamycin-derived phenol

Figure 1.4 Structures **23** to **35**; Non-Rifamycin Ansamycin Structures.

From the initial determination of its structure (Figure 1.4, **24**) natural product chemists wondered if the compound was microbial in origin, due to its similarity to the "ansa" antibiotics such as the rifamycins. In 1977, scientists at Takeda Chemical Industries reported the structures of the bacterial products, the ansamitocins, which very closely resembled the maytansenoids. Later work on compounds isolated from the bacterium, subsequently renamed as *Actinosynnema pretiosum*, demonstrated that they were in fact identical to those isolated from other plant genera. The work leading up to this determination has been well covered in a review by Kirchning *et al.* in 2008[19] and/or the chapter by Yu *et al.* in 2012,[20] as these cover the chemistry and biosynthesis of these microbial compounds.

As mentioned above, "precursors" of maytansine from microbial sources, specifically DM-1 (Figure 1.4, **25**) and DM-4 (Figure 1.4, **26**), with suitable chemical linkages, have been used as warheads linked to specific mono-clonal antibodies directed against tumor-linked epitopes. The utility of such antibody–drug conjugates has been discussed by Senter in 2009[21] and amplified the following year by both Alley[22] and Caravella and Lugovskoy.[23] The DM1-linked conjugates are specifically described in a 2010 review by Lambert (from Immunogen) covering these constructs and their clinical efficacies.[24] It is recommended that this article be read in conjunction with the 2011 paper by Kümler *et al.* covering the story of trastuzumab emtan-sine,[25] the combination of Herceptin® with a specific linkage to DM1 that is cleaved by enzymes on uptake into the tumor. The combination was ap-proved in 2012 and launched in 2013 in the USA. Recently, a clinical update was published by Barginear *et al.*, which provides detailed clinical reports, though it covers the period before the approval.[26]

Thus, a bioactive macrocycle that had failed clinical trials in the late 1970s, due to limited efficacy and substantial toxicity, has now become a potent and active treatment for specific breast cancers by repurposing it as a cytotoxic warhead on a targeted therapeutic.

1.3.4 Rhizoxin

This particular ansamycin (Figure 1.4, **27**) has quite a chequered past. It went into clinical trials in Europe as a tubulin interactive agent[27] but was dis-continued as a result of lack of activity.[28] It languished for many years until a report in 2005 identified the producing organism as an endophytic microbe, not the host fungus presumed to be the producer.[29,30] The story of the genetic dissection and the biosynthesis of the rhizoxin complex, plus a full analysis of the symbiotic bacterium was recently published by the Hertweck group who were responsible for the whole discovery of this unique biological interaction.[31] A total synthesis of another one of the rhizoxin analogues that also has bioactivity, WF-1360F (Figure 1.4, **28**), has recently been reported.[32]

1.3.5 Geldanamycin and Analogues/Hsp90 Inhibitors

In this section, apart from a very short historical introduction, the use of genetic modifications to biosynthetic pathways to biochemically produce and identify macrocyclic molecules that have Hsp90 binding activity, giving structures that have not yet been approached synthetically, will be presented. A much fuller story of the discoveries that led to the clinical development of a number of macrocyclic compounds as Hsp90 inhibitors using the basic geldanamycin skeleton will be presented in Chapter 2. It should be noted that there are also a wide variety of non-macrocyclic synthetic Hsp90 inhibitors, such as those from the Chiosis group at Memorial Sloan Kettering, which have been identified through intensive drug discovery programs, some of which have entered clinical trials for oncology.[33]

The benzoquinone ansamycin antibiotic geldanamycin (Figure 1.4, **29**) from *Streptomyces hygroscopicus* var *geldanus* was first reported by The Upjohn Company in 1970[34] and shown to have anti-parasitic activity. Subsequent studies demonstrated anti-tumor activity that was thought to be due to inhibition of the tyrosine specific kinase, *v-Src*, involved in regulating growth and cell proliferation as well as several signal transduction pathways.[35,36] In 1994 however, the compound was shown to bind to the ATPase heat shock protein 90 (Hsp90) by Whitesell and coworkers.[37] Then, three years later, Stebbins *et al.* reported that geldanamycin specifically bound to an ATP binding site at the N-terminus of Hsp90, altered its chaperone activity and indirectly led to cell death.[38] The history, predominantly from an NCI perspective of the various modifications of geldanamycin leading up to the initial development of tanespimycin (17-AAG; Figure 1.4, **30**), was described by Snader in 2005[39] with an interim report in 2005 on other details of the biological activity by Kingston and Newman,[40] and then further updated in 2012 by Snader.[41]

Using the knowledge derived from total genome sequences and the ability to "mix and match" genes within biosynthetic clusters and, in certain cases, to be able to add exogenous genes, potentially active structures produced from such efforts have been disclosed in the last few years. Thus analogues, such as thiazinogeldanamycin (Figure 1.4, **31**) and 19-hydroxy-4,5-dihydro-geldanamycin (Figure 1.4, **32**), have been reported from engineered strains of *S. hygroscopicus* JCM4427 together with other known derivatives,[42] though their bioactivities have not been fully delineated.

What is also of interest is that a close relative of geldanamycin, macbecin (Figure 1.4, **33**) was reported to be an Hsp90 inhibitor by researchers from Biotica in 2008. They demonstrated that this compound had both *in vitro* and *in vivo* activity in mice, and was more water soluble and less toxic than the geldanamycin derivatives in current clinical trials.[43] In a later paper the same year,[44] they reported the optimization and production of macbecin-based molecules that were derived by genetic modification of the macbecin biosynthetic complex in an *Actinosynnema pretiosum* subsp. *pretiosum*, nominally the same genus and species from which the ansamitocins were first isolated.

Since a number of reports attributed the "off-target" bioactivities of the base geldanamycin structure to the quinone moiety undergoing redox cycling, the Biotica team chose a molecule that had no quinonoid ring, as it was replaced by a phenol (Figure 1.4, **34**). The production of this compound was then further optimized to >200 mg L^{-1} by genetic manipulation in the same microbe. Further investigation demonstrated that it had activity *in vitro* and *in vivo* similar to that shown by 17-AAG, but was a tighter binder to Hsp90 and active at a lower molar dose in both cellular and murine assays.[44]

Somewhat similar modifications, but this time using the geldanamycin producer *S. hygroscopicus*, were reported in 2011 by Wu *et al.*, producing a molecule (Figure 1.4, **35**) similar to that optimized by the Biotica group, effectively differing only in two substituents from the phenol-containing macbecin analogue.[45] Thus, different modified ansamycin macrocycles with HSP90 activity are available for future screening.

1.4   Bryostatins (Protein Kinase C Inhibitors)

The isolation of this 20-membered class of macrolidic cytotoxins from the fouling invertebrate *Bugula neritina* over 30 years ago has led to massive collections of the nominal producing organism and to very elegant syntheses of various components.

The initial discovery of bryostatin 3 (Figure 1.5, **38**) was indirectly reported in 1970.[46] Subsequent developments leading to the report of the isolation

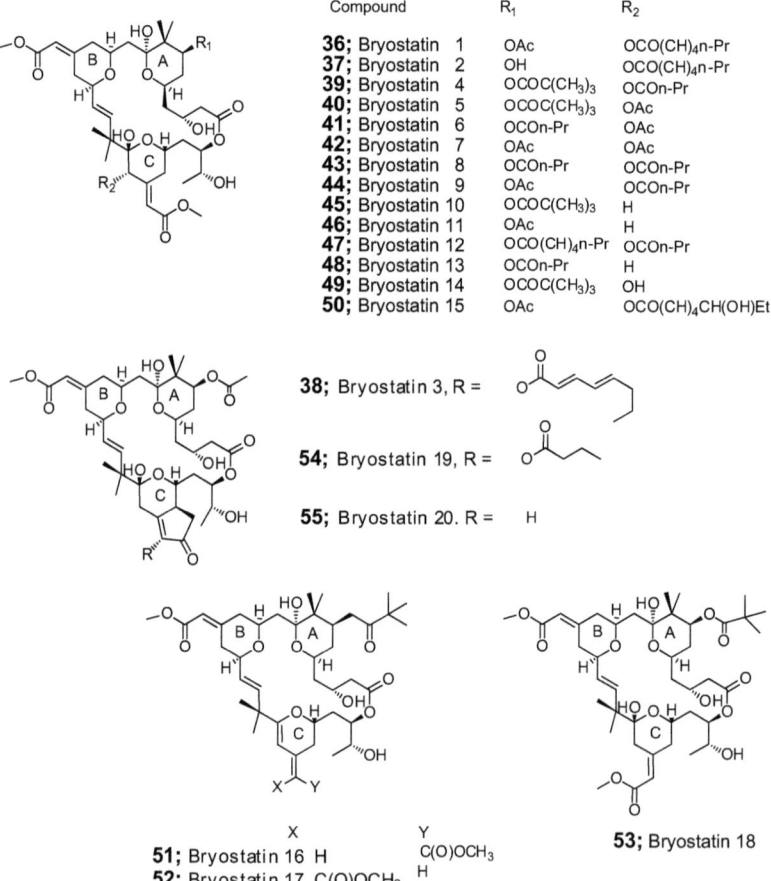

Compound	R₁	R₂
36; Bryostatin 1	OAc	OCO(CH)₄n-Pr
37; Bryostatin 2	OH	OCO(CH)₄n-Pr
39; Bryostatin 4	OCOC(CH₃)₃	OCOn-Pr
40; Bryostatin 5	OCOC(CH₃)₃	OAc
41; Bryostatin 6	OCOn-Pr	OAc
42; Bryostatin 7	OAc	OAc
43; Bryostatin 8	OCOn-Pr	OCOn-Pr
44; Bryostatin 9	OAc	OCOn-Pr
45; Bryostatin 10	OCOC(CH₃)₃	H
46; Bryostatin 11	OAc	H
47; Bryostatin 12	OCO(CH)₄n-Pr	OCOn-Pr
48; Bryostatin 13	OCOn-Pr	H
49; Bryostatin 14	OCOC(CH₃)₃	OH
50; Bryostatin 15	OAc	OCO(CH)₄CH(OH)Et

38; Bryostatin 3, R =

54; Bryostatin 19, R =

55; Bryostatin 20. R =   H

	X	Y
51; Bryostatin 16	H	C(O)OCH₃
52; Bryostatin 17	C(O)OCH₃	H

53; Bryostatin 18

Figure 1.5   Structures 36 to 55; Bryostatins.

and X-ray structure of bryostatin 1 (Figure 1.5, **36**) in 1982,[47] and the multi-year program that culminated in the isolation and purification of 18 bryostatins (Figure 1.5, **36–53**), have been well documented.[48–54]

All of the known bryostatins possess a 20-membered macrolactone ring with three remotely substituted pyran rings linked by a methylene bridge and an (*E*)-disubstituted alkene; all have geminal dimethyls at C_8 and C_{18}, and a four carbon sidechain (carbons 4–1) from the A ring to the lactone oxygen, with another four carbon chain (carbons 24–27) on the other side of the lactone oxygen to the C ring. Most have an exocyclic methyl enoate in their B and C rings, though bryostatin 3 (Figure 1.5, **38**), in particular, has a butenolide rather than the C-ring methyl enoate, and bryostatins 16 and 17 (Figure 1.5, **51** and **52**) have glycals in place of the regular C_{19} and C_{20} hydroxyl moieties.[54,55]

Work reported from the Peoples' Republic of China in 1998[56] and in 2004[57] gave the structure for bryostatin 19 (Figure 1.5, **54**), purified from a South China Sea collection of *Bugula neritina*. Then, in the same year, this report was followed by the publication by Lopanik *et al.* reporting the isolation of bryostatin 20 (Figure 1.5, **55**) from an Atlantic-sourced *Bugula neritina*.[58] Comparison with the structures of the other 18 bryostatins shows that these are closely related to bryostatin 3 in terms of their basic ring components.

Bryostatin 1 has been through well over 80 Phase I and Phase II clinical trials, with or without the addition of a cytotoxic agent in the protocol. One Phase I trial using bryostatin and temsirolimus was "actively recruiting" as of the beginning of July 2013 (NCT00112476) in the ClinicalTrials.gov web site, but in December, 2013, the status had moved to completed, but without any details published as of that date. One more trial, a potentially interesting Phase II trial investigating its use in Alzheimer's disease, is listed as "unknown status", with no information posted since 2008 (NCT00606164). The major dose-limiting toxicity for bryostatin appears to be very significant myalgia in patients. Whether this side effect can be ameliorated by alteration of dosing regimens is not clear.

Some excellent chemistry groups have synthesized a number of the bryostatins (regular structures are shown in Figure 1.5), and have devised simplified molecules based upon the basic skeleton that have much higher (orders of magnitude in some cases when compared to bryostatin 1) *in vitro* activities and can be produced by total synthesis (see discussion later in this section). An early synthetic example was the discussion of routes to bryostatin 1 by Masamune in 1988,[59] but it should be pointed out that with the exception of the Trost synthesis referred to later, none of these syntheses was a substitute for the isolation and purification of bryostatin 1 from natural sources. However, the first total synthesis of any bryostatin, was the enantiomeric synthesis of bryostatin 7 in 1990 by Masamune's group,[60] which was followed in 1998–99 by details of an enantiomeric synthesis of bryostatin 2 from the Evans' group.[61,62] The synthesis of bryostatin 3 was reported by Nishiyama and Yamamura in 2000[63] together with a fuller explanation of the strategies utilized by Ohmori in 2004.[64] These earlier syntheses along with the reported partial syntheses of other bryostatins were reviewed in detail through 2002 by Hale *et al.*[54] The total synthesis of bryostatin 7 using methodologies that would allow modifications to the base structure to be performed was reported in 2006 by the Hale group.[65] Two years later, in 2008, Trost and Dong published their elegant synthesis of bryostatin 16[66] involving some novel metal-linked catalysis steps[67] that included a ruthenium tandem alkyne-enone coupling, and then a palladium catalysed alkyne-ynoate macrocyclization to give the cyclized precursor of bryostatin 16.

A truly excellent compendium and thorough discussion of the chemistry efforts around the synthesis of the bryostatins was published in 2010 by Hale and Manaviazar covering the published results up to then.[55] It should be read by any chemists interested in the manifold methods and specific methodological differences that can be, and have been, used in both successful and unsuccessful syntheses of these agents. However, in spite of all of these methods, up to 2011, no *de novo* synthesis of bryostatin 1 had been published. Then, in 2011, the Keck group reported the first complete total synthesis of this agent.[68] This report was rapidly followed by a paper from Manaviazar and Hale with details of a shorter route[69] to the same compound. Later the same year, Trost *et al.* published on ring expanded versions of bryostatins obtained by total synthesis,[70,71] so the synthetic story of this class of macrocycles has not yet finished.

A number of simplified bryostatin analogues (often called "bryologs") have been synthesized using methods such as function-oriented synthesis. This technique was employed by Wender and other workers to develop simplified analogues with comparable or much improved activities, in some cases orders of magnitude in *in vitro* assays.[72–75] Further information was given in a review by Newman[76] and in a recent 2013 paper by the Keck group.[77] What is also of significant import is the recent report by the Wender group of *in vitro* anti-HIV activity for some of their newer analogues. It will be interesting to see if these can be further developed to provide *in vivo* activity.[78]

Thus, just as in the case of the erythromycin basic structure, the synthesis and biological activities of macrocyclic compounds first reported almost 45 years ago, are still being investigated, with perhaps more interesting biological discoveries to come, particularly as it is now almost certain that bryostatins are produced by an as yet uncultured microbe found initially in the larvae of the bryozoan. Current information can be obtained by inspection of the review by the Haygood group published in 2010.[79]

1.5   Epothilones

The epothilones are bioactive macrocycles that have led to very significant numbers of analogues being made by a variety of methods, including what was possibly the first example of genetic manipulation in the *Myxobacteriales* to optimize production of a desired molecule. A thorough review of the drug discovery effort surrounding this family of macrocycles and their subsequent clinical development can be found in Chapter 3 of this volume.

The initial identification by Reichenbach and Höfle of the 16-membered macrolides epothilones A and B (Figure 1.6, **56** and **57**) from *Sorangium cellulosum* So ce90, is covered in detail in reviews by Reichenbach and Höfle.[80–82] These discoveries, coupled to the report of their activity as tubulin stabilizers in 1995 by workers at Merck,[83] led to work in the USA and Germany on the production of these molecules and other variations from bioengineered organisms.

In 2000, workers at Kosan reported the isolation of the epothilone producing gene cluster from *Sporangium cellosum* strain SMP44 and expressed it in *Streptomyces coelicolor* CH999 together with expression of *EpoK*, the cytochrome P450 that epoxidizes epothilones C and D to A and B, respectively, in *E. coli*.[84] Contemporaneously, the original group at the GBH in Braunschweig also published their epothilone biosynthetic cluster from *S. cellulosum* So ce90.[85] Two years later, in 2002, Julien and Shah from Kosan demonstrated that the comparatively low yields seen in the *S. coelicolor* construct were materially improved by use of *Myxococcus xanthus* TA as a host, deleting *EpoK* and then using a variety of fermentation "tricks" including the well-known industrial technique of adding an adsorbent resin to the fermentations.[86] These and later reports on further fermentation optimization from the Kosan group should be consulted for specific information.[87–90] In addition, the work from the GBH concentrating on *Sorangium* species as a model organism should also be consulted from the original report from Gerth *et al.* in 2003[91] to the excellent review by Wenzel and Müller in 2009 on the impact of genomics on myxobacterial metabolomes.[92]

1.6   Rapamycins and "Rapalogs"

Rapamycin and its close chemical relatives can almost be called "a molecule for most diseases" since the rapamycins now cover molecules that have biological properties ranging from initial anti-fungal activities through immunomodulation to anti-tumor therapies, and even as a molecule to use in stents to avoid plaque formation in blood circulation.

In 1975, scientists at Ayerst laboratories reported the 31-membered macrocyclic antibiotic rapamycin (sirolimus; Figure 1.6, **58a**) to be a potential anti-fungal agent that was produced by the fermentation of a strain of *Streptomyces hygroscopicus* isolated from soil samples in Rapa Nui (Easter Island).[93–95] Rapamycin was unsuccessful as an anti-fungal agent due to its immunosuppressant effects, however its activity against syngeneic murine tumors was reported a few years later in 1984 by Sehgal and co-workers at Ayerst Research Laboratories.[96] At this time, the initial anti-tumor activity of rapamycin was not further developed, but as will be shown below, this parent structure (Figure 1.6, **58a**) has since led to the production of several

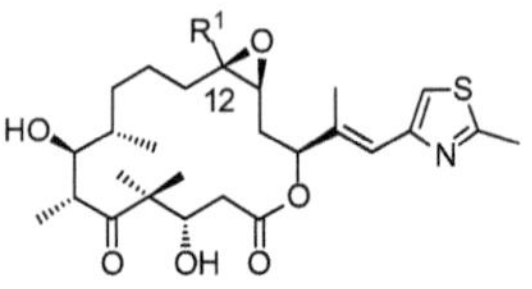

56. Epothilone A; R^1 = H
57. Epothilone B; R^1 = CH$_3$

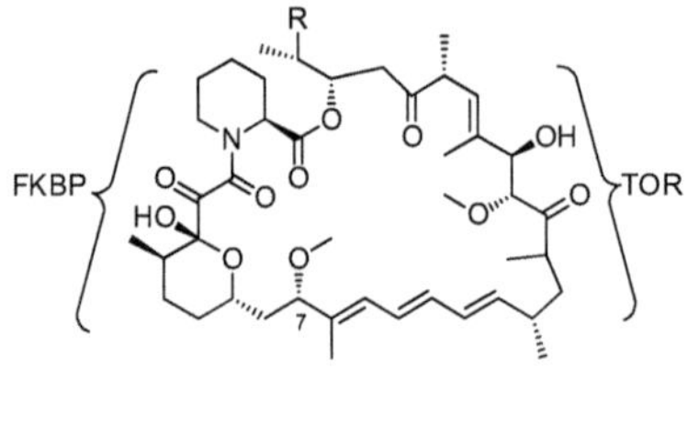

58 (a–e). Rapamycin Macrolide

R =

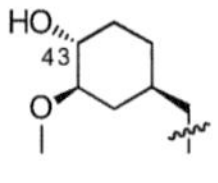

a. Sirolimus

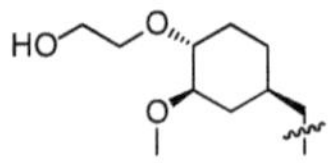

b. Everolimus

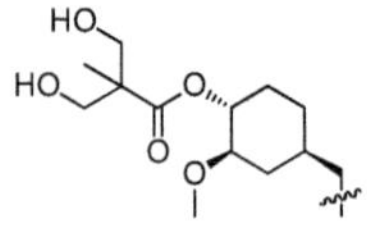

c. Temsirolimus

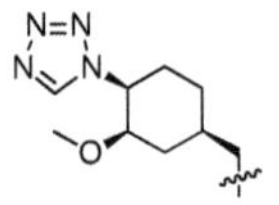

d. Zotarolimus

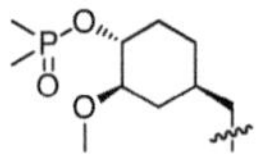

e. Ridaforolimus

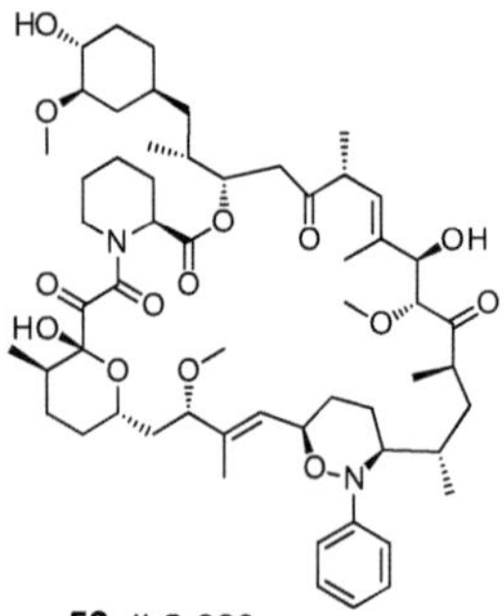

59. ILS-920

Figure 1.6   Structures **56** to **59**; Epothilones and Rapamycin-based Macrolides.

molecules with a variety of different pharmacological activities including, as mentioned above, anti-tumor activity. In the early 1990s, the molecular target of rapamycin in yeast was identified as TOR or "target of rapamycin",[97] followed three years later by the identification of the mammalian homolog, mTOR,[98] with these reports ultimately leading to the development of a wide variety of anti-cancer and other pharmacologic agents.

Initially, chemical modifications were made at the carbon atom at C^{43} on the rapamycin parent structure with numeration as in Zech *et al.*[99] rather than the alternative numbering system of McAlpine *et al.*,[100] which was based upon a comparison with FK506 (which would give a C^{40} substitution), ultimately leading to a total of four clinically approved drugs, rapamycin (sirolimus), everolimus, temsirolimus, and zotarolimus. In 1999, sirolimus (rapamycin) (Figure 1.6, **58a**) was approved as an immunosuppressive agent and is currently in Phase I/II trials for the treatment of various cancers. In a similar manner, everolimus (Figure 1.6, **58b**), was initially launched in 2004 as an immunosuppressive agent and it then was approved for the treatment of kidney, brain, pancreatic, and breast cancers in 2009, 2010, 2011, and 2012, respectively. Then, to add to the armamentarium of just this compound, in 2012 everolimus was released by Abbott to be used as a coating for stents in the treatment of coronary and peripheral arterial diseases. It is also currently in Phase III trials for treating diffuse large B-cell lymphoma (NCT00790036), liver (NCT01035229), and stomach (NCT00879333) cancers. Temsirolimus (CCI-779, Figure 1.6, **58c**) was first approved as a treatment for renal carcinoma in 2007, then in 2010 was approved in Japan and, as with its close chemical relatives, is currently in Phase II trials for the treatment of various carcinomas, mainly under the support of the NCI. Zotarolimus (Figure 1.6, **58d**) was launched in the USA in 2005 for the treatment of arterial restenosis, as a component of a stent, and recently the EU approved a stent containing novolimus, a metabolite of rapamycin that has a C^7-hydroxy group in place of the methoxyl in the parent molecule (*cf* Figure 1.6, **58a**).

Merck and Ariad Pharmaceuticals collaborated to develop another rapamycin derivative, ridaforolimus (AP-23573, Figure 1.6, **58e**), which is in Phase III clinical trials for the treatment of soft tissue carcinoma (NCT00538239) and bone cancer (NCT00538239). In contrast, from a chemical perspective, Wyeth Pharmaceuticals developed a rather interesting derivative of rapamycin, ILS-920, with a modified ring structure (Figure 1.6, **59**). By modification of the triene portion of the molecule mTOR binding would be disrupted. However, ILS-920 may have a different target as it is a non-immunosuppressive neurotrophic analogue reported to exhibit a binding affinity over 900-fold higher for FKBP52 than FKBP12. This analogue promotes neuronal survival and outgrowth *in vitro*, and binds to the β1 subunit of L-type calcium channels (CACNB1).[101] ILS-920 was under development for the treatment of stroke[102] with a Phase I clinical trial for the treatment of acute ischemic stroke completed (NCT00827190). Interestingly, FKBP52 inhibition is reported to affect tubulin interactions in cells[103] and this activity was exploited to screen natural products that inhibit the formation of a complex between FKBP52 and androgen receptors. Since this interaction may play a role in the progression of prostate cancer,[104] there is a possibility that ILS-920 may exhibit anti-tumor activity, although no reports of such activity have been published as yet. In addition to reports showing effects in the brain, there was a report in 2008 that demonstrated that rapamycin plus lithium may aid in the treatment of Huntingdon's disease, so this structure may advance into areas not envisioned in earlier days.[105]

Two prodrugs of rapamycin, Abraxis' ABI-009, a nanoparticle encapsulated formulation of rapamycin, and Isotechnika's TAFA-93 (structure not yet published), have also advanced into Phase I clinical trials. The structure of the latter molecule likely includes either the rapamycin core structure or may only have modifications at the C^{43} hydroxyl group, avoiding both the

FKBP-12 and TOR binding sites, as modifications anywhere else are thought to negate the intrinsic biological activity of these derivatives.[106,107]

Another area of the rapamycin story has to do with the use of bacterial "genetic engineering". In these programs, rapamycin derivatives are produced that are composed of biosynthetic gene clusters that have been modified, or expressed in unusual environments, with the aim of producing analogues with different structures and perhaps also different biological activities. Following on from the pioneering work of the Demain group at MIT,[108,109] one of the groups that spent many years studying the biosynthesis of rapamycin, and then developed methods of utilizing the information in order to produce novel compounds was the group led by Leadlay and Staunton at Cambridge University, which spawned the formation of the biotech company, Biotica.[110]

The methodologies and compounds developed since the 2004 review by Demain[109] have been presented by a number of authors in the last few years, commencing with a review by Graziani covering 2003 to 2008,[111] which should be read in conjunction with the 2010 review by Park *et al.*[112] These papers demonstrate the multiplicity of materials that can be produced by modification of biosynthetic units, and show the problems involved in the regulation of any biosynthetic process. Among the problems addressed is what is now realized to be the "Achilles Heel" of mutasynthetic processes designed to increase yields of desired molecules, namely the provision in the microbe used of sufficient precursors so as to be able to maintain growth and also increase production of the desired molecules. An excellent example of this, though not from rapamycin studies, is shown in the recent paper from Keasling's group discussing the production of artemisinic acid from a bioengineered yeast strain as a precursor for the semi-synthesis of artemisinin.[113]

The 2013 publications and patent applications from the Biotica group demonstrate the potential of these processes in producing engineered strains for producing novel rapalogs[114] and for utilizing the products for biosynthetic medicinal chemistry.[115–117] Using a combination of biosynthetic engineering and molecular modeling, multiple structural modifications were made to the rapamycin (sirolimus) scaffold (Figure 1.6, **58a**) to generate a series of rapalogs having various combinations of changes, including C6-demethylation, C7-O-demethylation, C14-carbonyl reduction to CH_2, C29-O-demethylation or reduction to CH_2, and C44-O-demethylation or reduction to CH_2.[116] The rapalog lacking the C6-methyl and 7-O methyl groups showed significantly enhanced cell line growth inhibition (mean IC_{70} = 7.4 µM) in a 37 cancer cell line screen, compared to rapamycin (mean IC_{70} = 16.3 µM).[116]

1.7 Peptidic Macrocycles

These agents can be either cyclic peptides with "regular" amino acids comprising their backbone, or molecules with what, at times, were thought to be non-proteinogenic (non-ribosomal) amino acid backbones. The discoveries in the last few years, particularly by the groups of Ireland and

Schmidt, (ref. 118 and publications cited therein), plus the recent review by Dunbar and Mitchell[119] have now demonstrated that a number of these (discussed later) are ribosomally encoded but then modified by other processing enzymes.

1.7.1 Gramicidin S (Antibiotic)

Although penicillins V and G are often touted in the West as being the first antibiotics to go into general use, in 1944 Gause and Brazhnikova reported on a variation of gramicidin, named as gramicidin S (Soviet).[120] Rather than being a linear peptide as were the earlier gramicidins A–C,[121,122] which are 15-mer peptides with alternating D and L amino acids, gramicidin S was subsequently shown to be a macrocycle (Figure 1.7, **60**). This initial report was followed the same year by a clinical paper showing efficacy in over 1500 patients in what was then the USSR.[123] Thus, this membrane-active cyclic peptide can also lay claim to being one of the first antibiotics to go into general use, though due to its "country of origin" the discovery may not have been given the credit that it deserved, though the publications were in two UK journals during the height of World War II. However, just to demonstrate that even today, almost 70 years after the initial report of its activity, variations are still being investigated. Thus the paper by Kapoerchan *et al.* in 2012 shows what can occur in terms of increased bioactivity when "inverted" analogues of the base molecule are produced.[124] For example, the analogue (Figure 1.7, **61**) shows increased antibacterial and reduced hemolytic activity compared to gramicidin S.

1.7.2 Ziconotide (Cone Snail Toxin)

Ziconotide (Figure 1.7, **62**), a peptidic cone snail toxin, has the distinction of being the first "direct from the sea" agent to be approved for any disease. In late December of 2004, the FDA approved this peptidic compound for treatment of intractable neuropathic pain, with "phantom limb pain" being a particular indication for this drug. Since the method of drug delivery is *via* an intra-thecal syringe from a reservoir in the peritoneum of the patient, the number of patients willing to tolerate the intricate delivery system is low, but there are studies in the literature demonstrating its value in very specific situations.[125]

This compound is the exact equivalent of the 25-residue peptide isolated from the venom of the cone snail *Conus magus* under the name of ω-conopeptide MVIIA.[126] Over 200 variations on the structure were made before the realization that the native peptide was the most effective. The Irish company Elan purchased the compound and rights and it was approved as stated earlier. In 2012 Olivera and collaborators published an excellent review in Biochemistry (Moscow)[127] covering these peptidic cone snail agents, which should be read in conjunction with a review a year earlier by Daly and Craik from the University of Queensland.[128]

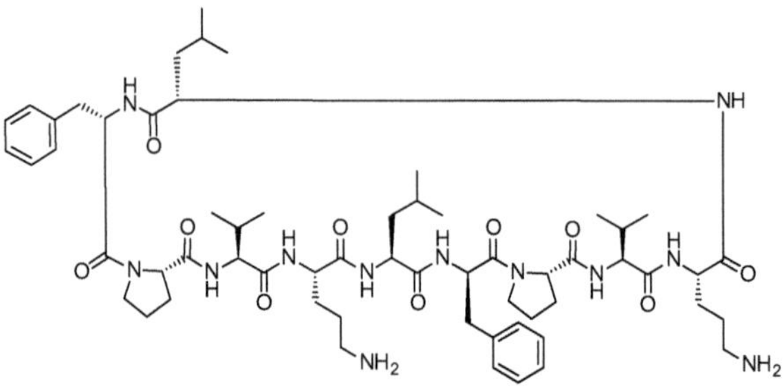

60. Gramicidin S

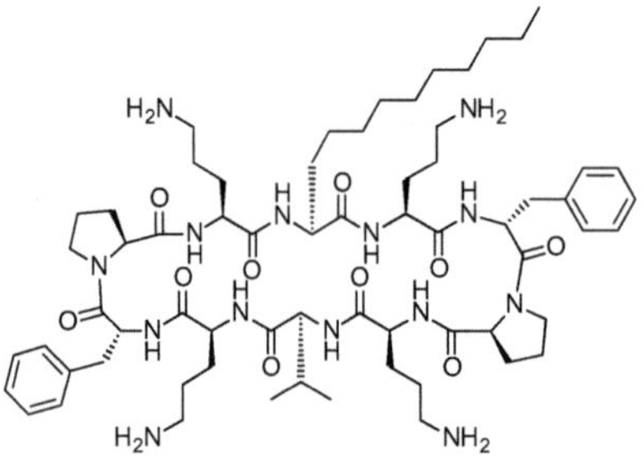

61. Gramicidin S Analogue

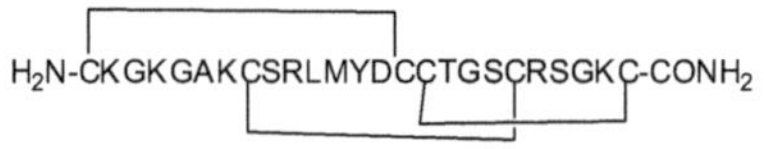

H$_2$N-CKGKGAKCSRLMYDCCTGSCRSGKC-CONH$_2$

62. Ziconotide / SNX-111 / Prialt$^{(R)}$

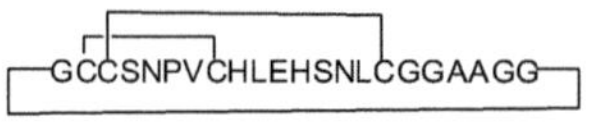

GCCSNPVCHLEHSNLCGGAAGG

63. cMII-6

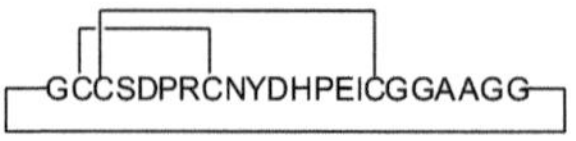

GCCSDPRCNYDHPEICGGAAGG

64. cVc1.1

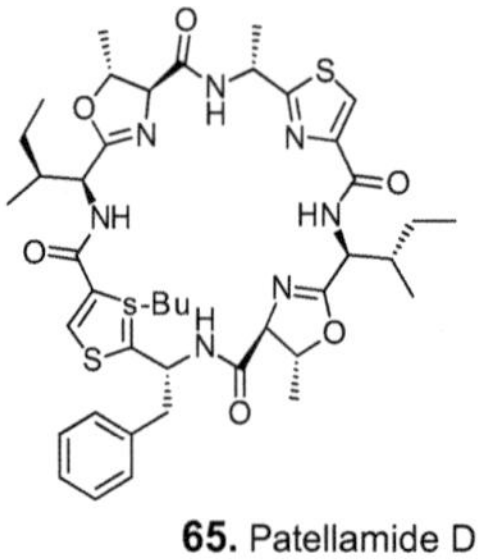

65. Patellamide D

Figure 1.7   Structures **60** to **65**; Mono- and Tri-cyclic Peptide-based Macrocycles.

This 2011 paper suggested that it might well be feasible to modify some of these toxins by linking their N and C termini together to obtain orally active molecules. In 2012 evidence for this methodology was published by the Queensland group, paving the way for agents in the future that may be orally dosed.[129,130] Thus, the cyclic analogue of α-conotoxin MII, cMII-6 (Figure 1.7, **63**), was synthesized and shown to have greatly enhanced proteolytic stability in human serum while retaining most of the activity of the parent peptide against the nicotinic acetylcholine receptor nAChRα6, a target of potential importance for treatment of Parkinson's disease.[129] In addition, Craik *et al.*

have reported the development of an orally active cyclic analogue of α-conotoxin Vc1.1 from the cone snail *Conus victoriae*, cVc1.1 (Figure 1.7, **64**), *via* cyclization of the peptide backbone.[131] The cyclic analogue was shown to be more stable in simulated intestinal fluid and human serum compared to linear Vc1.1, and it showed greater selectivity in the inhibition of calcium channels versus the α9α10nAChR. Testing in the rat CCI-model of neuropathic pain demonstrated that cVc1.1 produced analgesia when delivered orally, and was 120 times more potent than gabapentin, currently used for the treatment for neuropathic pain.[131]

1.7.3 Patellamides (Cytotoxic Cyclic Peptides)

The patellamide cyclic peptides are part of a large group of peptidic cytotoxins that were originally thought to be the products of non-ribosomal peptide synthetases. However, in a recent review[118] Schmidt *et al.*, utilizing new generation sequencing of the as yet uncultured cyanophyte *Prochloron* isolated from the tunicate, have demonstrated that these cyclic peptides, an example being Patellamide D (Figure 1.7, **65**), are the products of ribosomal peptide synthesis followed by "tailoring" to produce the oxazoles and thiazoles in their structures. These are formed by subsequent cyclization of the regular amino acids coded for in the initial sequences. The details of their discovery and the potential applications are given in detail in the review referenced above.

1.7.4 Cyclic Histone Deacetylase Inhibitors (HDACs)

The initial compounds, both from natural sources and synthesis were relatively simple structures consisting of a zinc-binding warhead (a hydroxamate or epoxide), a 4-carbon linker (mimicking the ε-amino side chain of lysine) and an aromatic "end". However, within the original natural product structures was a tetrapeptide known as trapoxin A (Figure 1.8, **66**), first reported by Itazaki *et al.* in 1990,[132] with recognition of the mechanism of action, irreversible inhibition of deacetylation of acetylated histone molecules, being published by Kijima *et al.* three years later.[133]

Following these identifications/MOAs, both new and old tetrapeptides were reported to demonstrate similar activities, with apicidins (Figure 1.8, **68** and **69**) being reported by the Merck group in 1996[134,135] and the much older tetrapeptides, chalmydocin and microsporin A also being identified as HDAC inhibitors.[136]

However, in 2006, a series of unusual tetrapeptides with three unnatural α-aminoacids were reported from the sponge *Mycale izuensis* and named as azumamides A–E.[137] Two of these compounds (azumamides A and E; Figure 1.8, **69** and **70**) were then synthesized together with a close analogue (Figure 1.8, **71**) that exhibited higher potency as an HDAC inhibitor,[138] a year after the report of the total synthesis of the A and E compounds by Izzo *et al.*[139] Very recently, the Olsen group at the Technical University of

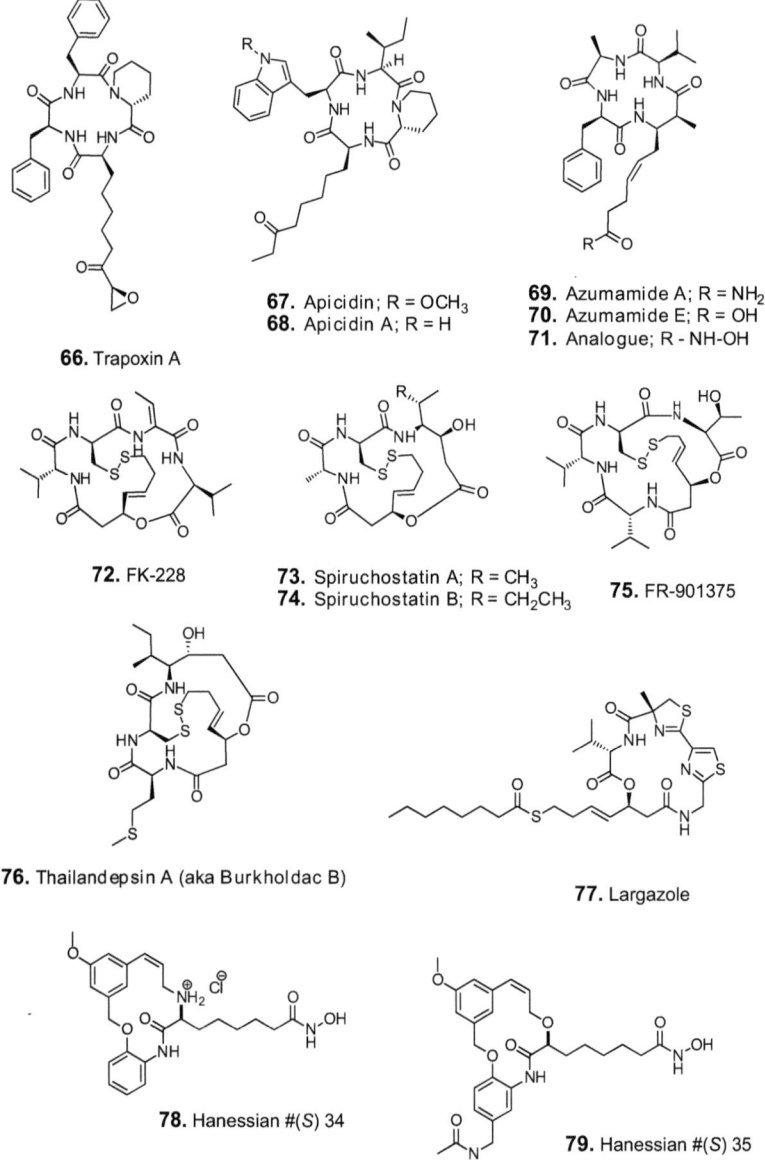

66. Trapoxin A

67. Apicidin; R = OCH₃
68. Apicidin A; R = H

69. Azumamide A; R = NH₂
70. Azumamide E; R = OH
71. Analogue; R - NH-OH

72. FK-228

73. Spiruchostatin A; R = CH₃
74. Spiruchostatin B; R = CH₂CH₃

75. FR-901375

76. Thailandepsin A (aka Burkholdac B)

77. Largazole

78. Hanessian #(S) 34

79. Hanessian #(S) 35

Figure 1.8   Structures **66** to **79**; Cyclic Histone Deacetylase Inhibitors.

Denmark reported on their synthetic work on the azumamide skeleton, which included the first synthesis of the B to D variants, confirming the original structural assignments, together with a full isotype profiling of this class of agents and identifying that the C and D analogues are potent and specific inhibitors of HDAC10 and 11.[140]

Contemporaneously with the determination of the MOA of trapoxin, a novel cytotoxic microbial agent was reported by Ueda *et al.* in 1994 from the phytotoxic bacterium *Chromobacterium violaceum*,[141] and its MOA was determined in 1998 by comparison to the activities of trichostatin A.[142] This compound, known nowadays by a variety of names, FK-228, depsipeptide, romidepsin or Istodax® (Figure 1.8, 72), can be thought of as the prototype structure for the cyclic agents (prodrugs) that contain a dithio bridge that when opened, will complex the zinc atom in the active site of the HDAC enzyme.[143] FK228 was recommended for FDA approval in September of 2009 as a treatment for cutaneous T-cell lymphoma and was launched in the USA in March, 2010.

However, FK228 was only the beginning of the isolation, identification and often, total synthesis of a number of depsipeptides all containing the dithio bridge and all acting as prodrugs for interaction with various isotypes of HDACs. In 2001, Masuoka *et al.* reported on the spiruchostatins A and B (Figure 1.8, 73 and 74) and in 2003, Chen *et al.*[144] reported the synthesis of FR-901375 (Figure 1.8, 75) a molecule closely related to FK228 that had only been reported in a Japanese patent in 1991. Spiruchostatin A was synthesized by the Ganesan group with a report in early 2004[145] and later, using the material synthesized by Ganesan, a group at the University of Southampton determined that this agent was a potent inhibitor of the Class 1 HDAC isotype.[146] Very recently a Japanese group reported on the synergistic activity of spiruchostatin A (under its code number, OBP-801) with the PI3K inhibitor LY294002 in an *in vitro* assay of human renal carcinoma cell lines; thus this agent may have potential in a tumor system that is resistant to most current therapies.[147]

In addition to the agents discussed above, a third set of microbial products have also been identified that have similar structures and activities. These are the thailandepsins, which were originally reported as a result of genomic analysis of a specific bacterium and whose original structures have undergone revision following total synthesis,[148] demonstrating that the compound known as burkholdac B (Figure 1.8, 76) is identical to the revised structure for thailandepsin A and has an activity against the MCF7 breast cancer cell line with an IC_{50} value of 60 pM. A recent paper from Wilson *et al.*, demonstrated activity against ovarian cell lines in the nanomolar range with thailandepsin A, thus extending the range of activities for this class of compounds.[149]

These is another microbial product, this time however, from a marine cyanophyte,[150] that also has a masked thiol group. However, rather than a dithio linkage, in this compound (largazole; Figure 1.8, 77), the thiol is masked as a thioester and requires hydrolysis to release the activated thiol for interaction with HDAC isotypes.[151] Following the report of the structure and its synthesis, a number of other groups have synthesized not only the base structure, but modifications thereon, including Ghosh and Kulkarni,[152] the Phillips group,[153] Luesch with synthetic modifications,[154] and Schreiber and Williams[155] all within 4 months of the presentation of the structure at an ACS Meeting, thus proving that if there is a novel and active agent from Nature, synthetic chemists are very willing to synthesize it and produce analogues.

Since that time, a number of other groups have extended the syntheses and activities, and these reports should be consulted by readers interested in modification of natural product structures.[156–159] In addition, expanded biological activities have also been reported for largazole and derivatives, including osteogenic activity,[160] sensitization of lymphoma cells to nucleosides,[161] proteosomal degradation,[162] and inhibition of liver fibrosis.[163]

Finally for this section there have been some very interesting reviews published in the last few years covering both syntheses from natural products or using combinatorial chemistry to provide different base structural molecules. Thus in 2009, Olsen and Ghadiri demonstrated how focused combinatorial libraries of cyclic α3β-tetrapeptides led to the identification of potent HDAC inhibitors, working from natural product scaffolds with modifications.[164] This work was followed in 2010 by the Hanessian group's demonstration how non-natural macrocyclic inhibitors of HDACs could be synthesized.[165] This later work gave synthetic molecules that demonstrated selectivity for the Class 6 HDAC isotype (Figure 1.8, **78** and **79**) depending upon their configuration at a given center. Then in 2013, there were three reviews published with one covering case studies on the synthesis of bioactive cyclodepsipeptide natural products by Stolze and Kaiser[166] and two that covered more of the biological aspects of these molecules.[167,168]

1.8   Buruli Toxins (Mycolactones A/B; Necrotic Contact Agents)

One of the simplest macrolides, mycolactone A/B, is a 12 membered ring with a pendant unsaturated polyhydroxy fatty acid ester and an upper un-saturated alkyl side chain (Figure 1.9, **80**) and it is one of the nastiest bioactive macrolides known from a physiological effect aspect.[169] This is the compound that causes the chronic necrotizing skin ulcer known as "Buruli Ulcer". The causative agent is a component of various strains of the myco-bacterium, *Mycobacterium ulcerans*, and until the recent total synthesis by Altmann's group at the ETH, studies were limited by the lack of pure com-pound(s) to work with.[170]

Mycolactone A/B (both *E* and *Z* isomers coexist in the purified microbial isolate) was difficult to obtain in pure form and therefore trying to determine its mechanism of action and thus potential treatments was very difficult. Soon after the publication by Altmann *et al.*, a group in France reported a diverted total synthesis of mycolactone A/B and analogues, thus providing

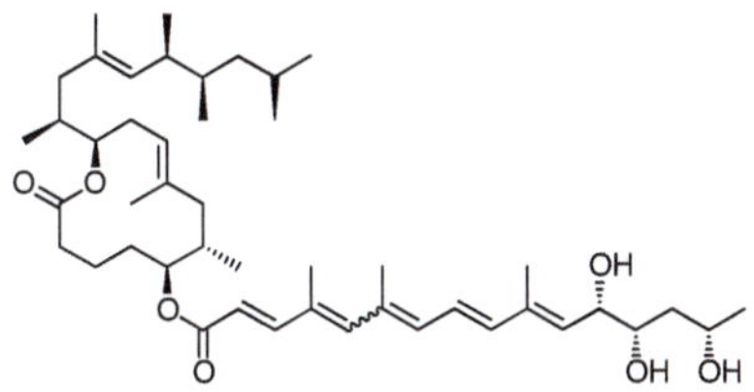

80. Mycolactone A/B

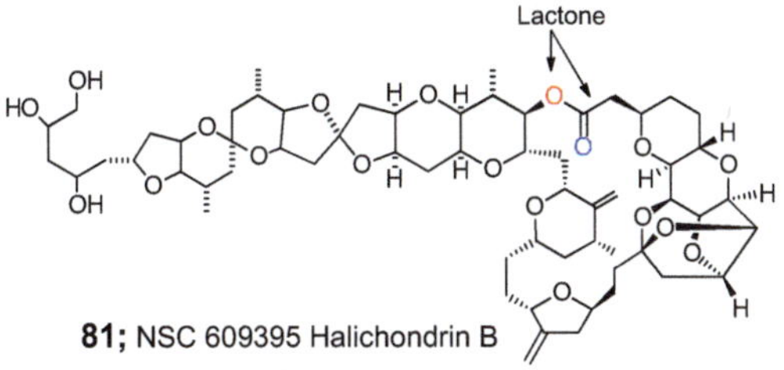

81; NSC 609395 Halichondrin B

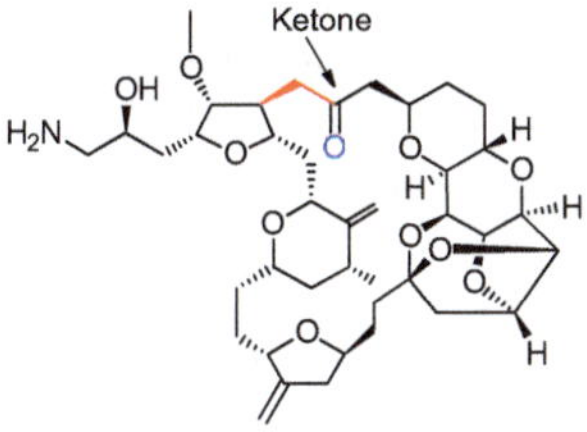

82; Eribulin; NSC 707389 [E7389]

Figure 1.9 Structures **80** to **82**; Mycolactones A/B, Halichondrin and Eribulin.

the potential to expand the SAR, though they found that the natural product was still the most toxic agent.[171]

In 2013, Altmann, working with a group of Swiss scientists including immunologists and tropical disease specialists, using mycolactones with differing lower side chains (the fatty acid esters) together with some changes on the upper side chain, have shown that the lactones have no antibiotic activities but are apoptotic, necrotic, and immunosuppressive in their interactions with mammalian cell types.[172] A derivative in which the lower side chain of mycolactone A/B was truncated to an acetyl residue was unique in strongly inhibiting the metabolism and cell proliferation of a murine L929 fibroblast cell line, while being non-cytotoxic at the highest concentrations used. Thus, through the use of total synthesis and techniques that permit "relatively" simple variations to the side chains, a series of these very toxic compounds can be obtained for future use by biologists and physicians investigating this very unpleasant disease.

1.9   Eribulin (Halaven®, E7389)

Due to its extraordinary anti-tumor activity, the antitubulin marine natural product halichondrin B (Figure 1.9, **81**) was chosen for preclinical development in 1992 by the Developmental Therapeutics Program (DTP) at the NCI. However, clinical development was severely impeded due to the limited amounts of compound available from natural sources.

Kishi's group reported the total synthesis for halichondrin B in 1992.[173] In collaboration with scientists at the Eisai Research Institute (ERI) in Woburn, MA, Kishi demonstrated that the right hand macrolide half of the molecule (approx MW of 600) retained all or most of the potency of the much larger parent compound. Chemists at the ERI, working very closely with Kishi's group, then synthesized over 200 analogues.[174,175]

In conjunction with the DTP, they demonstrated that the modified truncated macrocyclic ketone, eribulin (E7389; Figure 1.9, **82**), where the lactone in the macrocyclic ring was converted to a ketone and the ring pyran adjacent to the ketone was converted to a furan with a simple 3-carbon side chain, gave a molecule that had greater *in vivo* stability, possessed comparable bioactivity to and lower toxicity *in vivo* than halichondrin B (obtained by DTP in conjunction with New Zealand scientists).

Subsequently, the Eisai group has demonstrated that relatively minor changes to the "tail" of the eribulin molecule results in much lower propensity for inducing P-glycoprotein susceptibility while retaining *in vivo* potency.[176] Incorporation of a morpholine in the "tail" demonstrated oral activity in a subcutaneous LOX melanoma model,[177] and modification by ring closure at the "tail" yielded a different morpholino derivative that demonstrated intravenous *in vivo* activity in an orthotopic murine model of a human glioblastoma.[178]

The development of Eribulin (E7389), perhaps the most complex drug molecule yet produced by total synthesis, from a marine derived antitumor agent, halichondrin B, is a compelling example of the power of the DTS approach.

1.10   Conclusion

Although many more examples of bioactive macrocyclic compounds could be given, the molecules discussed above cover over 70 years of compound discovery, and are all based upon natural products. As was discussed in the Introduction, data reported in a 2013 review of macrocyclic drugs and clinical candidates indicated that the 68 registered macrocyclic drugs in use at the time were almost exclusively of natural origin. In the case of the 35 macrocyclic compounds in clinical trials that were considered, 25 were of natural origin, with 10 being of *de novo* design. Of significance was the observation that 43% of the clinical development candidates were orally administered, as compared to only 28% of the registered macrocyclic drugs. Even more noteworthy was the fact that 9 of the 10 *de novo* designed clinical candidates were orally bioavailable. These figures reflect a clear trend towards the increased development of orally bioavailable macrocyclic therapeutic agents, and suggest that synthetic and medicinal chemists are being guided by structural cues provided by bioactive natural macrocyclic agents in the design of synthetic mimics having the desired pharmacological properties, including oral bioavailability.

Two brief examples illustrating the utilization of macrocyclization by drug discovery programs to provide fully synthetic bioactive molecules are shown below. The first demonstrates the use of data from X-ray crystallography of the peptide KPF-pY-VNV bound to the Grb2-SH2 domain, to afford a lead series based upon a peptidomimetic structure that was pre-organized to give a β-turn configuration. This basic structure was then cyclized and slightly modified, yielding a potent *in vitro* active material. Further work by the same group produced a malonate derivative that is still biologically active (Figure 1.10, **83**).[179,180] The second example is the work of Zapf *et al.* on the synthesis of a series of Hsp90 inhibitors *via* use of the Buchwald-Hartwig cyclization reaction. Thus, starting from an acyclic clinical candidate and

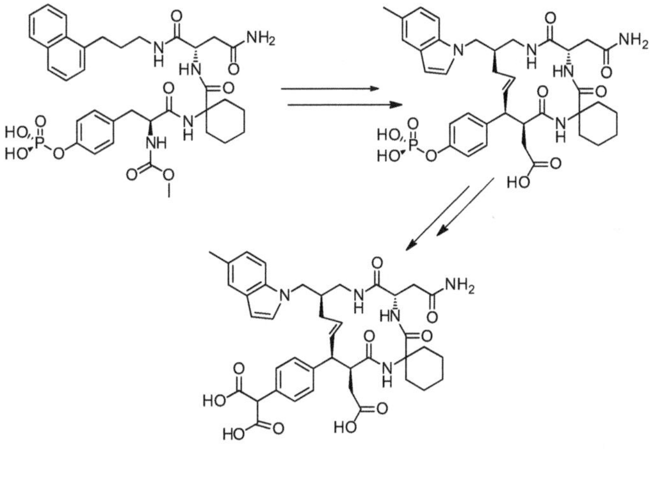

83. Cyclization; then Phosphate to Malonate

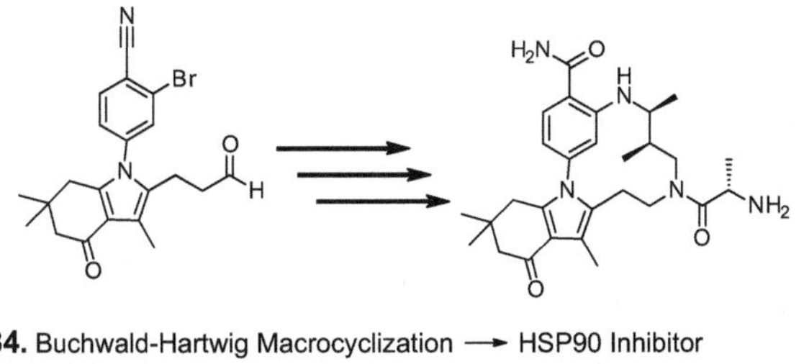

84. Buchwald-Hartwig Macrocyclization ⟶ HSP90 Inhibitor

Figure 1.10 Structures **83** to **84**; Syntheses of Totally Synthetic Bioactive Macrocycles.

leveraging a variety of synthetic methodologies to explore linkers with different functionalities, coupled to biological activity analyses at each stage, a potent orally dosed *in vivo* active Hsp90 inhibitor was identified (Figure 1.8, **84**).[181]

Finally, it has been the intent of this chapter to demonstrate the impressive variety of structures of bioactive natural product-based macrocycles, and also to show, albeit only with a few examples, that synthetic or quasi-synthetic macrocyclic compounds, derived from a natural product pharmacophore or close spatial relative, can provide drug-like structures on which to base the search for novel drug entities.

Thus, in the field of macrocyclic chemistry it is apparent that there can be a definite continuum from natural product structures to totally synthetic molecules that perform the same pharmacological tasks, aside from perhaps antibiotics, though that area may yet be conquered as shown by the success of the bicyclic, but not yet macrocyclic, quinolone-based antibacterial agents colloquially known as "floxacins".[182]

The area of macrocyclic chemistry thus offers an exciting and relatively new approach to effective drug discovery and development, substantially different to the focus on small molecules which, to date, has been favored by most medicinal chemistry drug discovery programs. This and subsequent chapters present promising evidence of a sustained and increasing interest in this field of drug discovery and development that augurs well for the availability of novel and more effective treatments for many of the serious diseases afflicting the global population.

References

1. F. Giordanetto and J. Kihlberg, *J. Med. Chem.*, 2014, **57**, 278.
2. E. M. Driggers, S. P. Hale, J. Lee and N. K. Terrett, *Nature Rev. Drug. Discov.*, 2008, **7**, 608.
3. E. Marsault and M. L. Peterson, *J. Med. Chem.*, 2011, **54**, 1961.
4. J. Mallinson and I. Collins, *Fut. Med. Chem.*, 2012, **4**, 1409.
5. S. A. Waksman and H. B. Woodruff, *Proc. Soc. Exptl. Biol. Med.*, 1940, **45**, 609.
6. C. Hackmann, *Z. Krebsforsch*, 1952, **58**, 607.
7. G. Schulte, *Z. Krebsforsch*, 1952, **58**, 500.
8. L. A. Garrett, D. C. Harmon and J. O. Schorge, *J. Clin. Oncol.*, 2013, **31**, e48.
9. A. B. Mauger and H. Lackner, in *Anticancer Agents from Natural Products*, ed. G. M. Cragg, D. G. I. Kingston and D. J. Newman, Taylor and Francis, Boca Raton, FL, 2nd edn, 2012, p. 363.
10. M. Gniazdowski, W. A. Denny, S. M. Nelson and M. Czyz, *Curr. Med. Chem.*, 2003, **10**, 909.
11. C.-H. Leung, D. S.-H. Chan, V. P.-Y. Ma and D.-L. Ma, *Med. Res. Revs.*, 2013, **33**, 823.
12. H.-J. Kang and H.-J. Park, *Biochemistry*, 2009, **48**, 7392.

13. P. P. Hung, C. L. Marks and P. L. Tardrew, *J. Biol. Chem.*, 1965, **240**, 1322.
14. C. J. B. Harvey, J. D. Puglisi, V. S. Pande, D. E. Cane and C. Khosla, *J. Am. Chem. Soc.*, 2012, **134**, 12259.
15. R. Mariani and S. I. Maffioli, *Curr. Med. Chem.*, 2009, **16**, 430.
16. D. Mitchison and G. Davies, *Int. J. Tuberc. Lung Dis.*, 2012, **16**, 724.
17. B. A. Chromy, M. Elsheikh, T. L. Christensen, D. Livingston, K. Petersen, J. P. Bearinger and P. D. Hoeprich, *Fut. Microbiol.*, 2012, **7**, 1011.
18. K. H. Jang, S.-J. Nam, J. B. Locke, C. A. Kauffman, D. S. Beatty, L. A. Paul and W. Fenical, *Angew. Chem., Int. Ed.*, 2013, **52**, 7822.
19. A. Kirschning, K. Harmrolfs and T. Knobloch, *C. R. Chimie*, 2008, **11**, 1523.
20. J.-W. Yu, H. G. Floss, G. M. Cragg and D. J. Newman, in *Anticancer Agents from Natural Products*, ed. G. M. Cragg, D. G. I. Kingston and D. J. Newman, Taylor and Francis, Boca Raton, FL, 2nd edn, 2012, pp. 407.
21. P. D. Senter, *Curr. Opin. Chem. Biol.*, 2009, **13**, 235.
22. S. C. Alley, N. M. Okeley and P. D. Senter, *Curr. Opin. Chem. Biol.*, 2010, **14**, 529.
23. J. Caravella and A. Lugovskoy, *Curr. Opin. Chem. Biol.*, 2010, **14**, 520.
24. J. M. Lambert, *Drugs Fut.*, 2010, **35**, 471.
25. I. Kümler, C. Ehlers Mortensen and D. L. Nielsen, *Drugs Fut.*, 2011, **36**, 825.
26. M. F. Barginear, V. John and D. R. Budman, *Mol. Med.*, 2013, **18**, 1473.
27. P. Lelieveld and H. R. Hendriks, *Can. Treat. Revs.*, 1990, **17**, 119.
28. A. R. Hanauske, G. Catimel, l. S. Aamda, W. ten Bokkel Huinink, R. Paridaens, N. Pavlidis, S. B. Kaye, A. te Velde, J. Wanders and J. Verweij, *Br. J. Cancer*, 1996, **73**, 397.
29. L. P. Partida-Martinez and C. Hertweck, *Nature*, 2005, **437**, 884.
30. L. P. Partida-Martinez, I. Groth, I. Schmitt, W. Richter, M. Roth and C. Hertweck, *Int. J. Sys. Evol. Microbiol.*, 2007, **57**, 2583.
31. K. Scherlach, B. Busch, G. Lackner, U. Paszkowski and C. Hertweck, *Angew. Chem., Int. Ed.*, 2012, **51**, 9615.
32. C. M. Neuhaus, M. Liniger, M. Stieger and K.-H. Altmann, *Angew. Chem., Int. Ed.*, 2013, **52**, 5866.
33. T. Taldone, D. Zatorska, H. J. Patel, W. Sun, M. R. Patel and G. Chiosis, *Heterocycles*, 2013, **87**, 91.
34. C. DeBoer, P. A. Meulman, R. J. Wnuk and D. H. Peterson, *J. Antibiot.*, 1970, **23**, 442.
35. Y. Uehara, M. Hori, T. Takeuchi and H. Umezawa, *Mol. Cell. Biol.*, 1986, **6**, 2198.
36. Y. Uehara, Y. Murakami, S. Mizuno and S. Kawalt, *Virology*, 1988, **164**, 294.
37. L. Whitesell, E. G. Mimnaugh, B. De Costa, C. E. Myers and L. M. Neckers, *Proc. Natl. Acad. Sci. USA*, 1994, **91**, 8324.

38. C. E. Stebbins, A. A. Russo, C. Schneider, N. Rosen, F. U. Hartl and N. P. Pavletich, *Cell*, 1997, **89**, 239.
39. K. M. Snader, in *Anticancer Agents from Natural Products*, ed. G. M. Cragg, D. G. I. Kingston and D. J. Newman, Taylor and Francis, Boca Raton, FL, 1st edn, 2005, p. 339.
40. D. G. I. Kingston and D. J. Newman, *Curr. Opin. Drug Discov. Develop.*, 2005, **8**, 207.
41. K. M. Snader, in *Anticancer Agents from Natural Products*, ed. G. M. Cragg, D. G. I. Kingston and D. J. Newman, Taylor and Francis, Boca Raton, FL, 2nd edn, 2012, p. 429.
42. W. Cheng-Zhu, J.-H. Jang, J.-S. Ahn, Y.-S. Hong and J. Microbiol, *Biotechnol.*, 2012, **22**, 1478.
43. C. J. Martin, S. Gaisser, I. R. Challis, I. Carletti, B. Wilkinson, M. Gregory, C. Prodromou, S. M. Roe, L. H. Pearl, S. M. Boyd and M.-Q. Zhang, *J. Med. Chem.*, 2008, **51**, 2853.
44. M.-Q. Zhang, S. Gaisser, M. Nur-E-Alam, L. S. Sheehan, W. A. Vousden, N. Gaitatzis, G. Peck, N. J. Coates, S. J. Moss, M. Radzom, T. A. Foster, R. M. Sheridan, M. A. Gregory, S. M. Roe, C. Prodromou, L. Pearl, S. M. Boyd, B. Wilkinson and C. J. Martin, *J. Med. Chem.*, 2008, **51**, 5494.
45. C.-Z. Wu, A. N. Moon, J.-H. Jang, D. Lee, S.-Y. Kang, J.-T. Park, J. S. Ahn, B. Y. Hwang, Y. H. Kim, H.-S. Lee and Y.-S. Hong, *J. Antibiot.*, 2011, **64**, 461.
46. G. R. Pettit, J. F. Day, J. L. Hartwell and H. B. Wood, *Nature*, 1970, **227**, 962.
47. G. R. Pettit, C. L. Herald, D. L. Doubeck, D. L. Herald, E. Arnold and J. Clardy, *J. Am. Chem. Soc.*, 1982, **104**, 6846.
48. M. Suffness, D. J. Newman and K. M. Snader, in *Bioorganic Marine Chemistry*, ed. P. Scheuer, Springer-Verlag, Berlin-Heidelberg, 1989, vol. **3**, p. 131.
49. G. R. Pettit, in *Progress in the Chemistry of Organic Natural Products*, ed. W. Hertz, G. W. Kirby, W. Steglich and C. Tamm, Springer-Verlag, New York, 1991, vol. **57**, p. 153.
50. G. R. Pettit, *J. Nat. Prod.*, 1996, **59**, 812.
51. D. J. Newman, in *Bryozoans in Space and Time*, ed. D. P. Gordon, A. M. Smith and J. A. Grant-Mackie, *NIWA*, Wellington, NZ, 1996, p. 9.
52. R. Mutter and M. Wills, *Bioorg. Med. Chem.*, 2000, **8**, 1841.
53. G. R. Pettit, C. L. Herald and F. Hogan, in *Anticancer Drug* Development, ed. B. C. Baguley and D. J. Kerr, Academic Press, San Diego, 2002, p. 203.
54. K. J. Hale, M. C. Hummersone, S. Manaviazar and M. Frigerio, *Nat. Prod. Rep.*, 2002, **19**, 413.
55. K. J. Hale and S. Manaviazar, *Chem. Asian J.*, 2010, **5**, 704.
56. H. Lin, X. Yao, Y. Yi, X. Li and H. Wu, *Zhongguo Haiyang Yaowu*, 1998, **17**, 1.
57. H. Lin, G. Liu, Y. Yi, X. Yao and H. Wu, *Dier Junyi Daxue Xuebao*, 2004, **25**, 473.

58. N. Lopanik, K. R. Gustafson and N. Lindquist, *J. Nat. Prod.*, 2004, **67**, 1412.

59. S. Masamune, *Pure Appl. Chem.*, 1988, **60**, 1587.

60. M. Kageyama, T. Tamura, M. H. Nantz, J. C. Roberts, P. Somfai, D. C. Whritenour and S. Masamune, *J. Am. Chem. Soc.*, 1990, **112**, 7407.

61. D. A. Evans, P. H. Carter, E. M. Carreira, J. A. Prunet, A. B. Charette and M. Lautens, *Angew. Chem., Int. Ed.*, 1998, **37**, 2354.

62. D. A. Evans, P. H. Carter, E. M. Carreira, A. B. Charette, J. A. Prunet and M. Lautens, *J. Am. Chem. Soc.*, 1999, **121**, 7540.

63. K. Ohmori, Y. Ogawa, T. Obitsu, Y. Ishikawa, S. Nishiyama and S. Yamamura, *Angew. Chem., Int. Ed.*, 2000, **39**, 2290.

64. K. Ohmori, *Bull. Chem. Soc. Japan*, 2004, **77**, 875.

65. S. Manaviazar, M. Frigerio, G. S. Bhatia, M. G. Hummersone, A. E. Aliev and K. J. Hale, *Org. Lett.*, 2006, **8**, 4477.

66. B. M. Trost and G. Dong, *Nature*, 2008, **456**, 485.

67. A. K. Miller, *Angew. Chem., Int. Ed.*, 2009, **48**, 3221.

68. G. E. Keck, Y. B. Poudel, T. J. Cummins, A. Rudra and J. A. Covel, *J. Am. Chem. Soc.*, 2011, **133**, 744.

69. S. Manaviazar and K. J. Hale, *Angew. Chem., Int. Ed.*, 2011, **50**, 8786.

70. B. M. Trost, H. Yang, C. S. Brindle and G. Dong, *Chem. - Eur. J.*, 2011, **17**, 9777.

71. B. M. Trost, H. Yang and G. Dong, *Chem. - Europ. J.*, 2011, **17**, 9789.

72. G. E. Keck, M. B. Kraft, A. P. Truong, W. Li, C. C. Sanchez, N. Kedei, N. E. Lewin and P. M. Blumberg, *J. Am. Chem. Soc.*, 2008, **130**, 6660.

73. B. M. Trost and G. Dong, *J. Am. Chem. Soc.*, 2010, **132**, 16403.

74. P. A. Wender, J. L. Baryza, S. E. Brenner, B. A. DeChristopher, B. A. Loy, A. J. Schrier and V. A. Verma, *Proc. Natl. Acad. Sci. U. S. A.*, 2011, **108**, 6721.

75. P. A. Wender and J. Reuber, *Tetrahedron*, 2011, **67**, 9998.

76. D. J. Newman, in *Anticancer Agents from Natural Products*, ed. G. M. Cragg, D. G. I. Kingston and D. J. Newman, Taylor and Francis, Boca Raton, FL, 2nd edn, 2012, p. 199.

77. N. Kedei, N. E. Lewin, T. Géczy, J. Selezneva, D. C. Braun, J. Chen, M. A. Herrmann, M. R. Heldman, L. Lim, P. Mannan, S. H. Garfield, Y. B. Poudel, T. J. Cummins, A. Rudra, P. M. Blumberg and G. E. Keck, *ACS Chem. Biol.*, 2013, **8**, 767.

78. B. A. DeChristopher, A. LoyBrian, M. D. Marsden, A. J. Schrier, J. A. Zack and P. A. Wender, *Nat. Chem.*, 2012, **4**, 705.

79. A. E. Trindade-Silva, G. E. Lim-Fong, K. H. Sharp and M. G. Haygood, *Curr. Opin. Biotechnol.*, 2010, **21**, 834.

80. G. Hoefle and H. Reichenbach, in *Anticancer Agents from Natural Products*, ed. G. M. Cragg, D. G. I. Kingston and D. J. Newman, Taylor and Francis, Boca Raton, FL, 2005, p. 413.

81. H. Reichenbach and G. Hoefle, *Drugs R&D*, 2008, **9**, 1.

82. G. Hoefle and H. Reichenbach, in *Anticancer Agents from Natural Products*, ed. G. M. Cragg, D. G. I. Kingston and D. J. Newman, Taylor and Francis, Boca Raton, Fl, 2nd edn, 2012, p. 513.

83. D. M. Bollag, P. A. McQueney, J. Zhu, O. Hensens, L. Koupal, J. M. Liesch, M. Goetz, E. Lazarides and C. M. Woods, *Cancer Res.*, 1995, **55**, 2325.

84. L. Tang, S. Shah, L. Chung, J. Carney, L. Katz, C. Khosla and B. Julien, *Science*, 2000, **287**, 640.

85. I. Molnar, T. Schupp, M. Ono, R. E. Zirkle, M. Milnamow, B. Nowak-Thompson, N. Engel, C. Toupet, A. Stratman, D. D. Cyr, J. Gorlach, J. M. Mayo, A. Hu, S. Goff, J. Schmid and J. M. Ligon, *Chem. Biol.*, 2000, **7**, 97.

86. B. Julien and S. Shah, *Antimicrob. Agents Chemother.*, 2002, **46**, 2772.

87. S. Frykman, H. Tsuruta, J. Lau, R. Regentin, S. Ou, C. Reeves, J. Carney, D. Santi and P. Licari, *J. Ind. Microbiol. Biotechnol.*, 2002, **28**, 17.

88. J. Lau, S. Frykman, R. Regentin, S. Ou, H. Tsuruta and P. Licari, *Biotechnol. Bioeng.*, 2002, **78**, 280.

89. C. M. Starks, Y. Zhou, F. Liu and P. J. Licari, *J. Nat. Prod.*, 2003, **66**, 1313.

90. R. Regentin, S. Frykman, J. Lau, H. Tsuruta and P. Licari, *Appl. Microbiol. Biotechnol.*, 2003, **61**, 451.

91. K. Gerth, S. Pradella, O. Perlova, S. Beyer and R. Müller, *J. Biotechnol.*, 2003, **106**, 233.

92. S. C. Wenzel and R. Müller, *Nat. Prod. Rep.*, 2009, **26**, 1385.

93. H. Baker, A. Sidorowicz, S. N. Sehgal and C. Vezina, *J. Antibiot.*, 1978, **31**, 539.

94. S. N. Sehgal, H. Baker and C. Vezina, *J. Antibiot.*, 1975, **28**, 727.

95. C. Vezina, A. Kudelski and S. N. Sehgal, *J. Antibiot.*, 1975, **28**, 721.

96. C. P. Eng, S. N. Sehgal and C. Vezina, *J. Antibiot.*, 1984, **37**, 1231.

97. J. Heitman, N. R. Movva and M. N. Hall, *Science*, 1991, **253**, 905.

98. E. J. Brown, M. W. Albers, T. Bum Shin, K. Ichikawa, C. T. Keith, W. S. Lane and S. L. Schreiber, *Nature*, 1994, **369**, 756.

99. S. G. Zech, M. Car, Q. K. Mohemmad, N. I. Narasimhan, C. Murray, L. W. Rozamus and D. C. Dalgarno, *J. Antibiot.*, 2011, **64**, 649.

100. J. B. McAlpine, S. J. Swanson, M. Jackson and D. N. Whittern, *J. Antibiot.*, 1991, **44**, 688.

101. B. Ruan, K. Pong, F. Jow, M. Bowlby, R. A. Crozier, D. Liu, S. Liang, Y. Chen, M. L. Mercado, X. Feng, F. Bennett, D. von Schack, L. McDonald, M. M. Zaleska, A. Wood, P. H. Reinhart, R. L. Magolda, J. Skotnicki, M. N. Pangalos, F. E. Koehn, G. T. Carter, M. Abou-Gharbia and E. I. Graziani, *Proc. Natl. Acad. Sci. USA*, 2008, **105**, 33.

102. M. Abou-Gharbia and W. Childers, *Pure Appl. Chem.*, 2012, **84**, 1543.

103. B. Chambraud, H. Belabes, V. Fontaine-Lenoir, A. Fellous and E. E. Baulieu, *J. Faseb.*, 2007, **21**, 2787.

104. J. T. De Leon, A. Iwai, C. Feau, Y. Garcia, H. A. Balsiger, C. L. Storer, R. M. Suro, K. M. Garza, S. T. Lee, Y. Sang Kim, Y. Chen, Y.-M. Ning, D. L. Riggs, R. J. Fletterick, R. K. Guy, J. B. Trepel, L. M. Neckers and M. B. Cox, *Proc. Natl. Acad. Sci. USA*, 2011, **108**, 11878.

105. S. Sarkar, G. Krishna, S. Imarisio, S. Saiki, C. J. O'Kane and D. C. Rubinsztein, *Hum. Mol. Genet.*, 2008, **17**, 170.

106. F. E. Koehn, *Curr. Opin. Biotech.*, 2006, **17**, 631.
107. D. J. Newman, *J. Med. Chem.*, 2008, **51**, 2589.
108. N. L. Pavia, A. L. Demain and M. F. Roberts, *J. Nat. Prod.*, 1991, **54**, 167.
109. A. L. Demain, *Annu. Rev. Microbiol.*, 2004, **58**, 1.
110. J. N. Andexer, S. G. Kendrew, M. Nur-e-Alam, O. Lazos, T. A. Foster, A. S. Zimmermann, T. D. Warneck, D. Suthar, N. J. Coates, F. E. Koehn, J. S. Skotnicki, G. T. Carter, M. A. Gregory, C. J. Martin, S. J. Moss, P. F. Leadlay and B. Wilkinson, *Proc. Nat. Acad. Sci. USA*, 2011, **108**, 4776.
111. E. I. Graziani, *Nat. Prod. Rep.*, 2009, **26**, 602.
112. S. R. Park, Y. J. Yoo, Y.-H. Ban and Y. J. Yoon, *J. Antibiot.*, 2010, **63**, 434.
113. C. J. Paddon, P. J. Westfall, D. J. Pitera, K. Benjamin, K. Fisher, D. McPhee, M. D. Leavell, A. Tai, A. Main, D. Eng, D. R. Polichuk, K. H. Teoh, D. W. Reed, T. Treynor, J. Lenihan, M. Fleck, S. Bajad, G. Dang, D. Dengrove, D. Diola, G. Dorin, K. W. Ellens, S. Fickes, J. Galazzo, S. P. Gaucher, T. Geistlinger, R. Henry, M. Hepp, T. Horning, T. Iqbal, H. Jiang, L. Kizer, B. Lieu, D. Melis, N. Moss, R. Regentin, S. Secrest, H. Tsuruta, R. Vazquez, L. F. Westblade, L. Xu, M. Yu, Y. Zhang, L. Zhao, J. Lievense, P. S. Covello, J. D. Keasling, K. K. Reiling, N. S. Renninger and J. D. Newman, *Nature*, 2013, **496**, 528.
114. S. G. Kendrew, H. Petkovic, S. Gaisser, S. J. Ready, M. A. Gregory, N. J. Coates, M. Nur-e-Alam, T. Warneck, D. Suthar, T. A. Foster, L. McDonald, G. Schlingman, F. E. Koehn, J. S. Skotnicki, G. T. Carter, S. J. Moss, M.-Q. Zhang, C. J. Martin, R. M. Sheridan and B. Wilkinson, *Metab. Eng.*, 2013, **15**, 167.
115. M. A. Gregory, S. Gaisser, H. Pelkovic and S. J. Moss, EP 2 277 896 A2, 24SEP2011.
116. M. A. Gregory, A. L. Kaja, S. G. Kendrew, N. J. Coates, T. Warneck, M. Nur-e-Alam, R. E. Lill, L. S. Sheehan, L. Chudley, S. J. Moss, R. M. Sheridan, M. Quimpere, M.-Q. Zhang, C. J. Martina and B. Wilkinson, *Chem. Sci.*, 2013, **4**, 1046.
117. M. A. Gregory, S. J. Moss and B. Wilkinson, WO 2013093493 A1, 27 JUN 2013.
118. E. W. Schmidt, M. S. Donia, J. A. McIntosh, W. F. Fricke and J. Ravel, *J. Nat. Prod.*, 2012, **75**, 295.
119. K. L. Dunbar and D. A. Mitchell, *ACS Chem. Biol.*, 2013, **8**, 473.
120. G. F. Gause and M. G. Brazhnikova, *Nature*, 1944, **152**, 703.
121. R. J. Dubos, *J. Exp. Med.*, 1939, **70**, 1.
122. R. J. Dubos, *J. Exp. Med.*, 1939, **70**, 11.
123. P. G. Sergiev, *Lancet*, 1944, **244**, 717.
124. V. V. Kapoerchan, A. D. Knijnenburg, P. Keizer, E. Spalburg, A. J. De Neeling, R. H. Mars-Groenendijk, D. Noort, J. M. Otero, L. S. A. L. M. J. van Raaji, G. A. van der Marel, H. S. Overkleeft and M. Overhand, *Bioorg. Med. Chem.*, 2012, **20**, 6059.
125. I. Alicino, M. Giglio, F. Manca, F. Bruno and F. Puntillo, *Pain*, 2012, **153**, 245.

126. B. M. Olivera, L. J. Cruz, V. De Santos, G. W. LeCheminant, D. Griffin, R. Zeikus, J. M. McIntosh, R. Galyean and J. Varga, *Biochemistry*, 1987, **26**, 2086.

127. A. E. Fedosov, S. A. Moshkovskii, K. G. Kuznetsova and B. M. Olivera, *Biochemistry (Moscow) Supp. Ser B, Biomed. Chem.*, 2012, **6**, 107.

128. N. L. Daly and D. J. Craik, *Drugs Fut.*, 2011, **36**, 25.

129. R. J. Clark, M. Akcan, Q. Kaas, N. L. Daly and D. J. Craik, *Toxicon*, 2012, **59**, 446.

130. C. I. Schroeder and D. J. Craik, *Fut. Med. Chem.*, 2012, **4**, 1243.

131. R. J. Clark, J. Jensen, S. T. Nevin, B. P. Callaghan, D. J. Adams and D. J. Craik, *Angew. Chem. Int. Ed.*, 2010, **49**, 6545.

132. H. Itazaki, K. Nagashima, K. Sugita, H. Yoshida, Y. Kawamura, Y. Yasuda, K. Matsumoto, K. Ishii, N. Uotani, H. Nakai, A. Terui, S. Yoshimatsu, Y. Ikenishi and Y. Nakagawa, *J. Antibiot.*, 1990, **43**, 1524.

133. M. Kijima, M. Yoshida, K. Sugita, S. Horinouchi and T. Beppu, *J. Biol. Chem.*, 1993, **268**, 22429.

134. S. J. Darkin-Rattray, A. M. Gurnett, R. W. Myers, P. M. Dulski, T. M. Crumley, J. J. Allocco, C. Cannova, P. T. Meinke, S. L. Colletti, M. A. Bednarek, S. B. Singh, M. A. Goetz, A. W. Dombrowski, J. D. Polishook and D. M. Schmatz, *Proc. Natl. Acad. Sci. USA*, 1996, **93**, 13143.

135. S. B. Singh, D. L. Zink, J. D. Polishook, A. W. Dombrowski, S. J. Darkin-Rattray, D. M. Schmatz and M. A. Goetz, *Tet. Lett.*, 1996, **37**, 8077.

136. L. A. Salvador and H. Luesch, in *Natural Products and Cancer Drug Discovery*, ed. F. E. Koehn, Humana Press, New York, 2013, p. 59.

137. Y. Nakao, S. Yoshida, S. Matsunaga, N. Shindoh, Y. Terada, K. Nagai, J. K. Yamashita, A. Ganesan, R. W. van Soest and N. Fusetani, *Angew. Chem. Int. Ed.*, 2006, **45**, 7553.

138. S. Wen, K. L. Carey, Y. Nakao, N. Fusetani, G. Packham and A. Ganesan, *Org. Lett.*, 2007, **9**, 1105.

139. I. Izzo, N. Maulucci, G. Bifulco and F. De Riccardis, *Angew. Chem. Int. Ed.*, 2006, **45**, 7557.

140. J. S. Villadsen, H. M. Stephansen, A. R. Maolanon, P. Harris and C. A. Olsen, *J. Med. Chem.*, 2013, **56**, 6512.

141. H. Ueda, H. Nakajima, Y. Hori, T. Fujita, M. Nishimura, T. Goto and M. Okuhara, *J. Antibiot.*, 1994, **47**, 301.

142. H. Nakajima, Y. B. Kim, H. Terano, M. Yoshida and S. Horinouchi, *Exp. Cell Res.*, 1998, **241**, 126.

143. R. Furumai, A. Matsuyama, N. Kobashi, K. H. Lee, M. Nishiyama, H. Nakajima, A. Tanaka, Y. Komatsu, N. Nishino, M. Yoshida and S. Horinouchi, *Cancer Res.*, 2002, **62**, 4916.

144. Y. Chen, C. Gambs, Y. Abe, P. Wentworth Jr and K. D. Janda, *J. Org. Chem.*, 2003, **68**, 8902.

145. A. Yurek-George, F. Habens, M. Brimmell, G. Packham and A. Ganesan, *J. Am. Chem. Soc.*, 2004, **126**, 1030.

146. S. J. Crabb, M. Howell, H. Rogers, M. Ishfaq, A. Yurek-George, G. K. Carey, B. M. Pickering, P. East, R. Mitter, S. Maeda, P. W. M. Johnson, P. Townsend, K. Shin-ya, M. Yoshida, A. Ganesan and G. Packham, *Biochem. Pharmacol.*, 2008, **76**, 463.
147. T. Yamada, M. Horinaka, M. Shinnoh, T. Yoshioka, T. Miki and T. Sakai, *Int. J. Oncol.*, 2013, **43**, 1080.
148. H. Benelkebir, A. L. Donlevy, G. Packham and A. Ganesan, *Org. Lett.*, 2011, **13**, 6334.
149. A. J. Wilson, Y.-Q. Cheng and D. Khabele, *J. Ovar. Res.*, 2012, **5**, 12.
150. K. Taori, V. J. Paul and H. Luesch, *J. Am. Chem. Soc.*, 2008, **130**, 1806.
151. Y. Ying, K. Taori, H. Kim, J. Hong and H. Luesch, *J. Am. Chem. Soc.*, 2008, **130**, 8455.
152. A. K. Ghosh and S. Kulkarni, *Org. Lett.*, 2008, **10**, 3907.
153. C. G. Nasveschuk, D. Ungermannova, X. Liu and A. J. Phillips, *Org. Lett.*, 2008, **10**, 3595.
154. Y. Ying, Y. Liu, S. R. Byeon, H. Kim, H. Luesch and J. Hong, *Org. Lett.*, 2008, **10**, 4021.
155. A. Bowers, N. West, J. Taunton, S. L. Schreiber, J. E. Bradner and R. M. Williams, *J. Am. Chem. Soc.*, 2008, **130**, 11219.
156. X. Zeng, B. Yin, Z. Hu, C. Liao, J. Liu, S. Li, Z. Li, M. C. Nicklaus, G. Zhou and S. Jiang, *Org. Lett.*, 2010, **12**, 1368.
157. J. A. Souto, E. Vaz, I. Lepore, A. C. Pöppler, G. Franci, R. Alvarez, L. Altucci and A. R. de Lera, *J. Med. Chem.*, 2010, **53**, 4654.
158. H. Benelkebir, S. Marie, A. L. Hayden, J. Lyle, P. M. Loadman, S. J. Crabb, G. Packham and A. Ganesan, *Bioorg. Med. Chem.*, 2011, **19**, 3650.
159. J. M. Guerra-Bubb, A. A. Bowers, W. B. Smith, R. Paranal, G. Estiu, O. Wiest, J. E. Bradner and R. M. Williams, *Bioorg. Med. Chem. Lett.*, 2013, **23**, 6025.
160. S. U. Lee, H. B. Kwak, S. H. Pi, H. K. You, S. R. Byeon, Y. Ying, H. Luesch, J. Hong and S. H. Kim, *ACS Med. Chem. Lett.*, 2011, **2**, 2011.
161. S. K. Ghosh, S. P. Perrine, R. M. Williams and D. V. Faller, *Blood*, 2012, **119**, 1008.
162. L. C. Wu, Z. S. Wen, Y. T. Qiu, X. Q. Chen, H. B. Chen, M. M. Wei, Z. Liu, S. Jiang and G. B. Zhou, *ACS Med. Chem. Lett.*, 2013, **4**, 921.
163. Y. Liu, Z. Wang, J. Wang, W. Lam, S. Kwong, F. Li, S. L. Friedman, S. Zhou, Q. Ren, Z. Xu, X. Wang, L. Ji, S. Tang, H. Zhang, E. L. Lui and T. Ye, *Liver Int.*, 2013, **33**, 504.
164. C. A. Olsen and M. R. Ghadiri, *J. Med. Chem.*, 2009, **52**, 7836.
165. L. Auzzas, A. Larsson, R. Matera, A. Baraldi, B. Deschenes-Simard, G. Giannini, W. Cabri, G. Battistuzzi, G. Gallo, A. Ciacci, L. Vesci, C. Pisano and S. Hanessian, *J. Med. Chem.*, 2010, **53**, 8387.
166. S. C. Stolze and M. Kaiser, *Molecules*, 2013, **18**, 1337.
167. H. Rajak, A. Singh, P. K. Dewangan, V. Patel, D. K. Jain, S. K. Tiwari, R. Veerasamy and P. C. Sharma, *Curr. Med. Chem.*, 2013, **20**, 1887.

168. F. F. Wagner, M. Weiwer, M. C. Lewis and E. B. Holson, *Neurotherap.*, 2013, **10**, 589.
169. K. M. George, D. Chatterjee, G. Gunawardana, D. Welty, J. Hayman, R. Lee and P. L. Small, *Science*, 1999, **283**, 854.
170. P. Gersbach, A. Jantsch, F. Feyen, N. Scherr, J.-P. Dangy, G. Pluschke and K.-H. Altmann, *Chem. - Eur. J.*, 2011, **17**, 13017.
171. A.-C. Chany, V. Casarotto, M. Schmitt, C. Tarnus, L. Guerin-Mace, C. Demangel, O. Mirguet, J. Eustache and N. Blanchard, *Chem. - Eur. J.*, 2011, **17**, 14413.
172. N. Scherr, P. Gersbach, J.-P. Dangy, C. Bomio, J. Li, K.-H. Altmann and G. Pluschke, *PLOS, Neg. Trop. Dis.*, 2013, **7**, e2143.
173. T. D. Aicher, K. R. Buszek, F. G. Fang, C. J. Forsyth, S. H. Jung, Y. Kishi, M. C. Matelich, P. M. Scola, D. M. Spero and S. K. Yoon, *J. Am. Chem. Soc.*, 1992, **114**, 3162.
174. M. J. Yu, Y. Kishi and B. A. Littlefield, in *Anticancer Agents from Natural Products*, ed. G. M. Cragg, D. G. I. Kingston and D. J. Newman, Taylor and Francis, Boca Raton, FL, 2nd edn, 2012, pp. 317.
175. M. J. Yu, W. Zheng and B. M. Seletsky, *Nat. Prod. Rep.*, 2013, **30**, 1158.
176. S. Narayan, E. M. Carlson, H. Cheng, H. Du, Y. Hu, Y. Jiang, B. M. Lewis, B. M. Seletsky, K. Tendyke, H. Zhang, W. Zheng, B. A. Littlefield, M. J. Towle and M. J. Yu, *Bioorg. Med. Chem. Lett.*, 2011, **21**, 1630.
177. S. Narayan, E. M. Carlson, H. Cheng, K. Condon, H. Du, S. Eckley, Y. Hu, Y. Jiang, V. Kumar, B. M. Lewis, P. Saxton, E. Schuck, B. M. Seletsky, K. Tendyke, H. Zhang, W. Zheng, B. A. Littlefield, M. J. Towle and M. J. Yu, *Bioorg. Med. Chem. Lett.*, 2011, **21**, 1634.
178. S. Narayan, E. M. Carlson, H. Cheng, K. Condon, H. Du, S. Eckley, Y. Hu, Y. Jiang, V. Kumar, B. M. Lewis, P. Saxton, E. Schuck, B. M. Seletsky, K. Tendyke, H. Zhang, W. Zheng, B. A. Littlefield, M. J. Towle and M. J. Yu, *Bioorg. Med. Chem. Lett.*, 2011, **21**, 1639.
179. Z.-D. Shi, K. Lee, H. Liu, M. Zhang, L. R. Roberts, K. M. Worthy, M. J. Fivash, R. J. Fisher, D. Yang and T. R. Burke Jr, *Biochim. Biophys. Res. Comm.*, 2003, **310**, 378.
180. Z.-D. Shi, C.-Q. Wei, K. Lee, H. Liu, M. Zhang, T. Araki, L. R. Roberts, K. M. Worthy, R. J. Fisher, B. G. Neel, J. A. Kelley, D. Yang and T. R. Burke Jr, *J. Med. Chem.*, 2004, **47**, 2166.
181. C. W. Zapf, J. D. Bloom, Z. Li, R. G. Dushin, T. Nittoli, M. Otteng, A. Nikitenko, J. M. Golas, H. Liu, J. Lucas, F. Boschelli, E. Vogan, A. Olland, M. Johnson and J. I. Levin, *Bioorg. Med. Chem. Lett.*, 2011, **21**, 4602.
182. L A. Mitscher, *Chem. Rev.*, 2005, **105**, 559.

CHAPTER 2

Recent Advances in Macrocyclic Hsp90 Inhibitors

D. M. RAMSEY,[a] R. R. A. KITSON,[b] J. I. LEVIN,[c] C. J. MOODY*[b] AND S. R. McALPINE*[a]

[a] School of Chemistry, University of New South Wales, Sydney, NSW 2052, Australia; [b] School of Chemistry, University of Nottingham, University Park, Nottingham, NG7 2RD, UK; [c] Boehringer Ingelheim Pharmaceuticals, Inc., Ridgefield, CT 06877, USA
*Email: C.J.Moody@nottingham.ac.uk; s.mcalpine@unsw.edu.au

2.1 Introduction

Medium (9–11 atoms) and large ($\geq$12 atoms) macrocycles are significant chemical weapons used by marine invertebrates, plants, and microorganisms to attack or defend.[1] The isolation and use of macrocycles as medicinal chemistry tools gained momentum during the Antibiotic Era (1940–1970), when synthesis and purification of large quantities of natural products were achieved, closing the "bench to bedside" gap that had plagued clinical drug development.[2] The discovery of cyclosporines, which target eukaryotic proteins, was one of the first novel macrocyclic inhibitors to be tested and clinically approved as a treatment for human disease.[3,4] As the focus of cancer research shifted towards targeting individual molecular pathways, the discovery and application of macrocycles as anticancer agents expanded.[4]

Tight binding interactions between a macrocycle and its oncogenic target rely on the size, flexibility, rigidity, binding energy, and functional group orientation of the macrocycle. An unsuitable "fit" occurs between the

RSC Drug Discovery Series No. 40
Macrocycles in Drug Discovery
Edited by Jeremy Levin
© The Royal Society of Chemistry 2015
Published by the Royal Society of Chemistry, www.rsc.org

molecule and target when any one of these properties is inadequately addressed and makes the molecule a poor binding partner.[5]

In spite of promising preclinical data, solubility problems and off-target effects can end the molecule's progress in early clinical studies. In this chapter we discuss how macrocycles are utilised within oncology to inhibit the heat shock response, specifically the molecular chaperone heat shock protein 90 (Hsp90). We describe what the clinical frontrunners (derivatives of the ansamycin antibiotic, geldanamycin) have taught us with regards to structural optimisation, solubility, and potency as a monotherapy. We then highlight how dual therapeutic approaches resurrect the clinical promise of these derivatives by lowering the effective dose and minimising off-target effects. Finally we discuss the next generation of macrocyclic Hsp90 inhibitors. These include promising lead structures derived from natural products, as well as synthetic derivatives modelled on structure-based designs that optimise the core contacts between Hsp90 and its bound ligands.

2.1.1   Macrocycles as Anticancer Agents

Anticancer drug development must optimise the thermodynamic properties of molecules to achieve the highest binding affinities to oncogenic targets (thereby lowering the effective dose), while minimising the properties that lead to biological instability or nonspecific binding events (reducing toxicity). Lipinski's Rule of Five established characteristics to measure a compound's drug "potential", including (a) no more than five hydrogen-bond donors and 10 hydrogen-bond acceptors; (b) a partition coefficient log P (Log P) score of less than five, indicating low lipophilicity; and (c) a molecular weight of less than 500 Daltons (Da).[6] Amendments to these characteristics rationalise why some compounds maintain oral bioavailability while not adhering to the Rule of Five, including: (a) having 10 or fewer rotatable bonds, and (b) 12 or fewer hydrogen-bond donors and acceptors combined.[7,8] Frequently, however, macrocycles do not adhere to Lipinski's rules nor the amendments, but they are successful clinical candidates and transition to the marketplace. A macrocycle's ability to overcome the issues of high molecular weight (>500 Da), more than 12 hydrogen bond donors and acceptors, and high Log P values is usually related to high binding affinity, stability, and specificity for a molecular target.

Medium-sized macrocycles contain 9–12 atoms organised in a ring. This structural pattern provides a special conformational constraint that, if utilised effectively, enhances binding to a specific domain (≥ 20 amino acids) of a biological target.[9] By providing a less flexible scaffold than the non-macrocyclic molecules, structures can be locked into a bioactive conformation that lowers entropy, reduces susceptibility to proteolytic cleavage and increases binding affinity relative to a structurally similar linear substrate.[10] Although membrane permeability is enhanced by cyclisation, macrocycles are often plagued by poor solubility issues due to hydrophobic residues that are typically incorporated within the structural backbone.[11] Scaling up syntheses of macrocycles from preclinical studies into early clinical trials is typically challenging if there are no repetitive elements or biosynthetic pathways to be utilised.[5] The advantages and disadvantages of the macrocyclic structure are prominently illustrated in Hsp90 research, where several macrocyclic Hsp90 inhibitors have been removed from further clinical study when the molecular promise was outweighed by the side-effects.[12]

Based on the structural similarities of each compound, macrocyclic inhibitors of Hsp90 can be organised into four classes:[1] Geldanamycin and its derivatives (Class I), radicicol and radanamycin (Class II), synthetic acyclic small molecule inhibitors (Class III), and macrocycles that target Hsp90's *N*-middle domain (Class IV) (Figure 2.1). Geldanamycin, a dominant representative of Class I inhibitors, was the first natural product inhibitor of Hsp90 to reach preclinical testing as a potential treatment for cancer.[13] Synthetic derivatives of geldanamycin continue to dominate clinical research, but new macrocycles based on other types of scaffolds have demonstrated preclinical promise and expanded the structures of *N*-terminal binding molecules.[14–16] Although the efficacy of the potent Class II inhibitor radicicol is diminished *in vivo* due to its metabolic instability, improvements incorporated into its synthetic derivatives and chimeras such as radanamycin have led to greater structural stability without loss of potency.[17–19] Class III inhibitors include the *o*-aminobenzamide SNX-2112 and the purine-class inhibitor BIIB021, which have been evaluated in several completed clinical trials.[20–22] Finally, natural products have supplied an alternative macrocyclic structure that binds to Hsp90 between the *N* and middle

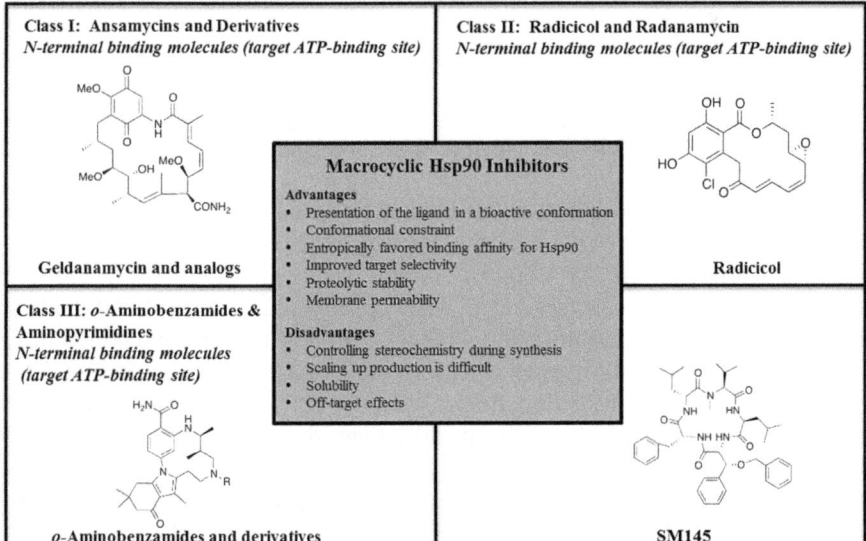

Figure 2.1 Four major classes of macrocyclic Hsp90 inhibitors.

domains (Class IV). This class of macrocyclic inhibitors allosterically modulate the *C*-terminus of Hsp90, and include the structures SM122 and SM145.[23–29]

2.1.2 Heat Shock Protein 90 (Hsp90) as an Oncogenic Target

The heat shock response contributes several key regulators of cellular homeostasis and protein stability.[30] Ranging in size from 20 to 100 kDa, heat shock proteins contribute to a number of vital support services that touch all aspects of cellular physiology, including transportation, migration, post-translational modification, signalling and protein recycling. Cancer cells accelerate these homeostatic processes due to the rapid division rates required for oncogenic growth, which leads to greater expression levels of heat shock proteins in tumours compared to normal cells.[31] Of particular interest to the cancer community is Hsp90, a molecular chaperone that stabilises and folds both intracellular and extracellular oncogenic proteins involved in metastasis, chemotherapeutic drug resistance, and cell growth.[32]

Highly active isoforms of Hsp90, Hsp90α and Hsp90β, contribute 3–5% of the total protein load in oncogenic cells (*vs.* 1–2% in normal cells).[33] Sharing 85% sequence homology both isoforms appear to have the same function within the cytosol. Cytosolic Hsp90α and Hsp90β fold and stabilize oncogenic proteins in conjunction with co-chaperones, without which Hsp90 would not function. The Hsp90 homologues located in the endoplasmic reticulum (glucose-related protein 94, GRP94) and mitochondria (tumour necrosis factor receptor-associated protein 1, TRAP1) appear to have ATP-dependent protein folding mechanisms, but no co-chaperones. Thus, unlike the cytosolic Hsp90 isoforms, it appears that neither of these isoforms, GRP94 and TRAP1, regulates oncogenic proteins. Instead, GRP94's main role is folding proteins that are involved in the immune response, and TRAP1 is responsible for protecting the integrity of the mitochondria under stress. Thus, Hsp90α and Hsp90β remain the main targets in developing Hsp90 inhibitors due to their association with oncogenic client proteins and pathways.

Interactions with over 400 client proteins and co-chaperones have established Hsp90's cellular role as a master regulator of multiple cellular pathways.[34,35] The majority of Hsp90's activity occurs in the cytosol, where it forms protein–protein interactions with approximately 60% of all cellular kinases and 30% of all ubiquitin ligases.[34,36] In addition, Hsp90 contributes to the maturation of hormone receptors and kinases that are essential for oncogenesis in hormone-dependent cancers.[37,38] Hsp90 also maintains protein quality control by facilitating the degradation of unfolded proteins through the ubiquitin/proteasome degradation pathway.[39] Disrupting these pathways through Hsp90 inhibition has catastrophic consequences for the cell and leads to the induction of cell death.

Hsp90 is a 732 amino acid protein organised into 3 domains:[40] an *N*-terminal 25 kDa domain that is responsible for ATP-binding; a 35 kDa middle domain (*M*-domain), which serves as the primary client protein docking site; and a 10 kDa *C*-terminal domain that serves as primary co-chaperone binding site and dimerisation hub (Figure 2.2).[40–43] The *N*-terminal and middle domains are connected by a short charged region (CR). A MEEVD (M = methionine, E = glutamic acid, V = valine, D = aspartic acid) amino acid sequence is located in the *C*-terminus, and binds to a subset of co-chaperones that contain repeating units of basic amino acids (tetratricopeptide-repeat or TPR regions). The MEEVD region overlaps with the dimerisation domain and it also facilitates the binding of numerous important co-chaperones and client proteins to Hsp90.[41,44]

The most common macrocyclic inhibitors (Classes I, II and III), as well as acyclic molecules currently in clinical trials (NVP-AUY922), are those that target Hsp90's N-terminal ATP-binding site.[37] Crosstalk between the *N*-terminal and *C*-terminal domains of Hsp90 affects the chaperone's ATPase activity, conformation, and client protein binding affinity. Inhibiting this pattern of allosteric communication by targeting the ATP-binding site alters the ability of Hsp90 to complete its enzymatic cycle (Figure 2.2).[45]

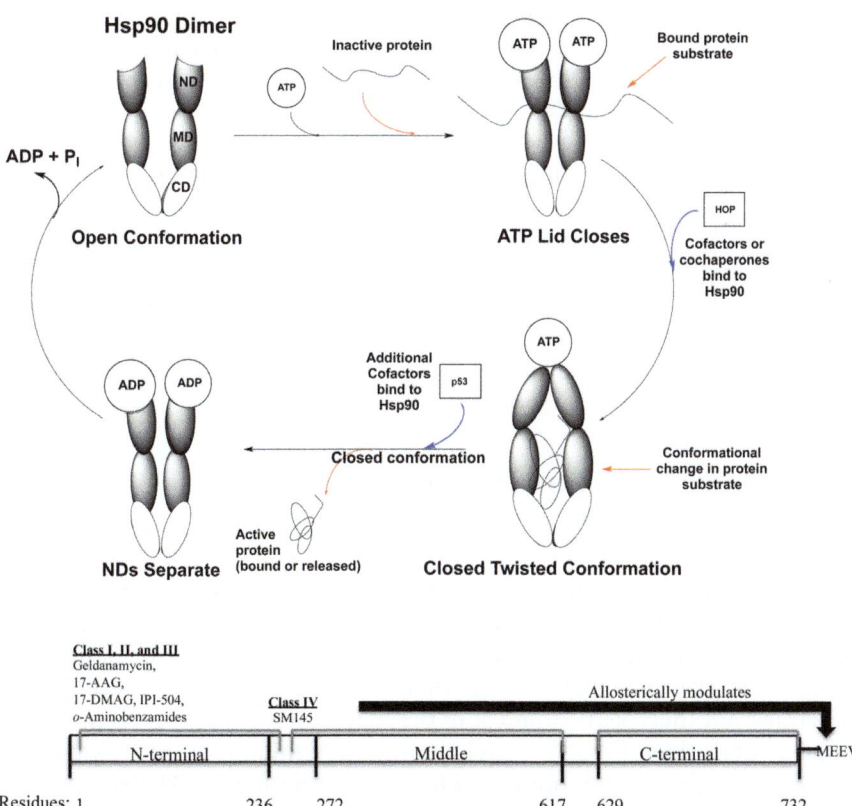

Figure 2.2 Hsp90 folding cycle and binding sites.[47]

Homodimerisation is the active conformation of Hsp90, which has led to the *C*-terminal dimerisation domain (with its nucleotide binding site and MEEVD co-chaperone binding region) becoming the focus of several Hsp90 inhibitors: Class IV (SM122 and 145), which show excellent Hsp90 inhibitory activity.[23–27,29,46] All four classes appear to modulate the allosteric cross talk between the *N*- and *C*- termini of Hsp90. However, each macrocyclic class of compounds impacts the clients and co-chaperone binding events uniquely.

Fluorescence resonance energy transfer (FRET) data of labelled Hsp90 dimers has revealed insights into the four allosteric conformations that Hsp90 assumes as a molecular chaperone (Figure 2.2).[48] The binding of two molecules of ATP to the *N*-terminal binding pockets is a rapid event, but the rate-limiting step is hydrolysis of ATP since Hsp90 must transition from an open to a closed complex before hydrolysis takes place (Figure 2.2).[49] ATP hydrolysis is accelerated by the binding of co-chaperone proteins to Hsp90, which reduces the flexibility of the chaperone and supports the formation of the closed-twisted conformation.[49] It is clear from FRET data that binding events have considerable structural implications across the entire scaffold of Hsp90. Inhibitors may target a specific domain, but their binding inter-action alters the Hsp90 dimer on a macro-scale level, preferentially binding to an open, transition (nucleotide binding) or closed state. For example, Class IV inhibitors bind to the *N*-middle domain, but they induce allosteric modifications that block the access of co-chaperones that target the MEEVD region of the *C*-terminus.[24–26,29]

Hsp90 inhibition can be assessed at three levels. At the biochemical level, direct and allosteric binding interactions between Hsp90 and macrocyclic inhibitors can be assessed for the modification of Hsp90 conformations. At the cellular level, Hsp90 inhibition will affect multiple cellular pathways at once, leading to observable changes in cell motility and survival. At the organismal level, dosage and efficacy of Hsp90 inhibitors are major land-marks that must be reached before macrocyclic therapies can make clinical progress. In this chapter we will discuss macrocyclic Hsp90 inhibitors at each of these three levels.

2.2 Class I: Ansamycins and Derivatives

2.2.1 Geldanamycin

The benzoquinone ansamycin antibiotic geldanamycin (NSC 122750) was isolated in 1970 by Peterson and colleagues from the bacteria *Streptomyces hygroscopicus* (Figure 2.3).[50] The biosynthesis, structure elucidation and antiproliferative activities of geldanamycin indicated drug development potential, but therapeutic interest in the macrocycle grew after its molecular targets were identified.[51,52] Geldanamycin inhibits DNA polymerases, tyrosine kinases, and multiple isoforms of mammalian Hsp90 (Hsp90α, Hsp90β, GP96/GRP94, TRAP-1), and inhibition of these molecular targets produces anticancer, anti-inflammatory, and antiviral effects.[15,51–55]

The reported potencies for geldanamycin against eukaryotic cell lines range between 20 nM and 5 μM,[19,45,51,56] and the observed variability has been shown to be both methodology-dependent as well as cell line dependent.[57]

Geldanamycin-based analogues compete with ATP/ADP for binding to the ATP-binding pocket of Hsp90.[58] The binding affinity (K_d) of geldanamycin (1) for the *N*-terminal domain of yeast Hsp90 is 1.2 μM,[59] and the crystal structure of geldanamycin bound to its *N*-terminal Hsp90 binding pocket has highlighted unique structural changes that occur at the binding interface.[59–61] Geldanamycin adopts a "C-clamp" conformation when bound to Hsp90, where the benzoquinone forms the top of the clamp and the aliphatic ansa ring, with *cis*-configured amide, forms the stem and base (Figure 2.3).[60] The benzoquinone contributes few contacts with Hsp90, but the ansa ring forms a network of van der Waals connections that nestles the macrocycle into the hydrophobic face of the ATP-binding pocket.[59] The C-12 methoxy group from geldanamycin forms hydrogen bonds with E88 and N92 amino acid residues in the ATP-binding pocket, and amino acid substitutions at these positions disrupt hydrogen bonding and lead to partial geldanamycin resistance in yeast.[58] Using targeted molecular dynamics (TMD) to simulate the conformational changes required for unbound geldanamycin to adopt its Hsp90-bound structure, Jez *et al.* revealed that a significant energy barrier exists for the molecule to adopt the less-stable C-clamp position ($\Delta G = 8.1$ kcal mol^{-1}), which may explain its slow association/dissociation rate with Hsp90.[62,63] In addition, several protein side chains of the amino acids within the ATP-binding pocket become more ordered upon binding of geldanamycin, which increases the overall entropic penalty of this binding interaction and reduces the binding affinity.

At the cellular level, Hsp90 inhibition by geldanamycin induces dramatic changes in the proteome, and metabolic processing of the compound also causes further cellular damage. Recent proteomic studies have shown that geldanamycin alters cellular protein levels through a decrease in *de novo* protein synthesis and a reduction in protein stability.[35,64] The complex and interlinking protein networks that are affected by geldanamycin form one arm of the apoptotic process, but the induction of metabolic stress through the reduction of the compound also contributes to cell death. Two enzymes metabolise the benzoquinone moiety of geldanamycin and enhance the macrocycle's potency or contribute to its toxicity. Solid tumours highly express NAD(P)H:quinone oxidoreductase enzyme 1 (NQO1), which uses NADH or NAD(P)H as catalysts for the 2-electron reduction of quinones to hydroquinones.[65] Reduction of the benzoquinone by NQO1 leads to enhanced cytotoxicity in ansamycin-treated breast cancer cell lines, and the cellular metabolism of geldanamycin explains its observed nanomolar to low micromolar potencies.[66] One-electron reductases present in cells can also metabolise quinones, generating unstable semiquinones and superoxide radicals that lead to cellular damage.[67] Liver cells express an abundance of one-electron reductases, and metabolism of geldanamycin by these enzymes

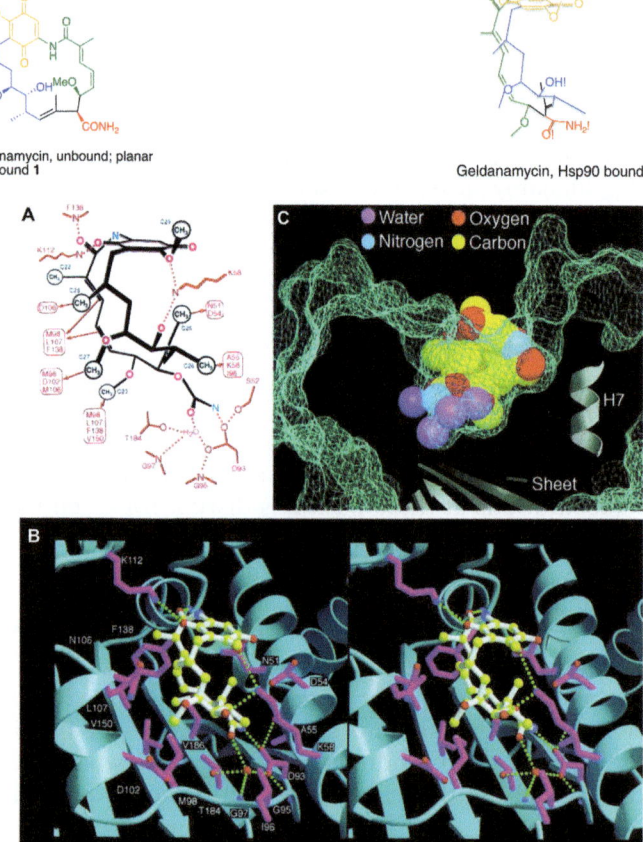

Geldanamycin, unbound; planar
Compound **1**

Geldanamycin, Hsp90 bound; C-clamp

Figure 2.3   Conformational changes of geldanamycin (**1**) when bound to Hsp90.[59–61]
Yellow indicates the benzoquinone, blue indicates the aliphatic ansa
ring, red indicates the C-7 carbamate group, and green indicates the
closing ring structure. The C-clamp conformation was reported by
Stebbens *et al.* (used with permission).[60] (A) Diagram of the bound
geldanamycin conformation summarising the hydrogen bond (dotted
lines) and van der Waals (arrows) contacts it makes with Hsp90 residues,
coloured brown. The oxygen atoms of geldanamycin are shown in red,
nitrogen atoms in blue, and methyl groups as closed circles; the
remaining carbon atoms are not explicitly shown. (B) Stereo view of the
geldanamycin–Hsp90-GBD interactions. Geldanamycin is coloured as
shown in structure above, and Hsp90 residues that make up the pocket
are coloured magenta. Hydrogen bonds are indicated by green dotted
lines, and the water molecule that bridges the geldanamycin carbamate
group with Asp93 is shown as a red sphere. (C) Geldanamycin, in space-
filling representation, adopts a structure that is, overall, complementary
to the pocket, shown as a blue molecular surface net. Although the fit is
extensive, there remains a buried cavity at the interface with three
trapped water molecules in it (coloured magenta), while a fourth water
molecule hydrogen bonds with the carbamate group and Asp93. The
reduced complementarity near the pocket entrance is evident as gaps
between the geldanamycin atoms and the Hsp90-GBD surface.

contributes significant hepatotoxicity compared to other clinical ansamycin derivatives.[68]

Poor solubility and hepatotoxicity led to removal of geldanamycin from further consideration as an anticancer therapy.[13] Although no longer considered an oral clinical candidate, recent preclinical data suggests that this macrocycle may hold therapeutic promise as a low-dose topical agent for the treatment of viral infections.[54] It is also noteworthy that ansamycin based-Hsp90 inhibitors are not limited to the geldanamycin family alone. Other potent inhibitors from the ansamycin family include the macbecins and herbimycins.[69] Indeed macbecin I itself has both a higher binding affinity for Hsp90 than geldanamycin ($K_d = 0.24$ μM $vs.$ 1.2 μM) and is more potent in some reported assays ($IC_{50} = 2$ μM).[69] Thus ansamycins have contributed not only a scaffold that has inspired numerous synthetic derivatives but also additional structural members that are new potential drug candidates.

Geldanamycin research has contributed three significant findings that were instrumental in optimising the SARs of ansamycin derivatives. First, the aliphatic ansa ring forms a network of bonds with the ATP-binding pocket of Hsp90, which are critical for ligand–protein stabilisation, but the entropic cost of binding to Hsp90 must be lowered in order to improve the binding affinity of ansamycin derivatives. Second, solubility must be improved to become a clinically viable candidate. Finally, cellular reduction and metabolism of ansamycins contributes significantly to potency and hepatotoxicity. Described below are ways in which derivatives of geldana-mycin were structurally modified in order to optimise potency, reduce toxicity, and thereby deliver a viable drug candidate into the clinical arena.

2.2.2 Geldanamycin Derivatives

2.2.2.1 17-Allyl-17-desmethoxygeldanamycin (17-AAG)

The first ansamycin-derived Hsp90 inhibitor to enter the clinic was 17-allylamino-17-desmethoxygeldanamycin, 2 (17-AAG; also known as KOS-953 or tanespimycin; Figure 2.4),[70–74] formed from the simple addition–elimination reaction of geldanamycin itself with allylamine.[15,75] Formation of toxic metabolites and poor solubility are two major drawbacks observed clinically when 17-AAG is used as an anticancer treatment. The liver enzyme CYP3A4 metabolises 17-AAG and produces the biologically active byproduct 17-amino-desmethoxygeldanamycin (17-AG, 5), which also inhibits Hsp90, as well as nephrotoxic epoxides and aldehydes such as acrolein.[72,76,77] To improve the solubility of the compound for patient administration, 17-AAG is dissolved in organic solvents such as dimethyl sulfoxide (DMSO), ethanol or Cremophor, or in a suspension of sucrose, lecithin and polysorbate 80.[78] The organic solvents themselves can be toxic or induce hypersensitivity in patients, which exacerbates the nephrotoxicity of 17-AAG's metabolic by-products and increases the overall toxicity profile

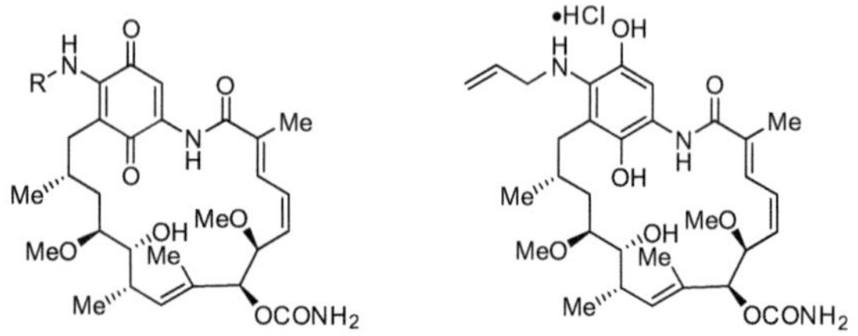

2 R = CH$_2$CH=CH$_2$: 17-AAG
3 R = CH$_2$CH$_2$NMe$_2$: 17-DMAG
5 R = H: 17-AG

4 17-AAG hydroquinone
hydrochloride (retaspimycin)

Figure 2.4   Structures of geldanamycin derivatives.

of the compound.[79,80] These issues paved the way for the development of 17-(dimethylaminoethylamino)-17-desmethoxygeldanamycin (17-DMAG, **3**).

A growing body of research has applied the therapeutic effects of 17-AAG in the treatment of non-cancer related disease models, including neurodegenerative disorders and infectious disease.[81–83] By enhancing the degradation of a mutant form of the androgen receptor, which requires Hsp90 for proper folding, 17-AAG reduces motor impairment in a mouse model of spinal and bulbar muscular atrophy (SBMA).[84] Hsp90 plays an important role in HIV-1 viral replication,[85] and 17-AAG demonstrates potency against HIV-infected primary blood mononuclear cells and reduces viral load at high nanomolar concentrations (IC$_{50}$ = 140 nM).[82] In addition to its potential use as an antiviral therapy, 17-AAG has shown promise in the treatment of certain intracellular parasites that rely on Hsp90 homologues for survival.[83,86] The Hsp90 homologue expressed by the malarial parasite *Plasmodium falciparum* (PfHsp90) exhibits 6-fold greater ATPase activity than human Hsp90, and 17-AAG inhibits growth of 50% of clinically isolated parasites in the mid-nanomolar range (IC$_{50}$ = 50–150 nM, depending on strain).[86] The genome of the protozoan that causes African sleeping sickness (*Trypanosoma brucei*) contains 10 tandem copies of an Hsp90 homologue, Hsp83, and treatment of parasites with 17-AAG (EC$_{50}$ = 30 nM) leads to cell cycle disruption, inhibition of cytokinesis, and sensitisation to heat shock.[83,87] These studies illustrate the clinical versatility of macrocyclic Hsp90 inhibitors and highlight the need for less toxic derivatives that can be tolerated by immunocompromised patients.

2.2.2.2   *17-Desmethoxy-N,N-dimethylethylenediaminogeldanamycin (17-DMAG)*

In view of the previously outlined adverse properties associated with 17-AAG, the more water-soluble and significantly less toxic geldanamycin derivative 17-desmethoxy-dimethylaminoethylaminogeldanamycin, **3** (17-DMAG; also known as KOS-1022 or alvespimycin), was developed.[88] The derivative is synthesised in an analogous fashion to 17-AAG, but using

N,*N*-dimethylethylenediamine as the nucleophile, rather than allylamine. The vastly increased aqueous solubility of 17-DMAG (1.4 mg mL^{-1} *vs.* 0.1 mg mL^{-1} for 17-AAG in 50 mM sodium phosphate buffer at pH 7.0)[88] allows formulation in saline or 5% aqueous dextrose when administering to patients.[88] Additionally, the quantitative metabolism of 17-DMAG was found to be significantly lower than that for 17-AAG, gauged by the urinary excretion percentage of un-metabolised drug of 10–15% (17-DMAG) *vs.* 2% (17-AAG).[89] However, despite these promising findings, the toxicity profile of 17-DMAG led to its discontinuation in the clinic, with significant hepatic, gastro-intestinal, and bone marrow toxicities observed, along with signs of nephro and gallbladder harm.[88]

2.2.2.3 *17-Allylamino-17-desmethoxygeldanamycin Hydroquinone Hydrochloride (IPI-504; Retaspimycin)*

Infinity Pharmaceuticals have developed a potent and highly soluble geldanamycin derivative: 17-allylamino-17-desmethoxygeldanamycin hydro-quinone hydrochloride, **4** (also known as IPI-504 or retaspimycin), which remains in clinical trials. The compound differs from the other related benzoquinone ansamycin drug candidates in that it is in the reduced hydroquinone form. This reduction can be effected either enzymatically, with quinone reductases such as NQO1,[66,90] or chemically with reducing agents such as sodium dithionite.[75] Despite the tendency for such electron-rich hydroquinones towards rapid oxidation back to the corresponding quinone, it appears that the formation of the salt (hydrochloride in the case of IPI-504) stabilises the reduced form, although an in-depth study of this has, to the best of our knowledge, yet to be reported. The aqueous solubility of benzoquinone ansamycins increases significantly upon reduction to the hydroquinone (1–3 mg mL^{-1} for 17-AAG hydroquinone *vs.* 35 µg mL^{-1} for 17-AAG)[91] and this is even more marked upon salt formation, with solubi-lities in excess of 200 mg mL^{-1} typical for salts of 17-AAG hydroquinone.[91] Despite its discontinuation for the treatment of refractory gastrointestinal stromal tumours following a high mortality rate of patients in a clinical trial,[91] retaspimycin continues to perform in the clinic, with accumulating evidence of efficacy against multiple myeloma, lung cancer, and other solid tumours.[91] In addition to retaspimycin, other non-quinone-based Hsp90 inhibitors have been discovered through biosynthetic engineering and can exhibit increased binding affinities compared to geldanamycin and macbecin, although oxidation to the quinone is still a potential source of toxicity for the analogues.[92]

2.2.2.4 *17-Amino-17-desmethoxygeldanamycin (17-AG; IPI-493)*

Infinity Pharmaceuticals also reported the highly soluble geldanamycin-derived 17-amino-17-desmethoxygeldanamycin **5** (17-AG; also known as

IPI-493), from the treatment of geldanamycin with ammonia.[93] 17-AG is also
the major metabolite of 17-AAG. This is thought to occur *via* C-oxidation
adjacent to the 17-nitrogen and elimination, with the release of acrolein,
adding to the toxicity profile of tanespimycin, as mentioned previously.[94]
Despite highly promising initial clinical evaluation against gastrointestinal
stromal tumours and investigations into the treatment of solid tumours, no
further developments in the clinical use of 17-AG have been reported.[91]

2.2.3 Modifications to C19

Despite the significant progression in geldanamycin-derived Hsp90 inhibitors described above, all of the candidates struggle with toxicity problems,
particularly hepatotoxicity. While this may be the lesser of two evils when
treating various cancers, for therapeutics of neurodegenerative conditions,
HIV/AIDS and parasitic diseases such as those outlined in Section 2.2.2.1,
these levels of toxicity are unacceptable. It therefore becomes an urgent
necessity to develop Hsp90 inhibitors with reduced toxicity, while maintaining or improving potency. The toxicity of benzoquinone ansamycins has
been postulated to arise from the conjugate addition of biological nucleophiles such as glutathione at the 19-position of the quinone ring.[68,95] While
19-substitution had been briefly investigated previously,[96] Moody, Ross,
Kitson and co-workers investigated the introduction of substituents at this
position (*via* the related 19-iodogeldanamycin[97] utilising Stille or Suzuki
cross-coupling reactions with various coupling partners) in order to suppress
this reaction and ameliorate the toxicity (Figure 2.5).[98,99]

   The 19-substituted geldanamycin derivatives were also treated with
amines to obtain the corresponding 17-AAG and 17-DMAG analogues. These
were analysed in several cellular systems to test their toxicity in comparison
to geldanamycin, 17-AAG and 17-DMAG. The data shown in Table 2.1
compare the toxicity profiles of the compounds against human umbilical

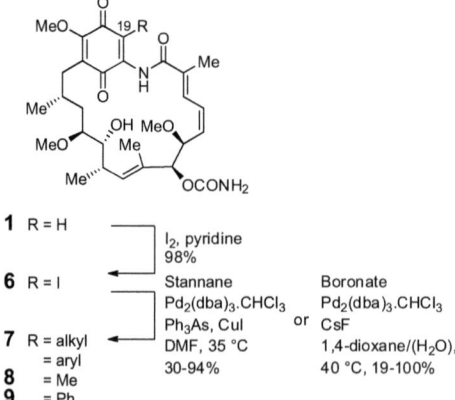

Figure 2.5   Position 19-substituted geldanamycin derivatives.

Table 2.1   Toxicity of benzoquinone ansamycins to human umbilical vein endothelial cells and ARPE-19 retinal cells.

Compound	HUVECs[a] IC$_{50}$/nM	ARPE-19 IC$_{50}$/nM
Geldanamycin (**1**)	0.041 ± 0.003	0.10 ± 0.04
19-Me-geldanamycin (**8**)	16.9 ± 3.3	> 20
19-Ph-geldanamycin (**9**)	2.1 ± 0.4	8.3 ± 0.7

[a]HUVEC are primary cells and ARPE-19 cells are a non-transformed human retinal pigmented epithelial cell line. Toxicity values were generated using the MTT assay. The values are represented as a mean $\pm$ standard deviation (n = 3). IC$_{50}$ (the dose leads to 50% cell death) of 19-substituted BQAs and their parent quinones.

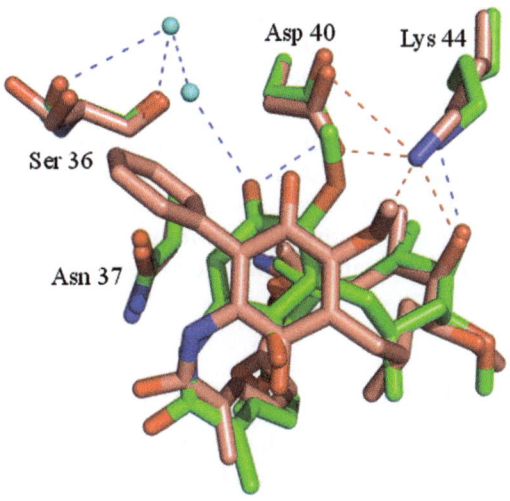

Figure 2.6   Overlay structures of geldanamycin, **1** (green), and 19-phenylgeldanamycin, 9 (salmon), bound in the ATP site of yeast Hsp90 as determined by protein X-ray crystallography. In general, in these geldanamycin analogues, the 19-substituents tend to alter binding to the protein through a positional change of the quinone group of the benzoquinone ansamycin.
Image from the article by Kitson *et al.*[98]

vein endothelial cells (HUVECs) and retinal pigmented epithelial cells (ARPE-19 cells). The results show conclusively that both 19-methyl (**8**) and 19-phenylgeldanamycin (**9**) are significantly less toxic than their parent quinones, thus 19-substitution markedly reduces the toxicity of benzoquinone ansamycins.[98]

Interestingly, a conformational switch was also observed upon introduction of a 19-substituent. The novel geldanamycin analogues were now found to adopt the well-documented C-clamp, *cis*-amide conformation, previously observed upon binding of benzoquinone ansamycins to Hsp90. With the aid of protein crystallography, the compounds were shown to bind to Hsp90 in an analogous fashion to the parent quinones, albeit with a slight shift in the position of the quinone (Figure 2.6). The Hsp90 inhibition of the 19-substituted analogues was analysed through assessment of the common biomarkers, client protein depletion with concomitant upregulation of other Hsps, and were found to be comparable to the parent compounds.[98] Additionally, studies in BT474 breast cancer cell lines showed that the 19-substituted benzoquinone ansamycins actually outperformed the parent quinones while being highly effective in Parkinsonian model SH-SY5Y human neuroblastoma cells.[98]

2.2.4   Combination Therapies

The use of Hsp90 inhibitors in combinatorial therapeutics is also a strategy that has been investigated in oncogenics. Given the resistance and toxicity issues with 17-AAG, it is not a successful "stand-alone" drug for the patient treatment of multiple cancers, yet it can be an effective therapeutic when used in combination with standard cancer treatments such as irinotecan, gemcitabine, docetaxel, trastuzumab, bortezomib and sorafenib.[12,91] In particular, the synergy of 17-AAG and bortezomib has been advanced to Phase III clinical trials following a successful Phase II study. The combination was found to be an effective treatment for multiple myeloma, while the addition of 17-AAG ameliorated known side-effects from bortezomib monotherapy.[91,100]

2.3   Class II: Radicicol and Radanamycin

The resorcylic acid lactone (RAL) radicicol **10** (also known as monorden), was first isolated in 1953 from *Monosporium bonorden*,[101] and it is the most potent *in vitro* natural product Hsp90 inhibitor found to date (IC$_{50}$ = 20–23 nM).[19,102] However, it is inactive *in vivo*, due to its metabolically sensitive functionalities (epoxide, Michael acceptor and macrolactone) (Figure 2.7).[17–19]

Radicicol binds to the ATP-binding site of Hsp90 with K$_d$ of 19 nM[59] and, despite similarities with geldanamycin (small aromatic head group, macrocycle with multiple H-bond acceptors and donors), the two molecules differ greatly in their binding to Hsp90. With radicicol, the resorcinol unit is positioned in an analogous fashion to the purine system of ATP/ADP, with H-bonding interactions with the L34, D79 and T171 amino acid residues of the protein, whereas the carbamate of geldanamycin satisfies these interactions and the quinone is located in the lower region of the binding pocket (Figure 2.8).[59]

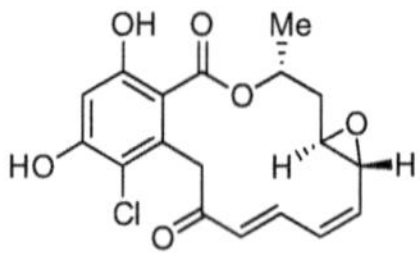

radicicol **10**

Figure 2.7   Structure of radicicol.

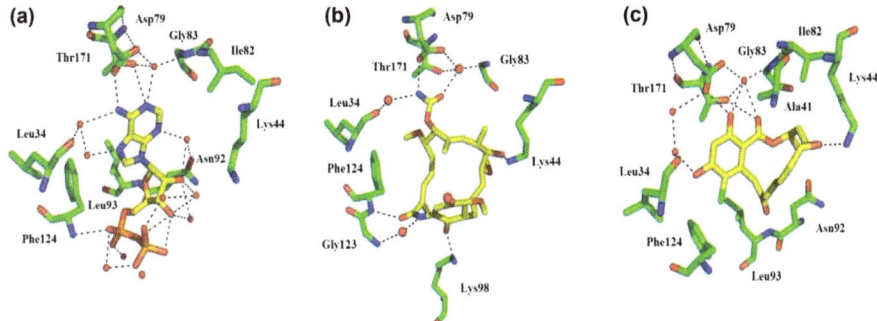

Figure 2.8 Crystal structures of (a) ADP, (b) geldanamycin (**1**) and (c) radicicol (**10**) co-crystallised with yeast Hsp90.
Images from the article by Pearl *et al.*[59]

In view of the high potency, yet poor stability of radicicol, the development of analogues where the sensitive functionalities have been removed in an attempt to improve *in vivo* activity has attracted considerable attention in the research community. The advances in radicicol analogues, including those in the clinic, are summarised below.

2.3.1 Direct Analogues of Radicicol

Much research effort has been devoted to the variation of the radicicol functionalities, through both semi and total synthesis, with ensuing structure–activity investigations. Alteration of the configuration or position of the methyl group has been shown to be detrimental for potency,[57,103] however de-methylated analogues retain their activity.[104] The hydrophobic interaction performed by the resorcinol chloride has also been shown to be critical for high activity, although this can be replaced successfully by an isopropyl group,[105–108] but not by bromide.[104] Variation of the macrocycle ring size has also been investigated, with 14 and 15-membered rings proving optimum.[104]

The C14–15 epoxide forms an interaction with the L44 residue of Hsp90, which is crucial for the high binding affinity. Indeed, Danishefsky has shown that merely inversion of the epoxide stereochemistry leads to a 40-fold drop in the activity of the compound.[57] Replacement of the epoxide with a cyclopropyl ring as in cyclopropradicicol, **11**, induced a lower penalty than inverting the stereochemistry of the epoxide, dropping the IC_{50} ∼ 8-fold (20 nM *vs.* 160 nM) (Figure 2.9, **11**). The inclusion of a cyclopropyl ring was a significant improvement as it provided a potent yet stable inhibitor. Similar to the epoxide analogues, inversion of the cyclopropyl group stereochemistry also gave a drop in activity.[57] Additionally, removal of the epoxide altogether,[104] or its replacement with rings such as a thiirane and cyclic carbonate[109] or other H-bonding moieties[110] gave much lower activity than radicicol itself, proposed to be due to the adoption of an alternative macrocycle conformation.[110,111]

Moody and Shinonaga have developed synthetic radicicol analogues in which the dienone moiety has been removed (**12** and **13**, Figure 2.9),[104,109,110] while Danishefsky has replaced the dienone of cyclo-proparadicicol with a triazole (**14**).[112] Moody has also incorporated a triazole into the macrocycle to give compound **15** in order to investigate the benefits of additional H-bonding potential.[103] Unfortunately, all of these analogues showed a significant drop in activity compared to radicicol itself, although potencies comparable to that of 17-AAG were achievable.[103]

In order to improve the metabolic stability of radicicol analogues, Moody and co-workers synthesised a series of fully synthetic resorcylic acid lactams, with or without substituents with extra H-bonding potential at C-10 adjacent to the macrocycle ketone. The unsubstituted macrolactam analogues (**16**, Figure 2.10) exhibited a drop in activity *vs.* radicicol in TR-FRET and FP assays, yet outperformed the corresponding macrolactone **12**.[113] Interestingly, the substituents at C-10 (**17** and **18**, Figure 2.10) were shown to displace a loop of residues in the Hsp90 ATP-binding site, enhancing activity by increasing the number of hydrophobic interactions between Hsp90 and the inhibitor. The macrolactams **17** and **18** were also indeed found to be more metabolically stable than both radicicol and the corresponding macrolactones through analysis in a human liver microsome assay with and without NADPH/NADH. After 30 minutes (with co-factors), 83% of

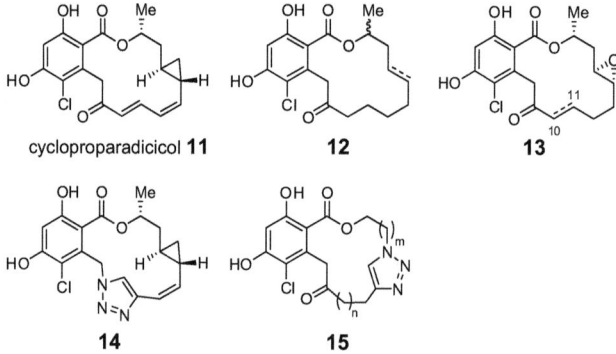

Figure 2.9 Radicicol analogues synthesised.

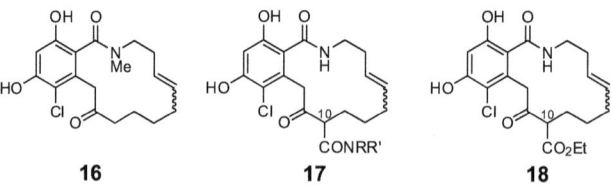

Figure 2.10 The structures of synthesised resorcylic acid lactams (RALs) 16, 17 and 18.

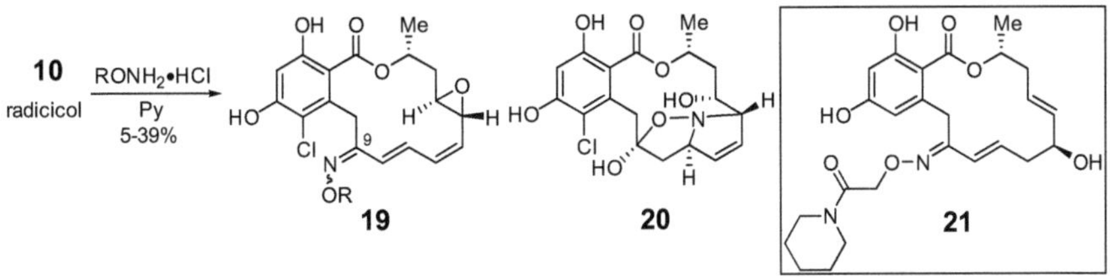

Scheme 2.1 The structures of radoxime derivatives **19** and **21**.[17,115]

radicicol and 90% of the macrolactone were metabolised, compared to 67% and 47% for macrolactams **17** and **18**, respectively. This percentage decreased to 5–10% metabolism with only the microsomes in the assay, compared to 33% for radicicol and 11% for the macrolactone.[114]

The treatment of radicicol with alkoxyamines gives the corresponding radoximes **19** in moderate yield (Scheme 2.1), increasing the *in vivo* activity of the compounds markedly, although the syntheses proceeded with significant quantities of by-products (**20**, Scheme 2.1).[17,115] Winssinger has also synthesised oxime analogues of the resorcylic acid lactones pochonins E and F.[116] The analogue *epi*-pochoxime F, **21** (Scheme 2.1) had an Hsp90 binding affinity greater than any of the natural pochonins or even radicicol ($K_D = 14$ nM).[116]

2.3.2 Radamide, Radester and Radanamycin

A series of "chimera" compounds with the pharmacophores from both radicicol and geldanamycin have been reported by Blagg and co-workers, known as radamide **22**,[117,118] radester **23**,[119–121] and radanamycin **24** (Figure 2.11).[19] Indeed radester **23** was found to be more potent than geldanamycin itself. A detailed SAR study was carried out for the radester and radanamycin analogues. For radesters **23**, a linker length of two carbon units and a methyl group α- to the ester oxygen were optimal, while a formamide-containing hydroquinone substituent proved superior for the geldanamycin-mimic. Intriguingly, the iodo-resorcinol derivative **23b** was found to be the most potent analogue.[121] For the radanamycin series, exemplified by macrocycle **24**, a carbon chain linker of three carbons connecting the reduced hydroquinone to the bottom phenyl moiety on the left side, and a two carbon chain on the right side were optimal, giving comparable potencies to the radester analogues (Figure 2.11).[121]

2.3.3 Radicicol-inspired Pyrazoles and Oxazoles

Workman and colleagues performed a high throughput screen of resorcinol-containing diaryl pyrazole Hsp90 inhibitors (Figure 2.12).[122] SAR analysis showed that a hydrophobic group at C5 (alkyl or halide), along with two free

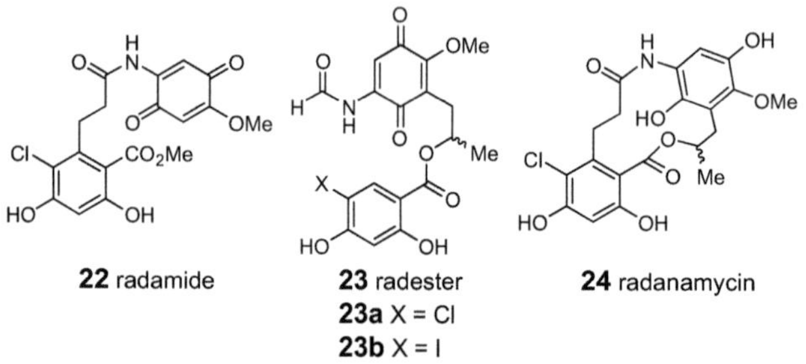

22 radamide

23 radester
23a X = Cl
23b X = I

24 radanamycin

Figure 2.11 Blagg's radicicol/geldanamycin "chimeras".[117–121]

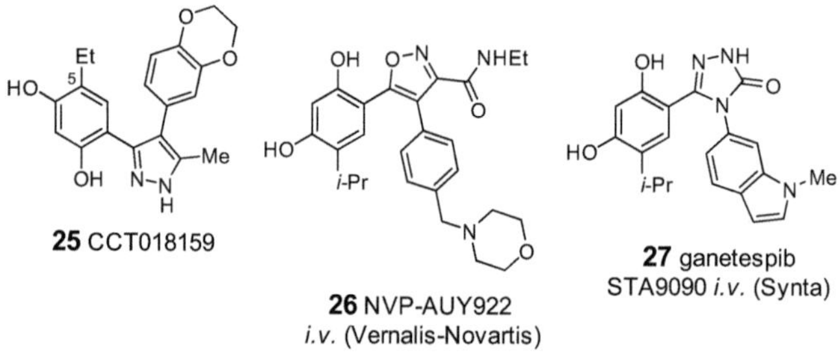

25 CCT018159

26 NVP-AUY922
i.v. (Vernalis-Novartis)

27 ganetespib
STA9090 *i.v.* (Synta)

Figure 2.12 Pyrazole and isoxazole-containing Hsp90 inhibitors.

phenols are essential for a high binding affinity. Lead optimisation gave compound CCT018159 (**25**, $IC_{50} = 7.1$ µM, Figure 2.12),[123,124] in which the pyrazole mimics the radicicol lactone unit. Similarly, isoxazoles, triazoles and benzisoxazole resorcinols were also potent Hsp90 inhibitors.[56,125–127] There are currently four related compounds in the clinic, including NVP-AU922, **26**, an intravenous drug from Vernalis-Novartis, currently in Phase II trials, and Synta's ganetespib (**27**), also administered intravenously, which has been evaluated in the clinic against advanced solid tumours and was progressed to Phase III clinical trials against non-small cell lung carcinoma.[96]

2.4 Class III: Macrocyclic *o*-Aminobenzamides and Aminopyrimidines

In addition to a variety of resorcinol-based acyclic inhibitors of Hsp90 with a structural similarity to the macrocyclic natural product radicicol, several other classes of synthetic acyclic small molecule inhibitors have been discovered and advanced to the clinic.[128] Among that group, two that have generated significant interest are the *o*-aminobenzamide SNX-2112 (**28**),[20–22] its pro-drug SNX-5422 (**29**, PF-04929113),[129] and the purine-class inhibitor BIIB021 (**30**, CNF2024),[130–132] all of which bind to the *N*-terminal ATP binding site of Hsp90 and have been evaluated in oncology clinical trials (Figure 2.13). Related to the purine inhibitor chemotype, numerous examples of aminopyrimidine Hsp90 inhibitors have been disclosed,[133–135] exemplified by the Phase I clinical compound **31** (NVP-HSP990),[134] which have binding modes to the protein that mimic the purines. Both the *o*-aminobenzamides and the aminopyrimidines have been the subject of drug discovery optimisation efforts involving the design and synthesis of macrocyclic analogues based on the acyclic leads.

The transformation of SNX-2112 (**28**) into a potent macrocyclic Hsp90 inhibitor with acceptable drug-like properties and potent *in vivo* activity began with an analysis of its key binding interactions to the protein, direct and water-mediated hydrogen bonds between the benzamide –NH$_2$ group and Asp93 and a hydrogen bond between the carbonyl of the tetra-hydroindazole of **28** and Tyr139 of the ATPase.[16] The requirement that both of these interactions be maintained for high affinity binding to the protein then defined a range of acceptable torsion angles between the benzamide and tetrahydroindolone ring, which further defined the size of the linker that could be accommodated connecting the two rings in a macrocycle (Figure 2.14). The physical properties of the linker, for example its polarity, were not expected to have a significant effect on potency given that it would be solvent exposed. Conversion of the tetrahydroindazole moiety of SNX-2112 (**28**) into a tetrahydroindolone was required in order to provide an at-tachment point for the macrocycle linker on the southern portion of the molecule (see **31** and **32**, Figure 2.14).

In the first iteration of macrocyclic inhibitor design, the SAR of a series of 11- to 14-membered ring benzamido-tetrahydroindolones was explored and

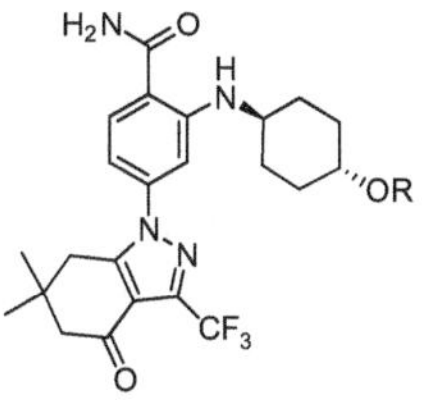

28 R = H (SNX-2112)
29 R = COCH$_2$NH$_2$(SNX-5422)

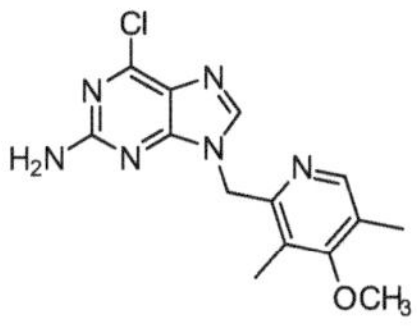

30 BIIB021

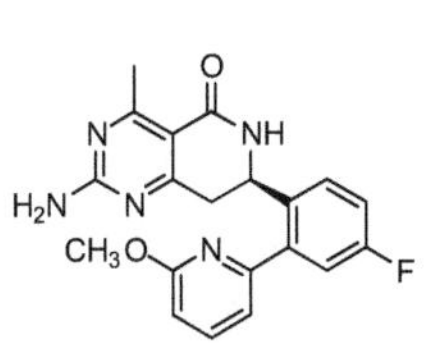

31 NVP-HSP990

Figure 2.13 Examples of acyclic *o*-aminobenzamide and aminopyrimidine Hsp90 inhibitors.

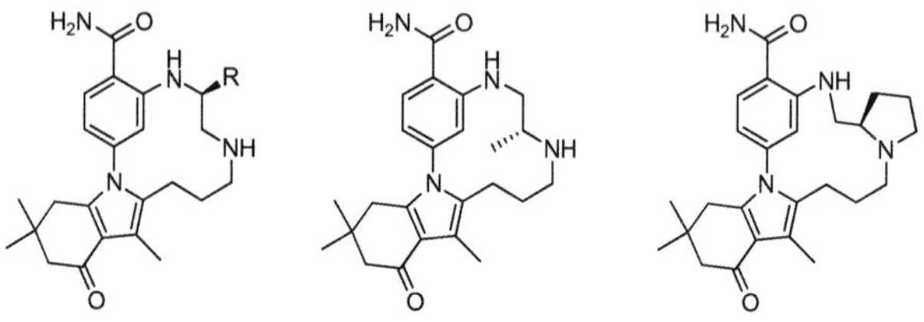

Figure 2.14   Initial iteration of amine-linked macrocyclic *o*-aminobenzamide Hsp90 inhibitors.

it was found, through the comparison of matched pairs, that 12-membered rings provided the best enzyme potency, presumably because this ring size provided the optimal torsion angle between the benzamide and tetra-hydroindolone rings, allowing both of the key ligand–protein binding interactions.[16] In addition, a rigidifying element, in the form of methyl substituents on the linker, was found to be beneficial for binding affinity and cellular activity. Thus, compound **31** (Figure 2.14), a 12-membered macrocycle with a basic amine in the linker and no additional substitution on the linking chain has an IC_{50} of 920 nM in an Hsp90 enzyme inhibition assay. The activity of compound **31** in a cell proliferation assay using the HCT116 colorectal cancer cell line is also in the high nanomolar range ($EC_{50} = 820$ nM). The 11-membered ring analogue (not shown) of **31** has an enzyme inhibition of IC_{50} 12.4 µM. The addition of a methyl group to the linker on the carbon adjacent to the aniline nitrogen to give compound **32** results in an 8-fold improvement in binding affinity ($IC_{50} = 110$ nM), as compared to **31**, with a parallel increase in activity in the HCT116 cell proliferation assay ($EC_{50} = 90$ nM). Analogue **32** (MW = 409; cLogP = 4.1) also has good kinetic aqueous solubility (>100 µg mL^{-1}) and is stable in rat liver microsomes ($t_{1/2} > 30$ min.), important parameters for the optimisation of oral pharmacokinetics. A more potent analogue could be obtained by appending a methyl group on the carbon next to the basic amine of the linker to give **33** with a binding IC_{50} of 91 nM and an HCT116 EC_{50} of 43 nM (geldanamycin HCT116 $EC_{50} = 30$ nM), while maintaining the solubility and microsomal stability of **32**.[136]

A variety of analogues in which an additional ring was fused to the macrocycle were also prepared in an effort to further rigidify the macrocycle linker and impact potency.[137] For example, pyrrolidine derivative **34** (Figure 2.14) has a binding IC_{50} of 96 nM and an EC_{50} of 30 nM in the HCT116 cell proliferation assay. It is notable that the (*S*)-enantiomer of **34** is more than 10-fold less active than **34** in the Hsp90 binding assay, indicative of the importance of this stereocentre for effective binding to Hsp90. When tested *in vivo* using a U87 glioma mouse xenograft model at 100 mg kg^{-1} *iv*, dosed twice per week (days 0 and 4), **34** almost completely suppressed tumour growth at day 8.

Although macrocycles **33** and **34** have attractive physical properties, and cell potency comparable to geldanamycin, both are relatively potent inhibitors of hERG, presumably due at least in part to the presence of a basic amine in the macrocycle linker. This liability was addressed by the design of amide linkers (Figure 2.15), thereby removing the basicity of the linker nitrogen.[136] Thus, lactam **35** has moderate Hsp90 enzyme activity ($IC_{50} = 214$ nM) and sub-micromolar cell proliferation activity (HCT 116 $EC_{50} = 815$ nM). It is notable that even with the significant linker rigidification through the incorporation of the amide, the angular methyl group in **35** is required for potency, as the corresponding desmethyl analogue is more than 30-fold less potent in the Hsp90 binding assay. A structurally related lactam, **36**, with the rigid amide closer to the aniline ring than the tetrahydroindolone, is significantly more potent than **35**, with a binding IC_{50} of 82 nM and an HCT116 EC_{50} of 56 nM. Importantly, **35** retains the solubility and rat microsomal stability of the amine-linked analogue **32** and is devoid of hERG activity (hERG $IC_{50} > 30$ μM). The methyl epimer of **36** (not shown) is 3-fold less potent in both binding and cell proliferation assays. Lactam **36** was active in a MDA-MB-361 xenograft biomarker study at 50 mg kg^{-1} p.o. As seen with other Hsp90 inhibitors that target the *N*-terminal ATP-binding site, it produced increases in both Hsp70 and Hsp90 levels that persisted more than 24 hours after dosing, at which time tumour levels of the drug remained high (1266 ng g^{-1}) even though plasma levels of **36** had declined to below 10 ng g^{-1}.

In an additional attempt to optimise potency with solubility, metabolic stability, and hERG activity, a series of amide-linked *o*-aminobenzamide macrocyclic Hsp90 inhibitors was prepared in which the amide carbonyl was exocyclic to the macrocycle, exemplified by **37** and **38** (Figure 2.15).[138] Alanine amide **37** is only moderately potent in the binding ($IC_{50} = 145$ nM) and HCT116 cell assays ($EC_{50} = 314$ nM), but it has excellent solubility, is stable in both rat and mouse microsomes ($t_{1/2} > 30$ min.) and has greatly improved stability in human microsomes ($t_{1/2} = 26$ min.) as compared to most *o*-aminobenzamide macrocyclic Hsp90 inhibitors. Interestingly, the addition of a second angular methyl group on the linker of **37**, to give **38**, results in significant improvements in enzyme potency ($IC_{50} = 83$ nM) and

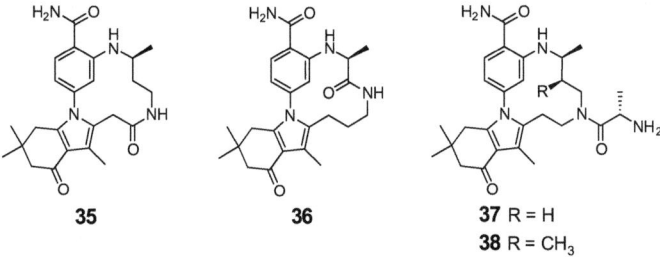

37 R = H
38 R = CH$_3$

Figure 2.15 Amide-linked macrocyclic macrocyclic *o*-aminobenzamide Hsp90 inhibitors.

HCT166 cell proliferation activity (EC_{50} = 63 nM) while maintaining some aqueous solubility (10 µg mL^{-1}), an optimal hERG inhibition profile (IC_{50} > 30 µM) and providing excellent stability in rat, mouse and human microsomes ($t_{1/2}$ > 30 min.). Compound **38** was tested in a H1975 mouse xenograft model and provided a substantial inhibition of tumour growth at a dose of 12.5 mg kg^{-1} *iv*, given once weekly, and reduced tumour volume from baseline at a once weekly dose of 25 mg kg^{-1} *iv*, after 25 days. Unfortunately, this macrocycle had poor bioavailability (F% = 4), perhaps due to its limited solubility, and no disclosure of an advancement into clinical trials has been made. Nevertheless, this drug discovery effort is an excellent example of the conversion of an acyclic small molecule Hsp90 inhibitor into a novel macrocyclic series with acceptable pharmacological and physical properties.

Another example of employing a macrocyclisation strategy to optimise an acyclic Hsp90 inhibitor began with the amino-triazine compound **39** (Figure 2.16), a high affinity binder to Hsp90 (K_D = 3.4 nM) with moderate anti-proliferative activity in HCT116 cells (IC_{50} = 460 nM) and poor bio-availability (F% = 5).[14] An X-ray crystal structure of **39** bound to the *N*-terminal domain of human Hsp90 indicates that it forms a single direct hydrogen bonding interaction with the protein, between the 2-amino group and Asp93 of Hsp90. The –SCH_3 group and chloro substituent of **39** provide hydrophobic interactions with the protein and there are multiple through-water interactions between the inhibitor and Hsp90, including those to the ether oxygen of **39** and two of its three triazine nitrogens. The macrocycle design strategy then focused on maintaining the interactions exhibited by **39** and engineering in additional interactions guided by the binding motif of geldanamycin with Hsp90.

The result of this exercise was the 16-membered macrocyclic amino-pyrimidine, **40** (CH5015765), with an amide linker (Figure 2.16).[14] This compound has a sub-nanomolar K_D (0.52 nM) and an IC_{50} of 150 nM in the HCT116 proliferation assay. The 17- and 18-membered analogues of **40**, with the linker extensions between the amides, are essentially equipotent to **40** in enzyme affinity and *in vitro* cell proliferation activity. An X-ray crystal structure of **40** with *N*-terminal Hsp90α shows an interaction between the benzamide carbonyl, through a water molecule, to Phe138 and Asn51, similar to the interaction between the ether oxygen of **39** and Hsp90. In

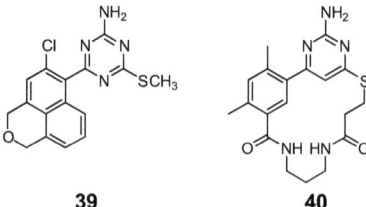

39   **40**

Figure 2.16   Acyclic aminopyrimidine hit and designed macrocyclic Hsp90 inhibitor analogue.

addition, the carbonyl of the alkyl amide of **40** forms a hydrogen bond to the side chain of Lys58 of the Hsp90 ATP binding site, mimicking an interaction of geldanamycin with the same residue. Macrocycle **40** has good solubility (125 μM) in fasted state simulated intestinal fluid (FaSSIF), good stability in human liver microsomes (CL = 0.28 μL min.$^{-1}$ mg^{-1} protein) and vastly improved bioavailability (F% = 71) as compared to **39**. In a HCT116 mouse xenograft model, **40** provided 83% tumour growth inhibition when dosed orally for 11 days, once a day, at 25 mg kg^{-1}. No clinical trials with CH5015765 have been reported to date.

2.5 Class IV: *N*-Middle Domain Hsp90 Macrocyclic Inhibitors

All current Hsp90 inhibitors in clinical development (including macrocyclic inhibitors from Classes I through III) bind to the ATP-binding pocket at the *N*-terminal domain.[128] Of the fifteen drugs currently under clinical review, twelve are structurally related to the geldanamycin derivative 17-AAG (Class I). The remaining three drugs bind to the same site as the other twelve, and impact the same cellular signalling pathways.[139,140] A significant problem with all *N*-terminal Hsp90 inhibitors is that they induce a heat shock response, which leads to an increase in a number of cellular maintenance proteins and chaperones including both Hsp70 and Hsp90.[141] Accumulation of Hsp70 rescues Hsp90-depleted cells by performing some of Hsp90's chaperone functions, such as maintaining the active conformation of certain Hsp90-regulated proteins, and can induce drug resistance in certain solid tumours.[142–146]

The therapeutic problems associated with molecules that bind to the *N*-terminus of Hsp90 have driven the search and discovery of molecules that bind other sites within the Hsp90 scaffold. Compounds that bind to Hsp90's *C*-terminus include coumermycin A1 (CA1, **41**, Figure 2.17) and its analogues (IC$_{50}$ ~ 3 μM) which control the same client proteins as those modulated by 17-AAG, with one exception: Ratajcak and co-workers showed that a millimolar concentration of the *C*-terminal inhibitor novobiocin disrupts several *C*-terminal co-chaperones from binding to Hsp90.[147–150] Further, compounds that modulate the *C*-terminus do not induce a heat shock response, providing the opportunity to avoid the resistance mechanism seen in the *N*-terminal ATP-binding molecules.[151] Optimisation and *in vivo* analysis of these small cyclic compounds will provide further insights into their therapeutic potential as anticancer agents.

The *C*-terminal domain of Hsp90 is known to interact with a specific subset of proteins that contain a tetratricopeptide-repeat (TPR) domain.[147] The TPR domain is a protein scaffold consisting of a semi-conserved sequence of 34 amino acids that occur in repeats throughout the protein.[152] Within the group of sixteen TPR proteins that interact with Hsp90, four are immunophilins: FK506 binding protein 52 (FKBP52), FKBP51, cyclophilin 40 (Cyp40), and

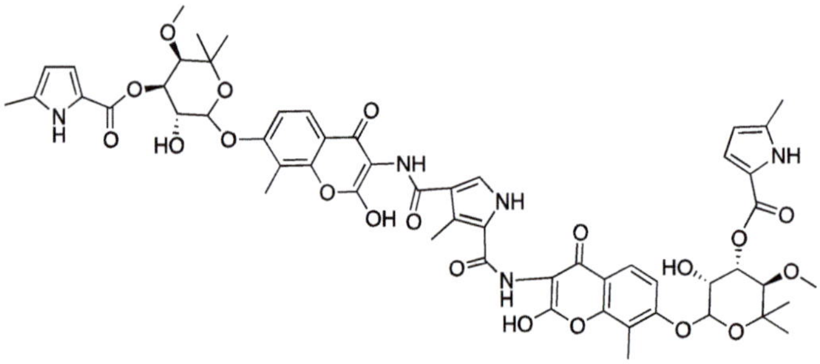

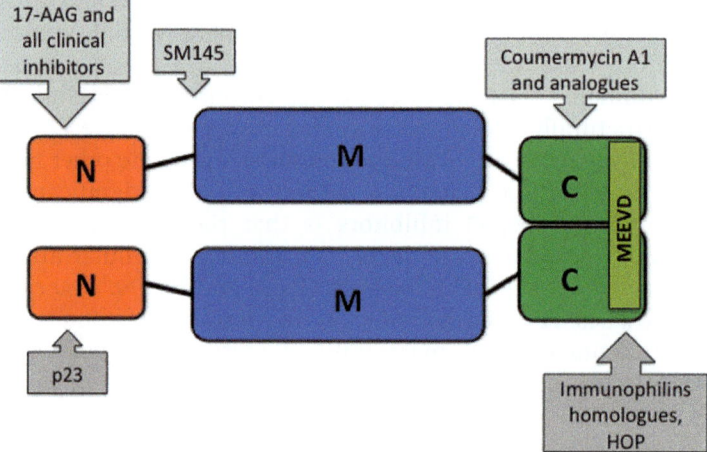

Coumermycin A1 (CA1) **41**

Figure 2.17 Structure of coumermycin A1 (**41**).

Figure 2.18 The Hsp90 dimer indicating where 17-AAG, coumermycin A1, SM145, and various co-chaperones important in hormone receptor development bind (M = methionine, E = glutamic acid, V = valine, D = aspartic acid).

FKBP38. Other TPR proteins that bind to Hsp90 include the *C*-terminus of Hsc70 interacting protein (CHIP), Unc45, and the mitochondrial import receptor of 70 kDa (Tom70).[153] In addition, a key co-chaperone that regulates Hsp90's function is the TPR-containing heat shock organising protein (HOP). These TPR-containing proteins are all regulated *via* their interaction with the MEEVD amino acids of Hsp90's *C*-terminus (Figure 2.18).

Three of the four immunophilins (FKBP51, FKBP52 and Cyp40) are well established to regulate cell growth through controlling hormone receptor (HR) interactions with Hsp90.[154] In addition, the homologs CHIP, Unc45 and Tom70 facilitate hormone receptor-regulated cell growth *via* Hsp90.[154] These co-chaperones regulate the maturation of hormone receptors by forming a multi-chaperone complex with Hsp90 and the co-chaperone p23. This complex induces a signalling cascade leading to cell growth.[154]

Since the interaction of Hsp90 with the immunophilins regulates steroid receptor function and development, blocking the interaction between the immunophilins' TPR domain and Hsp90's MEEVD region will likely affect HR protein levels and produce therapeutic benefits. A key question remains as to how Hsp90-regulated pathways can be inhibited without inducing the heat shock response and perpetuating undesirable effects such as drug resistance in hormone-responsive cancers.

Utilising pull-down assays the McAlpine lab have identified three structurally unique macrocycles, related to the naturally occurring penta-depsipeptide sansalvamide A, that bind to Hsp90: SM122 (43),[25,27] SM145 (44),[23,26,29,46,155] and SM185 (46)[23,28] (Figure 2.19) with GI_{50}s of 3.9 µM, 3.2 µM, and 7.6 µM,[23] respectively, in HCT116 colon cancer cells. Initial studies explored how modifications to the backbone of the macrocycle induced conformational changes that impacted binding to Hsp90.[156–161] It was discovered that several elements located within the backbone of the macrocycle were key to a potent Hsp90 inhibitor. First, at least a single D-phenylalanine, a second aromatic residue (D or L-phenyl alanine) and an *N*-methyl moiety were required to be placed within the backbone. Further, placement of these three elements within the scaffold was critical for the successful inhibition of Hsp90. For example, modifying the carbobenzyloxy (Cbz) group to a *tert*-butyloxycarbonyl (Boc) on the lysine in 43 resulted in complete loss of activity. SM145 (44) contains a benzylated phenyl serine moiety.

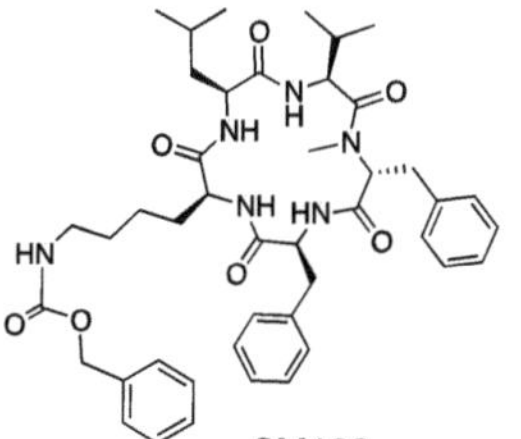

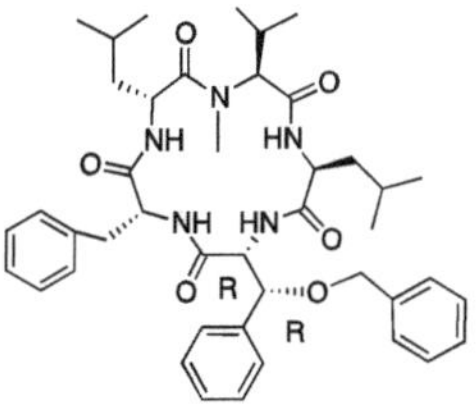

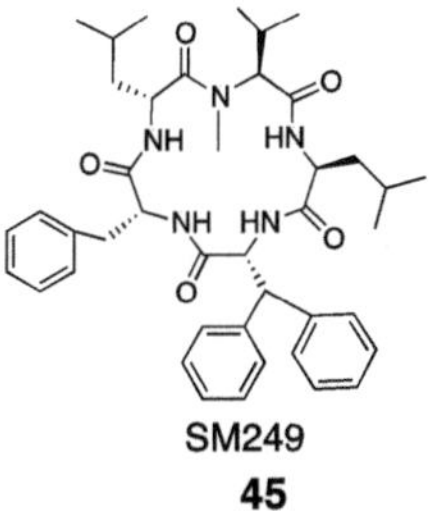

Figure 2.19 Structure of SM122 (**43**), SM145 (**44**), SM249 (**45**) and SM185 (**46**).

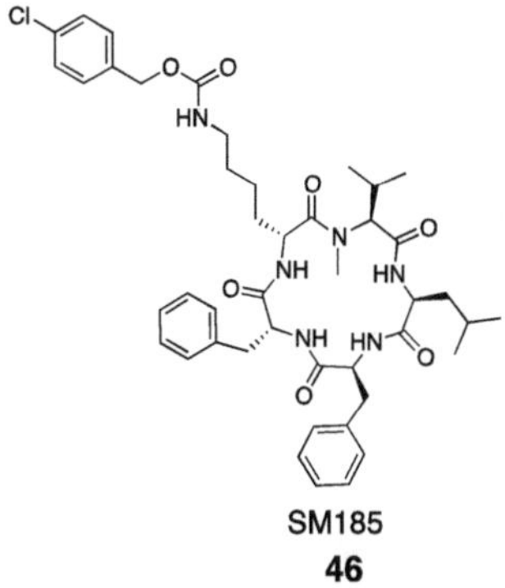

The stereochemistry of that moiety must be *R,R* as the *R,S* and *S,S*, and *S,R* combinations were 3-fold, 2.5-fold, and 1000-fold less active, respectively (with all other stereocentres and amino acids remaining the same).[23] Substitution of the benzylated phenyl serine for a benzhydryl group generates a molecule, **45**, that is just as active, but significantly less complicated to synthesise (GI$_{50}$ = 7 μM in HCT116 colon cancer cell lines). Finally, an interesting SAR study was done on SM185 (**46**) where replacing the chloro moiety from the ClCbz group with a hydrogen led to complete loss of activity. Altering the stereochemistry at the lysine residue, thus switching the D-lysine for an L-lysine, eliminated the compound's activity. Moving the *N*-methyl from the valine to the ClCbz-D-lysine also eliminated activity, but placing the *N*-methyl moiety on the D-phenyl alanine residue generated a compound that was as active as **46**.[23] Compounds **43**, **44**, and **46**, were all inactive if the Cbz, benzyl moiety, or ClCbz, respectively, were removed. Thus, a final assumption was that three aromatic moieties were useful in promoting activity.

Substitution of oxazoles, thiazoles and triazoles (Figure 2.20) showed no activity against any cancer cell lines.[46] It was surprising that the structures that were based on **43** (SM122), including **47** and **48**, which were identical to SM122 with the exception of inserting a thiazole or oxazole in place of a valine, did not have any biological activity. The same annihilation of activity was also observed when oxazoles were substituted into the SM145 backbone, as compounds **49**, **50**, and **51** (Figure 2.20) all had no activity. Thus, the

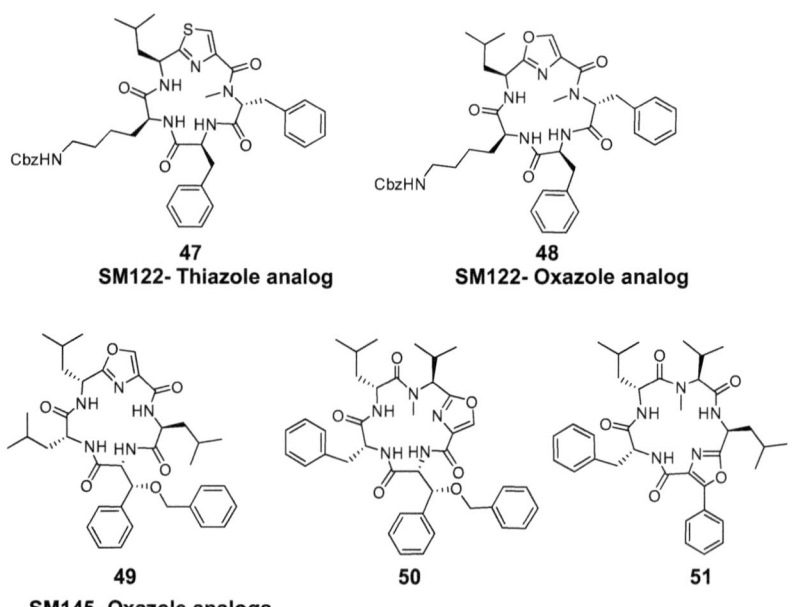

47
SM122- Thiazole analog

48
SM122- Oxazole analog

49
SM145- Oxazole analogs

50

51

Figure 2.20   Structure of SM122 (**43**), SM145 (**44**), SM249 (**45**) and SM185 (**46**).

inclusion of aromatic heterocycles detrimentally alters the macrocyclic ring conformation. These observations are in line with others, where the macrocyclic backbone is a scaffold that places the residues in the desired orientation. When the scaffold is modified, it disrupts the orientation and inhibits binding between the side-chains and the protein target (*i.e.* Hsp90).

2.5.1 SM122 *vs.* SM145 in Pull-down and Biochemical Assays

Utilising three tagged variants of SM122, the binding site on Hsp90 was evaluated. Pull-down assays using the *N*, *C*, *N*-Middle, and Middle-*C* mammalian Hsp90 domain truncations and each of the three variants demonstrated that **43** pulled down only the *N*-Middle domain, but not the *N* or middle domains separately (Figure 2.21).

Assays exploring how both SM122 and SM145 inhibited the client protein binding events between them and Hsp90 showed that SM122 inhibited both middle domain binding client proteins Akt and Her2 (Figure 2.22), as well as *C*-terminal clients and co-chaperones (FKBP52, HOP, and IP6K2). FKBP52 and HOP contain TPR regions that bind to the MEEVD sequence. Interestingly, SM145 has a different profile to SM122, where it inhibits all the *C*-terminal clients, including FKBP38, although it is less effective than

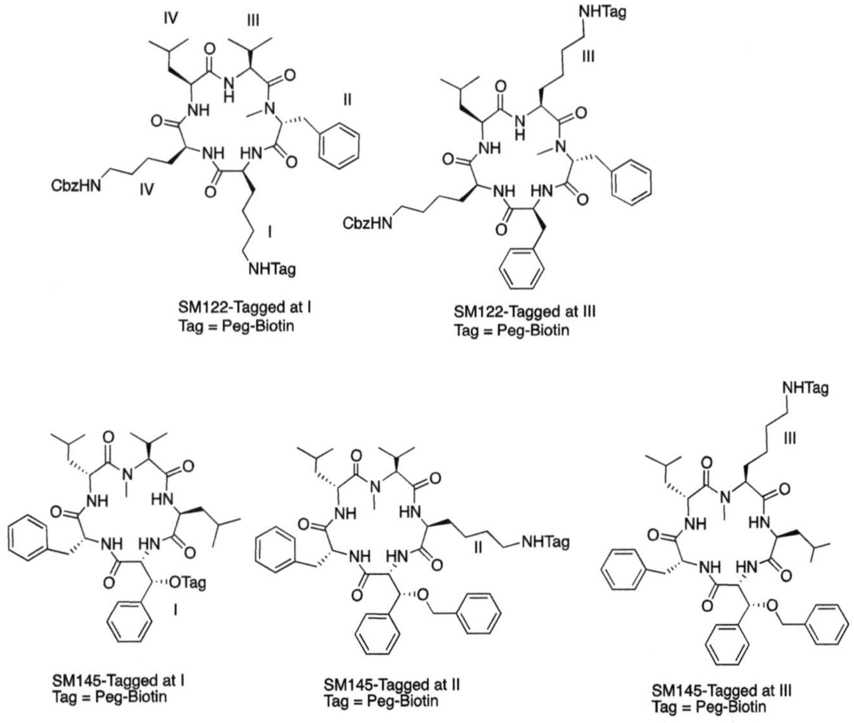

Figure 2.21 Pull-down molecules based on SM122 (**43**) and SM145 (**44**).

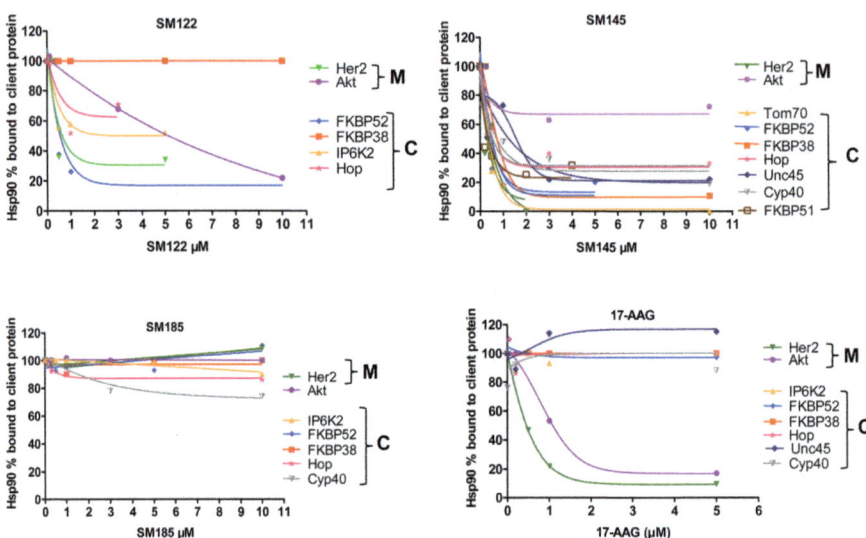

Figure 2.22 Client/co-chaperone binding assays with Hsp90 and the increased addition of: SM122 (**43**), SM145 (**44**), SM185 (**46**), and 17-AAG.

SM122 at inhibiting Akt from binding to Hsp90. It is important to note that although SM145 binds to the *N*-middle domain, it inhibits binding between Hsp90 and all co-chaperones that target the MEEVD region on Hsp90's *C*-terminus. Thus, it is an allosteric modulator of the *C*-terminus. SM185 was shown to pull-down Hsp90 at the *N*-middle domain,[28] but clearly it is modulating Hsp90's function in a manner that is unique from SM122 and SM145 as it does not block any of the client proteins and co-chaperones tested. Not unexpectedly, 17-AAG only blocks clients that bind to the Middle domain, but does not inhibit any of the *C*-terminal clients and co-chaperones from binding to Hsp90.

2.5.2 SM122 *vs.* SM145 in Cell-based Assays

Stresses within the cell induce a heat shock response (Figure 2.23). Under stress, Hsp27 picks up unfolded proteins that have started to aggregate, and it recruits Hsp90. This recruitment frees up the heat shock response regulator, HSF1. HSF1 is responsible for inducing up-regulation of all the heat shock proteins involved in protein folding, including Hsp70 and Hsp90. When Hsp90 inhibitors bind to the ATP-binding site, they trigger the release of HSF1, which is why they induce a heat shock response, up-regulate Hsp70 and Hsp90, and subsequently protect the cell. However, *C*-terminal inhibitors such as coumermycin A (CA1), **41**, do not trigger this event.

Comparing SM122 and SM145 in cell based assays allowed evaluation of how these molecules induced Hsp70, Hsp90, and HSF1. The impact on the protein of interest (Hsp70, Hsp90, and HSF1) of treating cell lysate with

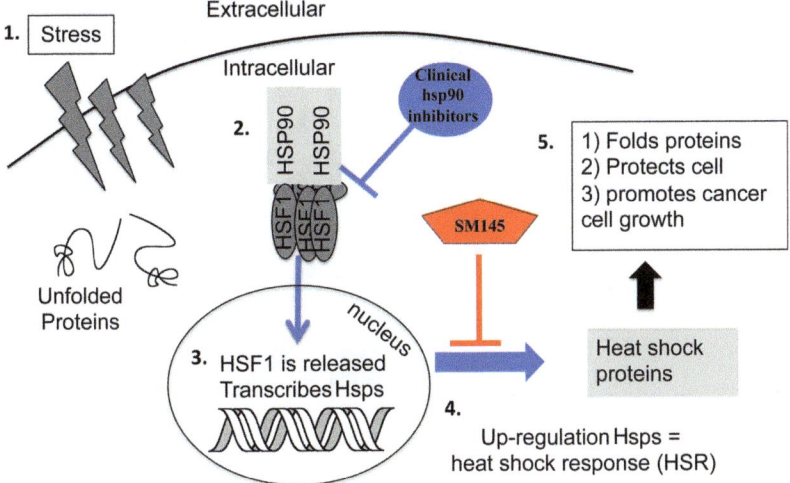

Figure 2.23 The heat shock response that is induced after the cell is stressed: 1. Stress induces unfolded proteins; 2. releasing Hsp90 from HSF1; 3. HSF1 transcribes heat shock proteins; 4. Inducing a heat shock response (HRS) with increased levels of Hsp27, Hsp40, Hsp70, Hsp90 and HSF1 proteins; and 5. leading to oncogenic growth. Clinical inhibitors block Hsp90-HSF1 interactions, inducing this response (blue arrows). SM145 stops the increase in hsps, inhibiting the HSR (red).[26,29,155]

levels of compound at or 10-fold over the IC_{50} value was examined by western blot analysis (Figure 2.24). It can been seen that with treatment of 17-AAG at 1 µM, Hsp70, Hsp90 and HSF1 are all induced to ∼3-fold over background. As reported by others, treatment with 50 µM of coumermycin A(1) (CA1, **41**) does not induce overexpression of any of these three proteins, nor does 50 µM of SM145. Thus, clearly SM145 is modulating the proteins that bind to the *C*-terminus of Hsp90, but is not inducing a heat shock response, whereas 17-AAG does induce a response. Although it is not clear if all compounds that target the *C*-terminus avoid inducing a heat shock response, it does appear that targeting the *C*-terminus will eliminate this clinical outcome.

Comparing the ability of 17-AAG *vs.* CA1 and SM145 to inhibit the induction of key immunophilins FKBP51 and FKBP52 shows that even at concentrations 10-fold over its IC_{50} value SM145 decreases the quantity of both immunophilins in cell lysate (Figure 2.25). Interestingly, 17-AAG induces FKBP51 protein expression by 2-fold and FKBP52 expression by 4-fold. Since both FKBPs are critical to hormone regulation, we evaluated the compound's impact on the glucocorticoid receptor (GR). Treatment with SM145 at 10-fold over its IC_{50} showed a decrease of 3-fold, whereas treatment with 17-AAG maintained the same level of GR as background. Thus, 17-AAG is not impacting downstream events that are connected to the immunophilins and hormone receptors, whereas SM145 not only avoids inducing a

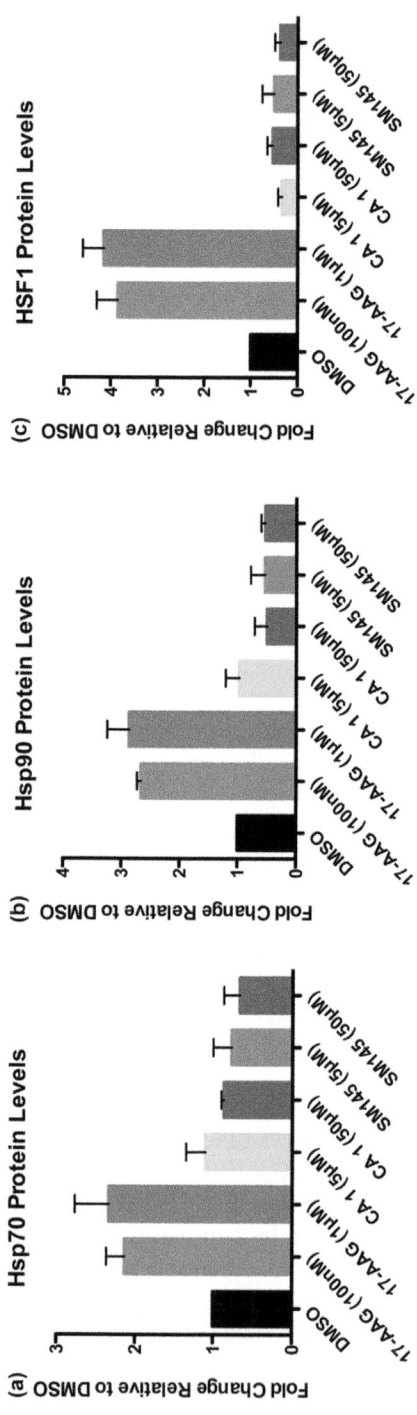

Figure 2.24 HeLa cell lysates were analysed for levels of HSR proteins: (a) Hsp70, (b) Hsp90, and (c) HSF1. Bands were quantitated with image j software, normalised to GAPDH levels and compared to the DMSO control (n $\geq$ 3, graph of mean $\pm$ SEM).

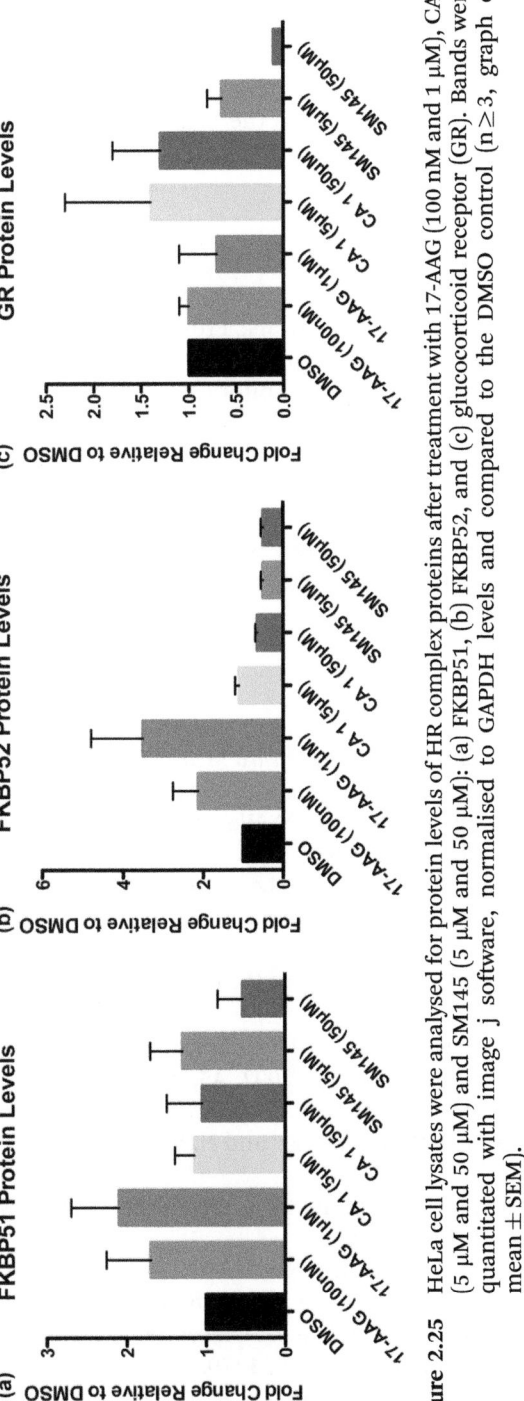

Figure 2.25 HeLa cell lysates were analysed for protein levels of HR complex proteins after treatment with 17-AAG (100 nM and 1 μM), CA1 (5 μM and 50 μM) and SM145 (5 μM and 50 μM): (a) FKBP51, (b) FKBP52, and (c) glucocorticoid receptor (GR). Bands were quantitated with image j software, normalised to GAPDH levels and compared to the DMSO control (n ≥ 3, graph of mean ± SEM).

heat shock response but it also decreases the GR receptor levels. SM145's ability to block the binding of FKBP51 and FKBP52 with Hsp90, is likely responsible for their degradation and subsequent reduction of GR production. Thus, Class IV compounds show tremendous promise as they target Hsp90 *via* a mechanism that avoids the heat shock response but maintains regulation of Hsp90's downstream functions.

2.6   Conclusion

Hsp90 inhibitors are facing intense scrutiny as potent anticancer therapies make progress through clinical trials. From competitive inhibitors of the ATP binding pocket (Classes I–III), to modulators of the *C*-terminal domain (Class IV), macrocyclic Hsp90 inhibitors have proven their value as lead compounds in spite of solubility and toxicity issues. Although these molecules may not follow all of Lipinski's Rules or amendments, their improved target selectivity and entropically favoured binding affinity have provided the necessary selectivity required for a targeted therapy. Further optimisation of lead structures and testing in both preclinical and clinical phases will establish macrocyclic Hsp90 inhibitors as the latest drugs in the arsenal of anticancer therapeutics.

References

1. J. Mallinson and I. Collins, *Future Med. Chem.*, 2012, **4**, 1409.
2. R. I. Aminov, *Front. Microbiol.*, 2010, **1**, 1.
3. S. Gaali, R. Gopalakrishnan, Y. Wang, C. Kozany and F. Hausch, *Curr. Med. Chem.*, 2011, **18**, 5355.
4. Y. K. Zee, B. C. Goh and S. C. Lee, *Future Oncol.*, 2012, **8**, 731.
5. L. A. Wessjohann, D. G. Rivera and O. E. Vercillo, *Chem. Rev.*, 2009, **109**, 796.
6. C. A. Lipinski, F. Lombardo, B. W. Dominy and P. J. Feeney, *Adv. Drug Dev. Rev.*, 1997, **23**, 3.
7. D. F. Veber, S. R. Johnson, H.-Y. Cheng, B. R. Smith, K. W. Ward and K. D. Kopple, *J. Med. Chem.*, 2002, **45**, 2615.
8. M. Rubinstein and M. Y. Niv, *Biopolymers*, 2009, **91**, 505.
9. E. M. Driggers, S. P. Hale, J. Lee and N. K. Terrett, *Nat. Rev. Drug Discov.*, 2008, 7, 608.
10. J. E. DeLorbe, J. H. Clements, B. B. Whiddon and S. F. Martin, *ACS Med. Chem. Lett.*, 2010, **1**, 448.
11. V. Jain, B. Jain, P. Tiwari, J. Saini, U. K. Jain, R. S. Pandey, M. Kumar, O. P. Katare, R. Chandra and J. Madan, *Anticancer Drugs*, 2013, **24**, 327.
12. Y. S. A. Kim, S. Lee, M.-J. Lee, G. Giaccone, L. Neckers and J. B. Trepel, *Curr. Top. Med. Chem.*, 2009, **9**, 1479.
13. J. G. Supko, R. L. Hickman, M. R. Grever and L. Malspeis, *Cancer Chemother. Pharmacol.*, 1995, **36**, 305.

14. A. Suda, H. Koyano, T. Hayase, K. Hada, K. Kawasaki, S. Komiyama, K. Hasegawa, T. A. Fukami, S. Sato, T. Miura, N. Ono, T. Yamazaki, R. Saitoh, N. Shimma, Y. Shiratori and T. Tsukuda, *Bioorg. Med. Chem. Lett.*, 2012, **22**, 1136.

15. R. C. Schnur, M. L. Corman, R. J. Gallaschun, B. A. Cooper, M. F. Dee, J. L. Doty, M. L. Muzzi, C. I. DiOrio, E. G. Barbacci, P. E. Miller, V. A. Pollack, D. M. Savage, D. E. Sloan, L. R. Pustilnik, J. D. Moyer and M. P. Moyer, *J. Med. Chem.*, 1995, **38**, 3813.

16. C. W. Zapf, J. D. Bloom, J. L. McBean, R. G. Dushin, T. Nittoli, C. Ingalls, A. G. Sutherland, J. P. Sonye, C. N. Eid, J. Golas, H. Liu, F. Boschelli, Y. Hu, E. Vogan and J. I. Levin, *Bioorg. Med. Chem. Lett.*, 2011, **21**, 2278.

17. S. Soga, L. M. Neckers, T. W. Schulte, Y. Shiotsu, K. Akasaka, H. Narumi, T. Agatsuma, Y. Ikuina, C. Murakata, T. Tamaoki and S. Akinaga, *Cancer Res.*, 1999, **59**, 2931.

18. S. Soga, Y. Shiotsu, S. Akinaga and S. V. Sharma, *Curr. Cancer Drug Targets*, 2003, **3**, 359.

19. M. Wang, G. Shen and B. S. Blagg, *Bioorg. Med. Chem. Lett.*, 2006, **16**, 2459.

20. S. Chandarlapaty, A. Sawai, Q. Ye, A. Scott, M. Silinski, K. Huang, P. Fadden, J. R. Partridge, S. Hall, P. Steed, L. Norton, N. Rosen and D. B. Solit, *Clin. Cancer Res.*, 2008, **14**, 240.

21. Y. Okawa, T. Hideshima, P. Steed, S. Vallet, S. Hall, K. Huang, J. Rice, A. Barabasz, B. Foley, H. Ikeda, N. Raje, T. Kiziltepe, H. Yasui, S. Enatsu and K. C. Anderson, *Blood*, 2009, **113**, 846.

22. K. H. Huang, J. M. Veal, R. P. Fadden, J. W. Rice, J. Eaves, J. P. Strachan, A. F. Barabasz, B. E. Foley, T. E. Barta, W. Ma, M. A. Sillinski, M. Hu, J. M. Partridge, A. Scott, L. G. DuBois, T. Freed, P. M. Steed, A. J. Ommen, E. D. Smith, P. F. Hughes, A. R. Woodward, G. J. Hanson, W. S. McCall, C. J. Markworth, L. Hinkley, M. Jenks, L. Geng, M. Lewis, J. Otto, B. Pronk, K. Verleysen and S. E. Hall, *J. Med. Chem.*, 2009, **52**, 4288.

23. R. P. Sellers, L. D. Alexander, V. A. Johnson, C.-C. Lin, J. Savage, R. Corral, J. Moss, T. S. Slugocki, E. K. Singh, M. R. Davis, S. Ravula, J. E. Spicer, J. L. Oelrich, A. Thornquist, C.-M. Pan and S. R. McAlpine, *Bioorg. Med. Chem.*, 2010, **18**, 6822.

24. R. C. Vasko, R. A. Rodriguez, C. N. Cunningham, V. C. Ardi, D. A. Agard and S. R. McAlpine, *ACS Med. Chem. Lett.*, 2010, **1**, 4.

25. L. D. Alexander, J. R. Partridge, D. A. Agard and S. R. McAlpine, *Bioorg. Med. Chem. Lett.*, 2011, **21**, 7068.

26. V. C. Ardi, L. D. Alexander, V. A. Johnson and S. R. McAlpine, *ACS Chem. Biol.*, 2011, **6**, 1357.

27. J. B. Kunicki, M. N. Petersen, L. D. Alexander, V. C. Ardi, J. R. McConnell and S. R. McAlpine, *Bioorg. Med. Chem. Lett.*, 2011, **21**, 4716.

28. D. Ramsey, M., J. McConnell, R., L. Alexander, D., K. Tanaka, W., C. Vera and M. and S. Mcalpine, R., *Bioorg. Med. Chem. Lett.*, 2012, **22**, 3287.

29. J. M. McConnell, L. D. Alexander and S. R. McAlpine, *Bioorg. Med. Chem. Lett.*, 2014, **24**, 661.
30. E. de Billy, J. Travers and P. Workman, *Oncotarget*, 2012, **8**, 741.
31. H. S. Oskay, B. Halacli and K. Altundag, *Med. Oncol.*, 2013, **30**, 575.
32. D. Stellas, A. El Hamidieh and E. Patsavoudi, *BMC Cell Biology*, 2010, **11**, 51.
33. L. Neckers, *Trends Mol. Med.*, 2002, **8**, S55.
34. M. Taipale, I. Krykbaeva, M. Koeva, C. Kayatekin, K. D. Westover, G. I. Karras and S. Lindquist, *Cell*, 2012, **150**, 987.
35. I. Fierro-Monti, P. Echeverria, J. Racle, C. Hernandez, D. Picard and M. Quadroni, *PLoS One*, 2013, **8**, e80425.
36. A. Finka and P. Goloubinoff, *Cell Stress Chaperones*, 2013, **18**, 591.
37. A. S. Reddy and S. Zhang, *Expert Rev. Clin. Pharmacol.*, 2013, **6**, 41.
38. A. Petrelli, in *Polypharmacology in Drug* Discovery, ed. J.-U. Peters, Wiley, Hoboken, NJ, 2012, ch. 8, pp. 149–165.
39. P. N. Münster, M. Srethapakdi, M. M. Moasser and N. Rosen, *Cancer Res.*, 2001, **61**, 2945.
40. P. Hawle, M. Siepmann, A. Harst, M. Siderius, H. P. Reusch and W. M. Obermann, *Mol. Cell. Biol.*, 2006, **26**, 8385.
41. S. F. Harris, A. K. Shiau and D. A. Agard, *Structure*, 2004, **12**, 1087.
42. H. Wegele, P. Muschler, M. Bunck, J. Reinstein and J. Buchner, *J. Biol. Chem.*, 2003, **278**, 39303.
43. D. R. Southworth and D. A. Agard, *Mol. Cell*, 2011, **42**, 771.
44. A. Carrello, E. Ingley, R. F. Minchin, S. Tsai and T. Ratajczak, *J. Biol. Chem.*, 1999, **274**, 2682.
45. B. Panaretou, C. Prodromou, S. M. Roe, R. O'Brien, J. E. Ladbury, P. W. Piper and L. H. Pearl, *EMBO J*, 1998, **17**, 4829.
46. M. R. Davis, E. K. Singh, H. Wahyudi, L. D. Alexander, J. Kunicki, L. A. Nazarova, K. A. Fairweather, A. M. Giltrap, K. A. Jolliffe and S. R. McAlpine, *Tetrahedron*, 2012, **68**, 1029.
47. F. U. Hartl, A. Bracher and M. Hayer-Hartl, *Nature*, 2011, **475**, 324.
48. M. Mickler, M. Hessling, C. Ratzke, J. Buchner and T. Hugel, *Nat. Struct. Mol. Bio.*, 2009, **16**, 281.
49. M. Hessling, K. Richter and J. Buchner, *Nat. Struct. Mol. Bio.*, 2009, **16**, 287.
50. C. DeBoer, P. A. Meulman, R. J. Wnuk and D. H. Peterson, *J. Antibiot. (Tokyo)*, 1970, **23**, 442.
51. H. Yamaki, H. Suzuki, E. C. Choi and N. Tanaka, *J. Antibiot. (Tokyo)*, 1982, **35**, 886.
52. R. D. Johnson, A. Haber and K. L. J. Rinehart, *J. Am. Chem. Soc.*, 1974, **96**, 3316.
53. K. L. Rinehart, K. Sasaki, G. Slomp, M. F. Grostic and E. C. Olson, *J. Am. Chem. Soc.*, 1970, **92**, 7591.
54. Y. H. Li, Q. N. Lu, H. Q. Wang, P. Z. Tao and J. D. Jiang, *J. Antibiot. (Tokyo)*, 2012, **65**, 509.

55. C. Chavany, E. Mimnaugh, P. Miller, R. Bitton, P. Nguyen, J. Trepel, L. Whitesell, R. Schnur, J. Moyer and L. Neckers, *J. Biol. Chem.*, 1996, **271**, 4974.
56. A. Gopalsamy, M. X. Shi, J. Golas, E. Vogan, J. Jacob, M. Johnson, F. Lee, R. Nilakantan, R. Petersen, K. Svenson, R. Chopra, M. S. Tam, Y. X. Wen, J. Ellingboe, K. Arndt and F. Boschelli, *J. Med. Chem.*, 2008, **51**, 373.
57. K. Yamamoto, R. M. Garbaccio, S. J. Stachel, D. B. Solit, G. Chiosis, N. Rosen and S. J. Danishefsky, *Angew. Chem., Int. Ed.*, 2003, **42**, 1280.
58. C. Prodromou, J. M. Nuttall, S. H. Millson, S. M. Roe, T. S. Sim, D. Tan, P. Workman, L. H. Pearl and P. W. Piper, *ACS Chem. Biol.*, 2009, **4**, 289.
59. S. M. Roe, C. Prodromou, R. O'Brien, J. E. Ladbury, P. W. Piper and L. H. Pearl, *J. Med. Chem.*, 1999, **42**, 260.
60. C. E. Stebbins, A. A. Russo, C. Schneider, N. Rosen, F. U. Hartl and N. P. Pavletich, *Cell*, 1997, **89**, 239.
61. C. Prodromou, S. M. Roe, R. O'Brien, J. E. Ladbury, P. W. Piper and L. H. Pearl, *Cell*, 1997, **90**, 65.
62. J. M. Jez, J. C. Chen, G. Rastelli, R. M. Stroud and D. V. Santi, *Chem. Biol.*, 2003, **10**, 361.
63. L. T. Gooljarsingh, C. Fernandes, K. Yan, H. Zhang, M. Grooms, K. Johanson, R. H. Sinnamon, R. B. Kirkpatrick, J. Kerrigan, T. Lewis, M. Arnone, A. J. King, Z. Lai, R. A. Copeland and P. J. Tummino, *Proc. Natl. Acad. Sci. U.S.A.*, 2006, **103**, 7625.
64. Z. Wu, G. A. Moghaddas and B. Kuster, *Mol. Cell. Proteomics*, 2012, **11**, M111.016675.
65. J. J. Cullen, M. M. Hinkhouse, M. Grady, A. W. Gaut, J. Liu, Y. P. Zhang, C. J. Weydert, F. E. Domann and L. W. Oberley, *Cancer Res.*, 2003, **63**, 5513.
66. W. Guo, P. Reigan, D. Siegel, J. Zirrolli, D. Gustafson and D. Ross, *Mol. Pharmacol.*, 2006, **70**, 1194.
67. G. Powis, *Free Radic. Biol. Med.*, 1989, **6**, 63.
68. W. Guo, P. Reigan, D. Siegel and D. Ross, *Drug Metab. Dispos.*, 2008, **36**, 2050.
69. C. J. Martin, S. Gaisser, I. R. Challis, I. Carletti, B. Wilkinson, M. Gregory, C. Prodromou, S. M. Roe, L. H. Pearl, S. M. Boyd and M. Q. Zhang, *J. Med. Chem.*, 2008, **51**, 2853.
70. U. Banerji, A. O'Donnell, M. Scurr, S. Pacey, S. Stapleton, Y. Asad, L. Simmons, A. Maloney, F. Raynaud, M. Campbell, M. Walton, S. Lakhani, S. Kaye, P. Workman and I. Judson, *J. Clin. Oncol.*, 2005, **23**, 4152.
71. M. P. Goetz, D. Toft, J. Reid, M. Ames, B. Stensgard, S. Safgren, A. A. Adjei, J. Sloan, P. Atherton, V. Vasile, S. Salazaar, A. Adjei, G. Croghan and C. Erlichman, *J. Clin. Oncol.*, 2005, **23**, 1078.

72. J. L. Grem, G. Morrison, X. D. Guo, E. Agnew, C. H. Takimoto, R. Thomas, E. Szabo, L. Grochow, F. Grollman, J. M. Hamilton, L. M. Neckers and R. H. Wilson, *J. Clin. Oncol.*, 2005, **23**, 1885.

73. R. K. Ramanathan, D. L. Trump, J. L. Eiseman, C. P. Belani, S. S. Agarwala, E. G. Zuhowski, J. Lan, D. M. Potter, S. P. Ivy, S. Ramalingam, A. M. Brufsky, M. K. K. Wong, S. Tutchko and M. J. Egorin, *Clin. Cancer Res.*, 2005, **11**, 3385.

74. D. B. Solit, S. P. Ivy, C. Kopil, R. Sikorski, M. J. Morris, S. F. Slovin, W. K. Kelly, A. DeLaCruz, T. Curley, G. Heller, S. Larson, L. Schwartz, M. J. Egorin, N. Rosen and H. I. Scher, *Clin. Cancer Res.*, 2007, **13**, 1775.

75. R. C. Schnur, M. L. Corman, R. J. Gallaschun, B. A. Cooper, M. F. Dee, J. L. Doty, M. L. Muzzi, J. D. Moyer and C. I. DiOrio, *J. Med. Chem.*, 1995, **38**, 3806.

76. M. J. Egorin, D. M. Rosen, J. H. Wolff, P. S. Callery, S. M. Musser and J. L. Eiseman, *Cancer Res.*, 1998, **58**, 2385.

77. T. W. Schulte and L. M. Neckers, *Cancer Chemother. Pharmacol.*, 1998, **42**, 273.

78. H. A. Burris, D. Berman, B. Murthy and S. Jones, *Cancer Chemother. Pharmacol.*, 2011, **67**, 1045.

79. D. Dye and J. Watkins, *Br. Med. J.*, 1980, **280**, 1353.

80. N. C. Santos, J. Figueira-Coelho, J. Martins-Silva and C. Saldanha, *Biochem. Pharmacol.*, 2003, **65**, 1035.

81. N. Fujikake, Y. Nagai, H. A. Popiel, Y. Okamoto, M. Yamaguchi and T. Toda, *J. Biol. Chem.*, 2008, **283**, 26188.

82. P. Joshi and C. A. Stoddart, *J. Biol. Chem.*, 2011, **286**, 24581.

83. K. J. Meyer and T. A. Shapiro, *J. Infect. Dis.*, 2013, **208**, 489.

84. M. Waza, H. Adachi, M. Katsuno, M. Minamiyama, C. Sang, F. Tanaka, A. Inukai, M. Doyu and G. Sobue, *Nat. Med.*, 2005, **11**, 1088.

85. B. O'Keeffe, Y. Fong, D. Chen, S. Zhou and Q. Zhou, *J. Biol. Chem.*, 2000, **275**, 279.

86. R. Pallavi, N. Roy, R. K. Nageshan, P. Talukdar, S. R. Pavithra, R. Reddy, S. Venketesh, R. Kumar, A. K. Gupta, R. K. Singh, S. C. Yadav and U. Tatu, *J. Biol. Chem.*, 2010, **285**, 37964.

87. J. C. Mottram, W. J. Murphy and N. Agabian, *Mol. Biochem. Parasitol.*, 1989, **37**, 115.

88. E. R. Glaze, A. L. Lambert, A. C. Smith, J. G. Page, W. D. Johnson, D. L. McCormick, A. P. Brown, B. S. Levine, J. M. Covey, M. J. Egorin, J. L. Eiseman, J. L. Holleran, E. A. Sausville and J. E. Tomaszewski, *Cancer Chemother. Pharmacol.*, 2005, **56**, 637.

89. M. J. Egorin, T. F. Lagattuta, D. R. Hamburger, J. M. Covey, K. D. White, S. M. Musser and J. L. Eiseman, *Cancer Chemother. Pharmacol.*, 2002, **49**, 7.

90. W. C. Guo, P. Reigan, D. Siegel, J. Zirrolli, D. Gustafson and D. Ross, *Cancer Res.*, 2005, **65**, 10006.

91. T. Kim, G. Keum and A. N. Pae, *Expert Opin. Ther. Pat.*, 2013, **23**, 919.

92. M. Q. Zhang, S. Gaisser, M. Nur-E-Alam, L. S. Sheehan, W. A. Vousden, N. Gaitatzis, G. Peck, N. J. Coates, S. J. Moso, M. Radzom, T. A. Foster, R. M. Sheridan, M. A. Gregory, S. M. Roe, C. Prodromou, L. Pearl, S. M. Boyd, B. Wilkinson and C. J. Martin, *J. Med. Chem.*, 2008, **51**, 5494.

93. Z.-Q. Tian, Y. Liu, D. Zhang, Z. Wang, S. D. Dong, C. W. Carreras, Y. Zhou, G. Rastelli, D. V. Santi and D. C. Myles, *Bioorg. Med. Chem.*, 2004, **12**, 5317.

94. J. R. Porter, J. E. Ge, J. Lee, E. Normant and K. West, *Curr. Top. Med. Chem.*, 2009, **9**, 1386.

95. R. L. Cysyk, R. J. Parker, J. J. Barchi, P. S. Steeg, N. R. Hartman and J. A. Strong, *Chem. Res. Toxicol.*, 2006, **19**, 376.

96. R. R. A. Kitson and C. J. Moody, *J. Org. Chem.*, 2013, **78**, 5117.

97. K. Sasaki and Y. Inoue, Kaken Chemical Co., Ltd., Tokyo, *Ger. Offen.* 3006097, 1980.

98. R. R. A. Kitson, C.-H. Chuan, R. Xiong, H. E. L. Williams, A. L. Davis, W. Lewis, D. L. Dehn, D. Siegel, S. M. Roe, C. Prodromou, D. Ross and C. J. Moody, *Nat. Chem.*, 2013, 307.

99. R. R. A. Kitson and C. J. Moody, *Chem. Commun.*, 2013, **49**, 8441.

100. P. G. Richardson, A. Z. Badros, S. Jagannath, S. Tarantolo, J. L. Wolf, M. Albitar, D. Berman, M. Messina and K. C. Anderson, *Br. J. Haematol.*, 2010, **150**, 428.

101. P. Delmotte and J. Delmotte-Plaque, *Nature*, 1953, **171**, 344.

102. S. V. Sharma, T. Agatsuma and H. Nakano, *Oncogene*, 1998, **16**, 2639.

103. J. E. H. Day, S. Y. Sharp, M. G. Rowlands, W. Aherne, P. Workman and C. J. Moody, *Chem. -Eur. J.*, 2010, **16**, 2758.

104. N. Proisy, S. Y. Sharp, K. Boxall, S. Connelly, S. M. Roe, C. Prodromou, A. M. Slawin, L. H. Pearl, P. Workman and C. J. Moody, *Chem. Biol.*, 2006, **13**, 1203.

105. P. A. Brough, W. Aherne, X. Barril, J. Borgognoni, K. Boxall, J. E. Cansfield, K.-M. Cheung, I. Collins, N. G. M. Davies, M. J. Drysdale, B. Dymock, S. A. Eccles, H. Finch, A. Fink, A. Hayes, R. Howes, R. E. Hubbard, K. James, A. M. Jordan, A. Lockie, V. Martins, A. Massey, T. P. Matthews, E. McDonald, C. J. Northfield, L. H. Pearl, C. Prodromou, S. Ray, F. I. Raynaud, S. D. Roughley, S. Y. Sharp, A. Surgenor, D. L. Walmsley, P. Webb, M. Wood, P. Workman and L. Wright, *J. Med. Chem.*, 2008, **51**, 196.

106. S. A. Eccles, A. Massey, F. I. Raynaud, S. Y. Sharp, G. Box, M. Valenti, L. Patterson, de Haven, A. Brandon, S. Gowan, F. Boxall, W. Aherne, M. Rowlands, A. Hayes, V. Martins, F. Urban, K. Boxall, C. Prodromou, L. Pearl, K. James, T. P. Matthews, K.-M. Cheung, A. Kalusa, K. Jones, E. McDonald, X. Barril, P. A. Brough, J. E. Cansfield, B. Dymock, M. J. Drysdale, H. Finch, R. Howes, R. E. Hubbard, A. Surgenor, P. Webb, M. Wood, L. Wright and P. Workman, *Cancer Res.*, 2008, **68**, 2850.

107. C. W. Murray, M. G. Carr, O. Callaghan, G. Chessari, M. Congreve, S. Cowan, J. E. Coyle, R. Downham, E. Figueroa, M. Frederickson,

B. Graham, R. McMenamin, M. A. O'Brien, S. Patel, T. R. Phillips, G. Williams, A. J. Woodhead and A. J. A. Woolford, *J. Med. Chem.*, 2010, **53**, 5942.

108. A. J. Woodhead, H. Angove, M. G. Carr, G. Chessari, M. Congreve, J. E. Coyle, J. Cosme, B. Graham, P. J. Day, R. Downham, L. Fazal, R. Feltell, E. Figueroa, M. Frederickson, J. Lewis, R. McMenamin, C. W. Murray, M. A. O'Brien, L. Parra, S. Patel, T. Phillips, D. C. Rees, S. Rich, D.-M. Smith, G. Trewartha, M. Vinkovic, B. Williams and A. J. A. Woolford, *J. Med. Chem.*, 2010, **53**, 5956.

109. H. Shinonaga, T. Noguchi, A. Ikeda, M. Aoki, N. Fujimoto and A. Kawashima, *Bioorg. Med. Chem.*, 2009, **17**, 4622.

110. J. E. H. Day, S. Y. Sharp, M. G. Rowlands, W. Aherne, W. Lewis, S. M. Roe, C. Prodromou, L. H. Pearl, P. Workman and C. J. Moody, *Chem. -Eur. J.*, 2010, **16**, 10366.

111. E. Moulin, V. Zoete, S. Barluenga, M. Karplus and N. Winssinger, *J. Am. Chem. Soc.*, 2005, **127**, 6999.

112. X. G. Lei and S. J. Danishefsky, *Adv. Synth. Catal.*, 2008, **350**, 1677.

113. J. E. H. Day, S. Y. Sharp, M. G. Rowlands, W. Aherne, A. Hayes, F. I. Raynaud, W. Lewis, S. M. Roe, C. Prodromou, L. H. Pearl, P. Workman and C. J. Moody, *ACS Chem. Biol.*, 2011, **6**, 1339.

114. Y. Xia, P. Rocchi, J. L. Iovanna and L. Peng, *Drug Discov. Today*, 2012, **17**, 35.

115. T. Agatsuma, H. Ogawa, K. Akasaka, A. Asai, Y. Yamashita, T. Mizukami, S. Akinaga and Y. Saitoh, *Bioorg. Med. Chem.*, 2002, **10**, 3445.

116. G. Karthikeyan, C. Zambaldo, S. Barluenga, V. Zoete, M. Karplus and N. Winssinger, *Chem. -Eur. J.*, 2012, **18**, 8978.

117. R. C. Clevenger and B. S. J. Blagg, *Org. Lett.*, 2004, **6**, 4459.

118. M. K. Hadden and B. S. J. Blagg, *J. Org. Chem.*, 2009, **74**, 4697.

119. V. D. Jadhav, A. S. Duerfeldt and B. S. J. Blagg, *Bioorg. Med. Chem. Lett.*, 2009, **19**, 6845.

120. G. Shen and B. S. J. Blagg, *Org. Lett.*, 2005, 7, 2157.

121. G. Shen, M. Wang, T. R. Welch and B. S. Blagg, *J. Org. Chem.*, 2006, **71**, 7618.

122. B. W. Dymock, X. Barril, P. A. Brough, J. E. Cansfield, A. Massey, E. McDonald, R. E. Hubbard, A. Surgenor, S. D. Roughley, P. Webb, P. Workman, L. Wright and M. J. Drysdale, *J. Med. Chem.*, 2005, **48**, 4212.

123. K. M. J. Cheung, T. P. Matthews, K. James, M. G. Rowlands, K. J. Boxall, S. Y. Sharp, A. Maloney, S. M. Roe, C. Prodromou, L. H. Pearl, G. W. Aherne, E. McDonald and P. Workman, *Bioorg. Med. Chem. Lett*, 2005, **15**, 3338.

124. M. G. Rowlands, Y. M. Newbatt, C. Prodromou, L. H. Pearl, P. Workman and W. Aherne, *Anal. Biochem.*, 2004, **327**, 176.

125. Y. H. Du, K. Moulick, A. Rodina, J. Aguirre, S. Felts, R. Dingledine, H. Fu and G. Chiosis, *J. Biomol. Screen.*, 2007, **12**, 915.

126. Y. L. Janin, *J. Med. Chem.*, 2005, **48**, 7503.
127. T. Taldone, W. L. Sun and G. Chiosis, *Bioorg. Med. Chem.*, 2009, **17**, 2225.
128. M. A. Biamonte, R. Van de Water, J. W. Arndt, R. H. Scannevin, D. Perret and W. C. Lee, *J. Med. Chem.*, 2010, **53**, 3.
129. A. Rajan, R. J. Kelly, J. B. Trepel, Y. S. Kim, S. V. Alarcon, S. Kummar, M. Gutierrez, S. Crandon, W. M. Zein, L. Jain, B. Mannargudi, W. D. Figg, B. E. Houk, M. Shnaidman, N. Brega and G. Giaccone, *Clin. Cancer Res.*, 2011, **17**, 6831.
130. K. Lundgren, H. Zhang, J. Brekken, N. Huser, R. E. Powell, N. Timple, D. J. Busch, L. Neely, J. L. Sensintaffar, Y. C. Yang, A. McKenzie, J. Friedman, R. Scannevin, A. Kamal, K. Hong, S. R. Kasibhatla, M. F. Boehm and F. J. Burrows, *Mol. Cancer Ther.*, 2009, **8**, 921.
131. M. A. Dickson, S. H. Okuno, M. L. Keohan, R. G. Maki, D. R. D'Adamo, T. J. Akhurst, C. R. Antonescu and G. K. Schwartz, *Ann. Oncol.*, 2013, **24**, 252.
132. S. R. Kasibhatla, K. Hong, M. A. Biamonte, D. J. Busch, P. L. Karjian, J. L. Sensintaffar, A. Kamal, R. E. Lough, J. Brekken, K. Lundgren, R. Grecko, G. A. Timony, Y. Ran, R. Mansfield, L. C. Fritz, E. Ulm, F. J. Burrows and M. F. Boehm, *J. Med. Chem.*, 2007, **50**, 2767.
133. J. Shi, R. Van de Water, K. Hong, R. B. Lamer, K. W. Weichert, C. M. Sandoval, S. R. Kasibhatla, M. F. Boehm, J. Chao, K. Lundgren, N. Timple, R. E. Lough, G. Ibanez, C. Boykin, F. J. Burrows, M. R. Kehry, T. J. Yun, E. K. Harning, C. Ambrose, J. Thompson, S. A. Bixler, A. Dunah, P. Snodgrass-Belt, J. Arndt, I. J. Enyedy, P. Li, V. S. Hong, A. McKenzie and M. A. Biamonte, *J. Med. Chem.*, 2012, **55**, 7786.
134. D. L. Menezes, P. Taverna, M. R. Jensen, T. Abrams, D. Stuart, G. K. Yu, D. Duhl, T. Machajewski, W. R. Sellers, N. K. Pryer and Z. Gao, *Mol. Cancer Ther.*, 2012, **11**, 730.
135. P. A. Brough, X. Barril, J. Borgognoni, P. Chene, N. G. Davies, B. Davis, M. J. Drysdale, B. Dymock, S. A. Eccles, C. Garcia-Echeverria, C. Fremont, A. Hayes, R. E. Hubbard, A. M. Jordan, M. R. Jensen, A. Massey, A. Merrett, A. Padfield, R. Parsons, T. Radimerski, F. I. Raynaud, A. Robertson, S. D. Roughley, J. Schoepfer, H. Simmonite, S. Y. Sharp, A. Surgenor, M. Valenti, S. Walls, P. Webb, M. Wood, P. Workman and L. Wright, *J. Med. Chem.*, 2009, **52**, 4794.
136. C. W. Zapf, J. D. Bloom, J. L. McBean, R. G. Dushin, T. Nittoli, M. Otteng, C. Ingalls, J. M. Golas, H. Liu, J. Lucas, F. Boschelli, Y. Hu, E. Vogan and J. I. Levin, *Bioorg. Med. Chem.*, 2011, **21**, 3411.
137. C. W. Zapf, J. D. Bloom, J. L. McBean, R. G. Dushin, J. M. Golas, H. Liu, J. Lucas, F. Boschelli, E. Vogan and J. I. Levin, *Bioorg. Med. Chem.*, 2011, **21**, 3627.
138. C. W. Zapf, J. D. Bloom, Z. Li, R. G. Dushin, T. Nittoli, M. Otteng, A. Nikitenko, J. M. Golas, H. Liu, J. Lucas, F. Boschelli, E. Vogan, A. Olland, M. Johnson and J. I. Levin, *Bioorg. Med. Chem.*, 2011, **21**, 4602.

139. J. Travers, S. Sharp and P. Workman, *Drug Discov. Today*, 2012, **17**, 242.
140. L. Neckers and P. Workman, *Clin. Cancer Res.*, 2012, **18**, 64.
141. M. V. Powers, K. Jones, C. Barillari, I. Westwood, R. L. van Montfort and P. Workman, *Cell Cycle*, 2010, **9**, 1542.
142. A. J. Massey, D. S. Williamson, H. Browne, J. B. Murray, P. Dokurno, T. Shaw, A. T. Macias, Z. Daniels, S. Geoffroy, M. Dopson, P. Lavan, N. Matassova, G. L. Francis, C. J. Graham, R. Parsons, Y. Wang, A. Padfield, M. Comer, M. J. Drysdale and M. Wood, *Cancer Chemother. Pharmacol.*, 2010, **66**, 535.
143. M. Kaiser, A. Kühnl, J. Reins, S. Fischer, J. Ortiz-Tanchez, C. Schlee, L. H. Mochmann, S. Heesch, O. Benlasfer, W. K. Hofmann, E. Thiel and C. D. Baldus, *Blood Cancer J.*, 2011, **1**, e28.
144. M. J. Braunstein, S. S. Scott, C. M. Scott, S. Behrman, P. Walter, P. Wipf, J. D. Coplan, W. Chrico, D. Joseph, J. L. Brodsky and O. Batuman, *J. Oncol.*, 2011, **2011**, 232037.
145. M. Chatterjee, M. Andrulis, T. Stühmer, E. Müller, C. Hofmann, T. Steinbrunn, T. Heimberger, H. Schraud, S. Kressmann, H. Einsele and R. C. Bargou, *Haematologica*, 2013, **98**, 1132.
146. J. R. McConnell and S. R. McAlpine, *Bioorg. Med. Chem. Lett.*, 2013, **23**, 1923–1928.
147. A. Donnelly and B. S. Blagg, *Curr. Med. Chem.*, 2008, **15**, 2702.
148. B. R. Kusuma, L. B. Peterson, H. Zhao, G. Vielhauer, J. Holzberlein and B. S. J. Blagg, *J. Med. Chem.*, 2011, **54**, 6234.
149. M. K. Hadden and B. S. Blagg, *Anticancer Agents Med. Chem.*, 2008, **8**, 807.
150. R. K. Allan, D. Mok, B. K. Ward and T. Ratajczak, *J. Biol. Chem.*, 2006, **281**, 7161.
151. J. D. Eskew, T. Sadikot, P. Morales, A. Duren, I. Dunwiddie, M. Swink, X. Zhang, S. Hembruff, A. Donnelly, R. A. Rajewski, B. Blad, J. R. Manjarrez, R. L. Matts, J. M. Holzbeierlein and G. A. Vielhauer, *Bio. Med. Central Cancer.*, 2011, **11**, 468.
152. A. S. Duerfeldt and B. S. J. Blagg, *Bioorg. Med. Chem. Lett.*, 2010, **20**, 4983.
153. W. B. Pratt and D. O. Toft, *Exp. Bio. Med.*, 2003, **228**, 111.
154. P. Echeverria and D. Picard, *Biochim. Biophys. Acta.*, 2010, **1803**, 641.
155. Y. C. Koay, J. R. McConnell, Y. Wang, S. J. Kim, L. K. Buckton, F. Mansour and S. R. McAlpine, *ACS Med. Chem. Lett.*, 2014, **5**, 771.
156. P. S. Pan, R. C. Vasko, S. A. Lapera, V. A. Johnson, R. P. Sellers, C.-C. Lin, C.-M. Pan, M. R. Davis, V. C. Ardi and S. R. McAlpine, *Bioorg. Med. Chem.*, 2009, **17**, 5806.
157. K. Otrubova, G. H. Lushington, D. Vander Velde, K. L. McGuire and S. R. McAlpine, *J. Med. Chem.*, 2008, **51**, 530.
158. P. S. Pan, K. McGuire and S. R. McAlpine, *Bioorg. Med. Chem. Lett.*, 2007, **17**, 5072.
159. K. Otrubova, K. L. McGuire and S. R. McAlpine, *J. Med. Chem.*, 2007, **50**, 1999.

160. T. J. Styers, A. Kekec, R. A. Rodriguez, J. D. Brown, J. Cajica, P.-S. Pan, E. Parry, C. L. Carroll, I. Medina, R. Corral, S. Lapera, K. Otrubova, C.-M. Pan, K. L. McGuire and S. R. McAlpine, *Bioorg. Med. Chem.*, 2006, **14**, 5625.
161. R. A. Rodriguez, P.-S. Pan, C.-M. Pan, S. Ravula, S. A. Lapera, E. K. Singh, T. J. Styers, J. D. Brown, J. Cajica, E. Parry, K. Otrubova and S. R. McAlpine, *J. Org. Chem.*, 2007, **72**, 1980.

CHAPTER 3

Epothilones

RAPHAEL SCHIESS AND KARL-HEINZ ALTMANN*

Department of Chemistry and Applied Biosciences, Institute of
Pharmaceutical Sciences, Swiss Federal Institute of Technology (ETH)
Zürich, HCI H405, Vladimir-Prelog-Weg 4, CH-8093 Zürich, Switzerland
*Email: karl-heinz.altmann@pharma.ethz.ch

3.1 Introduction

Epothilones A and B (Epo A and B) are naturally occurring 16-membered
macrolides that were first isolated in 1987 from the myxobacterium *Sorangium cellulosum Sc 90* (Figure 3.1)[1,2] and shown to exhibit potent *in vitro*
antiproliferative activity.

With the exception of a German patent application,[3] these findings remained unpublished, however; the scientific community at large became
aware of epothilones only in 1995, when studies at Merck Research Laboratories established that the pronounced *in vitro* antitumor activity of Epo
A and B involved the stabilization of cellular microtubules (MT) and the
suppression of MT dynamics.[4] This finding led to an immediate surge in
interest in these compounds, as the inhibition of cancer cell division by
interference with MT function was (and is) an important mechanistic principle in anticancer therapy. Compounds that either impair or promote MT
stability are essential anticancer drugs, such as the microtubule stabilizers
taxol and taxotere or the tubulin polymerization inhibitors vincristine and
vinblastine (among others).[5,6] Importantly at the time, epothilones represented the first non-taxane chemotype of microtubule-stabilizing agents
(MSA). In the meantime a growing number of additional natural products
have been recognized to be MSA (for reviews see ref. 7–10; for the most

RSC Drug Discovery Series No. 40
Macrocycles in Drug Discovery
Edited by Jeremy Levin
© The Royal Society of Chemistry 2015
Published by the Royal Society of Chemistry, www.rsc.org

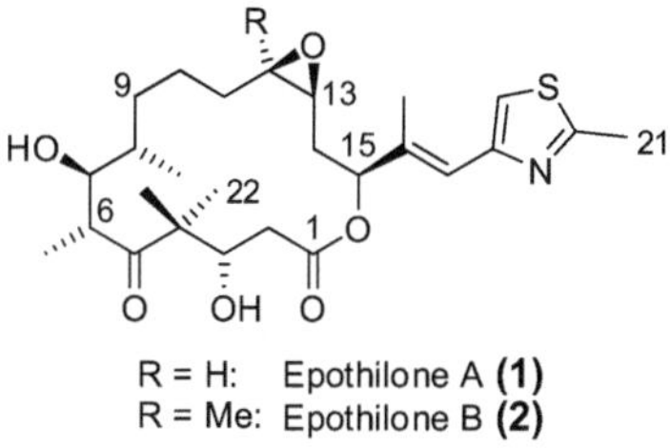

R = H: Epothilone A **(1)**
R = Me: Epothilone B **(2)**

Figure 3.1 Structure of naturally occurring Epo A and B.

recent example see ref. 11 and 12), of which the majority are macrolides of marine origin. In addition, numerous epothilone-type structures have been identified as minor components in fermentation broths from myxobacteria.[13–15]

In contrast to taxol, epothilones also potently inhibit the growth of multidrug-resistant cancer cells, including variants whose taxol resistance is mediated by specific tubulin mutations.[16–18] In addition, epothilones possess more favorable biopharmaceutical properties than taxol, for example, improved water solubility,[19] which offered a prospect for better tolerated clinical formulation vehicles than those required for taxol.[20]

Epo B and a number of its analogs have been demonstrated to possess potent *in vivo* antitumor activity,[18,21] and at least nine epothilone-type molecules have been advanced to clinical evaluation in humans. These include Epo B itself (EPO906, patupilone; developed by Novartis), Epo D (deoxy-Epo B, KOS-862; Kosan/Roche/BMS), BMS-247550 (ixabepilone, the lactam analog of Epo B; BMS), BMS-310705 (C21-amino-Epo B; BMS), ABJ879 (C20-desmethyl-C20-methylsulfanyl-Epo B; Novartis), 9,10-didehydro-Epo B (KOS-1584; Kosan/Roche/BMS)), the fully synthetic analog ZK-Epo (sagopilone, Bayer Schering),[22] and, most recently, 9,10-didehydro-12-desmethyl-12-trifluoromethyl-Epo D (iso-fludelone; Memorial-Sloan-Kettering Cancer Center)[23] and a compound of unknown structure that has been reported to be in Phase I studies in China (UTD1).[24] In addition, the folic acid conjugate BMS-753493 (BMS)[25] has been studied in Phase I clinical trials. Of these compounds, ixabepilone has been approved in the US for the treatment of advanced and metastatic breast cancer,[26,27] while approval has been denied by the European Medicines Agency (EMA) and is no longer being sought. Patupilone still appears to be under active development, although only on a very limited scale; phase III trials have been completed with patupilone in ovarian cancer, but Novartis did not apply for regulatory approval due to non-superiority over standard therapy.[28] The clinical development of ABJ879,[29] BMS-310705, KOS-862, KOS-1584, sagopilone, and BMS-753493[30] appears to have been terminated or at least put on hold.[31] However, MSA have recently become of interest for the possible treatment of neurodegenerative diseases[32] and Epo D (as BMS-241027) is currently undergoing Phase I clinical trials in Alzheimer disease patients.[33]

Epothilones have been widely pursued targets for total chemical synthesis (for reviews see ref. 34–39) and their structure–activity relationship (SAR) has been broadly evaluated; this research has been reviewed extensively (ref. 1, 34, 36, 38 and 40–46). It is not the objective of this chapter to provide yet another all-encompassing collection of SAR and synthetic data. Rather, after a brief summary of the *in vitro* and *in vivo* biological properties of Epo B, the discussion will focus on the chemistry of those modifications that have led to clinical development compounds and the most important preclinical features of these analogs.

3.2 Epothilone B

As indicated above, the antitumor activity of Epo B is based on its ability to bind to microtubules and to alter their intrinsic stability and dynamic properties. (For excellent reviews on microtubule structure and function see ref. 6 and 47–49.) Epothilones prevent the Ca^{2+} or cold-induced de-polymerization of pre-existing microtubule polymers in cell-free systems;[16] at the same time, they promote the polymerization of soluble tubulin into microtubule-like polymers under conditions that would normally destabilize microtubules.[4,16] As demonstrated by kinetic experiments, epothilones inhibit the binding of taxol to microtubules in a competitive manner and they bind to the taxol binding site on β-tubulin with affinities that exceed (Epo B) or are comparable (Epo A) to taxol affinity; likewise Epo B is a more potent tubulin-polymerizing agent than taxol or Epo A.[4,16,50,51] Structural studies on a complex between Zn^{2+}-stabilized tubulin polymer sheets and Epo A have confirmed that taxol and epothilones bind to the same site on β-tubulin (*vide infra*).[52] Interestingly, inhibition of cancer cell growth occurs at concentrations that are significantly lower than those required to induce tubulin polymerization.[41] This apparent discrepancy can be explained by the observation that Epo A and B accumulate inside cells several-hundred fold over external medium concentrations.[18,41,53] It also reflects the fact that growth inhibition by epothilones (and also other MSA) is a consequence of the suppression of microtubule dynamics rather than a shift in the equilibrium between soluble and polymerized tubulin towards the polymeric state.[6,54]

Treatment of human cancer cells with low nanomolar concentrations of Epo B produces aberrant mitotic spindles, results in cell cycle arrest in mitosis, and eventually leads to apoptotic cell death.[4,16] IC_{50}s for cancer cell growth inhibition are in the nanomolar or even sub-nanomolar range, depending on the specific cell type,[4,16,18] In addition, apoptosis induction by Epo B has been suggested to involve the formation of reactive oxygen species in mitochondria;[55] it has also been linked to the activation of the nuclear translocation of the transcription factor NFκB in a process that would be independent of the microtubule effects of the compound.[56] The true significance of these findings for the antitumor activity of Epo B still needs to be established.

Epo A/B, in contrast to taxol and other standard cytotoxic anticancer agents, are largely insensitive to phosphoglycoprotein-170 (Pgp)-mediated drug efflux *in vitro* in cellular systems,[4,16,18,50] and also in tumor models (*vide infra*). However, resistance to epothilones can arise through tubulin mutations that either affect ligand binding affinity or lead to hypostable microcutubules.[41,57,58] Similar observations have been reported for taxol and other MSA, but the clinical significance of this resistance mechanism has not been established.

Early experiments with Epo B at the Sloan-Kettering Cancer Center had suggested that the compound was too toxic to be a clinically useful anticancer agent.[59] In contrast, subsequent studies by the Novartis group clearly demonstrated potent antitumor activity in a number of human tumor models in mice[18,21,60,61] and also in syngeneic rat models.[21] Therapeutic effects were manifest either as profound tumor growth inhibition (*i.e.* stable disease) or significant tumor regression. In particular, regressions were observed in a HCT-15 colon carcinoma[21,61] and a KB-8511 cervix carcinoma[18,21] model, which are either poorly responsive or completely non-responsive to treatment with Taxol®. While Epo B treatment was accompanied by body weight loss, these effects were reversible and tumor growth inhibition could generally be achieved at tolerated dose levels. Low doses of Epo B have also been shown to have protracted effects on endothelial cell proliferation *in vitro*[62] and in tumor explants.[63] *In vivo*, Epo B has been found to induce vascular disruption in syngeneic tumors in rats.[64] Clinical trials with Epo B (patupilone) have recently been reviewed.[65]

3.3 Epothilone Analogs in Clinical Development and Related Structures

3.3.1 Side Chain-Modified Analogs

3.3.1.1 Sagopilone

Out of 350 epothilone analogs produced at Schering AG (now Bayer) by total synthesis up to 2006, the side chain-modified analog sagopilone (also known as ZK-EPO, 3; Figure 3.2) was chosen as a clinical candidate, since it combined high activity and efficacy with fast and efficient cellular uptake and

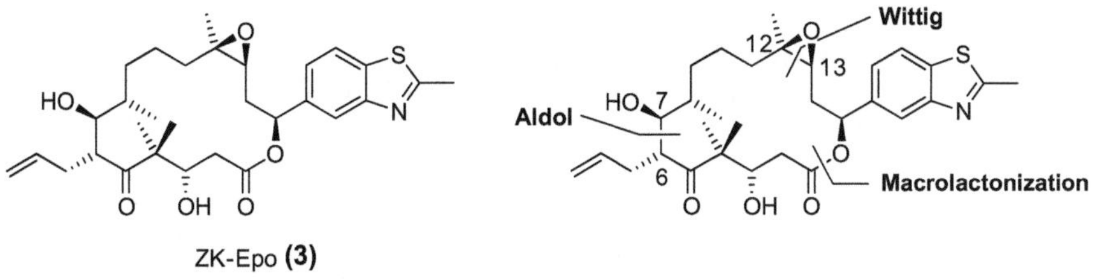

Figure 3.2 Structure of sagopilone (3) (left) and key retrosynthetic disconnections (right).

was not recognized by drug efflux pumps.[66,67] In comparison with natural Epo B, sagopilone (3) features a benzothiazole-derived side chain and an allyl substituent at position 6; the former type of modification has independently been investigated by the group at Novartis/ETH Zürich (*vide infra*).

Key steps in the synthesis of sagopilone (3) are a non-selective Wittig reaction (E/Z ratio of 1/1) between methyl ketone 4 and phosphonium salt 5 to install the double bond at C12–C13, a stereoselective aldol reaction between α-chiral aldehyde 6 and ketone 7 to establish the stereocenters at C6 and C7, and the macrolactonization of seco acid 9 (Figure 3.2, Scheme 3.1), to produce the fully protected macrolactone core structure.[66,67]

Overall, the synthesis of sagopilone (3) comprises 39 steps with the longest linear sequence being 22 steps. The synthesis depicted in Scheme 3.1 has been scaled up (with some modifications)[68] to deliver API (active pharmaceutical ingredient) for clinical studies. Sagopilone (3) exhibits highly potent antiproliferative activity with IC_{50} values of ≤ 1 nM against more than 100 cancer cell lines.[69] Against drug-sensitive cell lines sagopilone (3) is equipotent to, or even more potent than Epo B; it retains full activity against

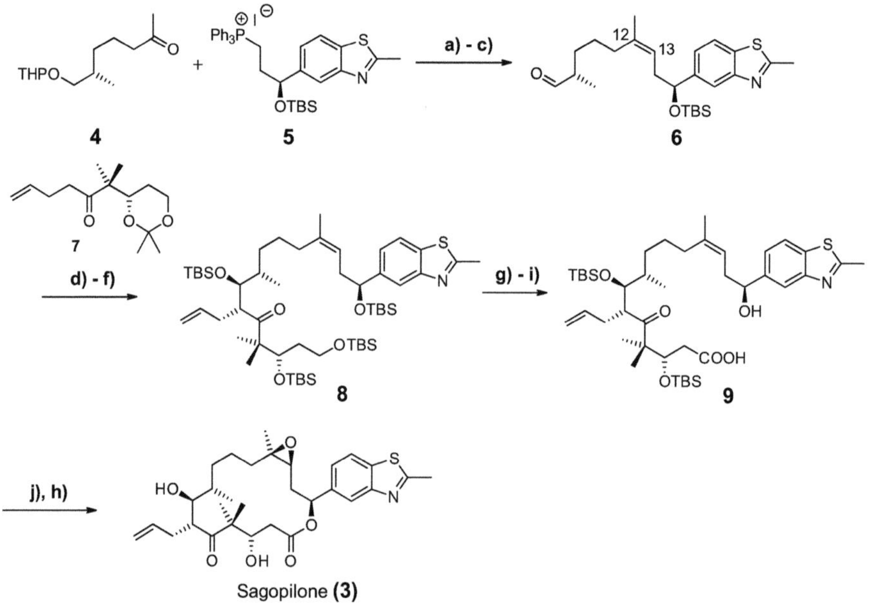

Sagopilone (3)

Scheme 3.1 (a) NaHMDS, THF, 0 °C→RT, 83% (1 : 1 mixture of Z and E isomers). (b) p-TsOH (cat.), EtOH, RT, 43% (86% for mixture of Z and E isomers). (c) (COCl)$_2$, DMSO, CH$_2$Cl$_2$, −78 °C; then Et$_3$N, −78 °C → 0 °C, crude. (d) 7, LDA, ZnCl$_2$, THF, −70 °C, then 6, THF, −70 °C, 64%. (e) p-TsOH (cat.), EtOH, RT, 97%. (f) TBSOTf, 2,6-lutidine, CH$_2$Cl$_2$, −70 °C → 0 °C, 96%. (g) CSA, CH$_2$Cl$_2$, MeOH, RT, 80%. (h) (1) (COCl)$_2$, DMSO, CH$_2$Cl$_2$, −78 °C; then Et$_3$N, −78 → 0 °C, crude; (2) NaOCl$_2$, NaH$_2$PO$_4$, 2-methyl-2-butene, THF, H$_2$O, tBuOH, 0 °C → 15 °C, 85 %. (i) (1) TBAF, THF, RT, crude; (2) 2,4,6-Cl$_3$C$_6$H$_2$C(O)Cl, Et$_3$N, THF, 0 °C, 60%. (j) HF · py, hexafluorosilicic acid, THF, RT, 87%. (h) DMDO, acetone/CH$_2$Cl$_2$, −78 °C, 71% + 10% β-epoxide. DMDO = 3,3-dimethyldioxirane.

multidrug-resistant cell lines, while the activity of Epo B is somewhat compromised in some cell lines and the activity of ixabepilone is significantly reduced.[70] This finding indicates that in contrast to taxol or other epothilones, sagopilone (3) is completely unrecognized by the Pgp-efflux pump. This is further supported by the fact that intracellular levels of the compound in multidrug-resistant cells are not affected by verapamil, a Pgp-inhibitor, while substantially different intracellular concentrations of taxol were observed in the presence or absence of the Pgp-blocker.[69] The potent *in vitro* activity of sagopilone (3) translates into high *in vivo* efficacy in human xenograft models in mice across different types of cancers, including models of breast, lung, ovarian, prostate, and pancreatic cancer and also models with resistance to taxol, in the absence of profound body weight loss (after iv administration of a single dose of 4–8 mg kg^{-1}).[71,72] In addition, sagopilone (3) crosses the blood – brain barrier and accumulates in brain tissue in both rats and mice, while taxol levels were below the limit of detection. As a result, sagopilone (3) showed significant growth inhibition of human glioblastoma in orthotopic mouse models, whereas taxol only displayed limited activity.[73] Sagopilone (3) could therefore be an attractive candidate for the treatment of brain metastases. Based on these promising preclinical results, sagopilone (3) entered clinical studies in 2003. These trials showed that the compound was well tolerated (for a cytotoxic drug), with peripheral neuropathy as the principal dose-limiting toxicity (DLT).[74–76] In 2008 sagopilone (3) entered Phase II clinical trials for the treatment of different cancers, such as platinum-resistant[77] and recurrent platinum sensitive ovarian cancer (in combination with carboplatin)[78] or androgen-independent prostate cancer (in combination with prednisone).[79] In the ovarian trial the primary efficacy end point was met (29 responders out of a total of 45 patients), while toxicities where manageable.[78] A PSA (prostate-specific antigen) response of 37% was observed in the prostate trial, but in the presence of significant neuropathy; the study would have been considered positive for a PSA response of 43%.[79] Phase II studies were also conducted in patients with non-small cell lung cancer (NSCLC)[80] or melanoma.[81] In contrast to other epothilones, sagopilone (3) was found to be active against melanoma even in pretreated patients with an objective response rate of 11.4% (one confirmed complete response, two confirmed partial responses, and one unconfirmed partial response). Only mild haematological toxicity and sensory neuropathy were observed in the melanoma trial.[81] In spite of these promising Phase II data, however, no further clinical development of the compound has been reported for several years, and it appears that the clinical development of sagopilone (3) has been discontinued.

3.3.1.2 ABJ879

A broad-based collaboration between the Nicolaou group at the Scripps Research Institute (TSRI) and the group at Novartis between 1996 and 2000 resulted in the identification of C20-desmethyl-C20-methylsulfanyl-Epo B (ABJ879, **10**; Figure 3.3) as a promising antitumor agent.[82] While Nicolaou

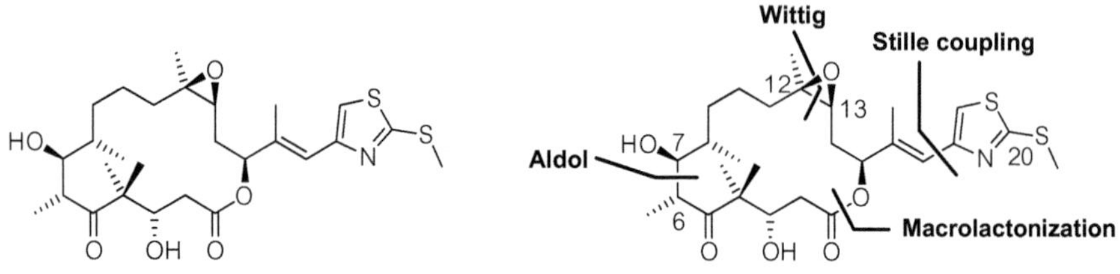

Figure 3.3   Structure of ABJ879 (**10**) (left) and key retrosynthetic disconnections (right).

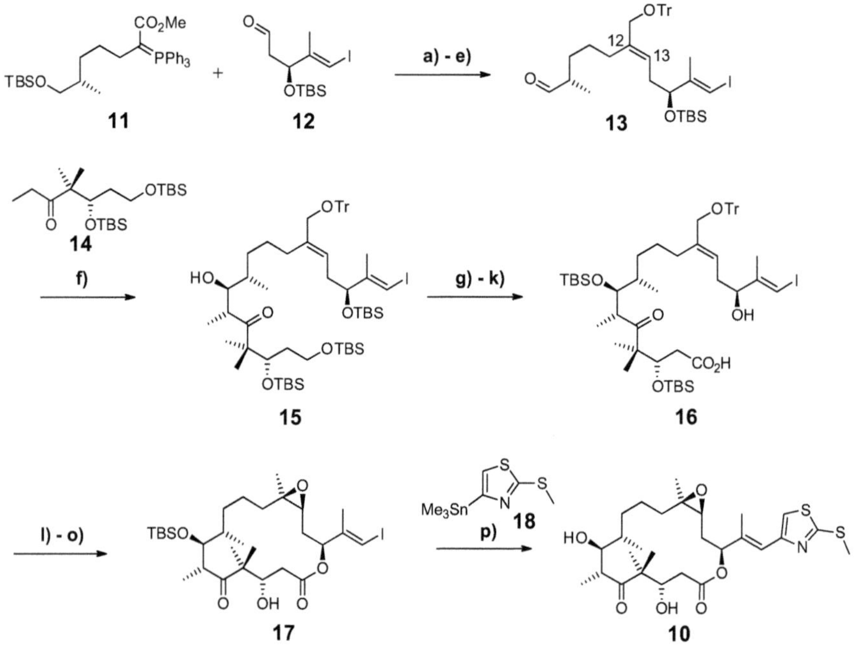

Scheme 3.2   (a) benzene, reflux, 92%. (b) DIBAL-H, THF, −78 °C, 71%. (c) TrCl, 4-DMAP, DMF, 80 °C, 94%. (d) HF · py, py/THF, 0 °C, 67%. (e) SO₃ · py, Et₃N, DMSO/CH₂Cl₂, 0 °C, 98%. (f) **14**, LDA, THF, −78 °C → -40 °C, then **13**, THF, −78 °C, then AcOH, −78 °C → 0 °C, 74%, dr 15:1. (g) TBSOTf, 2,6-lutidine, CH₂Cl₂, −20 °C → 0 °C. (h) HF · py, py/THF, 0 °C, 86%. (i) (COCl)₂, DMSO; then Et₃N, CH₂Cl₂, −78 °C → 0 °C, 98%. (j) NaOCl₂, NaH₂PO₄, 2-methyl-2-butene, THF, H₂O, *t*BuOH, RT, 100%. (k) TBAF, THF, 0 °C → RT, 95%. (l) 2,4,6-Cl₃C₆H₂C(O)Cl, Et₃N, THF, 0 °C, then DMAP in toluene, 0 °C → 75 °C, 84%. (m) HF · py, THF, 0 °C → RT, 86%. (n) (1) TsCl, Et₃N, 4-DMAP, CH₂Cl₂, 0 °C → RT. (2) NaI, aceteone, RT, 75%. (o) NaBH₃CN, DMPU, 45 °C, 70%. (p) Pd(dba)₂ · CHCl₃, CuI, AsPh₃, DMF, RT, 72%. DMPU = 1,3-dimethyl-3,4,5,6-tetrahydro-2(*1H*)-pyrimidinone.

eventually developed a *de novo* chemical synthesis of the compound, all profiling experiments and the Phase I clinical trials were performed with material obtained at Novartis by an undisclosed semisynthetic route from Epo B.

Key steps (Figure 3.3, Scheme 3.2) in the Nicolaou synthesis of ABJ879 (**10**) are the formation of the C12–C13 double bond *via* a selective Wittig reaction between phosphorane **11** and aldehyde **12**, the stereoselective aldol reaction of α-chiral aldehyde **13** and ketone **14**, macrolactonization of seco acid **16**, stereoselective Sharpless epoxidation, to afford the C12–C13 epoxide, and introduction of the heterocycle by means of Stille coupling.[82]

ABJ879 (**10**) was found to induce tubulin polymerization *in vitro* slightly more potently than Epo B, but proved to be a markedly more potent antiproliferative agent. The average IC_{50} value for growth inhibition across a panel of drug-sensitive human cancer cells lines was 0.09 nM.[83] Interestingly, the compound retained full activity against cancer cells overexpressing the drug efflux pump Pgp or harboring tubulin mutations. ABJ879 (**10**) was demonstrated to be a potent antitumor agent in experimental human xenograft models, where it produced transient regressions and inhibition of tumor growth in slow-growing NCI H-596 lung adenocarcinoma tumors and HT-29 colon tumors. In addition, inhibition of tumor growth in fast-growing, difficult to treat NCI H-460 large cell lung tumors was observed. A single dose administration of ABJ879 (**10**) induced long-lasting regressions and cures in Taxol®-resistant KB-8511 epidermoid carcinomas.[83] Based on these promising preclinical results, ABJ879 (**10**) entered Phase I clinical trials sponsored by Novartis in 2004. No clinical development has been reported since and no clinical data have ever been disclosed for the compound.

3.3.1.3   BMS-310705

C21-Amino Epo B (BMS-310705 (**19**); Figure 3.4) is a water soluble semisynthetic analog of Epo B with an *in vivo* antitumor and toxicity profile similar to that of ixabepilone (*vide infra*).[84]

The semisynthesis of BMS-310705 (**19**) in the first step involves conversion of Epo B into *N*-oxide **20** by oxidation with *m*-chloroperbenzoic acid. Treatment of **20** with trifluoroacetic acid (TFA) anhydride triggered a Polonovsky-type rearrangement that transposes the oxygen of the *N*-oxide moiety to C21 to give hydroxymethyl derivative **21**,[40,85] which is also naturally occurring

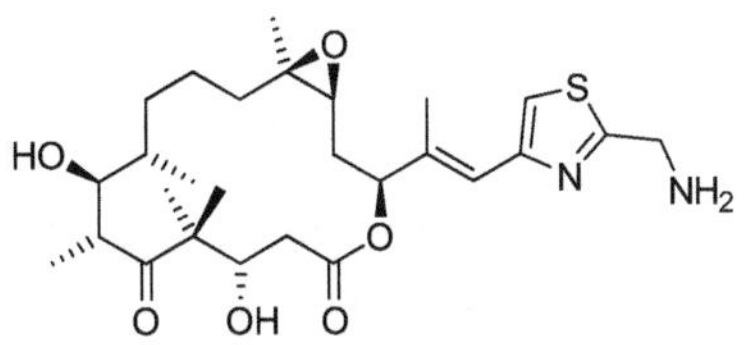

BMS-310705 (**19**)

Figure 3.4   Structure of BMS-310705 (**19**).

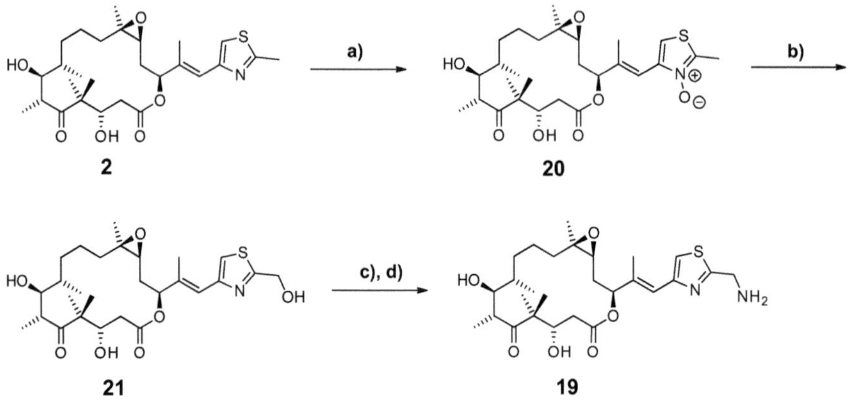

Scheme 3.3 (a) *m*-CPBA, CH$_2$Cl$_2$, RT, 48%. (b) 2,6-lutidine, TFA anhydride, CH$_2$Cl$_2$, 75 °C, then liquid NH$_3$, THF, 45 °C, 78%. (c) DPPA, DBU, THF, 94%. (d) P(CH$_3$)$_3$, THF/H$_2$O, RT, 91%. DPPA = diphenylphosphoryl azide.

and has been named epothilone F. Treatment of alcohol **21** with diphenyl-phosphoryl azide yielded an azide that was reduced under Staudinger conditions to afford amine BMS-310705 (**19**) (Scheme 3.3).[40,86]

Only limited preclinical data have been disclosed for BMS-310705 (**19**). In a patent application an IC$_{50}$ value of 0.8 nM for growth inhibition of the human cervix cancer cell line KB-31 has been reported[87] versus 1.2 nM for Epo B under comparable experimental conditions.[85] The compound was demonstrated to induce significant apoptosis in taxol- and platinum-refractive OC-2 ovarian cancer cells.[88] Activities of BMS-310705 (**19**) in human tumor xenograft models in mice were superior to those of taxol or Epo B.[89] Its improved water solubility enables the use of formulations not containing Cremophor-EL,[40] suggesting potential for development of BMS-310705 (**19**) as an oral anticancer drug.[88] The toxicity profile of the compound in humans appeared to be comparable to that of ixabepilone (*vide infra*), with diarrhoea, vomiting, and neutropenia as the dose limiting toxicities.[90] Two different dosing schedules were evaluated in Phase I studies and responses were documented for both, including partial responses in patients with breast, stomach, and ovarian cancer. A complete response was reported in a patient with non-small cell lung cancer.[40,91] No clinical development for BMS-310705 (**19**) has been reported for several years.

3.3.1.4   Other Potent Side Chain-Modified Analogs

In addition to the examples discussed above, many other potent side chain-modified epothilone analogs have been reported in the literature. Major advances in this area have resulted from the collaborative work between the Nicolaou group at the TSRI and the group at Novartis. For example, these groups discovered that pyridine-based analog **22** (Figure 3.5) is equipotent

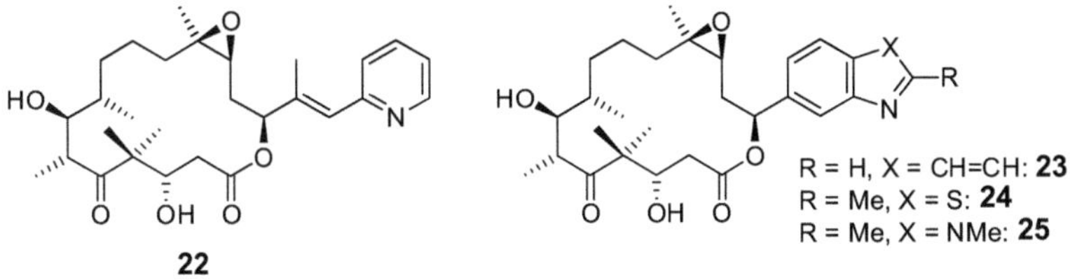

Figure 3.5 Epo B analogs with fused heterocyclic side chains.

with Epo B, thus demonstrating that the presence of a five-membered heterocycle is not required in order to maintain high biological activity.[92] In addition, it was shown that Epo B-like activity in pyridyl-epothilones is only observed if the ring N-atom is located adjacent to the attachment point of the linker connecting the pyridine ring and the macrocycle.

An intriguing class of side chain-modified epothilone analogs incorporating a fused phenyl moiety as a linker element between the heterocycle and the macrolactone core (in place of a trisubstituted double bond) (Figure 3.5), was developed independently by the groups at Schering (see above for the structure of sagopilone (**3**)) and Novartis/ETH Zürich. Analogs of this type, exemplified by quinoline **23**, benzothiazole **24** and benzimidazole **25**, consistently display enhanced *in vitro* activity over the corresponding parent epothilones, with the effect being particularly pronounced in the Epo D series.[93]

An epothilone analog with an isoxazole-bearing side chain has recently entered Phase I clinical trials; this compound (iso-fludelone (**52**)) will be discussed in Section 3.3.3.3.

3.3.2 Epoxide Modifications

3.3.2.1 KOS-862

Since the discovery of the epothilones a substantial amount of synthetic work has been expended on the modification of the epoxide moiety. These efforts were largely driven by the desire to elucidate the structural parameters that are essential to maintain biological activity; and the first structures to be investigated in this context were those that were intermediates in the total synthesis of Epo A or B. In particular, the natural product Epo D (deoxy-Epo B; KOS-862, **26**, Figure 3.6), the substrate for the final epoxidation step in the synthesis of Epo B, emerged as an important variant from early SAR studies. Scheme 3.4 summarizes Danishefsky's second generation synthesis of Epo D (**26**) that was developed in the context of extensive preclinical profiling of the compound.[101,102] (For the first generation Danishefsky approach to Epo B see ref. 94–96. For other early syntheses of Epo D see ref. 97–100).

In this improved synthesis of Epo D (**26**) the critical C6/C7 stereodiad was established by an aldol addition of ethyl ketone **27** to aldehyde **28**, which

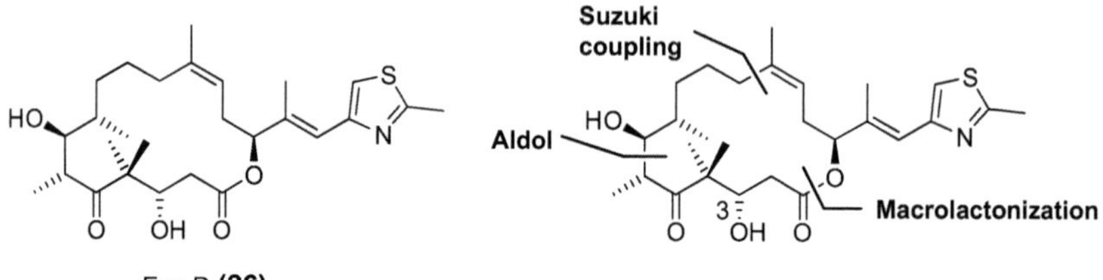

Figure 3.6   Structure of Epo D **26** (left) and key retrosynthetic disconnections (right).

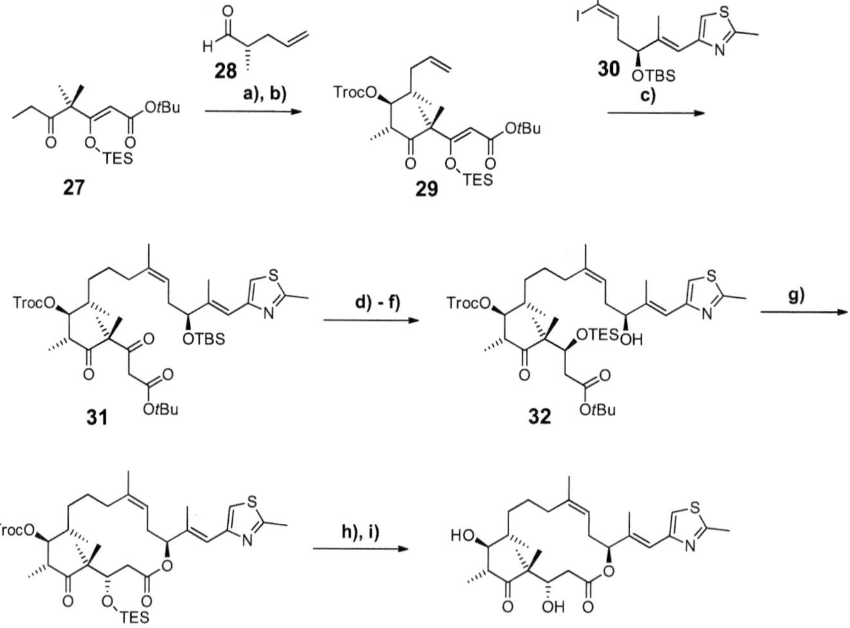

Scheme 3.4   (a) **27**, LDA, THF, −30 °C → −120 °C, then **28**, 60%, dr 5.5:1.
(b) TrocCl, pyridine, CH$_2$Cl$_2$, 0 °C → RT, then 0.5 N HCl in MeOH,
0 °C, 87%. (c) 9-BBN, THF, then **30**, [Pd(dppf)Cl$_2$], Ph$_3$As, Cs$_2$CO$_3$, H$_2$O,
DMF. (d) 0.4 N HCl in MeOH, RT, 50% (over two steps). (e) [(R)-
(binap)RuCl2], H$_2$ (83 bar), MeOH, HCl, RT, 88%, dr 95:5. (f) TESOTf,
2,6-lutidine, CH$_2$Cl$_2$, −78 °C → RT, then HCl/MeOH, 77%. (g) 2,4,6-
trichlorobenzoyl chloride, TEA, DMAP, toluene, RT, 78%. h) SmI$_2$, cat.
NiI$_2$, THF, −78 °C, 95%. i) HF-pyridine, THF, RT, 98%. LDA = lithium
diisopropylamide,   9-BBN = 9-borabicyclo[3.3.1]nonane,   dppf = 1,1′-
bis(diphenylphosphanyl)ferrocene,   binap = 2,2′-bis(diphenylphosphanyl)-1,1′-binaphtyl.

gave the desired aldol product with *ca.* 5.5:1 selectivity. Protection of the
secondary hydroxy group provided terminal olefin **29** which subsequently
underwent Suzuki coupling with vinyl iodide **30** to form the C12−C13 *Z*-
double bond selectively. A highly selective Noyori reduction of the C3-keto

group in **31** then produced the stereocenter at C3. In terms of the overall process optimization, efficient synthetic routes for the individual building blocks **27**, **28**, and **30** were elaborated. Obviously, this approach also provided improved access to Epo B.

The biological activity of Epo D (**26**) is somewhat lower than that of the epoxide-containing congeners, but the compound still is a highly potent antiproliferative agent;[96,103–106] it induces tubulin polymerization with the same potency as Epo B, it inhibits tumor cell growth with low nM IC$_{50}$s, and, like Epo B, it retains full activity against Pgp-overexpressing multidrug-resistant cells. The Sloan-Kettering group showed that the *in vitro* activity of Epo D is mirrored by potent *in vivo* efficacy and that the compound potently inhibits the growth of different types of solid tumors in mouse models of human cancer.[59,107] Epo D (**26**) has been investigated in a number of Phase I and Phase II clinical studies.[108,109] However, the clinical development of the compound in cancer has been discontinued, in spite of purportedly encouraging Phase II data.[110] As indicated in the Introduction, Epo D (**26**) (as BMS-241027) is currently undergoing Phase I clinical trials in Alzheimer disease patients.[33] (For the link between insufficient microtubule stability and Alzheimer's disease see ref. 32.)

3.3.2.2   Conjugation with Folic Acid

Receptor-specific targeting is an approach that enables selective delivery of cytotoxic drugs to cancer cells, thereby avoiding the collateral damage that accompanies their uptake by normal cells. The folate receptor is a cell surface glycoprotein that is expressed in relatively high levels in human epithelial cancers, but has limited expression in normal tissue.[111,112] It binds folic acid and conjugates tightly (folic acid $K_d = 10^{-9}$ M).[112] Upon binding the folic acid is internalized by endocytosis; therefore, conjugation of an antiproliferative agent to folic acid is a promising strategy to target drugs to tumors. Data from studies with cytotoxic folic acid conjugates in cell lines and tumor models are consistent with the selective targeting of cells overexpressing the folate receptor;[113,114] at the same time, it has been demonstrated repeatedly in a vast number of cases that conjugation of drugs to folic acid does not significantly affect folate receptor binding and receptor-mediated endocytosis.[115] Consequently, folic acid can be used for the targeted delivery of biologically active compounds. The Epo A analog-folic acid conjugate BMS-753493 (**34**) (Figure 3.7) resulted from a collaboration between Endocyte, Inc. and Bristol Myers Squibb.[116] The active drug entity is an *N*-hydroxyethyl aziridine analog of Epo A to which folic acid is attached through a disulfide cleavable self-immolative linker system. Based on previous fluorescence resonance energy transfer studies on other folate conjugates, the release of the drug upon reduction of the disulfide bond takes place within the endosomes of cancer cells.[117] The released *N*-hydroxyethyl-12α,13α-aziridinyl analog of Epo A inhibits the growth of human cancer cells about as efficiently as Epo B.[118]

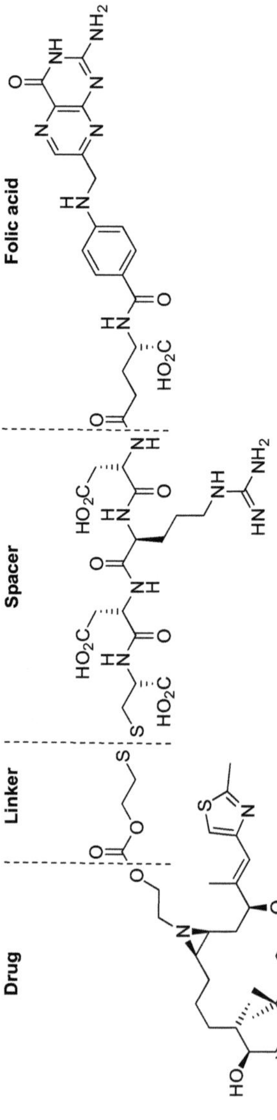

Figure 3.7   Structure of the epothilone-folate conjugate BMS-753493 (**34**).

The synthesis of 12α,13α-aziridinyl Epo A was based on the highly regio-selective opening of the epoxide ring in Epo A (**1**) with $MgBr_2 \cdot OEt_2$, subsequent inversion of the stereochemistry at the C12-position under Mitsunobu conditions and final *in situ* cyclization to afford the bis-TES-protected 12α,13α-azirdinyl Epo A derivative **37** (Scheme 3.5).[119] Treatment of **37** with 2-bromoethanol and deprotection resulted in *N*-hydroxyethyl-12α,13α-aziridinyl-Epo A (**38**).[25] This primary alcohol **38** was then reacted with activated carbonate **39** and the resulting disulfide underwent subsequent disulfide exchange to give the Epo A-folic acid conjugate BMS-753493 (**34**).[25]

BMS-753493 (**34**) showed potent cytotoxicity against folate receptor-positive human tumor cells *in vitro*. In the presence of an excess of folic acid the cells were no longer susceptible to the compound; likewise, BMS-753493 (**34**) was inactive against folate receptor negative cells. The conjugate showed antitumor activity *in vivo* in several different folate receptor positive tumor models. Furthermore, BMS-753493 (**34**) demonstrated excellent activity in

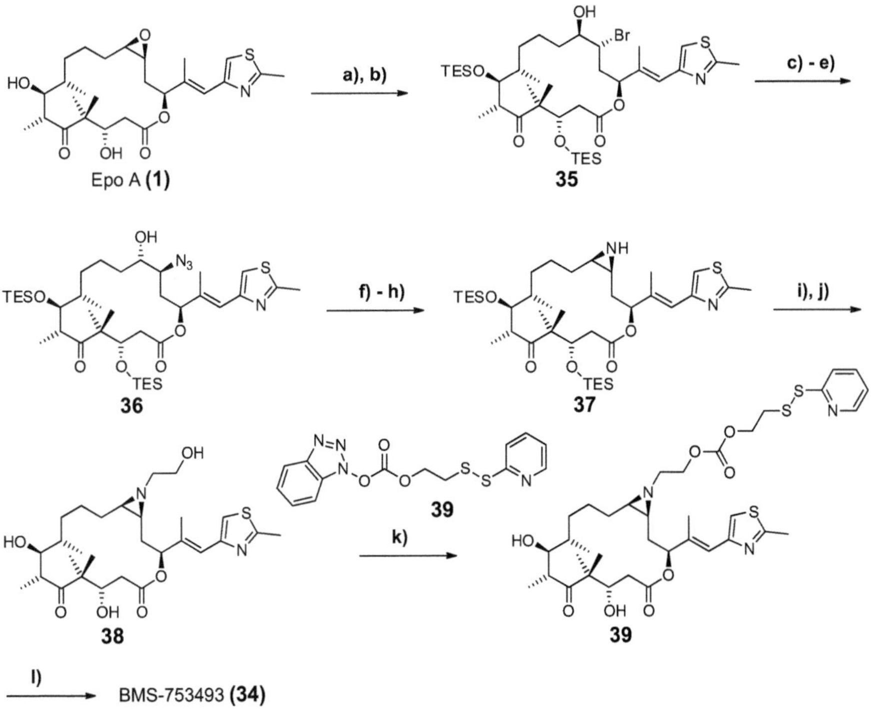

Scheme 3.5 (a) TESCl, DIPEA, DMF, RT, 90%. (b) $MgBr \cdot Et_2O$, CH_2Cl_2, $-20\,°C \rightarrow -5\,°C$, 45%, regioselectivity 20:1. (c) NaN_3, DMF, 42 °C, 60%. (d) *p*-NBA- DEAD, Ph_3P, RT, 99%. (e) NH_3, MeOH, RT, 88%. (f) Ph_3P, THF/H_2O, 45 °C, 85%. (g) MsCl, Et_3N, CH_2Cl_2, RT, 98%. (h) Me_3P, THF/H_2O, RT, 98%. (i) 2-bromoethanol, K_2CO_3, MeCN, 80 °C. (j) TFA/CH_2Cl_2, RT. (k) **39**, DMAP, CH_2Cl_2, RT. (l) thiol, H_2O, THF, RT. *p*-NBA = para-nitrobenzoic acid, DEAD = diethylazodicarboxylate.

combination with other chemotherapeutic agents. In analogy to the *in vitro* experiments, the antitumor activity of the conjugate was strongly reduced if an excess of folate was co-administered. These data strongly suggest that the activity of the conjugate is mainly mediated *via* the folate receptor.[116] BMS-753493 (**34**) was advanced to Phase I clinical trials, but does not seem to be under active development at this time.

3.3.3   9,10-Dehydroepothilones

3.3.3.1   KOS-1584

As first demonstrated by the Danishefsky group, the incorporation of an *E*-configured double bond between C9 and C10 in Epo D results in a significant increase in antiproliferative activity (KOS-1584 (**40**), Figure 3.8),[120,121] while the corresponding *Z*-isomer was markedly less active.[121] In earlier work, the latter had been thought to be the *E*-isomer **40**, but was later found to be (*Z*)-9,10-dehydroepothilone D.[122,123] This finding was in agreement with spectroscopic studies, which indicated that the bioactive conformation of epothilones is characterized by *anti*-periplanar conformations about the C9/C10 and C10/C11 bonds, respectively.[124] Based on its overall profile KOS-1584 (**40**) emerged as a very promising candidate for drug development and entered clinical trials.

The Danishefsky synthesis of KOS-1584 (**40**) made use of an aldol addition of ethyl ketone **41** to aldehyde **42**, giving the desired diastereomer in a 5.6:1 ratio, a second aldol addition to establish the chiral center at C3, an esterification to couple acid **46** and alcohol **47** and a ring-closing metathesis (RCM) to form the macrocycle; the latter yielding the *E*-isomer **49** exclusively. Finally, the heterocycle **50** was introduced *via* Horner – Wadsworth – Emmons (HWE) olefination to afford KOS-1584 (**40**) (Scheme 3.6).[120,121] It should be noted that this approach also allows the facile attachment of non-natural heterocycles at the final stage of the synthesis, a feature that was exploited by the Danishefsky group later in the synthesis of iso-fludelone (see Section 3.3.3.3).

In cell culture, the fully synthetic epothilone KOS-1584 (**40**) showed strong inhibitory activity against various drug-sensitive and MDR cancer cell lines. For example, the IC_{50} value of KOS-1584 (**40**) against the human leukaemia

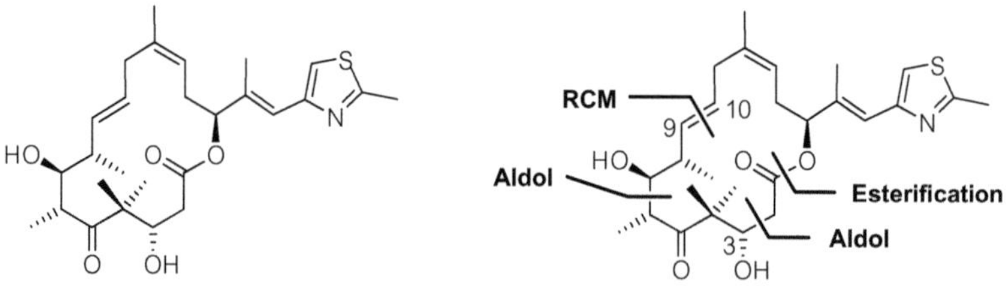

KOS-1584 (**40**)

Figure 3.8   Structure of KOS 1584 (**40**) and key retrosynthetic disconnections (right).

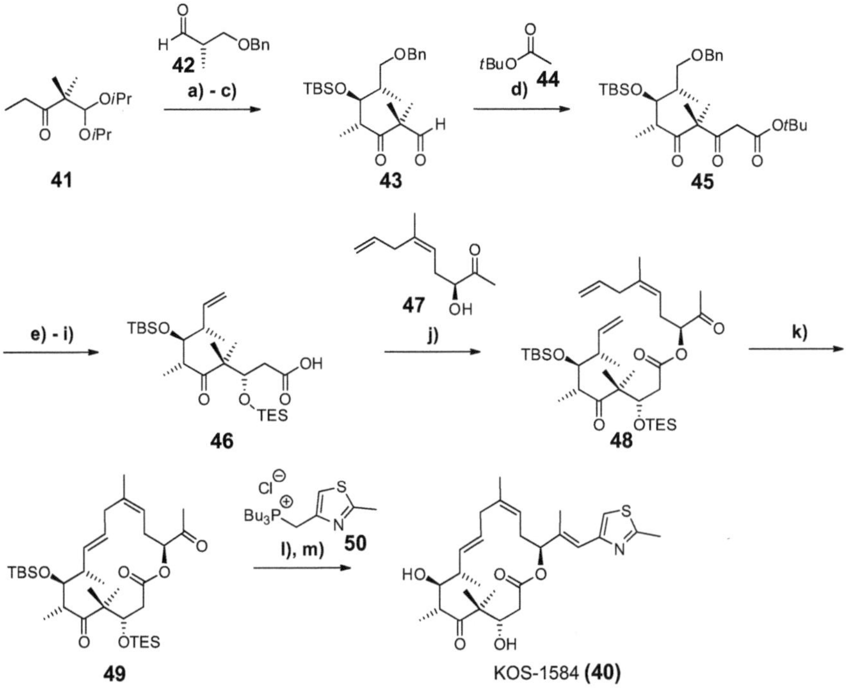

Scheme 3.6 (a) **41**, LDA, THF, −90 °C, then **42**, 78%, dr 85:15. (b) TBSOTf, 2,6-lutidine, CH$_2$Cl$_2$, −40 °C → −20 °C, 97%. (c) p-TsOH.H$_2$O (cat.), THF/H$_2$O (4:1), 64 °C, 98%. (d) **44**, LDA, cpTiCl(OR)$_2$, Et$_2$O, −78 °C, then **43**, 86%, dr 20:1. (e) TESCl, imidazole, DMF, 0 °C → RT, 98%. (f) H$_2$, Pd/C, EtOH, RT, 83%. (g) TPAP, NMO, CH$_2$Cl$_2$, RT, 95%. (h) MePPh$_3$I, n-BuLi, THF, −78 °C → −5 °C, 78%. (i) TESOTf, 2,6-lutidine, CH$_2$Cl$_2$, 0 °C → RT. (j) EDCI, DMAP, CH$_2$Cl$_2$, **47**, 0 °C → RT, 81% (over two steps). (k) Grubbs 2nd generation catalyst, toluene, 110 °C, 78%. (l) KHMDS, **50**, THF, −78 °C → −20 °C, 76%. (m) HF·pyridine, THF, RT, 97%. R = 1,2:5,6-di-O-isopropylidene-α-L-glucofuranos-3-O-yl.

cell line CCRF-CEM is 0.9 nM vs. 3.6 nM for Epo D.[120,121] Importantly, and rather surprisingly, compared to its 9,10-saturated congener the compound was found to be significantly more stable in mouse as well as human plasma.[125] The combination of cytotoxicity and plasma stability was sufficient reason for Danishefsky and co-workers to synthesize substantial amounts of KOS-1584 (**40**) to evaluate its in vivo efficacy. The compound was found to possess improved in vivo antitumor activity over Epo D (**26**) in a mouse model of human breast cancer MX-1, which was ascribed to its enhanced antiproliferative activity and, in particular, its improved plasma stability. However, along with its improved antitumor activity, the compound was also associated with significant toxicity.[125] Nevertheless, KOS-1584 (**40**) was advanced into clinical development and its safety, tolerability, and activity were evaluated in a Phase I dose escalation study.[109]

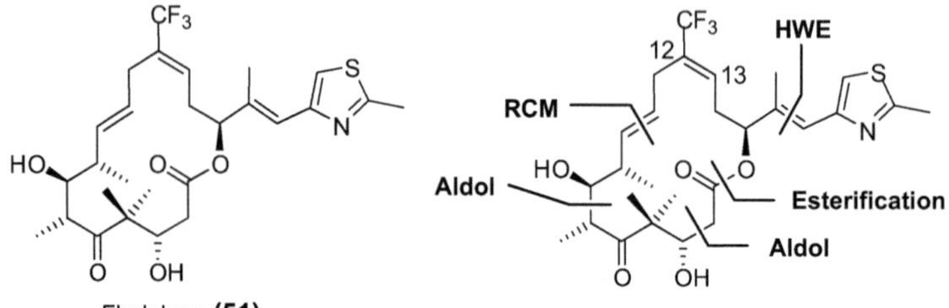

Figure 3.9   Structure of Fludelone (**51**) and key retrosynthetic disconnections (right).

3.3.3.2   *Fludelone*

In order to improve the therapeutic index of KOS-1584 (**40**), Danishefsky and co-workers explored replacing the three hydrogen atoms of the 26-methyl group with fluorine atoms. The underlying rationale for this design was that the presence of fluorine atoms would enhance the stability of the C12-C13 double bond towards oxidation, which was hypothesized to be responsible for the toxic side effects of KOS-1584 (**40**).[125,126]

The synthesis discussed above for KOS-1584 (**40**) (Scheme 3.6) could be directly applied to the desired fluorinated analog, which has been termed fludelone (**51**; Figure 3.9).[125] This compound indeed proved to be less toxic than KOS-1584 (**40**); at the same time it exhibits exquisite *in vivo* antitumor activity.[125,127,128] Treatment of nude mice bearing MX-1 human mammary carcinoma xenografts with **51** resulted in complete tumor disappearance without any relapse over several months after cessation of dosing. Strikingly, tumor remissions were achieved by both infusion and oral administration. Studies in human HCT-116 (colon), SK-OV-3 (ovary), PC-3 (prostate) and taxol-resistant CCRF-CEM (leukemia) xenografts revealed similar efficacy as in the initial MX-1 model.[128] Fludelone (**51**) proved to be superior not only over its non-fluorinated parent compound but also over taxol. The remarkable therapeutic index of fludelone (**51**) is thought to arise from a combination of cell killing activity and high plasma stability. In addition, the incorporation of the CF₃ group leads to a decrease in lipophilicity with an associated slight increase in water solubility and, hence, improved bioavailability.[128]

3.3.3.3   *Iso-Fludelone*

In an attempt to restore some of the potency that had been lost in the transition from KOS-1584 (**40**) to fludelone (**51**), the Danishefsky group designed an isoxazole-based analog of fludelone, which they named iso-fludelone (**52**, Figure 3.10).[129] This compound was also predicted to be more water-soluble than fludelone (**51**).

In fact, iso-fludelone (**52**) was found to be more potent *in vitro* than fludelone (**51**) and it is also more stable metabolically. *In vivo*, iso-fludelone (**52**) showed profound antitumor activity across a panel of different human

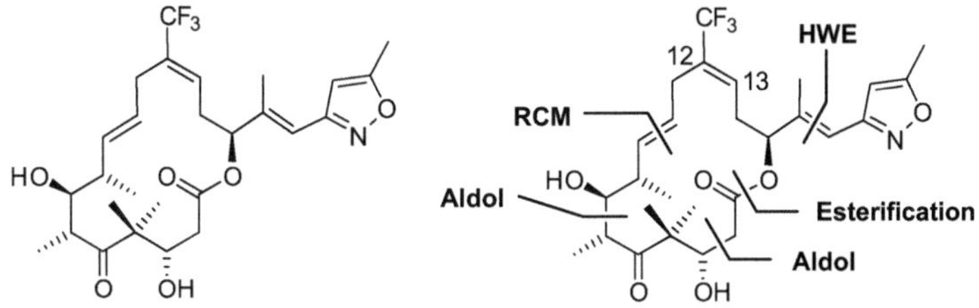

Figure 3.10 Structure of Iso-fludelone (52) and key retrosynthetic disconnections (right).

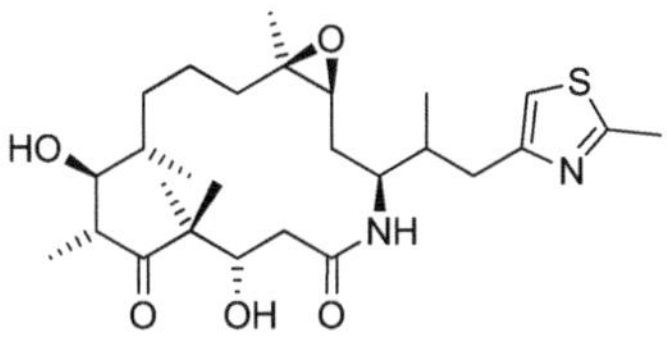

Ixabepilone (53)

Figure 3.11 Structure of Ixabepilone (53) (Ixempra®).

xenografts models, including mammary carcinoma MX-1, ovarian carcinoma SK-OV-3, and lung carcinoma A549 models; the compound was able to eradicate tumors without any sustained body weight loss.[129–131] Iso-fludelone (52) has been in Phase I clinical trials since 2011.

3.3.4 Ixabepilone

Early pharmacokinetic studies with epothilones in rodents pointed to a distinct vulnerability of the ester bond in the macrocycle to hydrolysis by (rodent) plasma esterases. Although esterase activity in rodent plasma is known to be substantially higher than in humans, these early findings also raised concerns about the metabolic stability of natural, macrolactone-based epothilones in humans. In response to these concerns the group at BMS conceived the metabolically more stable lactam analog of Epo B (53) as an alternative for future therapeutic applications.[132] This work has resulted in an efficient process for the preparation of the Epo B lactam,[132] a compound that was developed into a clinical anticancer drug and is marketed under the trade name Ixempra® (ixabepilone, 53, Figure 3.11).

Ixabepilone is produced by semisynthesis from Epo B (2) and the development of this process was critically dependent on BMS' collaboration with the Gesellschaft für Biotechnologische Forschung (now the Helmholtz Institute for Infectious Research) in Braunschweig, Germany, which provided the BMS group with an optimized Epo B producing strain of *S. cellulosum*. The semisynthesis of ixabepilone (53) exploits the allylic nature of the

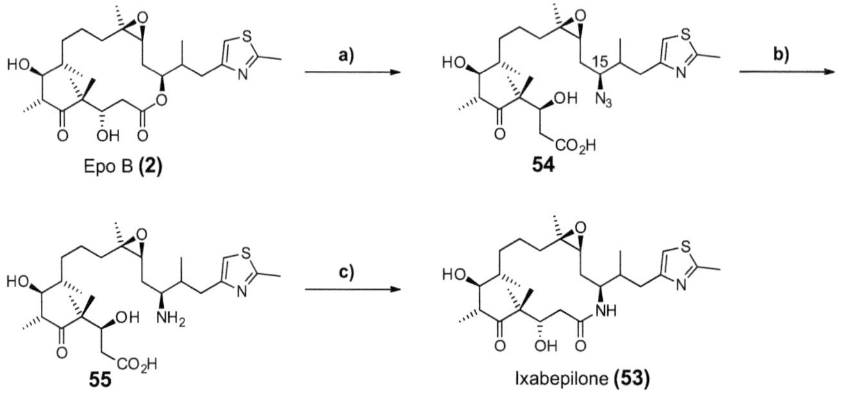

Scheme 3.7   (a) Pd(PPh$_3$)$_4$ (10 mol%), NaN$_3$, THF/H$_2$O, 45 °C, 70%. (b) PMe$_3$, THF/
H$_2$O, RT, 71%. (c) DPPA, NaHCO$_3$, DMF, 4 °C, 43% or EDCI, HOBt,
MeCN/DMF, RT 65%. DPPA = diphenylphophoryl azide.

epothilone lactone moiety, which can be opened by treatment with
Pd(PPh$_3$)$_4$; in the presence of sodium azide this leads to the formation of
azido acid **54** with complete retention of configuration at C15 (Scheme 3.7).
Subsequent reduction of the azide under Staudinger conditions followed by
macrolactamization gives ixabepilone (**53**). This semisynthetic route was
optimized into a one pot procedure, which yields ixabepilone in a single day
in 23% yield.[132] A full synthetic route to **53** has been reported by Danishefsky
and *co*-workers.[133]

Ixabepilone is a potent inducer of tubulin polymerization and exhibits
potent antiproliferative activity that is, however, about one order of magnitude lower than that of Epo B.[41] For example, IC$_{50}$ values against the human
colon carcinoma cell line HCT-116 are 3.6 nM and 0.42 nM, respectively, for
53 and Epo B.[132] In contrast to Epo B, **53** is less active against Pgp-overexpressing cell lines, which indicates that the compound is at least a moderate substrate for the Pgp efflux pump.[41] *In vivo*, ixabepilone (**53**) has
demonstrated efficacy in a wide range of human xenografts models in mice
with antitumor activity similar to that of Taxol® in Taxol®-sensitive tumor
models.[132,134,135] In spite of its limited activity against highly multidrug-resistant cell lines *in vitro*, ixabepilone (**53**) was shown to be superior to Taxol®
in Taxol®-resistant tumor models, demonstrating significant antitumor activity in HCT116/VM46 colon carcinoma, Pat-21 human breast carcinoma,
Pat-7 ovarian carcinoma, Pat-26 human pancreatic carcinoma and M5076
murine sarcoma models.[134] In addition, the compound has shown stronger
synergy with bevacizumab and sunitinib than Taxol®, especially in GEO and
HCT116/VM46 xenografts.[136]

Early clinical studies with ixabepilone (**53**) have been reviewed by Lin
et al.[137] and Pivot *et al.*[138] Objective responses to single-agent treatment were
observed in Phase I studies with the major DLT being neutropenia.[139] The
most comprehensive clinical evaluation of the compound was carried out in

metastatic breast cancer[140] in a multinational Phase III trial with 752 patients that had been anthracycline-pretreated and met pre-defined resistance criteria to taxanes.[27] These patients were randomly assigned to ixabepilone (40 mg per m² *iv* over three hours every three weeks) in combination with capecitabine (1000 mg per m² po bid q14d) and compared with capecitabine (1250 mg per m² po bid q14d) alone. The study demonstrated that the combination of ixabepilone and capecitabine was superior with "significant benefit being consistently maintained across predefined subgroups, including HER2-/ER-/PR- and HER2+."[141] As a result of that study ixabepilone (53) was approved by the FDA in 2007 for the treatment of metastatic or advanced breast cancer, either as single agent or in combination with capecitabine.[142]

3.4 Structural Studies and Pharmacophore Modeling

In spite of the longstanding clinical use of several MSA, the exact molecular interactions between any of these compounds (including those that are not used clinically) and their target protein, β-tubulin (or, perhaps, α-tubulin in the case of laulimalide and peloruside A),[143,144] had not been elucidated until very recently and neither had the molecular mechanisms by which they exert their microtubule-stabilizing effect. This was due to the lack of high-resolution structural information on tubulin/MSA complexes, a situation that has now changed (*vide infra*). Early attempts to develop a predictive pharmacophore model for epothilones[145–149] were based solely on the observation of a common tubulin binding site for epothilones and taxanes and tried to achieve the most appropriate alignment of common structural features between the two classes of ligands. These models then had to be re-assessed in light of the results of structural studies on the tubulin-bound conformation of Epo A, either by NMR spectroscopy on a soluble β-tubulin/Epo A complex,[124,150] or by electron crystallography (EC) of a complex between Epo A and a Zn²⁺-stabilized two-dimensional α,β-tubulin sheet (solved at 2.89 Å resolution).[52] Thus, while the EC-derived structure confirmed that taxol and Epo A indeed occupy the same binding pocket on β-tubulin, it also suggested a different binding mode for the two compounds, with different sets of hydrogen bonds and hydrophobic interactions being involved in the binding of each. Importantly, the tubulin-bound conformation of Epo A that was suggested based on the EC data is significantly different from any of the above computational models;[145–149] at the same time it also deviates significantly from the NMR structure of (soluble) tubulin-bound Epo A as determined by Carlomagno *et al.*[124] (Figure 3.12).

Attempts have been made to assess the validity of the various models by designing bridged epothilone analogs (Figure 3.13), which on the basis of the EC-derived model were anticipated to retain good activity (or even to show enhanced activity over the natural products). However, such compounds proved to be only poorly active.[152,153]

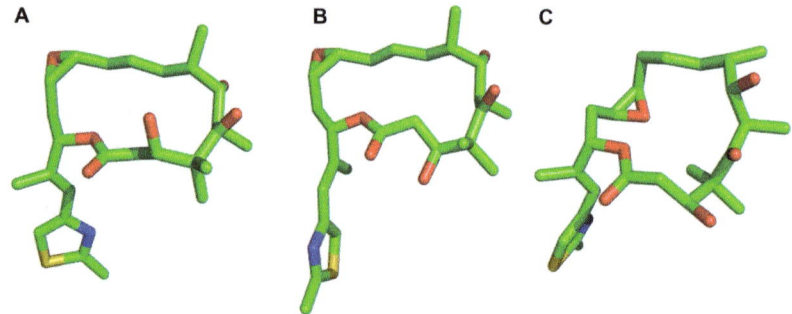

Figure 3.12   A: X-ray crystal structure of Epo A (crystals obtained from MeOH).[151] B: NMR-derived structure of tubulin-bound Epo A.[124] C: Electron crystal-lography-derived structure of tubulin-bound Epo A.[52]

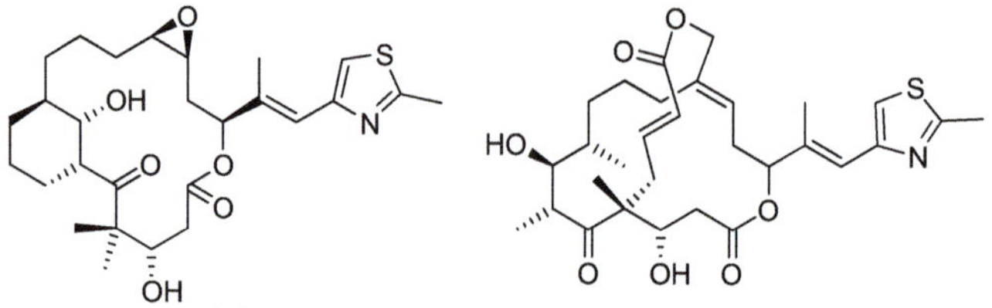

54   **55**

Figure 3.13   Structures of conformationally constrained epothilone analogs.

In addition, the EC-derived epothilone bioactive conformation is not compatible with several aspects of the SAR for this compound class, in-cluding the activity of 3-deoxy- and 3-deoxy-2,3-didehydro-epothilones. In contrast, recent NMR work by Erdélyi *et al.*[154] has shown that neither the removal of the 3-OH (3-deoxy-Epo A) group nor conformational restriction of the C2-C3 bond to a *trans* geometry (3-deoxy-2,3-didehydro-Epo A) sig-nificantly alter the overall conformation of the macrolide ring in the tubulin-bound state, relative to the NMR-derived bioactive conformation of Epo A. In a second study, they also showed that the NMR-derived tubulin-bound conformation of Epo A corresponds to a low energy conformation of the free ligand in aqueous solution.[155] Recent modeling studies by Botta and co-workers,[156] which were based on a previously developed pseudor-eceptor model for β-tubulin,[148,149] also support the validity of the NMR-derived bioactive conformation of epothilones (and, in addition, suggest the existence of a common pharmacophore between epothilones and taxol).

The question of the bioactive conformation of epothilones has also been addressed by density functional theory calculations.[157,158] One such study[157] has reached similar conclusions on the conformational preferences of the macrolactone ring as had been derived previously by Erdélyi *et al.* in their NMR work.[155]

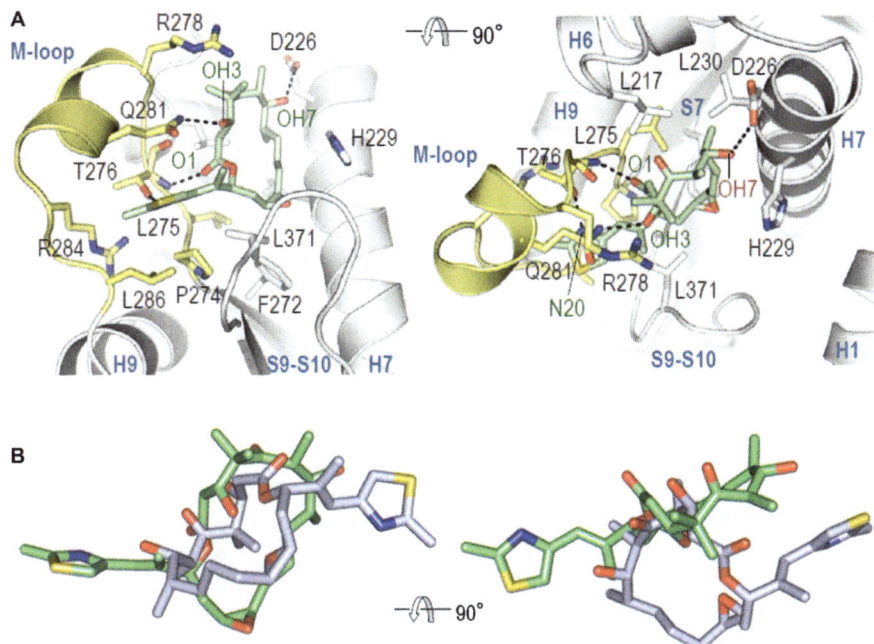

Figure 3.14 A: Structure of Epo A bound to the taxane binding pocket in β-tubulin in a T2R-TTL-Epo A complex. Interacting residues of β-tubulin are shown in stick representation. Oxygen and nitrogen atoms are colored in red and blue, respectively, carbon atoms in green (Epo A) or gray and yellow (β-tubulin). Hydrogen bonds are depicted as black dashed lines. B: Superimpostion of the structures of Epo A bound in the taxane-pocket in β-tubulin as derived by X-ray crystallography of a T2R-TTL-Epo A complex (light green) or by electron crystallography of zinc-stabilized tubulin sheets (cyan). T = tubulin; R = RB3, a microtubule binding protein; TTL = tubulin tyrosine ligase, a tubulin-processsing enzyme. Figure reproduced from ref. 159 with permission.

The most important development in the structural biology of the β-tubulin-epothilone complex is marked by the recent disclosure of a high-resolution X-ray crystal structure (at 2.6 Å) of a tetrameric protein complex between α/β-tubulin, the tubulin sequestering protein RB3 and the enzyme tubulin-tyrosine ligase with Epo A bound in the taxol site on β-tubulin.[159] The two most important conclusions derived from this structure are (1) that the orientation of the ligand in the binding site is opposite to what had been suggested by the EC data (and also the NMR work) (Figure 3.14A), but with a conformation of the ligand that is essentially identical with the NMR model of the bioactive conformation of Epo A; and (2) that ligand binding induces a partial structuring of the M-loop that may lead to enhanced inter-protofilament interactions (Figure 3.14B), which offers the first tangible molecular hypothesis on the mechanism of microtubule stabilization by epothilones (and also other MSA).[159]

3.5 Conclusions

After the discovery of their "taxol-like" mechanism of action in 1995, in combination with their activity against multidrug-resistant cells and tumors, epothilones were quickly and broadly embraced as highly attractive new lead structures for anticancer drug discovery. This has led to the synthesis and biological evaluation (including many *in vivo* studies) of hundreds of epothilone analogs and derivatives, thus establishing a comprehensive map of the structural elements associated with potent biological activity. While a number of other natural products (all of which had been known for many years prior) were recognized to be microtubule stabilizers subsequent to the crucial discovery of the epothilones' mechanism of action, epothilones (together with taxanes) today still represent the most widely explored leads for tubulin-directed anticancer drug discovery. However, only few new structures have emerged in more recent years, although interesting new analogs have still been reported (*cf.*, e.g. ref. 160).

At this point in time, nine epothilone-derived structures are known to have been advanced to clinical trials in humans; one of these, ixabepilone, has received FDA approval in 2007, which has provided final validation of the lead potential of epothilones for anticancer drug discovery. On the other hand, and with the exception of UTD1 and iso-fludelone, the development of all other candidate drugs in cancer is either uncertain (patupilone, sagopilone) or seems to have been terminated. However, Epo D is now in clinical trials for neurodegenerative diseases. Clearly, there are still numerous interesting preclinical candidates to be explored further, but it remains to be seen whether any of these will be taken into the clinic (either in cancer, or, perhaps, for neurodegenerative diseases) and, if so, whether any can be developed into a clinical drug.

References

1. G. Höfle and H. Reichenbach, *Epothilone, a myxobacterial metabolite with promising antitumor activity, in Anticancer Agents from Natural Products*, ed. G. M. Cragg, D. G. I. Kingston and D. J. Newman, Taylor & Francis, Boca Raton, FL, 2005, p. 413.
2. K. Gerth, N. Bedorf, G. Höfle, H. Irschik and H. Reichenbach, *J. Antibiot.*, 1996, **49**, 560.
3. G. Höfle, N. Bedorf, K. Gerth and H. Reichenbach, *Ger. Offen.* DE 4138042, 1993.
4. D. M. Bollag, P. A. McQueney, J. Zhu, O. Hensens, L. Koupal, J. Liesch, M. Goetz, E. Lazarides and C. M. Woods, *Cancer Res.*, 1995, **55**, 2325.
5. C. Dumontet and M. A. Jordan, *Nat. Rev. Drug Discov.*, 2010, **9**, 882.
6. M. A. Jordan and L. Wilson, *Nat. Rev. Cancer*, 2004, **4**, 253.
7. N. Agarwal, G. Sonpavde and O. Sartor, *Future Oncol.*, 2011, 7, 15.
8. K.-H. Altmann, *Curr. Opin. Chem. Biol.*, 2001, 5, 424.
9. K.-H. Altmann and J. Gertsch, *Nat. Prod. Rep.*, 2007, **24**, 327.

10. J. H. Miller, A. Jonathan Singh and P. T. Northcote, *Mar. Drugs*, 2010, **8**, 1059.

11. J. J. Field, A. J. Singh, A. Kanakkanthara, T. Halafihi, P. T. Northcote and J. Miller, *J. Med. Chem.*, 2009, **52**, 7328.

12. J. J. Field, B. Pera, E. Calvo, A. Canales, D. Zurwerra, C. Trigili, J. Rodríguez-Salarichs, R. Matesanz, A. Kanakkanthara, St. J. Wakefield, A. J. Singh, J. Jiménez-Barbero, P. Northcote, J. H. Miller, J. A. López, E. Hamel, I. Barasoain, K.-H. Altmann and J. F. Díaz, *Chem. Biol.*, 2012, **19**, 686.

13. I. H. Hardt, H. Steinmetz, K. Gerth, F. Sasse, H. Reichenbach and G. Höfle, *J. Nat. Prod.*, 2001, **64**, 847.

14. J.-D. Wang, N. Jiang, H. Zhang, L.-P. Ying, C.-X. Wang, W.-S. Xiang, B. Wu, H.-B. Wang and H. Bai, *Nat. Prod. Res.*, 2011, **25**, 1707.

15. Y.-J. Zhang, A.-W. Deng, H. Zhang, F.-Y. Xi, L.-P. Ying, J.-D. Wang and H. Bai, *J. Antibiot*, 2013, **66**, 285.

16. R. J. Kowalski, P. Giannakakou and E. Hamel, *J. Biol. Chem.*, 1997, **272**, 2534.

17. P. Giannakakou, D. L. Sackett, Y. K. Kang, Z. R. Zhan, J. T. M. Buters, T. Fojo and M. S. Poruchynsky, *J. Biol. Chem.*, 1997, **272**, 17118.

18. K.-H. Altmann, M. Wartmann and T. O'Reilly, *Biochim. Biophys. Acta, Rev. Cancer*, 2000, **1470**, M79.

19. G. H. Höfle, N. Bedorf, H. Steinmetz, D. Schomburg, K. Gerth and H. Reichenbach, *Angew. Chem. Int. Ed.*, 1996, **35**, 1567.

20. E. K. Rowinsky, *Annu. Rev. Med.*, 1997, **48**, 35.

21. T. O'Reilly, M. Wartmann, J. Brueggen, P. R. Allegrini, A. Flörsheimer, M. Maira and P. M. J. McSheehy, *Cancer Chemoth. Pharm.*, 2008, **62**, 1045.

22. For a review on clinical trials with epothilones see:H. M. Coley, *Cancer Treat. Rev.*, 2008, **34**, 378.

23. http://www.cancer.gov/clinicaltrials/search/view?cdrid=703047& version=HealthProfessional&protocolsearchid=11827469.

24. P. Zhang, M. Sun, R. Qiu, L. Tang, G. Dou and B. Xu, *Cancer Chemoth. Pharm.*, 2011, **68**, 971.

25. I. R. Vlahov, G. D. Vite, P. J. Kleindl, Y. Wang, H. K. R. Santhapuram, F. You, S. J. Howard, S-H. Kim, F. F. Y. Lee and C. P. Leamon, *Bioorg. Med. Chem. Lett.*, 2010, **20**, 4578.

26. E. Kaminskas, X. Jiang, R. Aziz, J. Bullock, R. Kasliwal, R. Harapanhalli, S. Pope, R. Sridhara, J. Leighton, B. Booth, R. Dagher, R. Justice and R. Pazdur, *Clin. Cancer Res.*, 2008, **14**, 4378.

27. For leading references on ixabepilone see: E. S. Thomas, H. L. Gomez, R. K. Li, H.-C. Chung, L. E. Fein, V. F. Chan, J. Jassem, X. B. Pivot, J. Klimovsky, F. Hurtado de Mendoza, B. Xu, M. Campone, G. L. Lerzo, R. A. Peck, P. Mukhopadhyay, L. T. Vahdat and H. H. Roche, *J. Clin. Oncol.*, 2007, **25**, 5210.

28. http://www.novartis.com/newsroom/media-releases/en/2010/1419057.shtml.

29. No publications for this compounds have appeared subsequent to the announcement of Phase I trials in a 2004 AACR meeting abstract: M. Wartmann, J. Loretan, R. Reuter, M. Hattenberger, M. Muller, J. Vaxelaire, S.-M. Maira, A. Flörsheimer, T. O'Reilly, K. C. Nicolaou and K.-H. Altmann, Proceedings of the American Association for Cancer Research, 2004, 45: Abstract 5440. The compound is no longer part of the (published) Novartis Oncology pipeline.

30. http://clinicaltrials.gov/ct2/results?intr=%22Epofolate%22.

31. BMS-310705, KOS-862, or KOS-1584 are not part of BMS' (published) development pipeline: http://www.bms.com/research/pipeline/Pages/default.aspx. While KOS-862 and KOS-1584 were initially developed by Kosan Biosciences, the company has been acquired by BMS. No active clinical trials could be identified for any of these compounds in the NCI webspace.

32. For a review see: C. Ballatore, K. R. Brunden, D. M. Huryn, J. Q. Trojanowski, V. M.-Y. Lee and A. B. Smith III, *J. Med. Chem.*, 2012, **55**, 8979.

33. http://clinicaltrials.gov/show/NCT01492374.

34. K. C. Nicolaou, F. Roschangar and D. Vourloumis, *Angew. Chem. Int. Ed.*, 1998, **37**, 2015.

35. C. R. Harris and S. J. Danishefsky, *J. Org. Chem.*, 1999, **64**, 8434.

36. K. C. Nicolaou, A. Ritzén and K. Namoto, *Chem. Commun.*, 2001, 1523.

37. J. Mulzer, *Monatsh. Chem.*, 2000, **131**, 205.

38. K.-H. Altmann, *Org. Biomol. Chem.*, 2004, **2**, 2137.

39. E. B. Watkins, A. G. Chittiboyina, J. C. Jung and M. A. Avery, *Eur. J. Org. Chem.*, 2006, **18**, 4071.

40. R. M. Borzilleri and G. D. Vite, *Drug. Future*, 2002, **27**, 1149.

41. M. Wartmann and K.-H. Altmann, *Curr. Med. Chem. Anticancer Agents*, 2002, **2**, 123.

42. K.-H. Altmann, *Mini Rev. Med. Chem.*, 2003, **3**, 149.

43. K.-H. Altmann, *Curr. Pharm. Design*, 2005, **11**, 1595.

44. K.-H. Altmann, B. Pfeiffer, S. Arseniyadis, B. A. Pratt and K. C. Nicolaou, *ChemMedChem*, 2007, **2**, 397.

45. R. Altaha, T. Fojo, E. Reed and J. Abraham, *Curr. Pharm. Design*, 2002, **8**, 1707.

46. For a recent book on epothilones *cf.*: K.-H. Altmann, G. Höfle, R. Müller, J. Mulzer and K. Prantz, *The Epothilones: An Outstanding Family of Anti-Tumor Agents*, ed. J. H. Mulzer, Springer, Progress in the Chemistry of Organic Natural Products, vol. 90, 2009.

47. E. Nogales, *Annu. Rev. Biophys. Biomol. Struct.*, 2001, **30**, 397.

48. O. Valiron, N. Caudron and D. Job, *Cell. Mol. Life Sci.*, 2001, **58**, 2069.

49. L. Amos, *Org. Biomol. Chem.*, 2004, **2**, 2153.

50. K.-H. Altmann, G. Bold, G. Caravatti, N. End, A. Flörsheimer, V. Guagnano, T. O'Reilly and M. Wartmann, *Chimia*, 2000, **54**, 612.

51. R. M. Buey, J. F. Diaz, J. M. Andreu, A. O'Brate, P. Giannakakou, K. C. Nicolaou, P. K. Sasmal, A. Ritzen and K. Namoto, *Chem. Biol.*, 2004, **11**, 225.

52. J. H. Nettles, H. L. Li, B. Cornett, J. M. Krahn, J. P. Snyder and K. H. Downing, *Science*, 2004, **305**, 866.

53. R. B. Lichtner, A. Rotgeri, T. Bunte, B. Buchmann, J. Hoffmann, W. Schwede, W. Skuballa and U. Klar, *Proc. Natl. Acad. Sci. U.S.A.*, 2001, **98**, 11743.

54. M. A. Jordan, *Curr. Med. Chem. Anticancer Agents*, 2002, **2**, 1.

55. N. R. Khawaja, M. Carré, H. Kovacic, M. A. Estève and D. Braguer, *Mol. Pharmacol.*, 2008, **74**, 1072.

56. S. H. Lee, S. M. Son, D. J. Son, S. M. Kim, T. Kim, S. Song, D. C. Moon, H. W. Lee, J. C. Ryu, D.-Y. Yoon and J. T. Hong, *Mol. Cancer Ther.*, 2007, **6**, 2786.

57. P. Giannakakou, R. Gussio, E. Nogales, K. H. Downing, D. Zaharevitz, B. Bollbuck, G. Poy, D. Sackett, K. C. Nicolaou and T. Fojo, *Proc. Natl. Acad. Sci. U.S.A.*, 2000, **97**, 2904.

58. L. He, C.-P. Yang and S. B. Horwitz, *Mol. Cancer Ther.*, 2001, **1**, 3.

59. T. C. Chou, X. G. Zhang, A. Balog, D. S. Su, D. F. Meng, K. Savin, J. R. Bertino and S. J. Danishefsky, *Proc. Natl. Acad. Sci. U.S.A.*, 1998, **95**, 9642.

60. T. O'Reilly, P. M. J. McSheehy, F. Wenger, M. Hattenberger, M. Muller, J. Vaxelaire, K.-H. Altmann and M. Wartmann, *Prostate*, 2005, **65**, 231.

61. J. Rothermel, M. Wartmann, T. L. Chen and J. Hohneker, *Semin. Oncol.*, 2003, **30**, 51.

62. G. Bocci, K. C. Nicolaou and R. S. Kerbel, *Cancer Res.*, 2002, **62**, 6938.

63. E. A. Woltering, J. M. Lewis, P. J. Maxwell 4th, D. J. Frey, Y.-Z. Wang, J. Rothermel, C. T. Anthony, D. A. Balster, J. P. O'Leary and L. H. Harrison, *Ann. Surgery*, 2003, **237**, 790.

64. S. Ferretti, P. R. Allegrini, T. O'Reilly, C. Schnell, M. Stumm, M. Wartmann, J. Wood, P. M. J. McSheehy and M. J. Paul, *Clin. Cancer Res.*, 2005, **11**, 7773.

65. B. Bystricky and I. Chau, *Exp. Opin. Investig. Drugs*, 2011, **20**, 107.

66. U. Klar, B. Buchmann, F. Schwede, W. Skuballa, J. Hofmann and B. Lichtner, *Angew. Chem.*, 2006, **118**, 8110.

67. U. Klar, B. Buchmann, F. Schwede, W. Skuballa, J. Hofmann and B. Lichtner, *Angew. Chem. Int. Ed.*, 2006, **45**, 7942.

68. U. Klar and J. Platzek, *Synlett*, 2012, 1291.

69. U. Klar, J. Hoffmann and M. Giurescu, *Expert Opin. Investig. Drugs*, 2008, **17**, 11.

70. S. Winsel, S. Hammer and J. Eschenbrenner, *Poster 720 presented at ECCO*, 2007, **14**, 23.

71. S. Hammer, A. Sommer and I. Fichtner, *Clin. Cancer Res.*, 2010, **16**, 1452.

72. J. Hoffmann, I. Vitale, B. Buchmann, L. Galluzzi, W. Schwede, L. Senovilla, W. Skuballa, S. Vivet, R. B. Lichtner, J. M. Vicencio, T. Panaretakis, G. Siemeister, H. Lage, L. Nanty, S. Hammer, K. Mittelstaedt, S. Winsel, J. Eschenbrenner, M. Castedo, C. Demarche, U. Klar and G. Kroemer, *Cancer Res.*, 2008, **68**, 5301.

73. J. Hoffmann, I Fichtner, M. Lemm, Ph. Lienau, H. Hess, A. Rotgeri, B. Hofmann and U. Klar, *Neuro. Oncol.*, 2009, **11**, 158.

74. P. Schmid, P. Kiewe, K. Possinger, A. Korfel, S. Lindemann, M. Giurescu, S. Reif, H. Wiesinger, E. Thiel and D. Kühnhardt, *Ann. Oncol.*, 2010, **21**, 633.

75. P. Fumoleau, B. Coudert, N. Isambert and E. Ferrant, *Ann. Oncol.*, 2007, **18**(Suppl 5), v9.

76. D. Arnold, W. Voigt and P. Kiewe, *Ann. Oncol.*, 2006, **17**(Suppl).

77. G J. Rustin, N. Reed and G. Jayson, *Abstract presented at the 15th International Meeting of the European Society for Gynaecological Oncology* 2007, Berlin, Germany.

78. S. McMeekin, R. Patel, C. Verschraegen, P. Celano, J. Burke, S. Plaxe, P. Ghatage, M. Giurescu, C. Stredder, Y. Wang and T. Schmelter, *Br. J. Cancer*, 2012, **106**, 70.

79. T. Beer, D. C. Smith, A. Hussain, M. Alonso, J. Wang, M. Giurescu, K. Roth and Y. Wang, *Br. J. Cancer*, 2012, **107**, 808.

80. U. Gatzemeier, J. V. von Pawel and E. Eschbach, *Eur. J. Cancer*, 2007, **5**, abstract 6538.

81. R. C. DeConti, A. P. Algazi, S. Andrews, P. Urbas, O. Born, D. Stoeckigt, L. Floren, J. Hwang, J. Weber, V. K. Sondak and A. I. Daud, *Br. J. Cancer*, 2010, **103**, 1548.

82. K. C. Nicolaou, A. Ritzen, K. Namoto, R. M. Buey, J. F. Diaz, J. M. Andreu, M. Wartmann, K.-H. Altmann, A. O'Brate and P. Giannakakou, *Tetrahedron*, 2008, **58**, 6413.

83. M. Wartmann, J. Loretan, R. Reuter, M. Hattenberger, M. Muller, J. Vaxelaire, S.-M. Maira, A. Floersheimer, T. O'Reilly and K.-H. Altmann, *Proc. Am. Assoc. Cancer Res.*, 2004, **45**, Abstract 5440.

84. F. Y. Lee, G. Vite, H. Gerhard, S.-H. Kim, J. Clark, K. Fager, K. Kennedy, R. Smykla, M.-L. Wen, K. Leavitt, K. Johnston, R. Peterson, A. Kamath, M. Franchini, G. Schulze, C. Fairchild, K. Raghavan, B. Long and R. Kramer, *Proc. AACR*, 2002, **43**, 792.

85. G. Höfle, N. Glaser, M. Kiffe, H.-J. Hecht, F. Sasse and F. Reichenbach, *Angew. Chem. Int. Ed.*, 1999, **38**, 1971.

86. G. Höfle, N. Glaser, T. Leibold, U. Karama, F. Sasse and H. Steinmetz, *Pure Appl. Chem.*, 2003, 75, 167.

87. G. Höfle, N. Glaser and T. Leibold, *Ger. Offen.* DE 19907588, 2000.

88. D. Uyar, N. Takigawa, T. Mekhail, D. Grabowski, M. Markman, F. Lee, R. Canetta, R. Peck, R. Bukowski and R. Ganapathi, *Gynecol. Oncol.*, 2003, **91**, 173.

89. A. V. Kamath, M. Chang, F. Y. Lee, Y. Zhang and P. H. Marathe, *Cancer Chemoth. Pharm.*, 2005, **56**, 145.

90. C. Sessa, A. Perotti, A. Llado, S. Cresta, G. Capri, M. Voi, S. Marsoni, I. Corradino and L. Gianni, *Ann. of Oncology*, 2007, **18**, 1548.

91. T. Mekhail, C. Chung and S. Holden, *Proc. Am. Soc. Clin. Oncol.*, 2003, **22**, 129, Abstract 515.

92. K. C. Nicolaou, R. Scarpelli, B. Bollbuck, B. Werschkun, M. Pereira, M. Wartmann, K.-H. Altmann, D. Zaharevitz, R. Gussio and P. Giannakakou, *Chem. Biol.*, 2000, 7, 593.

93. K.-H. Altmann, G. Bold, G. Caravatti, A. Flörsheimer, V. Guagnano and M. Wartmann, *Bioorg. Med. Chem. Lett.*, 2000, **10**, 2765.

94. A. Balog, D. Meng, T. Kamenecka, P. Bertinato, D. S. Su, E. J. Sorensen and S. J. Danishefsky, *Angew. Chem. Int. Ed.*, 1996, **35**, 2801.

95. D. Meng, P. Bertinato, A. Balog, D. S. Su, T. Kamenecka, E. J. Sorensen and S. J. Danishefsky, *J. Am. Chem. Soc.*, 1997, **119**, 10073.

96. D. S. Su, D. Meng, P. Bertinato, A. Balog, E. J. Sorensen, S. J. Danishefsky, Y. H. Zheng, T. C. Chou, L. He and S. B. Horwitz, *Angew. Chem. Int. Ed.*, 1997, **35**, 757.

97. K. C. Nicolaou, N. Winssinger, J. Pastor, S. Ninkovic, F. Sarabia, Y. He, D. Vourloumis, Z. Yang, T. Li, P. Giannakakou and E. Hamel, *Nature*, 1997, **387**, 268.

98. D. Schinzer, A. Bauer and J. Schieber, *Synlett*, 1998, 861.

99. S. A. May and P. A. Grieco, *Chem. Commun.*, 1998, 1597.

100. J. Mulzer, A. Montoulidis and E. Öhler, *J. Org. Chem.*, 2000, **65**, 7456.

101. A. Balog, C. Harris, K. Savin, X.-G. Zhang, T. C. Chou and S. J. Danishefsky, *Angew. Chem. Int. Ed.*, 1998, **37**, 2675.

102. C. R. Harris, S. D. Kuduk, A. Balog, K. Savin, P. W. Glunz and S. J. Danishefsky, *J. Am. Chem. Soc.*, 1999, **121**, 7050.

103. D. F. Meng, D. S. Su, A. Balog, P. Bertinato, E. J. Sorensen, S. J. Danishefsky, Y. H. Zheng, T. C. Chou, L. F. He and S. B. Horwitz, *J. Am. Chem. Soc.*, 1997, **119**, 2733.

104. D. S. Su, A. Balog, D. F. Meng, P. Bertinato, S. J. Danishefsky, Y. H. Zheng, T. C. Chou, L. F. He and S. B. Horwitz, *Angew. Chem. Int. Ed.*, 1997, **36**, 2093.

105. K. C. Nicolaou, D. Vourloumis, T. Li, J. Pastor, N. Winssinger, Y. He, S. Ninkovic, F. Sarabia, H. Vallberg, F. Roschangar, N. P. King, M. R. Finlay, P. Giannakakou, P. Verdier-Pinard and E. Hamel, *Angew. Chem. Int. Ed.*, 1997, **36**, 2097.

106. K. C. Nicolaou, N. Winssinger, J. Pastor, S. Ninkovic, F. Sarabia, Y. He, D. Vourloumis, Z. Yang, T. Li, P. Giannakakou and E. Hamel, *Nature*, 1997, **387**, 268.

107. T. C. Chou, X. G. Zhang, C. R. Harris, S. D. Kuduk, A. Balog, K. Savin, J. R. Bertino and S. J. Danishefsky, *Proc. Natl. Acad. Sci. U.S.A.*, 1998, **95**, 15798.

108. J. P. Monk, M. Villalona-Calero, J. Larkin, G. Otterson, D. S. Spriggs, A. L. Hannah, G. F. Cropp, R. G. Johnson and M. L. Hensley, *Invest. New Drug*, 2012, **30**, 1676.

109. E. T. Lam, S. Goel, L. J. Schaaf, G. F. Cropp, A. L. Hannah, Y. Zho, B. McCracken, B. I. Haley, R. G. Johnson, S. Mani and M. A. Villalona-Calero, *Cancer Chemoth. Pharm.*, 2012, **69**, 523.

110. http://phx.corporate-ir.net/phoenix.zhtml?c=121014&p=irol-newsArticle&ID=967533&highlight=.

111. M. D'Alincourt Salazar and M. Ratnam, *Cancer Metast. Rev.*, 2007, **26**, 141.

112. P. S. Low, W. A. Henne and D. D. Doorneweerd, *Acc. Chem. Res.*, 2007, **41**, 120.

113. C. A. Ladino, R. V. J. Chari, L. A. Bourret, N. L. Kedersha and V. S. Goldmacher, *Int. J. Cancer*, 1997, **73**, 859.

114. C. P. Leamon, *Curr. Opin. Invest. Drugs.*, 2008, **9**, 1277.

115. C. P. Leamon and J. Reddy, *Adv. Drug. Delivery Rev.*, 2004, **56**, 1127.

116. K. L. Covello, C. Flefleh, K. Menard, A. Wiebesiek, K. Mcglinchey, M. L. Wen, R. Westhouse, J. A. Reddy, I. R. Vlahov, J. Hunt, W. Rose, C. P. Leamon, G. D. Vite and F. Y. Lee, *Proceedings of the 99th Annual Meeting of AACR* 2008, San Diego, CA. Abstract #2326.

117. J. Yang, H. Chen, J. X. Cheng, I. R. Vlahov and P. S. Low, *Proc. Natl. Acad. Sci. U.S.A.*, 2006, **103**, 13872.

118. G. D. Vite, F. Y. Lee, C. P. Leamon and I. R. Vlahov, *U.S. Pat. Appl.* US2007276018, 2007.

119. A. Regueiro-Ren, M. Borzilleri, X. Zheng, S.-H. Kim, J. A. Johnson, C. R. Fairchild, F. Y. F. Lee, B. H. Long and G. D. Vite, *Org. Lett.*, 2001, **3**, 2693.

120. A. Rivkin, F. Yoshimura, A. E. Gabarda, T.-C. Chou, H. Dong, W. P. Tong and S. J. Danishefsky, *J. Am. Chem. Soc.*, 125, **2003**, 2899.

121. A. Rivkin, F. Yoshimura, A. E. Gabarda, Y. S. Cho, T. C. Chou, H. J. Dong and S. J. Danishefsky, *J. Am. Chem. Soc.*, 2004, **126**, 10913.

122. J. D. White, R. G. Carter, K. F. Sundermann and M. Wartmann, *J. Am. Chem. Soc.*, 2001, **123**, 5407.

123. J. D. White, R. G. Carter, K. F. Sundermann and M. Wartmann, *J. Am. Chem. Soc.*, 2003, **125**, 3190, [Erratum for J. Am. Chem. Soc., 123, 5407].

124. T. Carlomagno, M. J. J. Blommers, J. Meiler, W. Jahnke, T. Schupp, F. Petersen, D. Schinzer, K.-H. Altmann and C. Griesinger, *Angew. Chem. Int. Ed.*, 2003, **42**, 2511.

125. T.-C. Chou, H. Dong, A. Rivkin, F. Yoshimura, A. E. Gabarda, Y. S. Cho, W. P. Tong and S. J. Danishefsky, *Angew. Chem. Int. Ed.*, 2003, **42**, 4762.

126. B. E. Smart, *J. Fluorine Chem.*, 2001, **109**, 3.

127. K.-D. Wu, Y. S. Cho, J. Katz, V. Ponomarev, S. Chen-Kiang, S. J. Danishefsky and M. A. S. Moore, *Proc. Natl. Acad. Sci. U.S.A.*, 2005, **102**, 10640.

128. T.-C. Chou, H. Dong, X. Zhang, W. P Tong and J. S. Danishefsky, *Cancer Res.*, 2005, **65**, 9445.

129. T.-C. Chou, X. Zhang, Z.-Y. Zhong, Y. Li, L. Feng, S. Eng, D. R. Myles, R. Johnson, N. Wu, Y. I. Yin, R. M. Wilson and S. J. Danishefsky, *Proc. Natl. Acac. Sci. U.S.A.*, 2008, **105**, 13157.

130. Z. Zhong, L. Feng, S. Eng, D. Zhang, Y. Li, D. Craig, J. Gibson, T.-C. Chou, S. J. Danishefsky, J. Roberts, M. Simcox, P. Timmermans and R. Johnson, *Am. Assoc. Can. Res.*, 98th Annual Meeting in Los Angeles 2007, Abstract 1438.

131. T. C. Chou, X.-G. Zhang, H. Dong, Z. Zhong, L. Feng, Y. Li, M. Sherrill, P. Timmermanns, R. Johnson and S. J. Danishefsky, *Am. Assoc. Can. Res.*, 2008, 99th Annual Meeting in San Diego, Abstract 1402.

132. R. M. Borzilleri, X. Zheng, R. J. Schmidt, J. A. Johnson, S.-H. Kim, J. D. DiMarco, C. R. Fairchild, J. Z. Gougouts, F. Y. F. Lee, B. H. Long and G. D. Vite, *J. Am. Chem. Soc.*, 2000, **122**, 8890.

133. S. J. Stachel, C. B. Lee, M. Spassova, M. D. Chappell, W. G. Bornmann, S. J. Danishefsky, T.-C. Chou and Y. Guan, *J. Org. Chem.*, 2001, **66**, 4369.

134. F. Y. F. Lee, R. Borzilleri, C. R. Fairchild, A. V. Kamath, R. Smykla, R. A. Kramer and G. D. Vite, *Cancer Chemoth. Pharm.*, 2008, **63**, 157.

135. F. Y. F. Lee, R. Borzilleri, C. R. Fairchild, S.-H. Kim, B. H. Long, C. Reventos-Suarez, G. D. Vite, W. C. Rose and R. A. Kramer, *Clin. Cancer Res.*, 2001, **7**, 1429.

136. F. Y. F. Lee, K. L. Covello, S. Castaneda, D. R. Hawken, D. Kan, A. Lewin, M.-L. Wen, R.-P. Ryseck, C. R. Fairchild, J. Fargnoli and R. Kramer, *Clin. Cancer Res.*, 2008, **14**, 8123.

137. N. Lin, K. Brakora and M. Seiden, *Curr. Opin. Invest. Drugs.*, 2003, **4**, 746.

138. X. Pivot, A. Dufresne and C. Villanueva, *Clin. Breast Cancer*, 2007, **7**, 543.

139. J. Abraham, M. Agrawal, S. Bakke, A. Rutt, M. Edgerly, F. M. Balis, B. Widemann, L. Davis, B. Damle, D. Sonnichsen, D. Lebwohl, S. Bates, H. Kotz and T. Fojo, *J. Clin. Oncol.*, 2003, **21**, 1866.

140. E. Thomas, J. Tabernero, M. Fornier, P. Conté, P. Fumoleau, A. Lluch, L. T. Vahdat, C. A. Bunnell, H. A. Burris, P. Viens, J. Baselga, E. Rivera, V. Guarneri, V. Poulart, J. Klimovsky, D. Lebwohl and M. Martin, *J. Clin. Oncol.*, 2007, **25**, 3399.

141. L. T. Vahdat, E. Thomas, R. Li, J. Jassem, H. Gomez, H. Chung, R. Peck, P. Mukhopadhyay, J. Klimovsky and H. Roché, *J. Clin. Oncol.*, 2007, **25**(18S), 1006.

142. http://www.cancer.gov/cancertopics/druginfo/fda-ixabepilone.

143. O. Pineda, J. Farras, L. Maccari, F. Manetti, M. Botta and J. Vilarrasa, *Bioorg. Med. Chem. Lett.*, 2004, **14**, 4825.

144. J. Jiménez-Barbero, A. Canales, P. T. Northcote, R. M. Buey, J. M. Andreu and J. F. Díaz, *J. Am. Chem. Soc.*, 2006, **128**, 8757.

145. P. Giannakakou, R. Gussio, E. Nogales, K. H. Downing, D. Zaharevitz, B. Bollbuck, G. Poy, D. Sackett, K. C. Nicolaou and T. Fojo, *Proc. Natl. Acad. Sci. U.S.A.*, 2000, **97**, 2904.

146. I. Ojima, S. Chakravarty, T. Inoue, S. Lin, L. He, S. B. Horwitz, S. D. Kuduk and S. J. Danishefsky, *Proc. Natl. Acad. Sci. USA*, 1999, **96**, 4256.

147. M. Wang, X. Xia, Y. Kim, D. Hwang, J. M. Jansen, M. Botta, D. C. Liotta and J. P. Snyder, *Org. Lett.*, 1999, **1**, 43.
148. F. Manetti, S. Forli, L. Maccari, F. Corelli and M. Botta, *Il Farmaco*, 2003, **58**, 357.
149. F. Manetti, L. Maccari, F. Corelli and M. Botta, *Curr. Topics. Med. Chem.*, 2004, **4**, 203.
150. M. Reese, M. V. Sánchez-Pedregal, K. Kubicek, J. Meiler, M. J. J. Blommers, C. Griesinger and T. Carlomagno, *Angew. Chem. Int. Ed.*, 2007, **46**, 1864.
151. D. W. Heinz, W. D. Schubert and G. Höfle, *Angew. Chem. Int. Ed.*, 2005, **44**, 1298.
152. W. Zhang, Y. Jiang, P. J. Brodie, D. G. I. Kingston, D. C. Liotta and J. P. Snyder, *Org. Lett.*, 2008, **10**, 1565.
153. Q.-H. Chen, T. Ganesh, P. Brodie, C. Slebodnick, Y. Jiang, A. Banerjee, S. Bane, J. P. Snyder and D. G. I. Kingston, *Org. Biomol. Chem.*, 2008, **6**, 4542.
154. M. Erdélyi, B. Pfeiffer, K. Hauenstein, J. Fohrer, J. Gertsch, K.-H. Altmann and T. Carlomagno, *J. Med. Chem.*, 2008, **51**, 1469.
155. M. Erdélyi, A. Navarro-Vázquez, B. Pfeiffer, C. N. Kuzniewski, A. Felser, T. Widmer, J. Gertsch, B. Pera, J. F. Díaz, K.-H. Altmann and T. Carlomagno, *ChemMedChem*, 2010, **5**, 911.
156. S. Forli, F. Manetti, K.-H. Altmann and M. Botta, *ChemMedChem*, 2010, **5**, 35.
157. D. Rusinska-Roszak and M. Lozynski, *J. Mol. Model.*, 2009, **15**, 859.
158. V. A. Jiménez, *J. Chem. Inf. Model.*, 2010, **50**, 2176.
159. A. E. Prota, K. Bargsten, D. Zurwerra, J. J. Field, J. F. Díaz, K.-H. Altmann and M. O. Steinmetz, *Science*, 2013, **339**, 587.
160. F. Feyen, F. Cachoux, J. Gertsch, M. Wartmann and K.-H. Altmann, *Acc. Chem. Res.*, 2008, **41**, 21.

Macrocyclic Inhibitors of Zinc-dependent Histone Deacetylases (HDACs)

A. GANESAN

School of Pharmacy, University of East Anglia, Norwich Research Park, Norwich NR4 7TJ, UK
Email: a.ganesan@uea.ac.uk

4.1 Genetics Versus Epigenetics

In eukaryotic cells, the genome is encoded by DNA that is tightly wound around histone proteins in the nucleus. Packaging the DNA double helix in this manner enables it to be physically accommodated within a tiny space. Furthermore, it serves to protect the DNA and regulate the regions that undergo activation and gene transcription. The core DNA-histone structural unit is the nucleosome in which 146 base pairs of DNA are wrapped around an octamer consisting of four pairs of histone proteins H2A, H2B, H3 and H4 stapled together by the linker histone H1 (Figure 4.1).

In humans, single point mutations in DNA sequence can directly lead to diseases such as sickle cell anemia and cystic fibrosis or increase our susceptibility towards chronic multifactorial diseases such as cancer, inflammation, metabolic syndrome and neurodegenerative disorders. Genetics is the study of changes in the genome that then lead to changes in the observed phenotype. Such genomic mutations are life-long and transferred to the next generation; at present it is not possible to replace a defective genome by its normal counterpart.

RSC Drug Discovery Series No. 40
Macrocycles in Drug Discovery
Edited by Jeremy Levin
© The Royal Society of Chemistry 2015
Published by the Royal Society of Chemistry, www.rsc.org

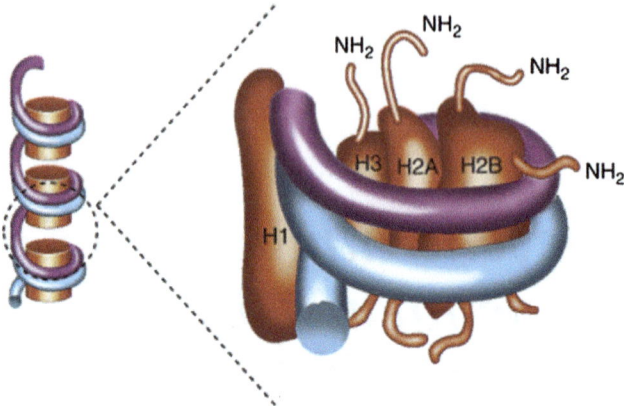

Figure 4.1   A representation of the nucleosome, with the DNA double helix colored
in blue and magenta and the histone proteins in ocher. The N-terminal
tails of the histones extend beyond the core and make interactions with
one another and with DNA.
(Reprinted with permission from Z. Amoura, S. Koutouzov and J. C.
Piette, *Curr. Opin. Rheumatol.*, 2000, **12**, 369.)

Recently, the science of genetics has been supplemented by epigenetics,
which is the study of heritable changes in an organism's phenotype without
an underlying change in the genome. The molecular basis for epigenetics is
the remodeling of the nucleosome due to covalent modifications of the DNA
and histone proteins.[1,2] These structural changes are dynamic unlike the
permanent genetic mutations and lead to alterations in DNA-histone affinity
and protein–protein interactions that influence the transcription machinery.
Overall, epigenetic modifications determine which genes become transcribed and which remain silent within a particular cell type. The introduction of these modifications is catalysed by a set of enzymes collectively
referred to as 'writers', while there is another set of 'eraser' enzymes that
reverses these reactions. Often, the writers and erasers are overexpressed or
mutated in diseased states suggesting that they are potential targets for drug
discovery. The activity of both the writers and erasers can be modulated by
small molecules, providing the opportunity to dynamically alter an aberrant
epigenome back to a normal state. The rest of this chapter describes the
chemical biology and drug discovery efforts directed against one particular
family of erasers, the zinc-dependent histone deacetylases (HDACs), with a
specific focus upon macrocyclic HDAC inhibitors. Additional material on
this topic can be found in two earlier reviews.[3,4]

4.2   Zinc-dependent Histone Deacetylases

The flexible N-terminal tails of histone proteins carry multiple positive
charges due to the presence of lysine and arginine residues. A key histone
post-translational   modification   is   the   acetylation   of   lysine   residues

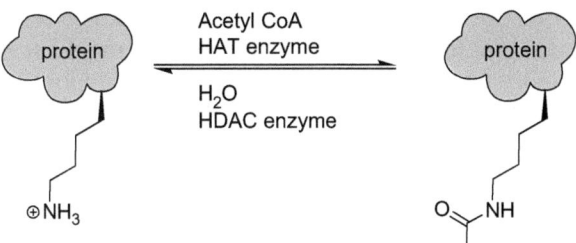

Figure 4.2 Reversible protein lysine acetylation catalysed by HATs and HDACs.

(Figure 4.2) by histone acetyltransferases (HATs). Acetylation converts the positively charged lysine side-chain to a neutral acetamide that has reduced affinity for DNA and allows the latter to unwind off the nucleosome to become transcribed. Furthermore, the acetyl-lysine side-chain serves as a chemical signal that is recognized by the bromodomain protein–protein interaction domain,[5] leading to the recruitment of specific histone binding partners such as transcription complexes. Last but not least, acetylation 'locks' the post-translational state of lysine, preventing it from undergoing other modifications that range in size from the addition of a single methyl group to the conjugation of proteins, such as ubiquitin or SUMO (small ubiquitin-like modifier), which have their own consequences with regards to gene activation or silencing.[6]

The reverse of lysine acetylation is the enzymatic hydrolysis of the acetamide by HDACs and it is the dynamic interplay between HATs and HDACs that regulates the acetylation state of the nucleosome and the switching on or off of specific genes. From a drug discovery perspective, inhibitors of both HATs and HDACs have been extensively pursued although HDACs have proved to be a more successful target. Numerous HDAC inhibitors have advanced to clinical trials as anticancer agents; among these, vorinostat[7] and romidepsin[8] received FDA approval in 2006 and 2009 respectively for the treatment of cutaneous T-cell lymphoma (CTCL). In terms of activity, vorinostat and romidepsin are nanomolar HDAC inhibitors with IC_{50} values of 288 and 24 nM respectively against HDACs purified from HeLa cells. HDAC inhibitors appear to be particularly suited for the treatment of CTCL as they act as immunosuppressants to reduce the production of pro-inflammatory cytokines that is a hallmark of this cancer.[9]

The human genome contains 18 HDACs that are classified according to their catalytic mechanism.[10] The focus of this chapter is the eleven zinc-dependent HDACs 1–11, which contain a zinc cation as the active site catalyst. In addition, there are seven sirtuins, SIRTs 1–7, which instead employ the cofactor NAD^+ for amide bond hydrolysis. The zinc-dependent HDACs are further subdivided into class I (HDACs 1, 2, 3 and 8), class IIa (HDACs 4, 5, 7 and 9), class IIb (HDACs 6 and 10) and class IV (HDAC 11) based on sequence homology and cellular localization. The class I HDACs are ubiquitously expressed and primarily located in the cell nucleus, where they do not bind to the nucleosome directly but are often found within transcriptional repressor complexes. The class IIa enzymes, HDACs 4, 5, 7 and 9, are tissue-specific and cytoplasmic in nature but shuttle to the nucleus upon activation, while the class IIb enzymes HDAC6 and 10 are predominantly cytoplasmic and unusually contain two catalytic domains. The remaining HDAC11 shares sequence homology with class I HDACs while being class II-like in cytoplasmic localization and, for that reason, it is placed separately in class IV.

The nuclear activity of class I and class II HDACs upon histones, reverting acetyl-lysine to lysine, is associated with gene silencing due to the increase in DNA-histone affinity and the loss of interactions with acetyl-lysine binding transcription factors and coactivators. In cancer cells, histone deacetylation serves to repress pathways that would normally prevent cell proliferation. The anticancer effect of HDAC inhibitors is due to the reactivation of these pathways that promote differentiation, cell cycle arrest or apoptosis instead of cell division.[11-13] Although this is the primary therapeutic outcome of HDAC inhibitors in cancer, the HDAC nomenclature is misleading as reversible lysine deacetylation is not exclusive to histones. It occurs in several thousand proteins, nuclear or otherwise, and some of the beneficial effects of HDAC inhibitors *in vivo*, as well as their side effects, are likely to arise from their impact upon nonhistone substrates.[14,15] While the interest in HDAC inhibition has largely focused on their anticancer properties, and this is the indication for which their application is most mature, HDAC inhibitors have demonstrated activity *in vitro*, and often in animal models, for practically all therapeutic areas including inflammation, central nervous system, cardiovascular and antimicrobial indications.[16,17] All of the eleven HDACs are linked to important biological processes (Table 4.1) and there is likely to be redundancy within their pathways, making it difficult to predict the ideal isoform selective inhibition profile for a particular disease state.

The X-ray structures of several human HDACs have been solved and reveal a catalytic mechanism akin to other metalloenzymes that carry out amide hydrolysis (Figure 4.3).[18] The acetyl-lysine substrate is positioned within a narrow channel that ends with a catalytic zinc cation. The metal serves to activate a water molecule to make it more nucleophilic and simultaneously coordinates to the acetyl group to make it a better electrophile. The attack of water results in a tetrahedral intermediate that collapses to give lysine and acetate, the latter leaving through an exit channel separate from the substrate binding pocket.

Typically, HDAC enzyme inhibitors are substrate mimics that can be described by a pharmacophore consisting of a warhead, spacer and cap.[19,20] The warhead is a reversible zinc binding functional group while the spacer occupies the hydrophobic substrate binding tunnel. At the other end of the molecule is the cap that serves to mimic the rest of the protein substrate and forms binding interactions with the surface exposed 'rim' of the HDAC. The zinc binding warhead is often a hydroxamic acid, ever since HDAC inhibition was demonstrated by Yoshida to be the molecular target of the natural

Table 4.1 A key role is indicated for individual HDAC isoforms (for simplicity, one is shown per enzyme whereas each performs multiple functions), together with the mouse knockout phenotype and the major potential therapeutic indications.

Isoform	Function	Knockout phenotype	Indication
Class I			
HDAC1	proliferation	embryonic lethal	cancer
HDAC2	proliferation	embryonic lethal	cancer
HDAC3	proliferation	embryonic lethal	cancer
HDAC8	proliferation	neural defects	cancer
Class II			
HDAC4	angiogenesis	bone defects	cancer, Huntington's
HDAC5	memory	cardiac defects	neurodegeneration
HDAC7	angiogenesis	embryonic lethal	autoimmune, inflammation
HDAC9	metabolism	cardiac defects	obesity, diabetes
HDAC6	migration, metastasis	viable	cancer, neurodegeneration
HDAC10	autophagy	knockout unknown	cancer
Class IV			
HDAC11	immune response	T-cell defects	cancer

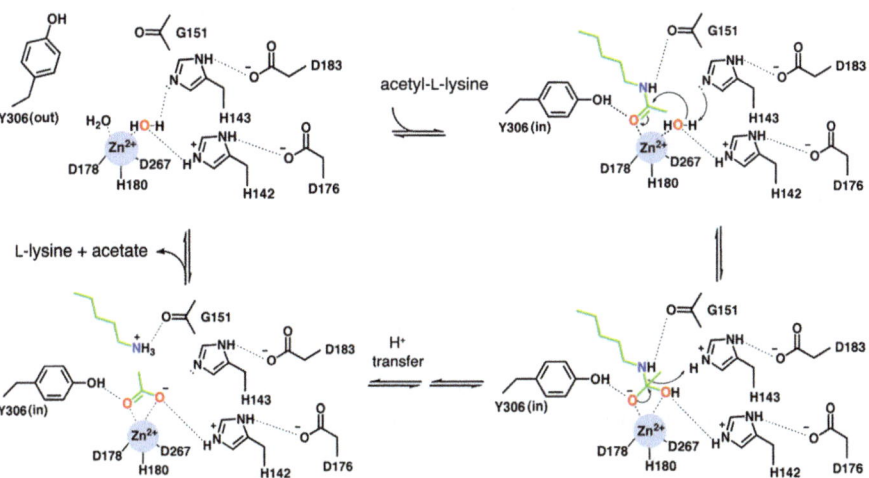

Figure 4.3 The catalytic mechanism proposed for human HDAC8. (Reprinted with permission from ref. 18.)

product hydroxamic acid trichostatin A (**1**, Figure 4.4) isolated from extracts of the bacterial species *Streptomyces hygroscopicus*.[21] The first X-ray structure of a HDAC inhibitor–enzyme complex, that of trichostatin A bound to a bacterial histone deacetylase-like protein (Figure 4.4), shows how the warhead and cap interact respectively with the active site and rim of the enzyme.[22] Meanwhile, at Columbia University, Breslow had independently

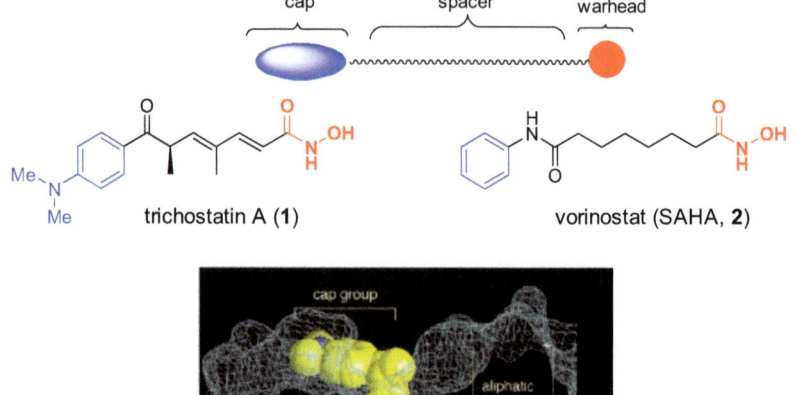

trichostatin A (**1**)   vorinostat (SAHA, **2**)

trichostatin A bound to a bacterial HDAC-like protein

Figure 4.4   Top: the warhead-spacer-cap pharmacophore typical of HDAC inhibitors illustrated by two classical examples with a hydroxamic acid warhead, the natural product trichostatin A and the synthetic approved drug vorinostat. Bottom: X-ray structure of trichostatin A bound to a bacterial HDAC-like protein.
(Bottom figure reprinted with permission from ref. 22.)

optimized a series of synthetic hydroxamic acids using a phenotypic screen involving cell differentiation. It was realized that these compounds, like trichostatin A, were HDAC inhibitors and the candidate vorinostat **2** (also known as suberoylanilide hydroxamic acid (SAHA)) was acquired by Merck and would go on to become the first-in-class HDAC inhibitor to be approved by the FDA with the trade name Zolinza®.[23]

In HDAC inhibitors, there is a 'yin and yang' relationship between the warhead and the cap. A warhead that tightly binds to the active site zinc will lead to enzyme inhibition even with a minimal spacer and cap. Examples include hydroxamic acids (as in Figure 4.4), benzamides and mercaptoketones – three functional groups that can engage in bidentate chelation with the zinc (Figure 4.5). Conversely, a weaker zinc binding warhead can be compensated for by a large cap that interacts extensively with the enzyme rim. For example, carboxylic acids, ketones and thiols are monodentate zinc binders and the most potent HDAC inhibitors featuring such relatively weak warheads all contain macrocyclic caps that engage in additional binding to the enzyme outside the zinc containing active site. Furthermore, the rim region of HDACs is less conserved compared to the active site and

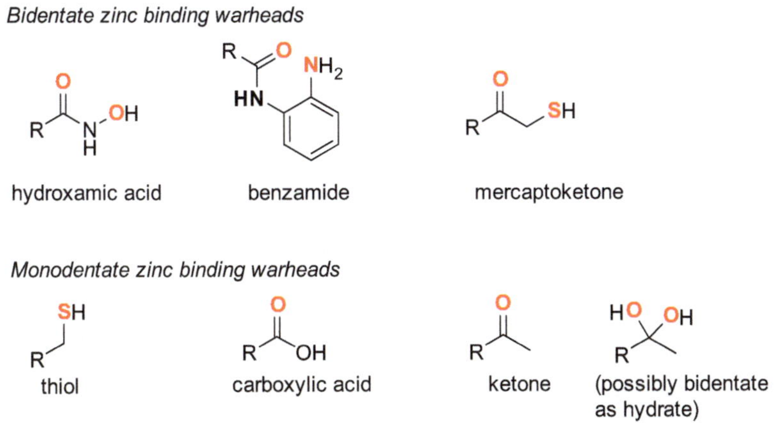

Bidentate zinc binding warheads

hydroxamic acid   benzamide   mercaptoketone

Monodentate zinc binding warheads

thiol   carboxylic acid   ketone   (possibly bidentate
                                                  as hydrate)

Figure 4.5   Examples of monodentate and bidentate zinc binding warheads found in HDAC inhibitors. Zinc binding atoms are shown in red.

hydrophobic tunnel and enzyme–inhibitor interactions in the rim can be discriminatory between isoforms. Even a minimal cap can be sufficient to achieve selectivity in isoform inhibition. In the case of vorinostat, the cap is only a phenyl ring but the drug is significantly more potent against class I HDACs compared to their class II counterparts. Such selectivity patterns can be enhanced in compounds with larger caps that engage in extended rim binding, as will be seen later in this chapter. Achieving subtype selectivity is currently an important goal in HDAC-directed drug discovery, as it should reduce side effects arising through inhibition of all eleven of the enzymes. In addition, the spacer and cap serve an important function in that they bind to features unique to HDACs, minimizing off-target effects arising from non-specific binding to other metalloenzymes.

Evaluating the activity of HDAC inhibitors is a complex process. The simplest mechanism-based assays involve partially purified HDACs extracted as a mixture from nuclear cell lysates. While this will provide a good indication of HDAC inhibition, it provides no information of isoform selectivity as the extracts are undefined in composition, albeit enriched in the class I nuclear HDACs. The determination of isoform selectivity requires assays with individual recombinant HDACs. However, as there are eleven of them, it is resource and cost intensive to profile compounds against the entire panel. An additional caveat is that enzyme assays with individual HDACs are a poor model for their cellular activity, as some HDACs have low stability or catalytic activity on their own whereas in cells they exist within multiprotein complexes. As a result, the literature is unfortunately replete with claims of class selective HDAC inhibitors that should be treated with caution as they are based on assaying only a few isoforms or assays performed under non-ideal conditions. There are relatively few inhibitors that have been fully characterized *and* display high selectivity; one example is the benzamide **3** (Figure 4.6) described by Merck which is the biphenyl analogue of Schering's

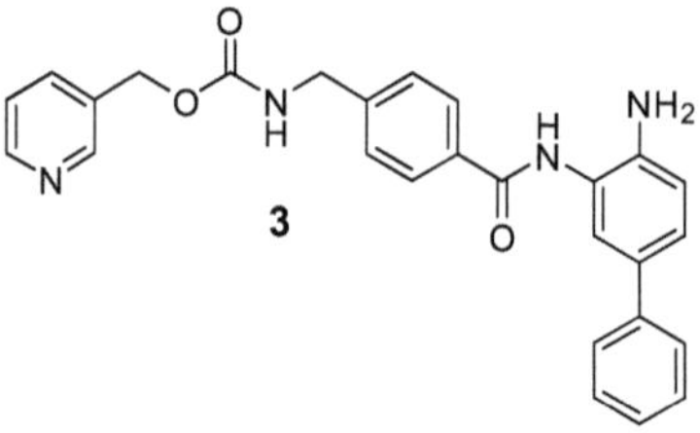

HDAC1	IC_{50} 10 nM	HDAC4	IC_{50} >50,000 nM
HDAC2	IC_{50} 72 nM	HDAC5	IC_{50} >50,000 nM
HDAC3	IC_{50} 6180 nM	HDAC7	IC_{50} >30,000 nM
HDAC8	IC_{50} >20,000 nM	HDAC6	IC_{50} >50,000 nM

Figure 4.6 A HDAC1/2 selective inhibitor reported by Merck.

clinical candidate MS-275 (entinostat). The additional phenyl ring binds to a deep buried pocket located beyond the active site zinc ion.[24] The size of this pocket can accommodate the phenyl group only in HDAC1/2 and not in the other isoforms, whereas MS-275 (with a hydrogen instead of the phenyl ring) equally inhibits HDAC2 and HDAC3. There may well be other HDAC inhibitors that are *more* selective than reported, because the compounds were not tested against all the isoforms.

In addition to enzyme assays, HDAC inhibitors are usually evaluated in cancer cell lines, where they potently inhibit growth proliferation to provide a cell-based phenotypic readout of activity. The cellular potency of HDAC inhibitors can exceed their activity in enzyme assays, as the precise HDAC isoforms that drive proliferation in a given cell type may be unknown. In any case, growth inhibition data should be supplemented with evidence to confirm that it is due to HDAC inhibition and not off-target effects. Typically, confirmatory evidence involves Western blotting of client proteins such as histones for nuclear HDACs or tubulin for HDAC6 to detect an increase in acetylation levels, or changes in a downstream biomarker such as induction of the cyclin-dependent kinase inhibitor p21.

4.3   The Cyclic Tetrapeptide Natural Products with a Ketone Warhead

In the 1970s and 1980s, a family of intriguing cyclic tetrapeptide natural products was isolated from fungal fermentations (Figure 4.7).[25–29] These natural products, 4–7, possessed potent biological activity with an unknown mechanism of action and contained a cyclic amino acid (proline or pipecolic acid), two other hydrophobic side-chains and a common unnatural amino acid bearing an epoxyketone side-chain. Within such cyclic tetrapeptides, there are severe transannular interactions between the side-chains if they are homochiral. Thus, cyclic tetrapeptides where all four residues are derived from L-amino acids are virtually unknown. The natural products obey this principle as they contain one or more D-amino acids and the incorporation of turn-inducing cyclic amino acids (proline/pipecolic acid or α-aminoisobutyric acid) that favor cyclization. A number of groups such as Rich,[30] Schmidt[31,32] and Baldwin[33] established methods for the total synthesis of the natural products and determined the preferred positions for

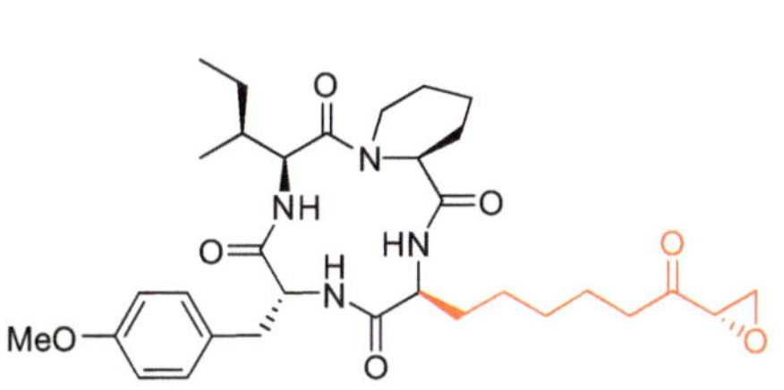

Cyl-2 (4)
Cylindrocladium scoparium

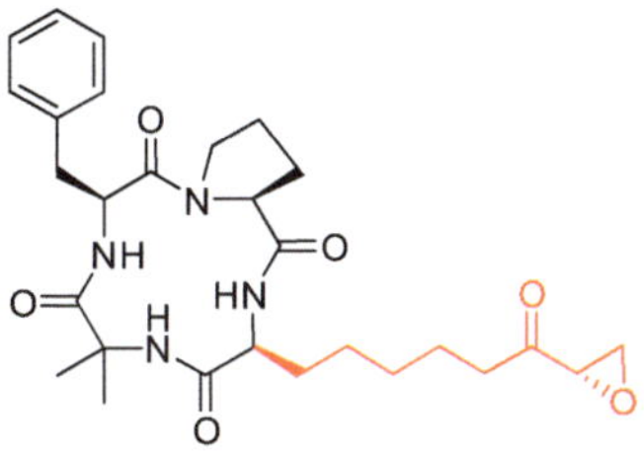

chlamydocin (5)
Diheterospora chlamydosporia

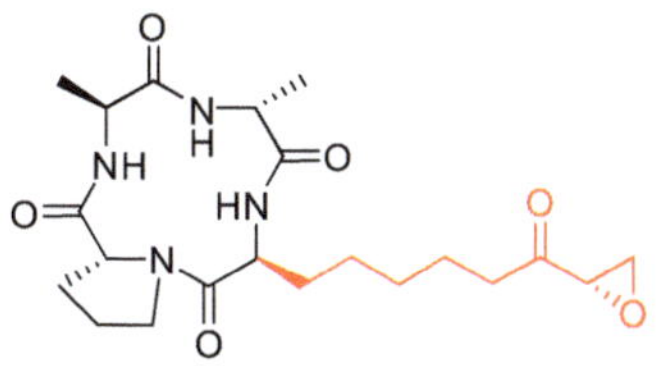

HC-toxin (6)
Helminthosporum carbonum

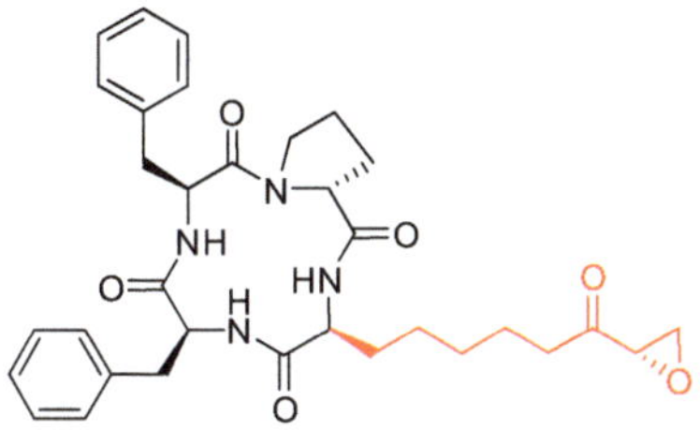

trapoxin B (7)
Helicoma ambiens

Figure 4.7 Structures of cyclic tetrapeptide HDAC inhibitors with a common epoxyketone zinc binding warhead.

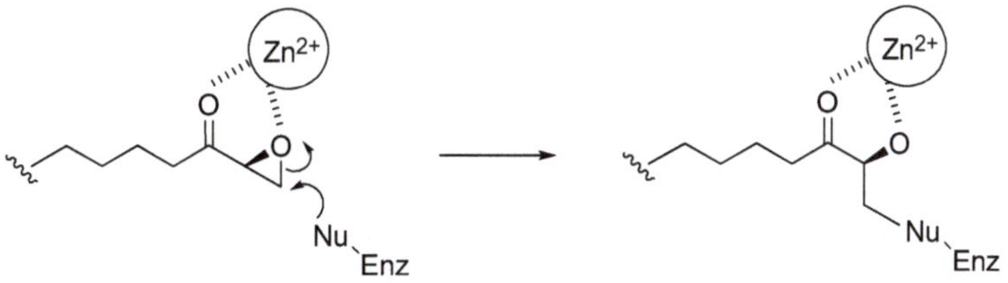

Figure 4.8 Irreversible inactivation of HDACs by epoxyketone natural products.

macrolactamization of linear precursors, setting the stage for later analogue synthesis by others.

A major breakthrough came about in 1993 with the discovery by Yoshida that the cyclic tetrapeptides, like the hydroxamic acid trichostatin A (**1**), were HDAC inhibitors.[34] While trichostatin A is a reversible inhibitor, trapoxin (**7**) is irreversible in its action, presumably due to ring opening of the epoxide by a nucleophilic residue at the enzyme active site to give a bidentate hydroxyketone zinc binding warhead (Figure 4.8). In support of this hypothesis, studies with the natural products showed that modification of the epoxyketone led to significant loss of activity: reduction of the Cyl-2 ketone to an alcohol (>1000 fold less active than Cyl-2),[26] reduction of the trapoxin epoxide to an alcohol (inactive at 100 nM)[34] or epoxide ring-opening of HC-toxin to a diol (inactive at 100 times the EC_{50} of the toxin).[35] Nevertheless, these results might be compound or assay specific, given the SAR of apicidin (**13**, *vide infra*).

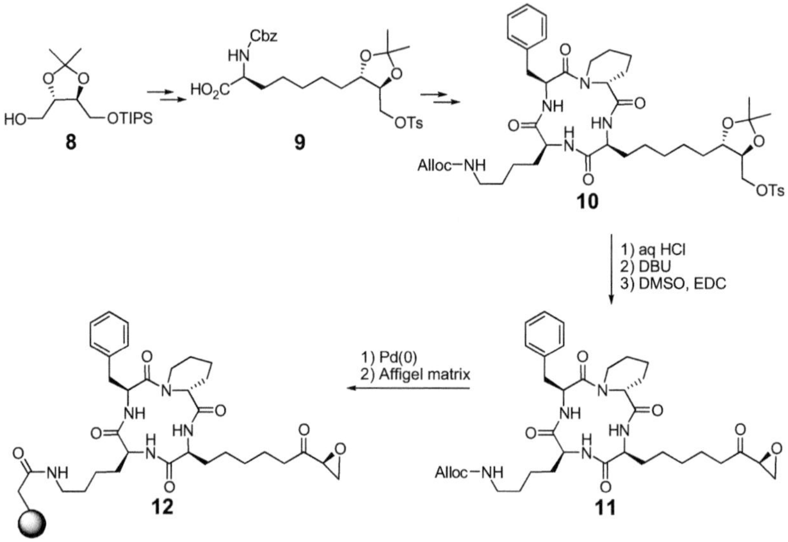

Scheme 4.1   The synthesis of an immobilized trapoxin analogue by Schreiber.

The covalent nature of trapoxin-HDAC inhibition was taken advantage of by Schreiber, who prepared an immobilized trapoxin analogue.[36] The tartrate-derived alcohol **8** (Scheme 4.1) was transformed by a series of steps to the protected unnatural amino acid **9**. This was then incorporated into a linear peptide that was cyclized to give **10**. The sequence of acetonide deprotection, tosylate displacement with epoxide formation and alcohol oxidation furnished the epoxyketone side-chain in trapoxin analogue **11**, which was covalently linked to a matrix to provide affinity reagent **12**. In-cubation of **12** with nuclear extracts followed by peptide microsequencing of the covalently bound component led to the first identification and cloning of HDAC1, the mammalian homologue of the yeast protein Rpd3p.[37]

While a nonselective hydroxamic acid such as trichostatin A (**2**) is equipotent against HDAC1 and HDAC6, the cyclic tetrapeptide natural products are nanomolar inhibitors of HDAC1 and >1000-fold less active against HDAC6 (Table 4.2).[37] Although these natural products have an epoxyketone warhead with the potential for covalent enzyme modification, a further twist came about with the discovery by Merck of the apicidin natural products.[39,40] The apicidins (Figure 4.9) are structurally related to the epoxyketone con-taining cyclic tetrapeptides but lack the epoxide in the side-chain. Apicidin (**13**) strongly inhibits HDACs from apicomplexan parasites with an IC_{50} of 1 nM against the partially purified HDACs from *Eimeria tenella*. In a malaria model with BALB/C mice infected by *Plasmodium berghei*, apicidin was effective at doses of 10 mg kg^{-1} (parenteral) and 25 mg kg^{-1} (oral).

Apicidin, unlike the epoxyketone natural products, is a reversible HDAC inhibitor and contains a ketone as the zinc binding warhead. It is possible that the ketone is present as the hydrate when bound to HDACs to enable

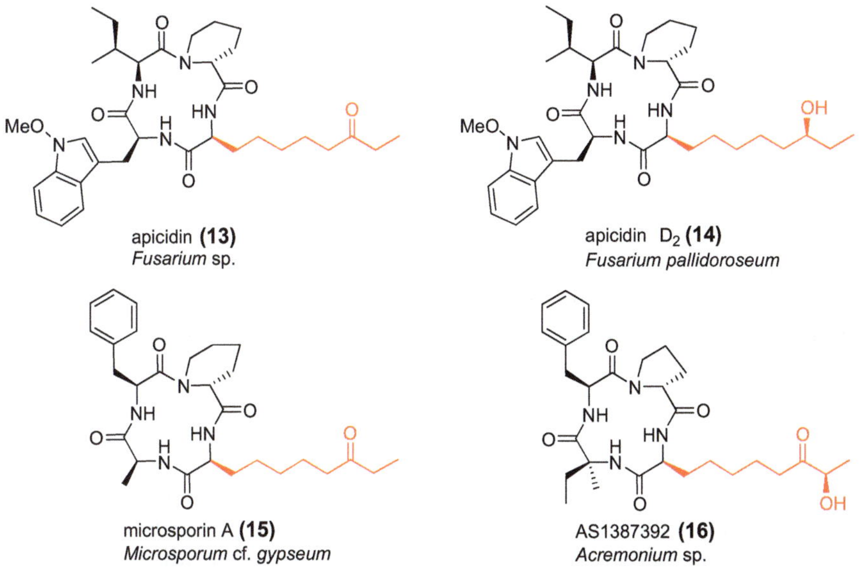

Figure 4.9 Examples of cyclic tetrapeptide HDAC inhibitors discovered subsequent to the epoxyketones in Figure 4.7.

Table 4.2 HDAC1 and HDAC6 inhibition by cyclic tetrapeptide natural products, with the IC_{50} values for trichostatin A given as a comparison.

Natural product	IC_{50} (nM) HDAC1	IC_{50} (nM) HDAC6
trichostatin A	6.0	8.6
Cyl-2	0.7	40 000
chlamydocin	0.15	1100
HC-toxin	1.0	na[a]
trapoxin B	0.11	360

[a]Not available.

tighter bidentate coordination to the metal. Interestingly, the alcohol analogue of apicidin has also been isolated as a natural product (apicidin D_2, **14**) and has a reduced IC_{50} of 400 nM against *E. tenella* HDACs. While this is a significant loss of activity compared to apicidin, it shows that even a monodentate alcohol can provide submicromolar potency with the aid of additional interactions between the macrocyclic cap and the enzyme rim. Recently, additional examples of natural products with ketone side-chains have been reported such as microsporin A[41] (**15**, IC_{50} of 140 nM against partially purified human HDACs) and AS1387392 disclosed by Astellas[42] (**16**, also known by the older code FR235225) with a hydroxy ketone side-chain. AS1387392 has an IC_{50} of 22 nM against human HDACs and displays good oral absorption in rats (C_{max} of 0.041 µg ml^{-1} after oral administration of 3.2 mg kg^{-1} and an area under the curve of 0.039 µg h ml^{-1} from 0 to 6 h after administration). The hydroxy ketone in **16** is likely to coordinate via bidentate zinc binding like the epoxyketone natural products (Figure 4.8), but without the need for covalent linkage to the enzyme and this contrasts with the loss of activity reported with earlier epoxide reductions or diol formation with HC-toxin and trapoxin.[26,38]

The potent biological activity of the cyclic tetrapeptides coupled with their unusual structures has sparked extensive synthetic investigation into these compounds to establish SAR and identify analogues with improved biological profiles. Typically, these syntheses are carried out in solution-phase as in Schreiber's approach to trapoxin (Scheme 4.1). An exception is the total synthesis of microsporin A by Silverman using a solid-phase approach (Scheme 4.2).[41] The Kenner 'safety-catch' sulfonamide resin[43] was used to assemble the linear tetrapeptide **17**, followed by resin activation towards nucleophilic attack by alkylation of the sulfonamide with iodoacetonitrile. Boc deprotection of the N-terminus then induced macrocyclization to cleave the natural product from the resin.

Merck have reported a series of apicidin analogues that were assayed against partially purified HDACs from the parasite *E. tenella* and human HeLa cells.[44,45] A linear version of apicidin generated by acidic methanolysis of the natural product and capping the N-terminus with an acetyl group was inactive, thus highlighting the importance of the macrocyclic scaffold. Replacement of the tryptophan residue by basic heterocycles as in **18** increased activity and the quinoline **19** showed selectivity towards the parasite enzyme. With the ethyl ketone warhead, replacement of the ethyl by methyl and *n*-propyl was tolerated whereas the bulkier *i*-propyl and phenyl groups led to loss of activity. Introducing an α-fluoro substituent in **20** did not increase potency although it should increase ketone hydration, whereas a hydroxy-ketone group with potential bidentate coordination as in **21** (and the later discovered natural product **16**) was beneficial.

Merck explored a variety of alternative warheads to the ketone side-chain. The carboxylic acid methyl ester **22** was surprisingly potent compared to the carboxylic acid **23** and the hydroxamic acid **24** although the latter would be expected to be superior zinc binding groups. The high activity of thiol ester **25** was attributed to hydrolysis during the assay to release a thiol warhead. Perhaps the most intriguing result was that of the saturated side-chain **26**, passed over without comment by Merck. While this compound is certainly

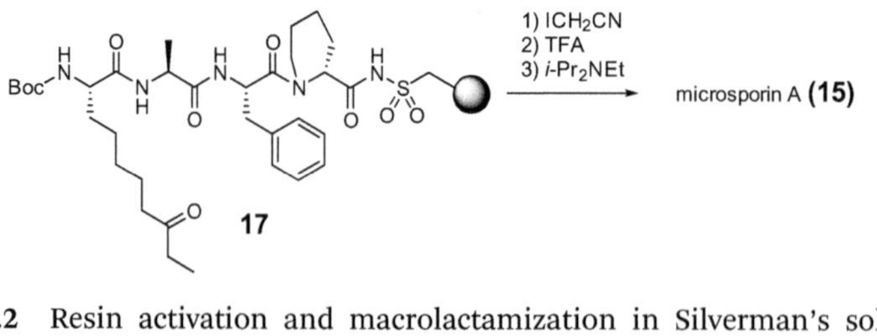

Scheme 4.2   Resin activation and macrolactamization in Silverman's solid-phase total synthesis of microsporin A.

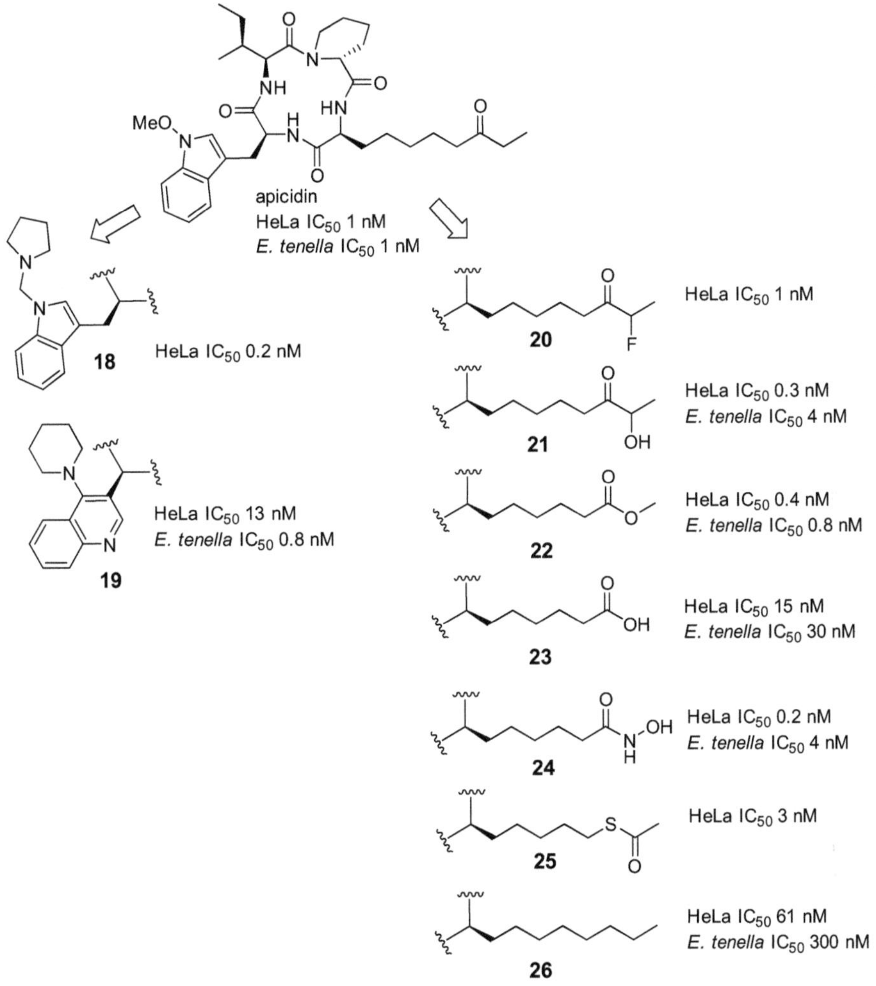

Figure 4.10 Summary of Merck's SAR of apicidin, with IC_{50} values for HDACs purified from HeLa cells and the parasite *E. tenella*.

less potent than the others in Figure 4.10, the nanomolar level of activity is high given the complete absence of a warhead and is indeed better than that observed with Merck's approved drug vorinostat (**2**, IC_{50} 288 nM, Section 4.2).

In the Merck studies, the hydroxamic acid analogue of apicidin **24** had significant activity against the human HDACs. Nishino and Yoshida extended this work by preparing hydroxamic acid versions of the epoxyketone natural products, and these CHAPs (= cyclic hydroxamic acid containing peptide) were nanomolar HDAC inhibitors.[46] The lead CHAP31 (**27**, Figure 4.11) has an IC_{50} of 1.4 nM against HDACs purified from the B16/BL6 cell line and inhibited proliferation of these cells with an IC_{50} of 5.4 nM.[47]

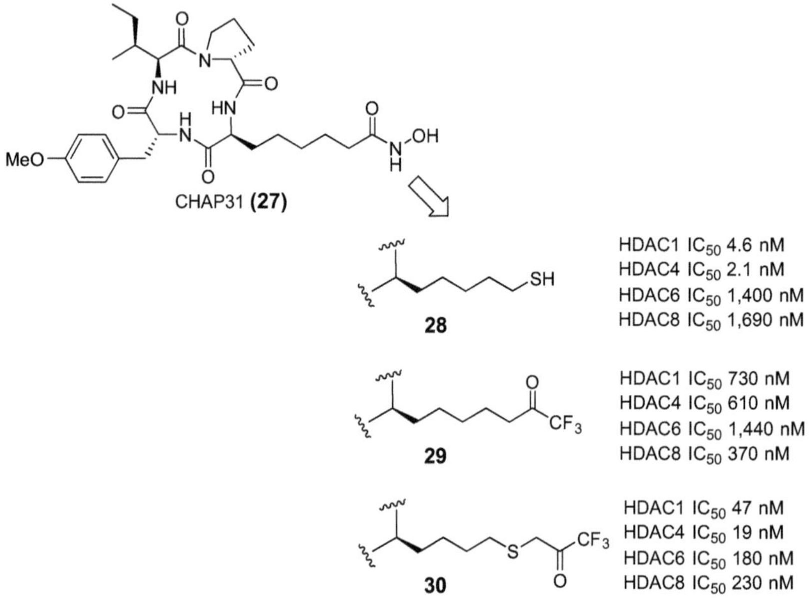

CHAP31 **(27)**

28

HDAC1 IC_{50} 4.6 nM
HDAC4 IC_{50} 2.1 nM
HDAC6 IC_{50} 1,400 nM
HDAC8 IC_{50} 1,690 nM

29

HDAC1 IC_{50} 730 nM
HDAC4 IC_{50} 610 nM
HDAC6 IC_{50} 1,440 nM
HDAC8 IC_{50} 370 nM

30

HDAC1 IC_{50} 47 nM
HDAC4 IC_{50} 19 nM
HDAC6 IC_{50} 180 nM
HDAC8 IC_{50} 230 nM

Figure 4.11   Examples of Nishino and Yoshida's synthetic cyclic tetrapeptide analogues.

Unlike the natural products, CHAP31 contains alternating L- and D-amino acids. In general, stereochemical changes in these cyclic tetrapeptides are tolerated as long as the zinc binding warhead is of L-stereochemistry to match the L-stereochemistry of the acetyl-lysine HDAC substrates that they mimic. Besides hydroxamic acids, several other zinc binding warheads were explored by Nishino and Yoshida such as thiol **28** and trifluoromethyl ketones **29** and **30** (Figure 4.11).[48,49] Compounds **28** and **30** potently inhibit HDAC1 although they have a different chain length in the spacer and it was speculated that **30** might achieve bidentate coordination by involving the thioether for metal binding. Like the natural products, all these compounds are poor inhibitors of HDAC6.

Nishino and Yoshida investigated the effect of introducing a second macrocycle by tethering two of the peptide side-chains. This was accomplished by synthesizing tetrapeptides with pendant alkenes that were subjected to ring-closing metathesis and hydrogenation.[50,51] The example **31** (Figure 4.12) displays an improved potency against HDAC1 and HDAC4 compared to the linear model compound **32**.

Recently, Ghadiri has reported modified cyclic tetrapeptides with alterations in the peptide backbone.[52] It was proposed that the most bioactive conformation of apicidin contains a *cis* amide rotamer and this was probed by incorporating a triazole isostere for the amide. The 1,5-triazole **33** (Figure 4.13) showed decreased isoform selectivity compared to apicidin, more potently inhibiting HDAC6 and HDAC8 than the natural product.

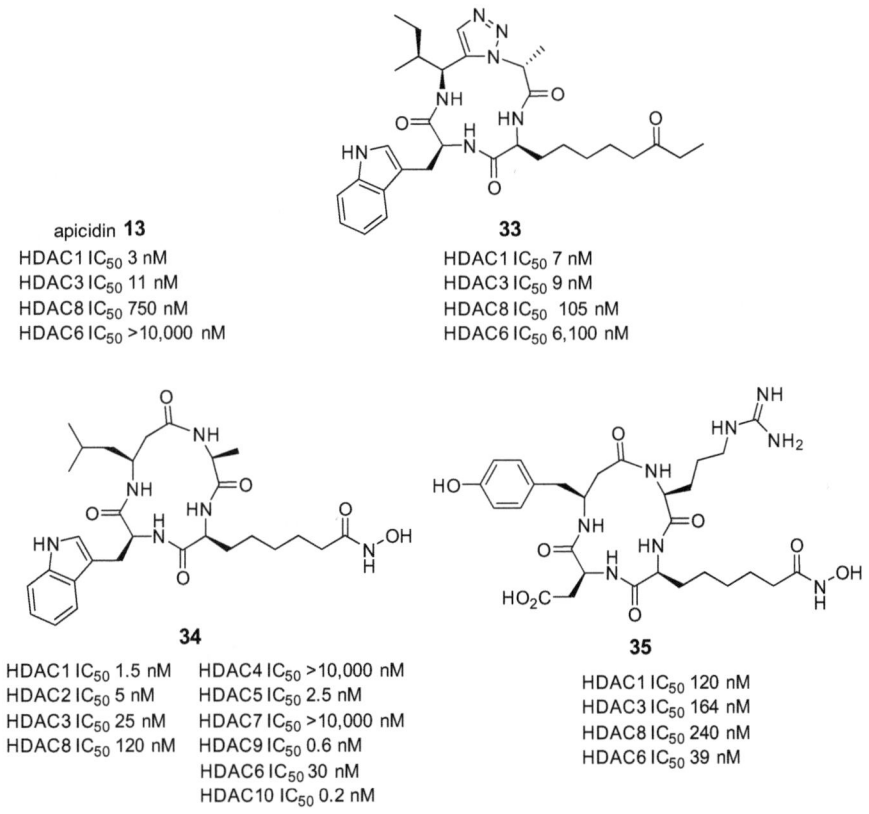

Figure 4.12   A bis-macrocyclic HDAC inhibitor **31** together with a linear macrocyclic control **32**.

31   HDAC1 IC_{50} 9.1 nM
HDAC4 IC_{50} 5.5 nM
HDAC6 IC_{50} 410 nM

32   HDAC1 IC_{50} 25 nM
HDAC4 IC_{50} 12 nM
HDAC6 IC_{50} 340 nM

apicidin **13**
HDAC1 IC_{50} 3 nM
HDAC3 IC_{50} 11 nM
HDAC8 IC_{50} 750 nM
HDAC6 IC_{50} >10,000 nM

33
HDAC1 IC_{50} 7 nM
HDAC3 IC_{50} 9 nM
HDAC8 IC_{50} 105 nM
HDAC6 IC_{50} 6,100 nM

34

HDAC1 IC_{50} 1.5 nM   HDAC4 IC_{50} >10,000 nM
HDAC2 IC_{50} 5 nM   HDAC5 IC_{50} 2.5 nM
HDAC3 IC_{50} 25 nM   HDAC7 IC_{50} >10,000 nM
HDAC8 IC_{50} 120 nM   HDAC9 IC_{50} 0.6 nM
                           HDAC6 IC_{50} 30 nM
                           HDAC10 IC_{50} 0.2 nM

35

HDAC1 IC_{50} 120 nM
HDAC3 IC_{50} 164 nM
HDAC8 IC_{50} 240 nM
HDAC6 IC_{50} 39 nM

Figure 4.13   Examples of apicidin analogues **33–35** reported by Ghadiri, with activities against HDAC isoforms compared to that of apicidin.

In addition, Ghadiri examined the effect of macrocycle size by preparing a series of apicidin analogues in which one α-amino acid is replaced by a β-amino acid.[53,54] Among these less conformationally restrained compounds, compound **34** showed some improvement in growth inhibition of cancer cell lines relative to apicidin (IC_{50} of 0.6 nM against the MCF7 breast cancer cell line compared to 7 nM for apicidin). The compound's isoform selectivity was profiled against the full set of HDACs (Figure 4.13) and it is interestingly a potent HDAC6 inhibitor unlike most of the natural products or synthetic analogues discussed above. By introducing polar and ionizable side-chains that are quite different to the hydrophobic residues present in the natural products, Ghadiri was able to further reverse this trend; analogue 35 inhibits HDAC6 more potently than the class I HDACs. However, in growth proliferation assays, the compound was only micromolar in activity presumably due to issues with cell permeability.

As a class, the cyclic tetrapeptide natural products were among the earliest compounds to be identified as HDAC inhibitors. They have led to important insights into HDAC function and the first recombinant cloning of a human HDAC, while apicidin and trapoxin continue to be widely used as chemical probes. Nevertheless, despite the high potency of the natural products as well as the many analogues prepared by industry, including examples with efficacy in animal models, none has thus far advanced to clinical development. Merck appear to have focused on antiparasitic applications and did not declare an advanced candidate compound. More recently, academic groups have concentrated on exploiting these as anticancer agents via the inhibition of human HDACs. This has generated a variety of interesting analogues and demonstrated that the scaffold tolerates changes in macrocycle size, stereochemistry, substituents and zinc binding warhead, and that such alterations influence isoform selectivity.

4.4 The Depsipeptide Natural Products with a Thiol Warhead

After the cyclic tetrapeptides, the bicyclic depsipeptides were the second class of macrocyclic natural product HDAC inhibitor to be discovered. The first and foremost example is FK228 (36, Figure 4.14), discovered by high-throughput screening at Fujisawa using a phenotypic assay for compounds with the ability to revert the morphology of *ras*-transformed cancer cells and

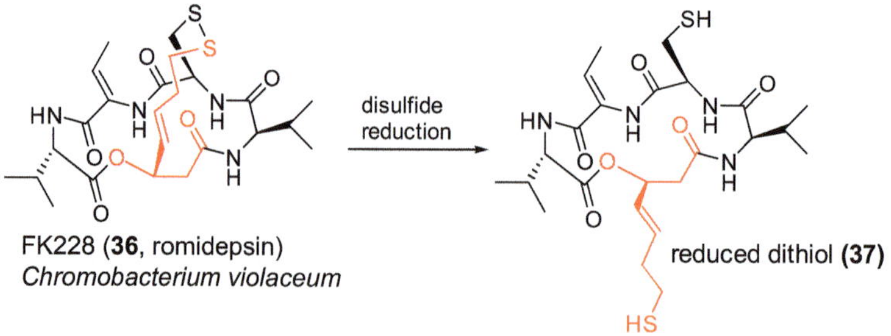

Figure 4.14   The bicyclic depsipeptide prodrug FK228 and the active form produced by disulfide reduction, with the zinc binding thiol unit shown in red.

disclosed in 1994.[55,56] FK228 was isolated from an extract of the bacterial species *Chromobacterium violaceum* and reported as having high antitumor activity in cell-based assays and ascitic and solid tumour xenograft models by intravenous and intraperitoneal administration.[57] Four years later, Yoshida demonstrated that FK228's mechanism of action is via HDAC inhibition.[58,59]

A zinc binding warhead is not discernible within the structure of FK228; however, within the reducing environment of the cell, the natural product undergoes reductive cleavage of the disulfide bridge to release the free dithiol (**37**) that reversibly binds to the HDAC active site zinc. Recent evidence for this binding mode can be found in the X-ray structure of largazole (**40**, *vide infra*) thiol, another depsipeptide HDAC inhibitor with an identical zinc binding warhead, bound to human HDAC8.[60] The X-ray structure (Figure 4.15) shows the thiol coordinated to the zinc atom within the enzyme active site, while distortions of the enzyme side-chains take place to accommodate the natural product's macrocyclic cap.

The macrocycle in these depsipeptides is similar in size to a pentapeptide and as such not bound by the steric constraints of the smaller cyclic tetrapeptides of the previous section. Of the four chiral side-chains in FK228, three are of D-stereochemistry which is consistent with the natural product acting as a retro-inverso peptide[61] when bound to HDACs. For this reason, the side-chain bearing the zinc binding thiol (in red in Figure 4.14) needs to maintain D-stereochemistry, whereas in the ketone bearing cyclic tetrapeptides, the warhead should be of L-stereochemistry to mimic a natural protein. Studies with unnatural analogues indicate that the other side-chains in depsipeptide HDAC inhibitors are tolerant of stereochemical switches

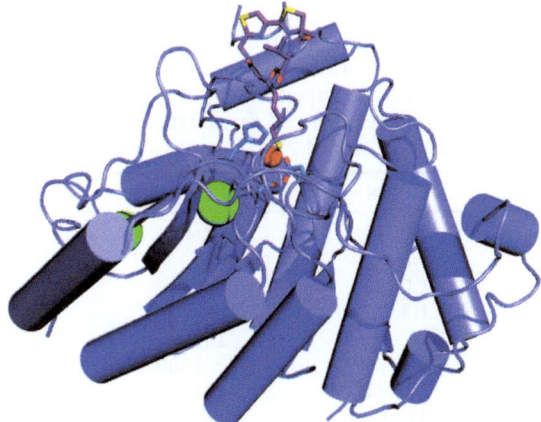

Figure 4.15 X-ray structure of largazole thiol bound to human HDAC8. The thiol is shown as a stick figure in magenta. The active site Zn^{2+} ion (red sphere) is coordinated by D178, H180 and D267 residues. Structural K^+ ions appear as green spheres.
(Reprinted with permission from ref. 60.)

although the D-stereochemistry present in the natural products is likely to be beneficial *in vivo* as it avoids hydrolysis by endogenous proteases.

The high activity of FK228 led to its progression as a preclinical candidate. Compared to the synthetic bidentate hydroxamic acids such as vorinostat (Figure 4.4), FK228 is more potent although its zinc binding warhead is a monodentate thiol. Like the cyclic tetrapeptides, the gain of potency arises from FK228's macrocyclic scaffold and its ability to engage in additional binding interactions with the enzyme. The size of the scaffold also enables FK228 to discriminate between isoforms; the reduced thiol **37** potently inhibits the class I HDACs (Table 4.3. IC_{50}: HDAC1 0.8 nM; HDAC2 1.0 nM; HDAC3 1.3 nM; HDAC8 26 nM) and is relatively poor in the inhibition of the tissue-specific class IIa HDACs and HDAC6. FK228 was out-licensed by Fujisawa to Gloucester Pharmaceuticals who named it romidepsin and began Phase I clinical trials in 2004. Romidepsin received FDA approval for the treatment of cutaneous T-cell lymphoma in 2009 and is marketed by Celgene under the trade name Istodax®. It is administered by intravenous infusion, although oral dosing in rats at 50 mg kg^{-1} gave a respectable 15.6% bioavailability given the peptidic nature of the molecule.[62] At the time of writing, romidepsin is the only HDAC inhibitor besides vorinostat to receive FDA approval.

Since the isolation of FK228, the family of depsipeptide natural product HDAC inhibitors that share an identical β-hydroxy acid subunit bearing a thiol zinc binding warhead has grown to over ten members. In the spiruchostatins isolated from *Pseudomonas* strains and exemplified by spiruchostatin A (**38**, Figure 4.16), disclosed by Yamanouchi,[63] the warhead is tied up as an internal disulfide as in FKK28. The spiruchostatins contain a statine β-amino acid instead of the unsaturated dehydrobutyrine (Dhb) amino acid residue present in FK228. Recently, genome mining experiments

Table 4.3 IC_{50} values (nM) for inhibition of HDACs from HeLa nuclear extracts and individual HDAC isoforms (where available) by thiol forms of members of the FK228 family of depsipeptide natural products and growth inhibition of the MCF7 breast cancer cell line by the prodrug natural products (data taken from ref. 68, 74 and 75).

Assay	FK228	Largazole	Thailandepsin A
HeLa HDACs	24	0.04	5
HDAC1	0.8	0.4	14
HDAC2	1.0	0.9	3.5
HDAC3	1.3	0.7	4.8
HDAC8	26	102	1200
HDAC4	470	>1000	42 000
HDAC5	>1000	>1000	
HDAC7	3200	>1000	11 000
HDAC9	12 000	>1000	12 000
HDAC6	330	42	380
HDAC10	0.9	0.5	
HDAC11	0.3	>1000	
MCF7	1	5	0.06

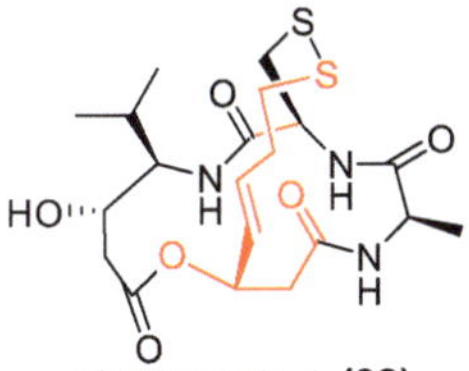

spiruchostatin A (38)
Pseudomonas sp.
HeLa HDACs (thiol) IC_{50} 5 nM

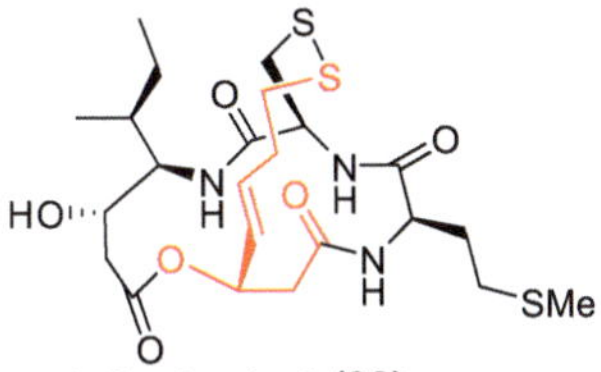

thailandepsin A (39)
Burkholdac thailandensis
HeLa HDACs (thiol) IC_{50} 5 nM

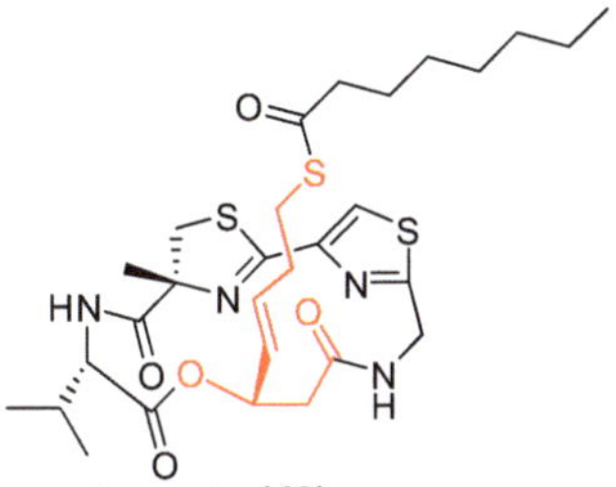

largazole (40)
Symploca sp.
HeLa HDACs (thiol) IC_{50} 0.04 nM

Figure 4.16 Examples of the FK228 family of depsipeptide HDAC inhibitors. Enzyme inhibition values are given for the free thiol.

by Cheng based on the FK228 gene cluster[64,65] have led to the identification of additional spiruchostatin examples from *Burkholderia thailandensis* named thailandepsins, such as thailandepsin A (39).[66–68] Meanwhile, largazole (40) isolated from the marine cyanobacterium *Symploca* sp. has some unique features.[69] In largazole, the zinc binding thiol is masked as a metabolically labile ester rather than a disulfide and the peptide backbone has undergone cyclization with the side-chains to form thiazole and thiazoline heterocycles.

Among the newer depsipeptides, largazole is exceptionally potent in enzyme assays with an IC_{50} of 40 pM against HeLa HDACs and subnanomolar IC_{50} values against HDAC1, 2 and 3 (Table 4.3). The activity in cell proliferation assays is lower, which might be partially due to the thiol ester prodrug nature of the natural product. Thailandepsin A, on the other hand, is similar in enzyme activity to FK228 (Table 4.3) but significantly more potent in the cell assay and this may be due to subtle differences in isoform selectivity between the two natural products. As they were discovered more recently, it is too early to tell if the spiruchostatins or largazole, or analogues thereof, will progress to clinical trials as FK228 did.

There have been many total syntheses of the depsipeptide HDAC inhibitors by academic groups. In the first, by Simon,[70] macrolactonization of the linear *seco*-hydroxy acid **41** (Scheme 4.3) to the FK228 precursor **43** proved to be challenging under the usual conditions of carboxylic acid activation due to competing elimination of the allylic alcohol. Instead, the cyclization was accomplished by alcohol inversion under Mitsunobu conditions using large

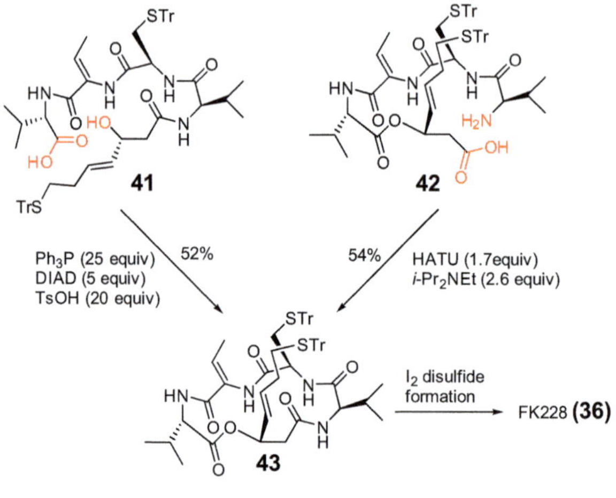

Scheme 4.3 Macrolactonization and macrolactamization routes to FK228.

excesses of reagents. Subsequent total syntheses by Williams[71] and Ganesan[72] found the macrolactonization to proceed with poor yields, and Ganesan instead adopted a macrolactamization strategy to FK228 via the intermediate **42**. Similarly, total syntheses of largazole have also relied on macrolactamization; in both FK228 and largazole, the steric hindrance caused by the α-isopropyl side-chain of the carboxylic acid hinders macrolactonization whereas it has been successful in approaches to the spiruchostatins[73] and thailandepsins[74] that lack this alkyl group.

All of the macrocyclic depsipeptide natural products contain the identical zinc binding thiol side-chain. Various syntheses of this subunit have been reported; that by Ganesan involves an asymmetric acetate aldol reaction of aldehyde **44** (Scheme 4.4) using the Fujita-Nagao thiazolidinethione chiral auxiliary to give protected β-hydroxy acid **45**.[73] Others such as Luesch have carried out the aldol reaction with acrolein to give the simpler product **46**.[75] The vinyl compound is incorporated into the macrocycle, and the thiol side-chain later introduced by alkene cross-metathesis. This approach has the advantage that a variety of zinc binding groups or chain lengths can be appended at a late stage for SAR studies, and confirmed that the natural products contain the optimal chain length for HDAC inhibition. A quite different route to the vinyl carboxylate was recently reported in Breit's synthesis of homolargazole.[76] Rhodium-catalysed hydrocarboxylation of allene **47** gave the protected ester **48** in high yield and diastereoselectivity.

The total syntheses and SAR studies, notably by Ganesan[77] with FK228 and Williams[78,79] with largazole, have identified the key features within depsipeptide HDAC inhibitors that are required for HDAC inhibition (Figure 4.17). The macrocyclic backbone is essential as linear uncyclized compounds are inactive. Within the macrocycle, the zinc binding thiol warhead needs to be of D-stereochemistry and the epimer is virtually inactive, while the other amino acid residues present can be varied without loss in activity. The

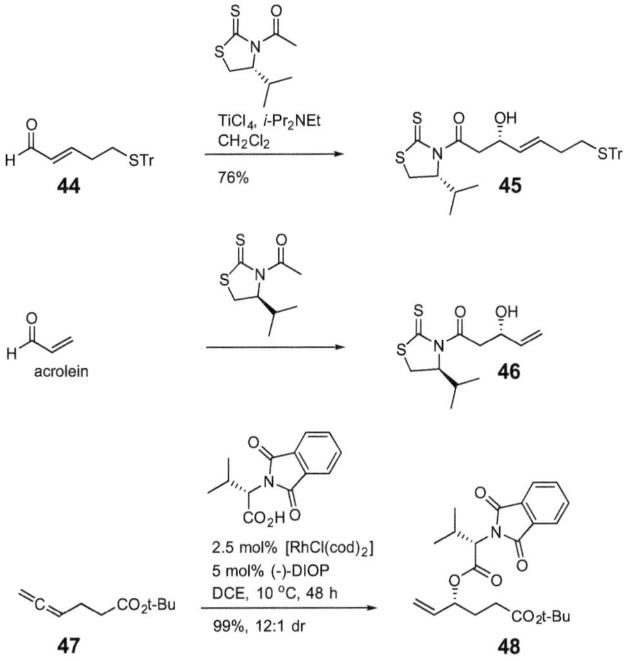

Scheme 4.4 Synthesis of the β-hydroxy-γ,δ-unsaturated acid present in the depsi-peptide natural products.

dehydrobutyrine Michael acceptor is not needed and it is speculated that its function is to tie up the thiol from the cysteine side-chain upon disulfide ring opening. The zinc binding thiol warhead needs to be protected to ensure efficient cell uptake, whether as a disulfide as in FK228 or a thioester as in largazole and synthetic analogues. Cleavage of the octanoyl ester in largazole by liver microsomes was found to be very rapid ($t_{1/2} < 5$ minutes), suggesting that other esters should be preferred for *in vivo* applications.[80]

Among the depsipeptide analogues that illustrate the above SAR trends are compounds **49–51**. In compound **49**, reported by Ganesan, the FK228 scaffold has been simplified without loss of activity (HeLa HDACs IC$_{50}$ 5 nM) by (i) replacing the dehydrobutyrine residue with a chemically inert valine and (ii) replacing a second valine residue by glycine.[77] The largazole analogue **50** synthesized by Williams features a thiazole-pyridine switch and is among the most potent depsipeptides in terms of enzyme inhibition (HDAC1 IC$_{50}$ 0.32 nM).[78] Meanwhile, Ganesan's analogue **51** shows that replacement of the thiazoline ring in largazole by a simpler achiral α-aminoisobutyric acid residue is tolerated (HeLa HDACs IC$_{50}$ 1 nM).[80]

A different approach was taken by Ahn, who redesigned the spacer present in the depsipeptide natural products by employing an isosteric thiol. Instead of the β-hydroxy acid unit that needs to be obtained by total synthesis (Scheme 4.4), Ahn linked differentially protected aspartic acid to cysteamine

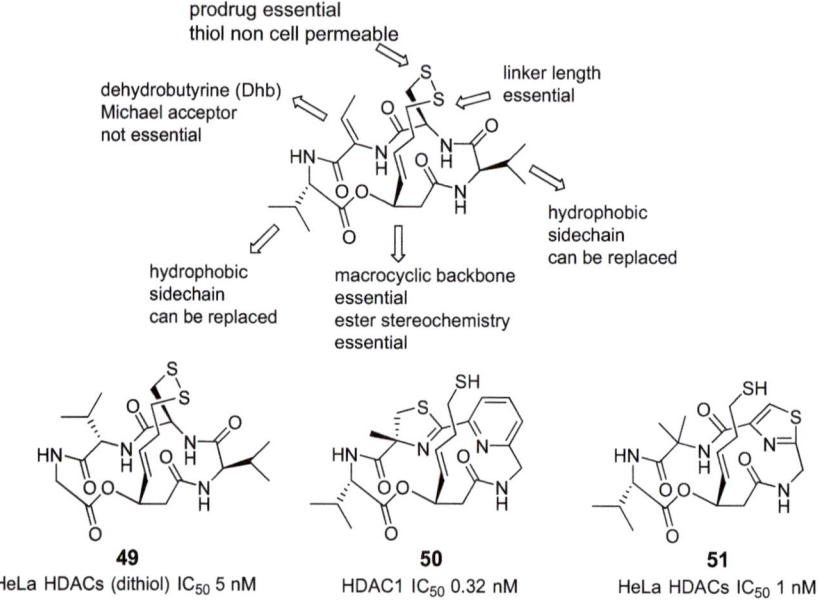

Figure 4.17 Key SAR of FK228 and examples of potent synthetic depsipeptide analogues **49–51**.

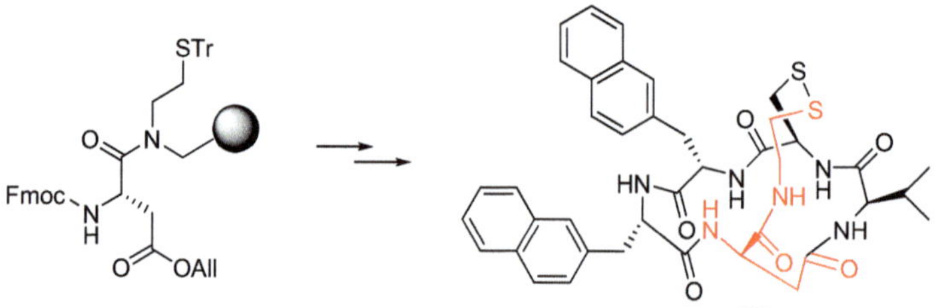

Figure 4.18 Synthesis of an analogue **52** of the depsipeptide natural products with an isosteric substitution of the zinc binding warhead.

immobilized on the backbone amide linker (BAL) resin (Figure 4.18). Solid-phase synthesis and disulfide bridging with a cysteine residue led to a series of cyclic peptide isosteres of the depsipeptides such as **52**.[81,82] Although these analogues were growth inhibitors of cancer cell lines and induced fetal haemoglobin in erythroid progenitors, detailed investigation of their HDAC inhibitory activity has not been published.

4.5 The Azumamide Natural Products with a Carboxylic Acid Warhead

The azumamides are a family of natural product HDAC inhibitors isolated from the marine sponge *Mycale izuensis* (Figure 4.19).[83] Interestingly, the

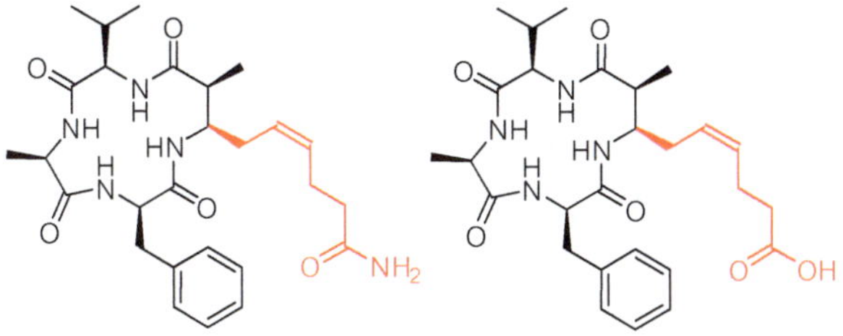

azumamide A (**53**)
HeLa HDACs IC$_{50}$5800 nM

azumamide E (**54**)
HeLa HDACs IC$_{50}$110 nM

Figure 4.19   Structures of azumamides A and E.

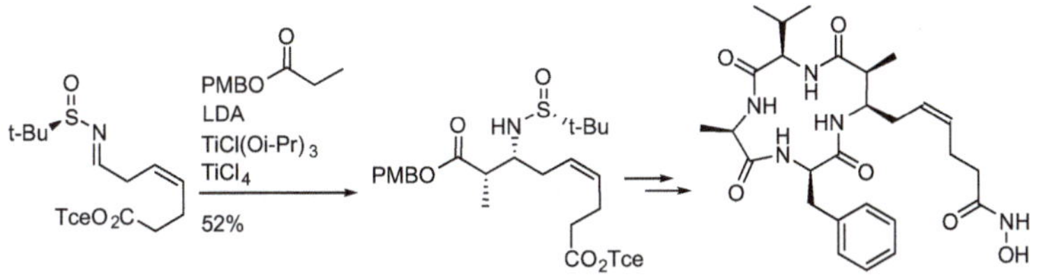

55   **56**   **57**

HeLa HDACs IC$_{50}$ 7 nM

Scheme 4.5   Synthesis of the azumamide β-amino acid via stereoselective imino aldol reaction and further conversion to the unnatural hydroxamic acid analogue **57**.

zinc binding warhead in these natural products is either a carboxamide (azumamide A, **53**) or a carboxylic acid (azumamide E, **54**). In the literature, the azumamides are often grouped together with the cyclic tetrapeptides in Section 4.3. However, this is incorrect as the azumamide scaffold is composed of three α-amino acids and one β-amino acid. Thus, the macrocycle contains an additional atom compared to the trapoxin or apicidin tetra-peptides and this is sufficient to relax the stereochemical requirements and permit all side-chains to be homochiral. In this regard, the D-stereo-chemistry of the azumamide residues results in a retro-inverso peptide and in terms of both chirality and macrocycle size the azumamides are closer to the FK228 depsipeptides than the cyclic tetrapeptides.

Several academic groups have accomplished the total synthesis of the azumamides. In Ganesan's route,[84] the unnatural β-amino acid was prepared by an imino aldol reaction between imine **55** (Scheme 4.5) containing Ellman's *tert*-butylsulfinyl chiral auxiliary[85] and a propionate enolate to afford **56** as a single diastereomer. This was carried forward to a linear peptide followed by macrolactamization to accomplish the total synthesis of azu-mamides A and E. Biological assays established that azumamide A (HeLa HDACs IC$_{50}$ = 5800 nM) was a significantly poorer HDAC inhibitor compared to azumamide E (HeLa HDACs IC$_{50}$ = 110 nM), as would be predicted based on the weaker zinc binding affinity of a neutral carboxamide relative to an ionized carboxylic acid. Besides the azumamides, the unnatural analogue **57** with a hydroxamic acid warhead was prepared and shown to be significantly more active (HeLa HDACs $IC_{50} = 7$ nM) than the natural products. Like the cyclic tetrapeptides and depsipeptides in the previous sections, the azumamides are relatively poor in the inhibition of HDAC6; for example **57** had an IC_{50} of 3 and 143 nM respectively against HDAC1 and HDAC6.

4.6 Synthetic Macrocyclic HDAC Inhibitors

The previous sections have shown that Nature has evolved a variety of macrocyclic HDAC inhibitors using peptide and depsipeptide scaffolds. Throughout, a common motif has been potent enzyme inhibition achieved by augmenting the zinc binding warhead by additional binding interactions with the macrocyclic cap. In a similar vein, a number of fully synthetic HDAC inhibitors have been designed that incorporate a macrocyclic cap. In the earliest example, from Abbott,[86] intramolecular Mitsunobu alkylation of **58** (Figure 4.20) gave the macrocycle **59** that was carried forward to hydroxamic acid **60**. Compound **60** had an IC_{50} of 38 nM against HDACs isolated from the K562 cell line; however, the importance of the macrocycle is unclear as the uncyclized version **61** was equipotent in HDAC inhibition.

Starting from a differentially protected *bis*-amino acid, Etzkorn assembled the peptidomimetic macrocyclic hydroxamic acid **62** (Figure 4.21).[87] This compound had an IC_{50} of 46 nM against HeLa HDACs compared to 167 nM for the linear peptide **63**, indicating that the conformational rigidity imposed by the macrocycle was beneficial for biological activity. Using a

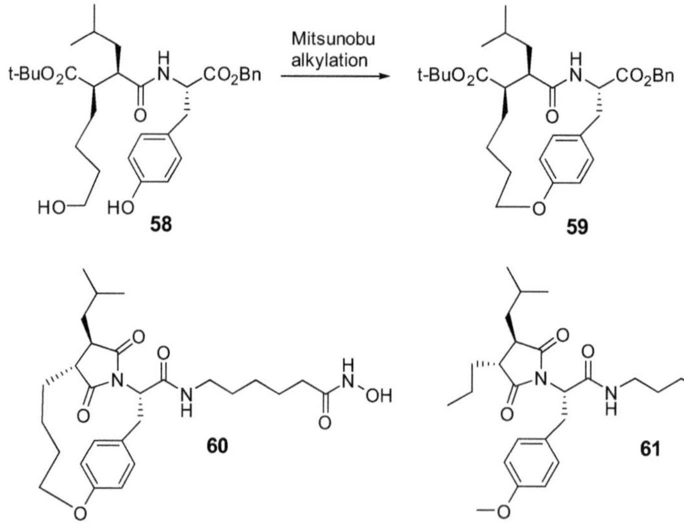

Figure 4.20 Synthesis of the macrocyclic scaffold **59** leading to HDAC inhibitor **60** and a linear analogue **61**.

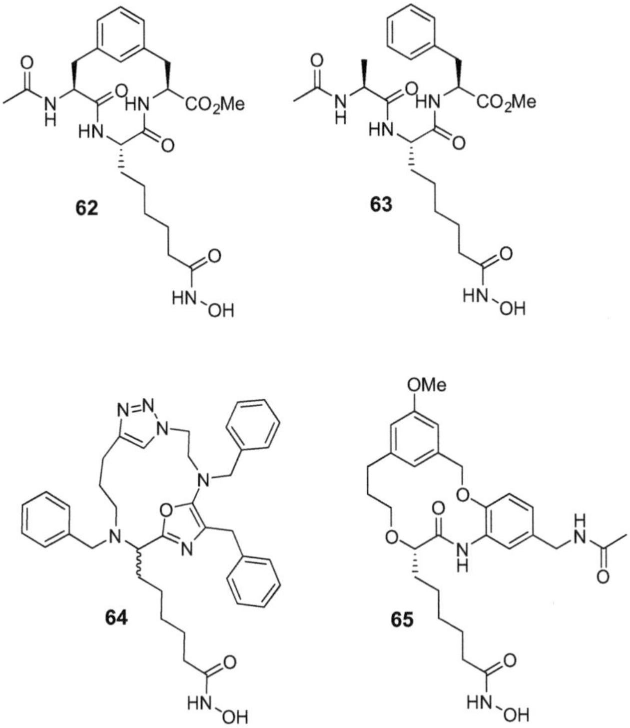

Figure 4.21 Examples of peptidomimetic HDAC inhibitors, together with a linear peptide **63** used as a control for **62**.

three-component condensation between isonitrile, amine and aldehyde, Bifulco and Tron constructed an oxazole core that was elaborated to the macrocycle **64** by copper-catalysed Huisgen alkyne-azide 1,3-dipolar 'click' cycloaddition.[88] The racemic macrocycle was active in a cell-based HDAC assay with an IC_{50} of 4.3 μM although results from an *in vitro* enzyme assay were not reported. More recently, Hanessian has prepared a library of macrocyclic HDAC inhibitors.[89] The lead compound, **65**, was a nanomolar inhibitor of class I, II and IV HDACs and displayed isoform selectivity for the cytoplasmic HDAC6 (IC_{50} of 0.4 nM versus, for example, 41 nM against HDAC1).

In the application of macrocyclic scaffolds for drug discovery, a major bottleneck is synthetic tractability and the need to make multiple analogues to explore each scaffold. To address these issues, Tang and Schreiber designed a series of aldehyde bearing macrocycles that are obtained by ring-closing metathesis from readily accessible precursors.[90] These caps were then condensed in microtitre plates with hydrazines connected to a spacer and hydroxamic acid warhead to generate a library of potential HDAC inhibitors in situ, followed by enzymatic assay without purification. From this library, macrocycle **66** (Figure 4.22) was found to be HDAC8 selective

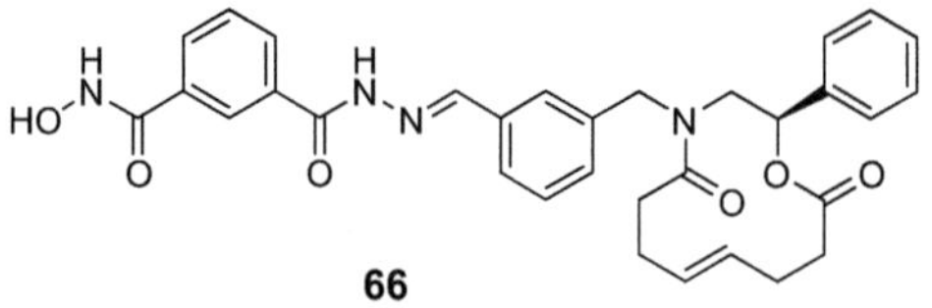

66

HDAC1 3600 nM
HDAC3 15,000 nM
HDAC8 23 nM

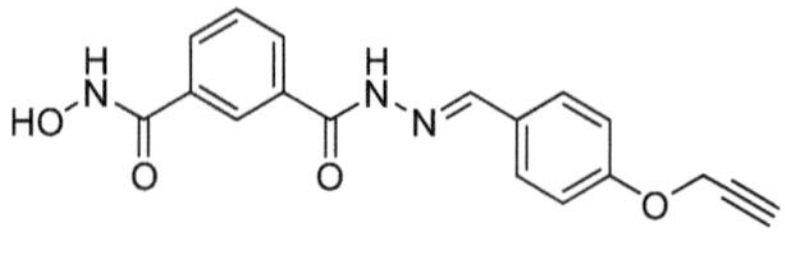

67

HDAC1 6300 nM
HDAC3 6200 nM
HDAC8 29 nM

Figure 4.22 Structure of two HDAC inhibitors obtained by aldehyde–hydrazine condensation, with IC_{50} values against specific HDAC isoforms indicated.

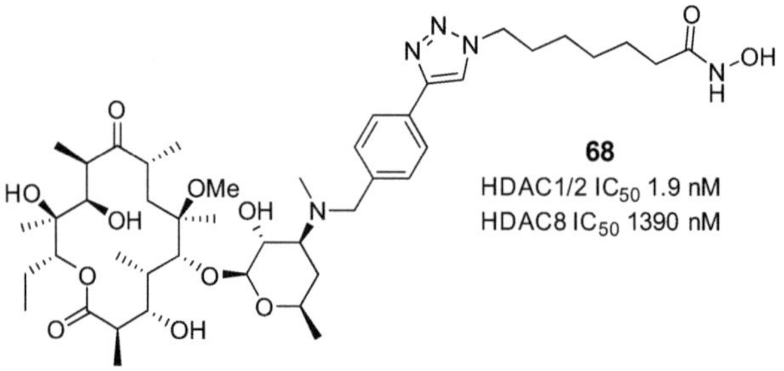

68

HDAC1/2 IC_{50} 1.9 nM
HDAC8 IC_{50} 1390 nM

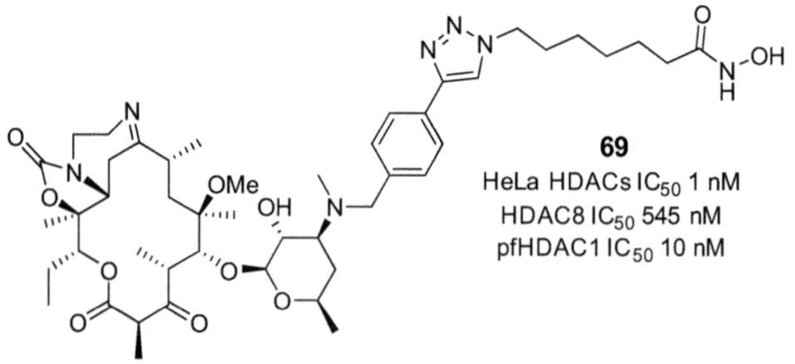

69

HeLa HDACs IC_{50} 1 nM
HDAC8 IC_{50} 545 nM
pfHDAC1 IC_{50} 10 nM

Figure 4.23 Examples of HDAC inhibitors with a cap derived from macrolide antibiotics.

($IC_{50} = 23$ nM) in its inhibition profile. Nevertheless, the linear hydroxamic acid **67** from the same library had a similar activity against HDAC8 ($IC_{50} = 29$ nM) and an improved HDAC1/HDAC8 isoform selectivity.

Up to now, the synthetic macrocycles discussed in this section are all peptidomimetic in nature and prepared by multistep sequences. A radically different strategy was taken by Oyelere, who grafted the hydroxamic acid zinc binding warhead and a spacer onto macrocycles that are readily available from other biologically active molecules. A series of scaffolds was prepared from the macrolide family of antibacterial agents and derivatized with pendant alkynes.[91,92] 'Click' cycloaddition with hydroxamic acids containing a terminal azide produced a library of potential HDAC inhibitors that illustrate how changes in the macrocycle can influence activity even when the spacer and warhead are identical. Compounds **68** and **69** (Figure 4.23) respectively feature macrocycles derived from erythromycin and the tricyclic ketolide TE-802. Both compounds inhibit human HDACs, and **69** was a nanomolar inhibitor of HDAC1 from *Plasmodium falciparum*. In cell proliferation assays, these compounds had a reduced micromolar level of activity.

4.7 Summary

The warhead-spacer-cap pharmacophore for HDAC inhibition does not obligatorily require a macrocyclic scaffold; indeed the compounds that have reached clinical trials do not contain a macrocycle with the single (but important) exception of FK228. Nevertheless, the many natural and synthetic HDAC inhibitors discussed in this chapter highlight the value of macrocycles in general to increase target affinity and selectivity – features that are of importance in applications ranging from *in vitro* profiling and chemical biology to *in vivo* models and drug discovery. We may draw some general conclusions from the experience gained by the study of macrocyclic HDAC inhibitors:

1. Each macrocyclic scaffold has a preferred length of the spacer and warhead to promote optimal interaction with the enzyme active site; shorter or longer spacers then lead to loss of activity.
2. Each macrocyclic scaffold has a characteristic pattern of isoform selectivity. However, within a scaffold, further refinements in selectivity are possible (*e.g.* compare FK228 **36**, thailandepsin A **39** and largazole **40** in Table 4.3) and in certain cases the selectivity can be overturned by the choice of substituents (*e.g.* apicidin **13** versus analogue **35**).
3. Each macrocyclic scaffold can tolerate some variation in zinc binding warhead, with bidentate chelators often providing the highest activity.
4. The importance of the macrocyclic scaffold, whether in HDAC inhibitors or other areas of drug discovery, may not always be clear. It is important to compare the activity of macrocycles with linear analogues to define the contributions specific to the macrocycle and this should be ideally backed up by X-ray crystallography of enzyme–inhibitor complexes.
5. Macrocycles have the potential to display more chemical information and engage in additional target binding interactions compared to linear or smaller ring containing congeners while the additional rigidity imposed by the macrocycle can improve physicochemical properties. The challenge lies in juggling these gains with the ease of macrocycle synthesis and improving ligand efficiency compared to a non-macrocyclic smaller molecule.

The macrocyclic HDAC inhibitors have already culminated in one approved drug (FK228, romidepsin) and have greatly aided our understanding of the target and its physiological relevance. Further success stories can be anticipated with the knowledge that has been accumulated and the increased availability of HDAC X-ray structures and homology models to aid inhibitor design. The future is likely to see an even greater importance placed on HDACs as drug discovery targets as their biology becomes better understood and inhibitors become valuable in multiple therapeutic applications, either as single agents or in combination therapy.

4.8   Notes

This review covers published material up to March 2014. In doing so, patents have deliberately been excluded as source material, since it is not always possible to match biological data to specific compounds or substantiate claims that have not been peer-reviewed. Even with this qualification, the primary literature on macrocyclic HDAC inhibitors is extensive. For reasons of space, this chapter is focused on examples with biological data and only the most potent compounds within a series are discussed. I apologize to those scientists whose elegant accomplishments have been presented in abridged form or omitted entirely but interested readers will be able to find further details in the references.

References

1. P. Chi, C. D. Allis and G. G. Wang, *Nat. Rev. Cancer*, 2010, **10**, 457.
2. C. M. Rivera and B. Ren, *Cell*, 2013, **155**, 39.
3. T. L. Newkirk, A. A. Bowers and R. M. Williams, *Nat. Prod. Rep.*, 2009, **26**, 1293.
4. S. C. Mwakwari, V. Patil, W. Guerrant and A. K. Oyelere, *Curr. Top. Med. Chem.*, 2010, **10**, 1423.
5. S. Knapp, *Med. Chem. Commun.*, 2014, **5**, 288.
6. G. E. Zentner and S. Henikoff, *Nat. Rev. Struct. Mol. Biol.*, 2013, **20**, 259.
7. S. Grant, C. Easley and P. Kirkpatrick, *Nat. Rev. Drug Discov.*, 2007, **6**, 21.
8. K. M. VanderMolen, W. McCulloch, C. J. Pearce and N. H. Oberlies, *J. Antibiot.*, 2011, **64**, 525.
9. C. E. Tiffon, J. E. Adams, L. van der Fits, S. Wen, P. A. Townsend, A. Ganesan, E. Hodges, M. H. Vermeer and G. Packham, *Br. J. Pharmacol.*, 2011, **162**, 1590.
10. X. J. Yang and E. Seto, *Nat. Rev. Mol. Cell. Biol.*, 2008, **9**, 206.
11. A. Ganesan, L. Nolan, S. J. Crabb and G. Packham, *Curr. Cancer Drug Tar.*, 2009, **2**, 963.
12. H. J. Kim and S. C. Bae, *Am. J. Transl. Res.*, 2011, **3**, 166.
13. K. Ververis, A. Hiong, T. C. Karagiannis and P. V. Licciardi, *Biologics: Tar. Ther.*, 2013, **7**, 47.
14. X. J. Yang and E. Seto, *Mol. Cell*, 2008, **31**, 449.
15. B. N. Singh, G. H. Zhang, Y. L. Hwa, J. P. Li, S. C. Dowdy and S. W. Jiang, *Expert Rev. Anticancer Ther.*, 2010, **10**, 935.
16. C. A. Dinarello, G. Fossati and P. Mascagni, *Mol. Med.*, 2011, **17**, 333.

17. J. Tang, H. Yan and S. Zhuang, *Clin. Sci.*, 2013, **124**, 651.
18. P. M. Lombardi, K. E. Cole, D. P. Dowling and D. W. Christianson, *Curr. Opin. Struct. Biol.*, 2011, **6**, 735.
19. M. Paris, M. Porcelloni, M. Binaschi and D. Fattori, *J. Med. Chem.*, 2008, **51**, 1505.
20. P. Jones, *Med. Chem. Commun.*, 2012, **3**, 135.
21. M. Yoshida, M. Kijima, M. Akita and T. Beppu, *J. Biol. Chem.*, 1990, **265**, 17174.
22. M. S. Finnin, J. R. Donigian, A. Cohen, V. M. Richon, R. A. Rifkind, P. A. Marks, R. Breslow and N. P. Pavletich, *Nature*, 1999, **401**, 188.
23. P. A. Marks and R. Breslow, *Nat. Biotechnol.*, 2007, **25**, 84.
24. D. J. Witter, P. Harrington, K. J. Wilson, M. Chenard, J. C. Fleming, B. Haines, A. M. Kral, J. P. Secrist and T. A. Miller, *Bioorg. Med. Chem. Lett.*, 2008, **18**, 726.
25. A. Hirota, A. Suzuki, K. Aizawa and S. Tamura, *Agric. Biol. Chem.*, 1973, **37**, 955.
26. A. Closse and R. Huguenin, *Helvet. Chim. Acta*, 1974, **57**, 533.
27. J. Liesch, C. Sweeley, G. Staffled, M. Anderson, D. Weber and R. Scheffer, *Tetrahedron*, 1982, **38**, 45.
28. K. Umehara, K. Nakahara, S. Kiyoto, M. Iwami, M. Okamoto, H. Tanaka, M. Kohsaka, H. Aoki and H. Imanaka, *J. Antibiot.*, 1983, **36**, 478.
29. H. Itazaki, K. Nagashima, K. Sugita, H. Yoshida, Y. Kawamura, Y. Yasuda, K. Matsumoto, K. Ishii, N. Uotani, H. Nakai, A. Terui, S. Yoshimatsu, Y. Ikenishi and Y. Nakagawa, *J. Antibiot.*, 1990, **43**, 1524.
30. M. Kawai and D. H. Rich, *Tetrahedron Lett.*, 1983, **24**, 5309.
31. U. Schmidt, A. Lieberknecht, H. Griesser and F. Bartkowiak, *Angew. Chem. Int. Ed. Engl.*, 1984, **23**, 318.
32. U. Schmidt, U. Beutler and A. Lieberknecht, *Angew. Chem. Int. Ed. Engl.*, 1989, **28**, 333.
33. J. E. Baldwin, R. M. Adlington, C. R. A. Godfrey and V. K. Patel, *Tetrahedron*, 1993, **49**, 7837.
34. M. Kijima, M. Yoshida, K. Sugita, S. Horinouchi and T. Beppu, *J. Biol. Chem.*, 1993, **268**, 22429.
35. L. M. Ciuffetti, M. R. Pope, L. D. Dunkle, J. M. Daly and H. W. Knoche, *Biochemistry*, 1983, **22**, 3507.
36. J. Taunton, J. L. Collins and S. L. Schreiber, *J. Am. Chem. Soc.*, 1996, **118**, 10412.
37. J. Taunton, C. A. Hassig and S. L. Schreiber, *Science*, 1996, **272**, 408.
38. R. Furumai, Y. Komatsu, N. Nishino, S. Khochbin, M. Yoshida and S. Horinouchi, *Proc. Natl. Acad. Sci. USA*, 2001, **98**, 87.
39. S. J. Darkin-Rattray, A. M. Gurnett, R. W. Myers, P. M. Dulski, T. M. Crumley, J. J. Allocco, C. Cannova, P. T. Meinke, S. L. Colletti, M. A. Bednarek, S. B. Singh, M. A. Goetz, A. W. Dombrowski, J. D. Polishook and D. M. Schmatz, *Proc. Natl. Acad. Sci. USA*, 1996, **93**, 13143.
40. S. B. Singh, D. L. Zink, J. M. Liesch, R. T. Mosley, A. W. Dombrowski and G. F. Bills, *J. Org. Chem.*, 2002, **67**, 815.

41. W. Gu, M. Cueto, P. R. Jensen, W. Fenical and R. B. Silverman, *Tetrahedron*, 2007, **63**, 6535.

42. S. Sasamura, K. Sakamoto, S. Takagaki, T. Yamada, S. Takase, H. Mori, T. Fujii, M. Hino and M. Hashimoto, *J. Antibiot.*, 2010, **63**, 633.

43. A. Ganesan, in *Linker Strategies in Solid-phase Organic Synthesis*. ed. P. J. H. Scott, Wiley, 2009, pp. 135–150.

44. S. L. Colletti, R. W. Myers, S. J. Darkin-Rattray, A. M. Gurnett, P. M. Dulski, S. Galuska, J. J. Allocco, M. B. Ayer, C. Li, J. Lim, T. M. Crumley, C. Cannova, D. M. Schmatz, M. J. Wyvratt, M. H. Fisher and P. T. Meinke, *Bioorg. Med. Chem. Lett.*, 2001, **11**, 107.

45. S. L. Colletti, R. W. Myers, S. J. Darkin-Rattray, A. M. Gurnett, P. M. Dulski, S. Galuska, J. J. Allocco, M. B. Ayer, C. Li, J. Lim, T. M. Crumley, C. Cannova, D. M. Schmatz, M. J. Wyvratt, M. H. Fisher and P. T. Meinke, *Bioorg. Med. Chem. Lett.*, 2001, **11**, 113.

46. R. Furumai, Y. Komatsu, N. Nishino, S. Khochbin, M. Yoshida and S. Horinouchi, *Proc. Natl. Acad. Sci. USA*, 2001, **98**, 87.

47. Y. Komatsu, K. Y. Tomizaki, M. Tsukamoto, T. Kato, N. Nishino, S. Sato, T. Yamori, T. Tsuruo, R. Furumai, M. Yoshida, S. Horinouchi and H. Hayashi, *Cancer Res.*, 2001, **61**, 4459.

48. N. Nishino, B. Jose, S. Okamura, S. Ebisusaki, T. Kato, Y. Sumida and M. Yoshida, *Org. Lett.*, 2003, **5**, 5079.

49. B. Jose, Y. Oniki, T. Kato, N. Nishino, Y. Sumida and M. Yoshida, *Bioorg. Med. Chem. Lett.*, 2004, **14**, 5343.

50. N. Nishino, G. M. Shivashimpi, P. B. Soni, M. P. Bhuiyan, T. Kato, S. Maeda, T. G. Nishino and M. Yoshida, *Bioorg. Med. Chem.*, 2008, **16**, 437.

51. N. M. Islam, T. Kato, N. Nishino, H. J. Kim, A. Ito and M. Yoshida, *Bioorg. Med. Chem. Lett.*, 2010, **20**, 997.

52. W. S. Horne, C. A. Olsen, J. M. Beierle, A. Montero and M. R. Ghadiri, *Angew. Chem. Int. Ed.*, 2009, **48**, 4718.

53. A. Montero, J. M. Beierle, C. A. Olsen and M. R. Ghadiri, *J. Am. Chem. Soc.*, 2009, **131**, 3033.

54. C. A. Olsen and M. R. Ghadiri, *J. Med. Chem.*, 2009, **52**, 7836.

55. H. Ueda, H. Nakajima, Y. Hori, T. Fujita, M. Nishimura, T. Goto and M. Okuhara, *J. Antibiot.*, 1994, **47**, 301.

56. N. Shigematsu, H. Ueda, S. Takase, H. Tanaka, K. Yamamoto and T. Tada, *J. Antibiot.*, 1994, **47**, 311.

57. H. Ueda, T. Manda, S. Matsumoto, S. Mukumoto, F. Nishigaki, I. Kawamura and K. Shimomura, *J. Antibiot.*, 1994, **47**, 315.

58. H. Nakajima, Y. B. Kim, H. Terano, M. Yoshida and S. Horinouchi, *Exp. Cell Res.*, 1998, **241**, 126.

59. R. Furumai, A. Matsuyama, N. Kobashi, K.-H. Lee, N. Nishiyama, H. Nakajima, A. Tanaka, Y. Komatsu, N. Nishino, M. Yoshida and S. Horinouchi, *Cancer Res.*, 2002, **62**, 4916.

60. K. E. Cole, D. P. Dowling, M. A. Boone, A. J. Phillips and D. W. Christianson, *J. Am. Chem. Soc.*, 2011, **133**, 12474.

61. M. D. Fletcher and M. M. Campbell, *Chem. Rev.*, 1998, **98**, 763.
62. K. K. Chan, R. Bakhtiar and C. Jiang, *Invest. New Drugs*, 1997, **15**, 195.
63. K. Masuoka, A. Nagai, K. Shin-ya, K. Furihata, K. Nagai, K.-I. Suzuki, Y. Hayakawa and H. Seto, *Tetrahedron Lett.*, 2001, **42**, 41.
64. Y. Q. Cheng, M. Yang and A. M. Matter, *Appl. Environ. Microbiol.*, 2007, **73**, 3460.
65. V. Y. Potharla, S. R. Wesener and Y. Q. Cheng, *Appl. Environ. Microbiol.*, 2011, **77**, 1508.
66. J. B. Biggins, C. D. Gleber and S. F. Brady, *Org. Lett.*, 2011, **13**, 1536.
67. C. Wang, L. M. Henkes, L. B. Doughty, M. He, D. Wang, F. J. Meyer-Almes and Y. Q. Cheng, *J. Nat. Prod.*, 2011, **74**, 2031.
68. C. Wang, C. J. Flemming and Y. Q. Cheng, *Med. Chem. Commun.*, 2012, **3**, 976.
69. K. Taori, V. J. Paul and H. Luesch, *J. Am. Chem. Soc.*, 2008, **130**, 1806.
70. K. W. Li, J. Wu, W. Xing and J. A. Simon, *J. Am. Chem. Soc.*, 1996, **118**, 7237.
71. T. J. Greshock, D. M. Johns, Y. Noguchi and R. M. Williams, *Org. Lett.*, 2008, **10**, 613.
72. S. Wen, G. Packham and A. Ganesan, *J. Org. Chem.*, 2008, **73**, 9353.
73. A. Yurek-George, F. Habens, M. Brimmell, G. Packham and A. Ganesan, *J. Am. Chem. Soc.*, 2004, **126**, 1030.
74. H. Benelkebir, A. M. Donlevy, G. Packham and A. Ganesan, *Org. Lett.*, 2011, **13**, 6334.
75. J. Hong and H. Luesch, *Nat. Prod. Rep.*, 2012, **29**, 449.
76. C. Schotes, D. Ostrovskyi, J. Senger, K. Schmidtkunz, M. Jung and B. Breit, *Chem. Eur. J.*, 2014, **20**, 2164.
77. A. Yurek-George, A. Cecil, A. H. K. Mo, S. Wen, H. Rogers, F. Habens, S. Maeda, M. Yoshida, G. Packham and A. Ganesan, *J. Med. Chem.*, 2007, **50**, 5720.
78. A. Bowers, N. West, T. Newkirk, A. Troutman-Youngman, S. L. Schreiber, O. Wiest, J. E. Bradner and R. M. Williams, *Org. Lett.*, 2009, **11**, 1301.
79. J. M. Guerra-Bubba, A. A. Bowers, W. B. Smith, R. Paranal, G. Estiu, O. Wiest, J. E. Bradner and R. M. Williams, *Bioorg. Med. Chem. Lett.*, 2013, **23**, 6025.
80. H. Benelkebir, S. Marie, A. L. Hayden, J. Lyle, P. M. Loadman, S. J. Crabb, G. Packham and A. Ganesan, *Bioorg. Med. Chem.*, 2011, **19**, 3650.
81. S. Di Maro, R. C. Pong, J. T. Hsieh and J. M. Ahn, *J. Med. Chem.*, 2008, **51**, 6639.
82. L. Makala, S. Di Maro, T. F. Lou, S. Sivanand, J. M. Ahn and B. S. Pace, *Anemia*, 2012, Article ID 428137.
83. Y. Nakao, S. Yoshida, S. Matsunaga, N. Shindoh, Y. Terada, K. Nagai, J. K. Yamashita, A. Ganesan, R. W. M. van Soest and N. Fusetani, *Angew. Chem. Int. Ed.*, 2006, **45**, 7553.
84. S. Wen, K. L. Carey, Y. Nakao, N. Fusetani, G. Packham and A. Ganesan, *Org. Lett.*, 2007, **9**, 1105.

85. M. T. Robak, M. A. Herbage and J. A. Ellman, *Chem. Rev.*, 2010, **110**, 3600.

86. M. L. Curtin, R. B. Garland, H. R. Heyman, R. R. Frey, M. R. Michaelides, J. Li, L. J. Pease, K. B. Glaser, P. A. Marcotte and S. K. Davidsen, *Bioorg. Med. Chem. Lett.*, 2002, **12**, 2919.

87. T. Liu, G. Kapustin and F. A. Etzkorn, *J. Med. Chem.*, 2007, **50**, 2003.

88. T. Pirali, V. Faccio, R. Mossetti, A. A. Grolla, S. D. Micco, G. Bifulco, A. A. Genazzani and G. C. Tron, *Mol. Divers.*, 2010, **14**, 109.

89. L. Auzzas, A. Larsson, R. Matera, A. Baraldi, B. Deschênes-Simard, G. Giannini, W. Cabri, G. Battistuzzi, G. Gallo, A. Ciacci, L. Vesci, C. Pisano and S. Hanessian, *J. Med. Chem.*, 2010, **53**, 8387.

90. W. Tang, T. Luo, E. F. Greenberg, J. E. Bradner and S. L. Schreiber, *Bioorg. Med. Chem. Lett.*, 2011, **21**, 2601.

91. A. K. Oyelere, P. C. Chen, W. Guerrant, S. C. Mwakwari, R. Hood, Y. Zhang and Y. Fan, *J. Med. Chem.*, 2009, **52**, 456.

92. S. C. Mwakwari, W. Guerrant, V. Patil, S. I. Khan, B. L. Tekwani, Z. A. Gurard-Levin, M. Mrksich and A. K. Oyelere, *J. Med. Chem.*, 2010, **53**, 6100.

CHAPTER 5

Designed Macrocyclic Kinase Inhibitors

ANDERS POULSEN,*[a] ANTHONY D. WILLIAM[b] AND
BRIAN W. DYMOCK[c]

[a] Experimental Therapeutics Centre, A*STAR, 11 Biopolis Way, #03-10/11
The Helios, 138667, Singapore; [b] Institute of Chemical and Engineering
Sciences, A*STAR, 11 Biopolis Way, The Helios #03-08, 138667, Singapore;
[c] Department of Pharmacy, National University of Singapore, 18 Science
Drive 4, 117543, Singapore
*Email: apoulsen@etc.a-star.edu.sg

5.1 Introduction

5.1.1 Introduction to Macrocyclic Kinase Inhibitors

For the last decade kinases have become one of the most intensively pursued
classes of drug targets, primarily for the treatment of cancer.[1,2] De-regulation
of kinase function has also been implicated in other disorders such as
immunological, neurological, and infectious diseases.[3] These studies generated considerable interest in the development of small molecule kinase
inhibitors. To date, with over 500 known kinases identified, the biological
consequences of multi-kinase inhibition are still poorly defined. Hence, for
new kinase inhibitors it is important to understand the relationship between
selectivity, efficacy, and safety and then to adopt rational strategies to
identify inhibitors with desirable selectivity profiles.[4,5] However, it is important to appreciate that the high degree of structural homology among
and within kinase families poses a particular challenge for the development

RSC Drug Discovery Series No. 40
Macrocycles in Drug Discovery
Edited by Jeremy Levin
© The Royal Society of Chemistry 2015
Published by the Royal Society of Chemistry, www.rsc.org

of selective small molecule inhibitors.[6] One chemistry driven approach to address this challenge is to take advantage of the unique intrinsic chemical features of macrocycles as an alternative lead finding strategy from the high throughput screening of large compound libraries. Restricting the conformation of acyclic multi-kinase inhibitor scaffolds generates novel molecular scaffolds and could increase selectivity.[7–11] This focused rational approach opens up relatively under-explored chemical space. Macrocycles can possess high selectivity, attributable to their well defined three-dimensional shape, allowing them to fit into the DFG-in conformation of the ATP-binding site of target kinases. Furthermore, macrocycle formation may reduce conformational freedom thereby reducing the entropy cost of binding and increasing the free energy of binding. This can result in unique selectivity profiles that may offer potential in a wide range of therapeutic areas. Such applications range from both hematological malignancies and solid tumors to autoimmune disorders such as rheumatoid arthritis (RA) and psoriasis. Industry analysts predict that the world market for small molecule kinase inhibitor drugs will reach \$32.7 billion worldwide in the coming years and small molecule macrocycles have the potential to play an increasing and significant role in this challenging therapeutic space.[12]

5.1.2   Literature Survey of Macrocyclic Kinase Inhibitors

In general, macrocycles are chemically defined as ring structures of at least 12 atoms, typically 500 to 2000 daltons in size. Macrocyclic natural products are generally chemically complex and challenging to synthesize, making it difficult and resource intensive to build structure activity relationships (SAR). Macrocycles are often not drug-like and tend to violate the 'rule-of-five' affecting aqueous solubility, lipid-membrane permeability, and oral absorption, hence limiting their adoption in drug discovery and development.[13] Recently, there has been intense interest in small molecule macrocycles of molecular weight less than 500 daltons, as evident from several reports and reviews published in the last three years,[14–17] and recent summaries of macrocycles at various stages of development.[18] The design and synthesis of macrocyclic inhibitors of kinases, in particular, has been ongoing for almost 20 years and has encompassed a wide range of chemotypes, from innovative analogs of the natural product staurosporine and large peptidic structures to macrocyclic variants of aminopyrimidines. Short summaries of these studies are presented herein followed by an in-depth description of the design, structure–activity relationships, physical properties, synthesis, preclinical pharmacology, and early clinical data for the three most advanced macrocyclic kinase inhibitors. Discovered by S*BIO in Singapore, these three clinical stage compounds are pacritinib (SB1518, **1**), a dual JAK2/FLT3 inhibitor,[9] SB1578 (**2**), a more selective JAK2 inhibitor,[11] and TG02 (SB1317, **3**), a CDK2/JAK2/FLT3/ERK5 inhibitor[10] (Figure 5.1).

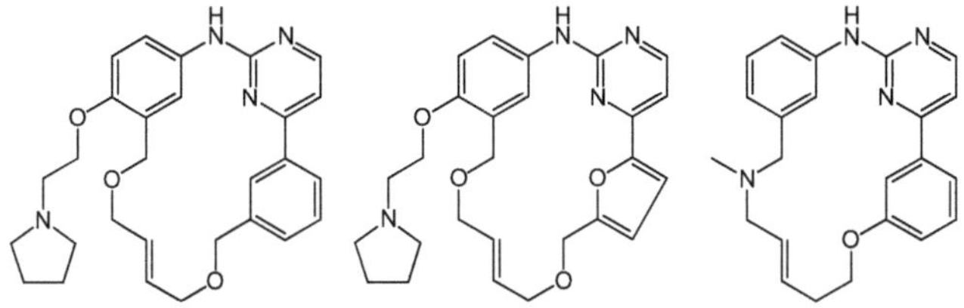

Figure 5.1 The 3 macrocyclic kinase inhibitors currently in clinical development. These compounds were first synthesized by S*BIO and are now being developed by CTI Biopharma Corp. (SB1518 and SB1578) and Tragara Pharmaceuticals (TG02/SB1317).

The first examples of macrocyclic small molecule kinase inhibitors designed from a non-macrocyclic lead were members of a novel class of macrocyclic bisindolylmaleimides. These compounds are ATP competitive inhibitors of Protein Kinase C (PKC), based on the staurosporine core, reported by Lilly in the mid-1990s (Table 5.1). Arising conceptually from the cleavage of the bridging C–O bonds of the natural product, compounds 4–9 exhibited a range of activities against rat brain PKC, a mixture of at least four PKC family isozymes. Amine derivatives 4–6 and alcohol 9 displayed sub-micromolar IC$_{50}$s in this assay. Profiling against individual isozymes in the PKC family revealed that analogs 4 and 5 were both single-digit nanomolar inhibitors of PKCβI and II with selectivity of approximately 50-fold over PKCα and from 6 to more than 1000-fold over other PKC family members. Primary amine 6 and alcohol 9 were five to 10-fold less potent than 4 against PKCβI and II, while macrocycles 7 and 8 bearing larger substituents had PKCβI IC$_{50}$s of 120 and 170 nM, respectively. Of the analogs 4–9, only amines 4, 5, and 7 had sub-micromolar activity in an endothelial cell-based plasminogen activator assay. Compound 4 (LY333531) was also several orders of magnitude more selective for inhibition of PKCβ in comparison to other protein kinases such as calcium calmodulin (1060-fold selective) or Src tyrosine kinase (2200-fold selective). Staurosporine, on the other hand, is a potent inhibitor of PKA, calcium calmodulin, Src tyrosine kinase, and casein kinase in addition to PKC.[19]

In an example of a series of macrocyclic kinase inhibitors designed by the cyclization of an acyclic lead molecule, a series of crown ether-fused anilinoquinazoline analogs has been reported by Betapharma as novel epidermal growth factor receptor (EGFR) tyrosine kinase inhibitors. Inspired by Iressa™ (gefitinib) and Tarceva™ (erlotinib), both approved for the treatment of lung and other cancers (Table 5.2),[20] these fused anilinoquinazoline analogs showed potent EGFR kinase inhibition with IC$_{50}$ values as low as 2 nM. A ring size of 12 or more atoms was preferred for the ring fused to the quinazoline as evidenced by the dramatic increase in potency for analogs 11–13, with 12 and 13-membered rings, as compared to the 8-membered

Table 5.1 ATP Dependent kinase IC$_{50}$ values for staurosporine derivatives selectively inhibiting PKC isoforms.

Compound	Structure	Kinase IC$_{50}$ (µM)							
		PKCα	PKCβI	PKCβII	Rat Brain-PKC	PKA	Ca (calmodulin)	Casein Kinase	Src
Staurosporine		0.045	0.023	0.019	0.19	0.10	0.0004	14	0.001
4 (LY333531)	LY333531	0.36	0.0047	0.0059	0.32	>100	6.2	>100	>100

Compound								
5	NT	>100	2.2	49	0.16	0.005	0.005	0.24
6	89	>100	2.7	83	0.79	0.033	0.048	1.1
7	11	>100	5.3	>100	1.9	0.044	0.12	3.5

Table 5.1 (*Continued*)

Compound	Structure	Kinase IC$_{50}$ (μM)							
		PKCα	PKCβI	PKCβII	Rat Brain-PKC	PKA	Ca (calmodulin)	Casein Kinase	Src
8		>5.0	0.17	0.044	10	>100	56	>100	>100
9		0.72	0.073	0.028	0.63	>100	6.0	>100	>100

Table 5.2 Fused anilino-quinazoline analogues are EGFR kinase inhibitors.

Compound	Structure	EGFR IC$_{50}$ (nM)[a]	Cell Tyrphos IC$_{50}$ (nM)[b]
10		85	N.D.[c]
11		5	50
12		2	55
13 Icotinib		2	45
14		8	>1000
15		150	N.D.

[a]*In vitro* kinase assay.
[b]EGFR-mediated intracellular tyrosine phosphorylation assay.
[c]Not determined.

ring analog **10**. Ether linkages in the macrocycle provided the best biochemical and cell potency as compared to those incorporating a thioether or sulfonamide linker (**14** and **15**). Amongst the series, icotinib (**13**), was progressed into the clinic and has undergone Phase III studies. Icotinib was found to be non-inferior to gefitinib with similar tolerability in non-small cell lung carcinoma (NSCLC) patients that were previously treated with chemotherapy agents.[20,21]

A series of peptidic macrocycles has been published by researchers from Harvard and Stony Brook University who reported highly specific, bisubstrate-competitive proto-oncogene tyrosine protein kinase Src inhibitors

Table 5.3   Cyclic peptides and their IC_{50} values against Akt Isoforms.

Compound	Structure	IC_{50} (nM)		
		Akt2	Akt1	Akt3
17 (Pakti-L1)	Ac-Tyr-Ile-Leu-Val-Arg-Asn-Arg-Leu-Leu-Arg-Val-Asp-Cys-Gly-NH2	110	> 25000	4200
18	Ac-Tyr-Trp-Ile-Val-Leu-Thr-Trp-Pro-Ile-Val-Thr-Arg-Arg-Cys-Gly-NH2	92	~ 1000	~ 1000

from DNA-templated macrocycles. They identified a library of peptide macrocycles that inhibited Src with IC_{50} values down to 680 nM. Two of the macrocyclic compounds showed a remarkable level of specificity, inhibiting only Src kinase and not Abelson murine leukemia (Abl) kinase or hemopoietic cell kinase (Hck). The development of second-generation macrocycles, based on the initial findings, enabled optimization to potencies less than 4 nM (**16**) (Figure 5.2).[22]

Researchers from The University of Tokyo have described another class of peptidic macrocyclic kinase inhibitors, linked by a thioether functionality and produced in library format from random sequences of mRNA. This led to the identification of Akt isoform-selective inhibitors (Table 5.3), a challenging task due to mechanistic and structural similarities of the Akt kinase isoforms. Thus, cyclic peptide **18** is a moderately potent inhibitor of Akt2 with an IC_{50} around 100 nM and approximately 10-fold selectivity over Akt1 and Akt3. One of the inhibitors, Pakti-L1 (**17**, Figure 5.2 and Table 5.3) showed very high isoform-selectivity for Akt2 over Akt1 (>225-fold) and Akt3 (38-fold).[23]

Other notable macrocyclic kinase inhibitors are the quinoxalinone pan-CDK inhibitors, exemplified by compound **19**, from the Banyu Tsukuba Research Institute (Figure 5.3).[24] The pyrrolidine-based linker was inserted in order to constrain the dihedral angle between the two bicyclic ring systems of **19**. Compound **19** is more than 1000-fold selective against a panel of 62 kinases outside of the CDK family. It inhibits CDK1, 2, 4, 5, 6, and 9 with equal potency, in the low nanomolar range, and is also a potent inhibitor of GSK 3β ($IC_{50} = 13$ nM) (Table 5.4). The methyl substituent at the 2-position of the pyrrolidine sits in a lipophilic pocket of the protein and significantly improves potency against CDK4 ($IC_{50} = 6.4$ nM). Compound **19** also showed anti-tumor efficacy at a tolerated dose in a nude rat xenograft tumor model. An 8 hour constant infusion of the compound inhibited retinoblastoma phosphorylation (pRb) and induced apoptosis in tumor cells at ~ 30 nM that led to the inhibition of tumor growth.[24]

Based on the crystallographic analysis of a complex of checkpoint kinase 1 (Chk1) with an acyclic pyrazinyl urea-based inhibitor, and molecular modeling, a class of macrocyclic Chk1 inhibitors was designed by Abbott (Figure 5.4).[25] These novel Chk1 inhibitors exhibited excellent selectivity over a panel of more than 70 kinases. The 14- and 15-membered macrocycles, **20** and **21**, were equipotent while the 16-membered analog was approximately 4-fold less active ($IC_{50} = 28$ nM) presumably due to reduced

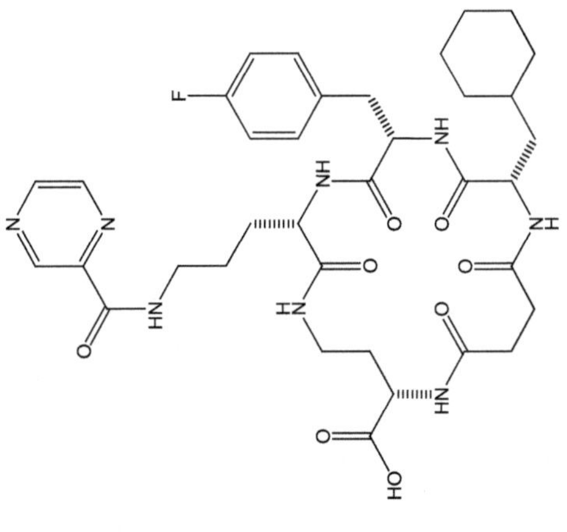

16

Src IC$_{50}$ = 4 nM

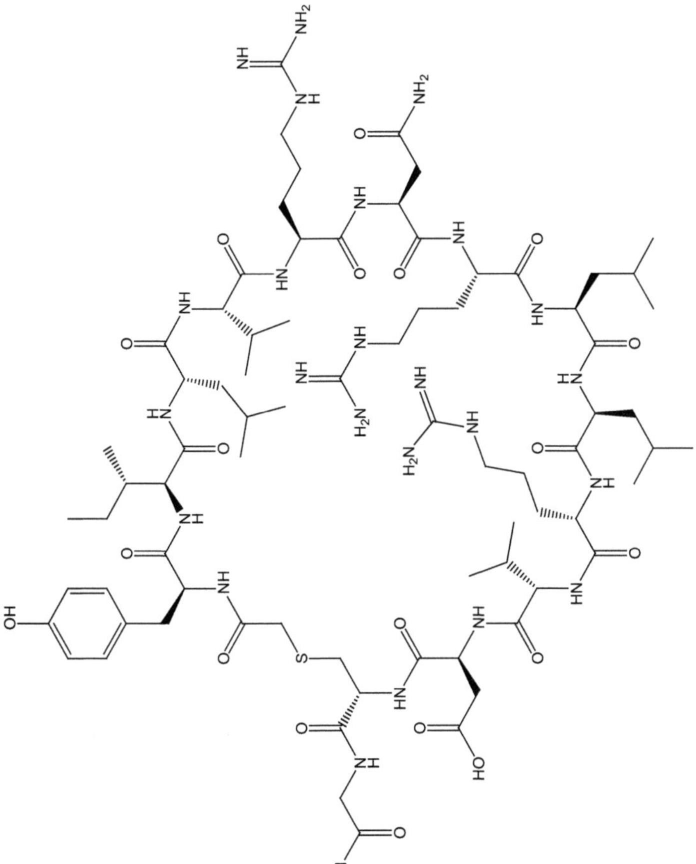

17

Pakti-L1

Figure 5.2 DNA template macrocycle from Stony Brook University (**16**) and thioether macrocyclic peptide Akt-2 Selective inhibitor (Pakti-L1, **17**) from The University of Tokyo.

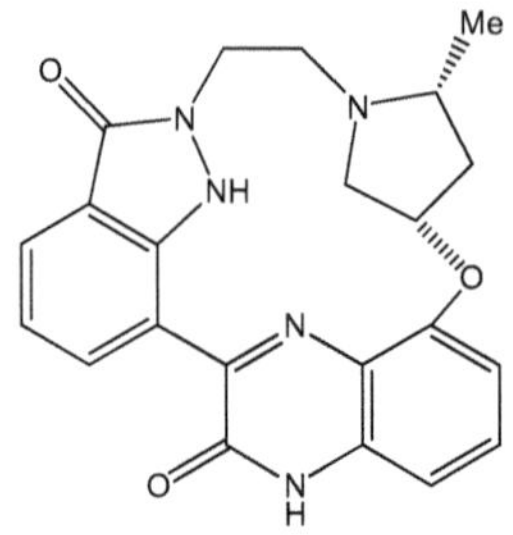

19

Figure 5.3 Quinoxalinone macrocycle based pan-CDK inhibitor from the Banyu Tsukuba Research Institute.

Table 5.4 Activity against the Cdk family and other kinases for compound **19**.

Kinases	IC_{50} (nM)	Selectivity
CDK4	6.4	1
CDK6	12	
CDK2	3.4	
CDK1	1	
CDK5	4.5	
CDK7	660	
PKA, PKC, ERK 1& 2, p38, KDR, FLT1&4, FGFR1&2, Src, Tie-2, PDGF, EGFR		>100

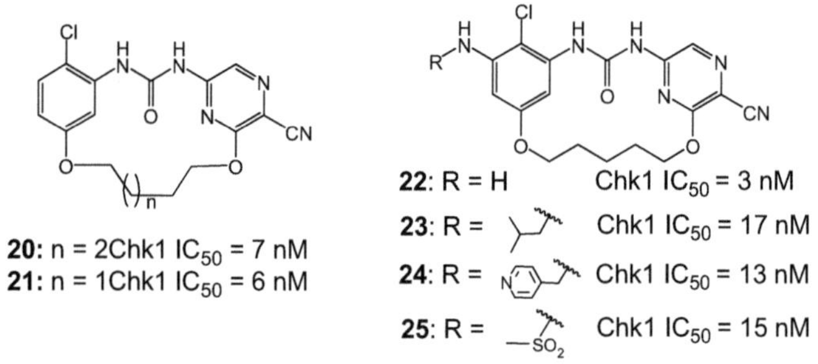

20: n = 2 Chk1 IC_{50} = 7 nM
21: n = 1 Chk1 IC_{50} = 6 nM

22: R = H   Chk1 IC_{50} = 3 nM
23: R =   Chk1 IC_{50} = 17 nM
24: R =   Chk1 IC_{50} = 13 nM
25: R =   Chk1 IC_{50} = 15 nM

Figure 5.4 Macrocyclic Chk1 inhibitors designed by Abbott.

rigidity. Compounds **22–25**, in which a polar amino functionality has been placed at the solvent exposed 4-position of the phenyl ring, were identified as ideal Chk1 inhibitors. These analogs showed no single-agent activity but significantly potentiated the cytotoxicity of the DNA-damaging anti-tumor agents doxorubicin and camptothecin *in vitro* in a cervical cancer cell line.

Another instance of an acyclic kinase inhibitor being transformed into a series of macrocyclic inhibitors was based on the high throughput screening hit **26**. This diaminopyrimidine inhibitor is equipotent against CDK1 and CDK2 ($IC_{50} = 100$ nM) with modest cellular activity. Schering developed the first macrocyclic aminopyrimidines as inhibitors of CDK1/2 and vascular endothelial growth factor (VEGF) receptor 2 tyrosine kinase after X-ray crystallography of **26** showed that the phenyl ring and terminal carbon of the alkyne were in close proximity when bound to CDK2. Although the initial macrocyclic target, **27**, was considerably less potent than **26**, replacement of the ether linker of **27** with a sulfonamide to give **28** provided a potent inhibitor of CDK1/2 and VEGF-R2 with improved activity over **26** in the MCF7 cell line. Compound **28** was also orally active in a HeLa-MaTu (Hormone-independent MaTu human mammary tumor cells) xenograft model at 50 and 100 mg/kg giving 70 and 90% tumor growth inhibition, respectively. A new binding interaction revealed by co-crystallization experiments was reported for CDK2 inhibitor **28** in which one oxygen of the sulfonamide and the sulfonamide NH form three hydrogen bonds with the protein. These compounds displayed potent antiproliferative activities against MCF7 human breast tumor cells *in vitro* (Figure 5.5).[26] According to the authors the macrocyclic approach stabilized the bioactive conformation of acyclic **26**.

A similar design strategy was used by Polaris to identify macrocyclic CK2 inhibitors based on the X-ray co-crystal structures of pyrazolo[1,5-*a*][1,3,5]triazines such as **29** with corn casein kinase-2 (cCK2) protein. Acyclic pyrazolo[1,5-*a*][1,3,5]triazine **29** is a potent inhibitor of protein kinase CK2 ($K_i < 1$ nM). However, it exhibits relatively weak cellular activity against prostate and colon cancer cell lines, presumably a consequence of poor membrane permeability due to the near planar nature of the molecular structure for this class of compounds, as observed in the X-ray co-crystal structure. Macrocyclic analog of **29**, compound **30**, was nearly 100-fold less active against CK2 but the change proved beneficial as the alkyl chain forced the molecule to adopt a non-planar conformation, thereby improving cell membrane permeability. Compound **30** strongly inhibited cancer cell

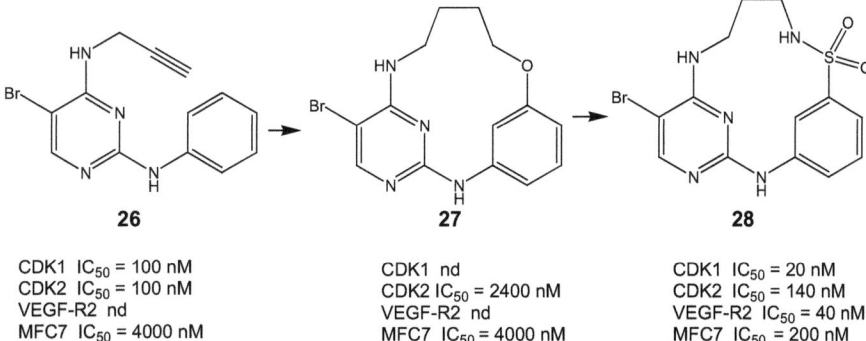

26

CDK1 IC_{50} = 100 nM
CDK2 IC_{50} = 100 nM
VEGF-R2 nd
MFC7 IC_{50} = 4000 nM

27

CDK1 nd
CDK2 IC_{50} = 2400 nM
VEGF-R2 nd
MFC7 IC_{50} = 4000 nM

28

CDK1 IC_{50} = 20 nM
CDK2 IC_{50} = 140 nM
VEGF-R2 IC_{50} = 40 nM
MFC7 IC_{50} = 200 nM

Figure 5.5 Schering's macrocyclic aminopyrimidines as inhibitors of CDK1/2 and VEGF kinases.

proliferation with an IC_{50} of 290 nM in HCT116 colon cancer cells (Figure 5.6), an improvement of almost 100-fold over **29**. In a prostate cancer cell line (PC3) **30** gave an IC_{50} of 880 nM, a 5-fold improvement over **29**.[27]

Another series of macrocyclic bis(indolyl)maleimide kinase inhibitors, conceptually derived from the staurosporine scaffold and the Lilly PKC inhibitors **4–9**, have been reported by Johnson & Johnson. These novel macrocycles of bis(indolyl)maleimide pyridinophanes, **31–35**, were screened against a panel of 100 kinases and found to be potent and selective inhibitors of glycogen synthase kinase-3 beta (GSK-3β) (Figure 5.7).[28] Notably, the activity of these pyridinophanes against PKC-β is greatly reduced relative to compounds **4–9**, perhaps due to their increased ring size (17–19 atoms). Simply by changing the attachment point of the propyl linkers to the aminopyridine group from 3,6 in **32/33** to 4,6 in **34/35**, potency was increased 3–5 fold. It was suggested that the conformation of the macrocyclic linker of these analogs may be governed to some degree by the

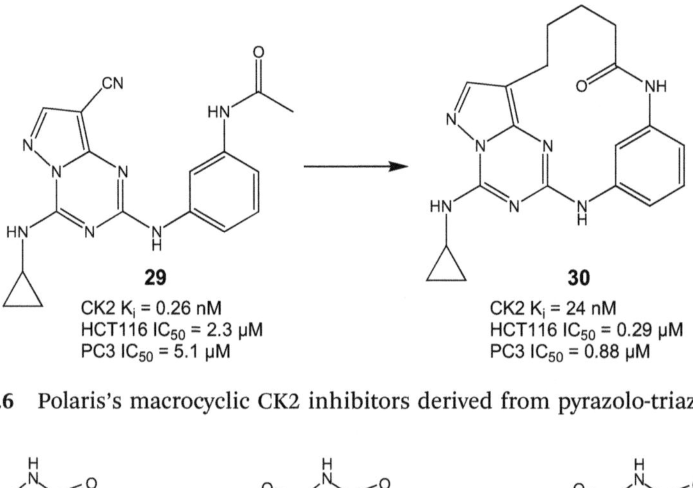

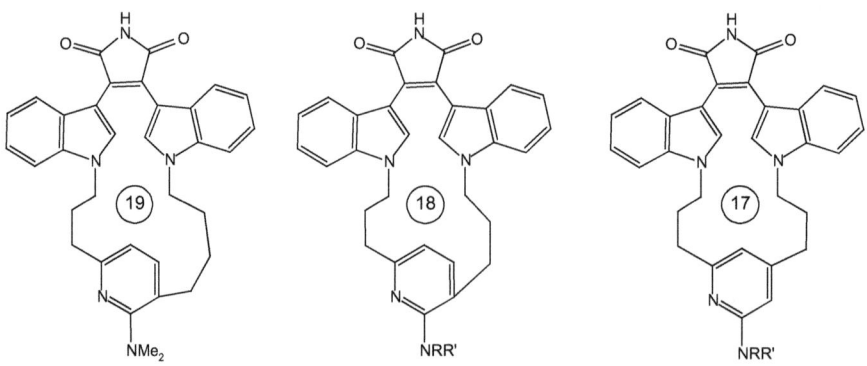

29

CK2 K_i = 0.26 nM
HCT116 IC_{50} = 2.3 µM
PC3 IC_{50} = 5.1 µM

30

CK2 K_i = 24 nM
HCT116 IC_{50} = 0.29 µM
PC3 IC_{50} = 0.88 µM

Figure 5.6 Polaris's macrocyclic CK2 inhibitors derived from pyrazolo-triazines.

31: GSK-3β IC_{50} = 0.003 µM   **32**: R=R'=Me; GSK-3β IC_{50} = 0.037 µM   **34**: R=R'=Me; GSK-3β IC_{50} = 0.007 µM
                                        33: R,R'=(CH₂)₄; GSK-3β IC_{50} = 0.030 µM   **35**: R,R'=(CH₂)₄ ; GSK-3β IC_{50} = 0.011 µM

Figure 5.7 Johnson & Johnson's selective inhibitors of GSK-3β based on novel macrocycles of bis(indolyl)maleimide pyridinophanes.

pyridinophane unit, which may impart the high inhibitory potency for GSK-3β and the selectivity over many other kinases. Interestingly, an X-ray crystal structure of **31** shows that the aminopyridine moiety is solvent exposed and does not reveal any key interactions between this part of the macrocycle linker and the protein.

In yet another demonstration of the potential benefits of converting an acyclic diaminopyrimidine kinase inhibitor into a macrocyclic template, Cephalon has reported a novel set of 13 macrocycles as potential anaplastic lymphoma kinase (ALK) inhibitors (Figure 5.8).[29] As in previous instances in which this strategy has been undertaken it is proposed that this macrocyclization rigidly locks the molecules into a low energy bioactive conformation similar to that adopted by the acyclic diaminopyrimidine scaffold. The comparison of ALK biochemical potency for **36** relative to the analogous constrained macrocycle **37** shows ALK activity to be significantly improved for the macrocycle although these compounds were equipotent in a cellular assay. It was also noted that if the 2-carbon linker of the macrocycle was olefinic (macrocyclization *via* a Pd-catalysed Heck coupling) instead of a saturated ethyl linker (made *via* hydrogenation of the vinyl linker), enzyme activity was eroded, perhaps due to the effect of the added rigidity on the torsion angles between the phenyl rings. Of the 13 analogs reported, **38**, in which a *N*-methylsulfonamide group has been appended on the aniline at the 4-position of the pyrimidine ring, exhibited low nanomolar NPM-ALK (nucleophosmin-ALK) cellular activity ($IC_{50} = 10$ nM) and was more potent in enzymatic and cellular assays as compared to the desmethoxy analog **39** ($IC_{50} = 3.4$ nM; cell $IC_{50} = 120$ nM). Macrocycle **38** also exhibits an excellent selectivity preference for inhibition of ALK relative to insulin receptor (IR) kinase (IR/ALK ratio of 173). A docking analysis of compound **38** bound to ALK revealed that the sulfonamide moiety forms an interaction with the conserved lysine in the ATP binding pocket, perhaps rationalizing its effect on potency.

Radicicol (compound **40**, Figure 5.9) and related resorcinol acid lactones from Université Louis Pasteur have also been described as tyrosine kinase inhibitors as well as Hsp90 inhibitors (see Chapter 2).[31]

In summary, numerous examples of designed macrocyclic kinase inhibitors have been reported to bind to the active DFG-in conformations of kinases.[19,20,24–29] Several of these type 1 kinase inhibitors were evolved from acyclic leads that often adopt a semi circular conformation when bound to the active kinase. This is opposed to type 2 inhibitors that bind to the inactive DFG-out conformation in which the inhibitors adopt a rod shape.[30] No macrocyclic kinase inhibitors binding to the DFG-out conformation have been reported. Through their restricted conformations these macrocycles can offer improved control of molecular shape and the ability to bind specifically to a smaller array of biological targets as compared to their acyclic comparators. This untapped potential is only beginning to be properly explored and now represents a growing and exciting field of drug research. Reports of preclinical research where macrocyclic kinase inhibitors have

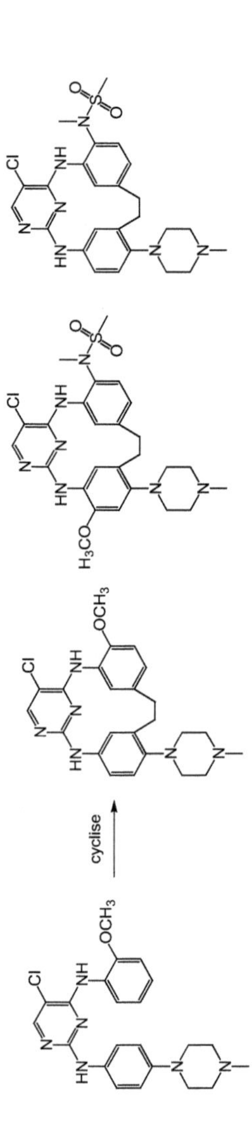

36 ALK IC_{50} = 22 nM

37 ALK IC_{50} = 3.1 nM

38 ALK IC_{50} = 0.5 nM
NMP-ALK Cell IC_{50} = 10 nM

39 ALK IC_{50} = 3.4 nM
NMP-ALK Cell IC_{50} = 120 nM

Figure 5.8 Cephalon Inc.'s anaplastic lymphoma kinase (ALK) macrocycles derived from diaminopyrimidine.

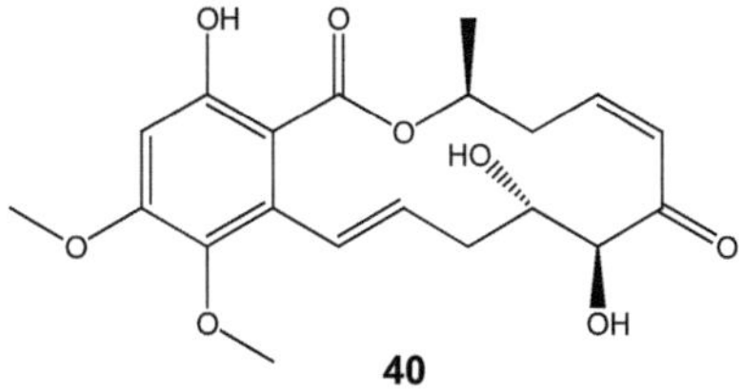

40

Flt3 IC_{50} = 7 nM
VEGF-R3 IC_{50} = 7 nM
VEGF-R2 IC_{50} = 7 nM
PDGFR beta IC_{50} = 7 nM

Figure 5.9 Radicicol related resorcinol acid lactones from Université Louis Pasteur.

been specifically targeted range from orally available synthetic small molecules to natural-product inspired templates to cyclic and stapled peptides. In the following sections the design criteria, both in terms of medicinal chemistry and biology, pharmacology and clinical data surrounding the most advanced macrocyclic kinase inhibitors now in clinical trials will be discussed in detail.

5.2 Biology Rationale

Inhibition of a single kinase, or small number of kinases, has been shown in multiple oncology indications to give rise to rapid emergence of resistance. Patients who respond to initial therapy cruelly experience devastating relapse raising the question of how to add value to highly targeted kinase inhibitor therapy. Inhibition of *more than one* signaling pathway known to be important in disease is one potential answer. Such selected multiple pathway inhibitions must be synergistic so as to ensure increased efficacy with acceptable tolerability. A small number of clinical stage macrocyclic kinase inhibitors have attempted to explore such a concept in a controlled way, taking advantage of the restrained conformation of the macrocyclic structure. Synergy of the JAK–STAT axis with mutated FLT3 is discussed herein for pacritinib for oncology indications. The additional c-FMS activity of SB1578 provides an attractive kinase inhibition profile for the treatment of RA. A cyclin dependent kinase inhibition profile with additional JAK/FLT and ERK5 inhibition, a highly attractive combination for the treatment of multiple tumor types, is demonstrated by TG02.

5.2.1 Janus Kinases (JAKs)

Comprising a family of four cytoplasmic tyrosine kinase enzymes, JAK1, JAK2, JAK3, and tyrosine kinase 2 (TYK2), the Janus kinases (JAKs) are important cell-signaling mediators in myeloid malignancies,[32] inflammatory, and autoimmune diseases.[33] Discovery of the V617F mutation in JAK2 in myeloproliferative neoplasm (MPN) patients catalysed rapid advances in JAK therapeutic research.[34-37] Within only 5 years two pivotal Phase III trials led to the approval of the JAK1/2 selective inhibitor ruxolitinib[38] (Jakafi/INCB018424, Incyte/Novartis) for the treatment of myelofibrosis.[39,40] Even more recently, the pan-JAK inhibitor tofacitinib[41] (Xeljanz/CP690,550, Pfizer) was approved in November of 2012 for the treatment of RA.[42-44]

Detailed reviews of JAK pathway biology are available.[32,33,45] In brief, specific cytokines trigger receptor signaling cascades driven by specific JAK family enzymes through the signal transducers and activators of transcription (STAT) intracellular enzymes. JAK–STAT signals are negatively regulated by the suppressors of cytokine signaling (SOCS).[46] Given the specific nature of these cascades, selective inhibitors of specific family members are expected to have different therapeutic applications.

JAK1 knockout mice die shortly after birth and analysis of JAK1 deficient cells revealed that JAK1 signals through the class I receptors, cytokines that activate the gp130 subunit or the γ_c receptor.[47] On the other hand JAK2 deficiency in mice is embryonic lethal due to a lack of erythropoiesis.[48,49] Following receptor stimulation by erythropoietin, thromobopoeitin, GM-CSF, IL-3, or IL-5, among others, JAK2 phosphorylates the intracellular receptor protein where STAT3/5 bind and are themselves phosphorylated by JAK2, whereupon phospho-STAT3/5 dimerises and translocates to the nucleus where they activate gene transcription.[33] When JAK2 is permanently 'switched on' (constitutively activated) it is a driver for some neoplasias. A mutation in JAK2, V617F, was found to be a major player in MPNs, especially in polycythemia vera (PV) where the mutation rates were over 90%.[34-37] Primary myelofibrosis (PMF) and essential thrombocythemia (ET) patients possess less mutated JAK2 protein (usually at least 50% of patients) hence the role of mutant JAK2 appears to still be significant in these patient populations. The role of JAK2 in lymphoma has been reviewed in detail.[50] JAK2 is frequently over-expressed and activated in lymphomas (Hodgkin's Lymphoma (HL) and Non-Hodgkin's Lymphoma (NHL)). JAK2 activation has been reported to be associated with mutation of the suppressor of cytokine signaling (SOCS)-1 gene in both HL and primary mediastinal large cell NHL.[51-53] The inhibition of JAK2 is associated with anti-proliferative activity in a variety of lymphoma cell lines.[54,55]

Inactivating JAK3 mutations reported in humans with severely compromised immunodeficiency (SCID) syndrome are characterized by a loss of T and NK cells, abnormal B cell function, and hypoplasia of lymphoid tissues.[56,57] JAK3 genetic mouse knockouts are SCID, consistent with the consequences of the mutation in humans.[58] Inhibition of JAK3 by non-selective kinase inhibitors such as tofacitinib, has contributed to their efficacy in treating RA but potentially at the expense of immunosuppression inviting opportunistic infections.[59] Rates of serious infections with tofacitnib will be closely watched as more post-marketing patient data is obtained. Recently Pfizer challenged the recent non-approval notice from the European authorities but failed to overturn the verdict.[60]

Further rationale supportive of the application of JAK inhibitors in RA has been demonstrated through the contribution of IL-6 to rheumatoid synovitis through the activation of the JAK–STAT pathway. Tofacitinib is known to inhibit this IL-6 stimulated activation.[61]

TYK2 is also a potential target for immune-inflammatory diseases.[62] TYK2 signals through the IL-12 and IL-23 cytokines, important mediators of STAT3/4 signaling unregulated in RA.[63,64] Kinase inactivating mutations in TYK2 in mice[65] show that the kinase activity is required for type I interferon mediated activation of STATs. TYK2 deficient mice were found to be protected against antibody-induced arthritis.[66] Therefore, TYK2 kinase inhibitor therapy may provide a highly targeted approach to autoimmune diseases.

Ubiquitous expression of JAK family enzymes raises the question of the toxicity of inhibitors, potentially limiting doses of the clinically tested drugs. Selective inhibitors are clearly required to delineate the various roles played by each JAK family member and wild type versus mutant enzymes. Macrocycles are well placed to exploit their conformational properties to this aim.

5.2.2 FMS-like Tyrosine Kinase 3 (FLT3)

FLT3 (FMS-like tyrosine kinase-3), a class III receptor tyrosine kinase (RTK), is the most frequently mutated gene in acute myeloid leukemia (AML).[67] FLT3 plays an important role in the maintenance, growth, and development of hematopoietic and non-hematopoietic cells. Internal tandem duplication (ITD) of the juxtamembrane domain-coding sequence of the FLT3 gene is a common gain-of-function mutation causing constitutively active FLT3 signaling leading to activation of STAT5 downstream. FLT3-ITD AML is associated with poor response to FLT3 inhibitor therapy and ultimately drug resistance.[68] Following FLT3 inhibitor therapy emergence of drug resistance is rapid. Mutations in the tyrosine kinase domain (TKD), particularly of the D835 residue,[68] which are rare in untreated populations, emerge under drug treatment generating resistant FLT3-ITD/TKD double mutants.[69] These mutants are highly resistant to FLT3 inhibitors resulting in rapid disease progression. Strategies to overcome this resistance onset have focused recently on combinations of FLT3 inhibitors with inhibition of additional kinases either in a single molecule or with two different drugs. Therefore macrocycles such as pacritinib (1) and TG02 (3), discussed herein, with their JAK2/FLT3 inhibitor profile are attractive for the treatment of AML.

5.2.3 Cyclin-dependent Kinases (CDKs)

CDKs are central mediators of cell proliferation and their roles in various aspects of cell growth and development have been extensively characterized and explored for the treatment of various oncological conditions.[70] CDKs 1, 2, 4, and 6 are associated with cell division and control the cell cycle through the G1, S, G2, and M phases.[71] Other cellular functions controlled by specific

CDKs include transcription (CDKs 7, 8, 9, 11), differentiation (CDKs 2, 5, 6, 9) and neuronal cell death (CDK5). Cells undergo apoptosis when exposed to inhibitors of CDKs.[71] Selective inhibition of a single kinase is often readily compensated by cancer cells, but inhibition of CDKs 1, 2, and 9 has been shown to have significant consequences *via* cell cycle arrest and apoptosis.[72] CDKs are serine–threonine kinases and are therefore challenging to inhibit selectively. This has led to difficulties in reaching efficacious exposures at tolerated doses in clinical trials with multi-CDK inhibiting drugs such as flavopyridol (alvocidib) and purines such as roscovitine/CYC202 (seliciclib).[73] Recently, an agent combining CDK4 and CDK6 inhibition, exemplified by palbociclib (PD-0332991, Pfizer), which has entered Phase III clinical trials for the treatment of breast cancer, has broken through the efficacy/tolerability stalemate to give patients new hope. Macrocyclization of kinase inhibitor pharmacophores may offer opportunities in accessing required conformations to inhibit desirable CDKs, such as CDKs 1, 2, and 9 while having improved pharmacokinetic properties offering oral dosing options for clinicians.

5.2.4   Other Kinases

Increased signaling through c-FMS, a tyrosine kinase receptor, occurs in diseases involving activation of tissue macrophages. Levels of macrophage colony-stimulating factor (M-CSF), the c-FMS ligand, are increased in the joints of RA patients, leading to bone erosion *via* macrophage and osteoclast cell development.[74] Inhibition of c-FMS by small molecules inhibits disease progression in animal models of RA indicating that it may play a pivotal role in the pathogenesis of the disease.[75,76] SB1578 (compound 2), discussed below, is a macrocycle that demonstrates c-FMS activity as well as potency against JAK2/FLT3 making it a unique candidate for small molecule RA therapy.[77]

Evidence that the ERK5 (extracellular-signal-regulated kinase-5)-MEK5 (MAPK mitogen-activated protein kinase-5) signaling pathway is important in cancer disease progression is beginning to emerge.[78] Expression of MEK5 is up-regulated by constitutively active STAT3, important in breast cancer,[79] and increased expression of ERK5 is associated with poor survival in early breast cancer.[80] A selective inhibitor of ERK5, XMD8-92, has anti-proliferative effects on HeLa cells and inhibited the growth of human tumour xenografts providing further support for ERK5 inhibition as a potential new cancer therapy.[81] Inhibition of ERK5 by TG02 (compound 3), potently inhibited proliferation of triple negative breast cancer cell lines and exerted strong anti-tumor activity in the MDA-MB-231 breast cancer xenograft model.[82] In multiple myeloma cell lines TG02 inhibited proliferation, survival, and induced apoptosis in patient-derived primary malignant plasma cells. Both single-agent activity and enhancement of bortezomib activity in combination were shown in two multiple myeloma xenograft models.[83] TG02 is in Phase I clinical trials (*vide infra*).

In summary, strong rationales exist for the clinical testing of molecules offering combination inhibitory profiles against CDKs, JAK2, FLT3, and other relatively unexplored targets, including c-FMS and ERK5, for a variety of therapeutic indications both oncologic and immunologic. For example, the blockade of specific multiple pathways, such as the JAK–STAT axis and FLT3-ITD in AML, and CDK with ERK5 are suggested to be synergistic therefore leading to enhanced antitumor activity. Furthermore, these desirable multi-kinase inhibitory profiles are achievable *via* small molecule macrocycles, structures that could offer new hope for the development of breakthrough therapies. Herein we discuss the first generation of clinical stage macrocyclic kinase inhibitors exhibiting such profiles, their design, synthesis, structure activity relationships, and assessment of the latest clinical data in a range of oncologic conditions.

5.3 Medicinal Chemistry

5.3.1 Macrocycle Design

In a high throughput screen (HTS) for Aurora A inhibitors several hits were identified having a 2-aniline-4-phenyl-pyrimidine scaffold, as exemplified by compound **41** (Figure 5.10a). These compounds generally had inhibitory constants in the low nanomolar range in an Aurora A biochemical assay.[84] Upon docking of compound **41** into the ATP-binding site of an Aurora A X-ray structure[8] the aniline hydrogen bond donor and the 1-position pyrimidine hydrogen bond acceptor were found to form hydrogen bonds to Ala213 in the kinase hinge region. The three aromatic rings of the ligand form hydrophobic contacts with Leu139, Val147, Ala160, and Leu210 in the N-terminal domain, as well as Leu194, Leu263, and Ala273 of the C-terminal domain (Figure 5.10b). It was observed that the inhibitor was binding in a semi-circular shape and that the substituents in the 3-positions of both phenyl rings were pointing towards each other. This scaffold is ubiquitous in the kinase inhibitor literature having been reported in numerous papers and patents.[85] To achieve novelty, macrocycle formation was proposed by connecting the 3-position substituents *via* a macrocyclic linker formed by ring closing metathesis (Figure 5.10c). Each side of the linker was connected by a heteroatom to the phenyl 3-position directly or by a benzylic methylene. These are designated X and Y in Figure 5.10c. Heteroatoms compatible with the metathesis reaction are an ether oxygen, amine nitrogen, and amide nitrogen. The chain length for the tether connecting rings A and C could be controlled in the four positions designated m, n, o, and p. Initially linkers containing a basic amine and ether oxygen, as in compound 3 (Table 5.5), were investigated. Compounds with all possible chain lengths were generated and subjected to a conformational search. The resulting conformational ensembles were then docked into Aurora A. Poses of 3 were found to have the same interactions with Aurora A as those described for **41** with

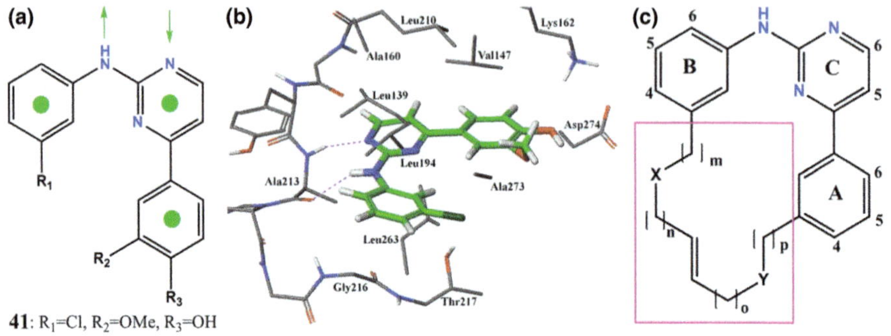

Figure 5.10 (a) The scaffold of the HTS leads. **41** had an Aurora A IC_{50} of 0.012 μM. The arrows indicate hydrogen bond interactions with the kinase hinge region. Solid dots indicate important hydrophobic interactions with the ATP-binding site. (b) Compound **41** docked into Aurora A showing the hydrogen bonds to Ala213 as purple dotted lines. (c) The structure of the proposed macrocycles. The three aromatic rings in the compounds discussed here will be referred to as the A, B, or C-ring, respectively. The part of the macrocycle shown inside the magenta box will be referred to as the linker. Macrocycles compatible with our synthetic route and proposed binding mode could have m,p = 0–1, n,o = 1–3, and X,Y = NR, O, CONH, NHCO. If X is a basic nitrogen, the compound will be referred to as 'N-linked' and compounds wherein X is an ether oxygen as 'O-linked'.

Figure 5.10a and c reproduced with kind permission from Springer Science + Business Media, *J. Mol. Model.*, 2013, **19**, 119, Figure 1.

an additional hydrogen bond to Thr217 formed by the basic nitrogen in the macrocyclic linker. Unfortunately, when **3** was synthesized it displayed disappointing activity against Aurora A with an IC_{50} of 1μM, approximately 100-fold lower than the initial hit, **41**.

5.3.2 SAR and Structural Biology

A kinase panel screen revealed that although **3** is a weak inhibitor of Aurora A, it is a potent pan-CDK, FLT3, and JAK2 inhibitor with inhibitory constants in the low nanomolar range. To investigate the reason for its activity against CDK2 and FLT3 compound **3** was docked into X-ray structures of these kinases.[8] In addition to the usual hydrogen bonds to the kinase hinge and hydrophobic interactions with residues in the N- and C-terminal domains, a salt bridge to Asp86 and Asp689, in the CDK2 and FLT3 C-terminal domains, respectively, was observed (Figure 5.11). Due to their *in vitro* potency, the enormous potential utility for molecules that selectively inhibit this combination of kinases and their excellent intellectual property (IP) position these macrocycles entered lead optimization for CDK/FLT3 and JAK2/FLT3 projects aiming to optimize potency, selectivity, and drug-like properties. The first region of the inhibitor to be investigated was the macrocyclic linker.[9,10]

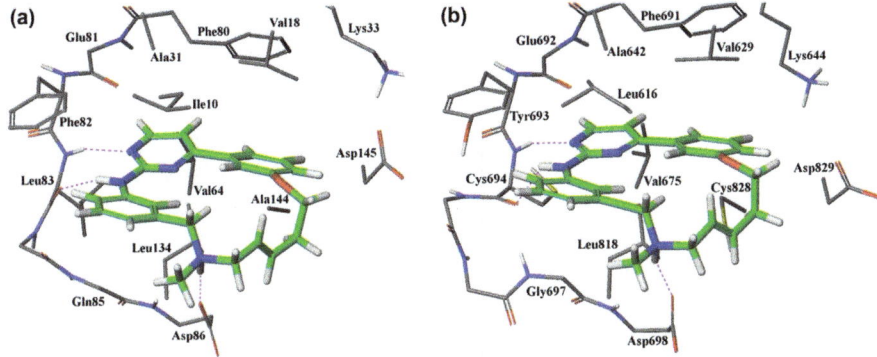

Figure 5.11 Multikinase inhibition by N-linked macrocycles. (a) Compound **3** docked into CDK2 and (b) FLT3. The binding mode is similar to that of **41** docked into Aurora A (Figure 5.10b). The basic nitrogen of the macrocyclic linker forms an additional salt bridge to Asp86 in CDK2 and the homologous residue Asp698 in FLT3.

The effect of the linker heteroatoms on activity and selectivity was investigated with compounds **42–47** (Table 5.5). Aniline-linked analog **42** was 13-fold less active against CDK2 than compound **3** but its FLT3 and JAK2 activity only decreased by a factor of two. Similar profiles were observed with the bis-phenol-linked derivative **43** and the benzyl ether **44**. Generally, CDK2 activity decreased at least 10-fold when the basic amine of **3** was replaced with a non-basic atom or functional group, whereas FLT3 and JAK2 activity decreased less. When the phenolic oxygen in **3** was replaced by the more rigid amides, as in **45** and **46**, activity against all kinases investigated was greatly reduced. Compound **47**, where the linker is reversed as compared to **3**, had a profile similar to **42**. Varying the linker composition is clearly important but attempts to study these compounds in cells were hampered by poor solubility. In an effort to increase solubility, substitution of the B-ring with metabolically robust short basic side chains led to the synthesis of compound **1**. Prior SAR (not shown) confirmed that a dibenzylic linker was preferred: substitution of the B-ring with methoxy in this series gave a compound with JAK2 IC_{50} of 70 nM and CDK2 IC_{50} of 0.86 μM. Extension of the methoxy to a pyrrolidinylethoxy, as in **1**, increased solubility and cellular potency (see below). Possessing a di-benzylic ether linker, **1** was found to be a potent JAK2 and FLT3 inhibitor with over 150-fold selectivity for CDK2. Furthermore, **1** showed selectivity within the JAK family for the JAK2 and TYK2 subtypes, consistent with a desirable target profile for myeloproliferative diseases and lymphoid malignancies. At this point it became clear that the oxygen-linked macrocycles were excellent leads for the selective JAK2/FLT3 inhibitors project whereas the nitrogen-linked compounds were developed as leads for the multikinase CDK inhibitor project.

Compound **48**, the *cis* isomer of *trans*-olefin analog **1**, formed as the minor isomer during the ring closing metathesis (RCM) to provide the macrocycle, was found to be less potent against JAK2 and FLT3. However, against CDK2

Table 5.5 Exploration of macrocyclic linkers.[a]

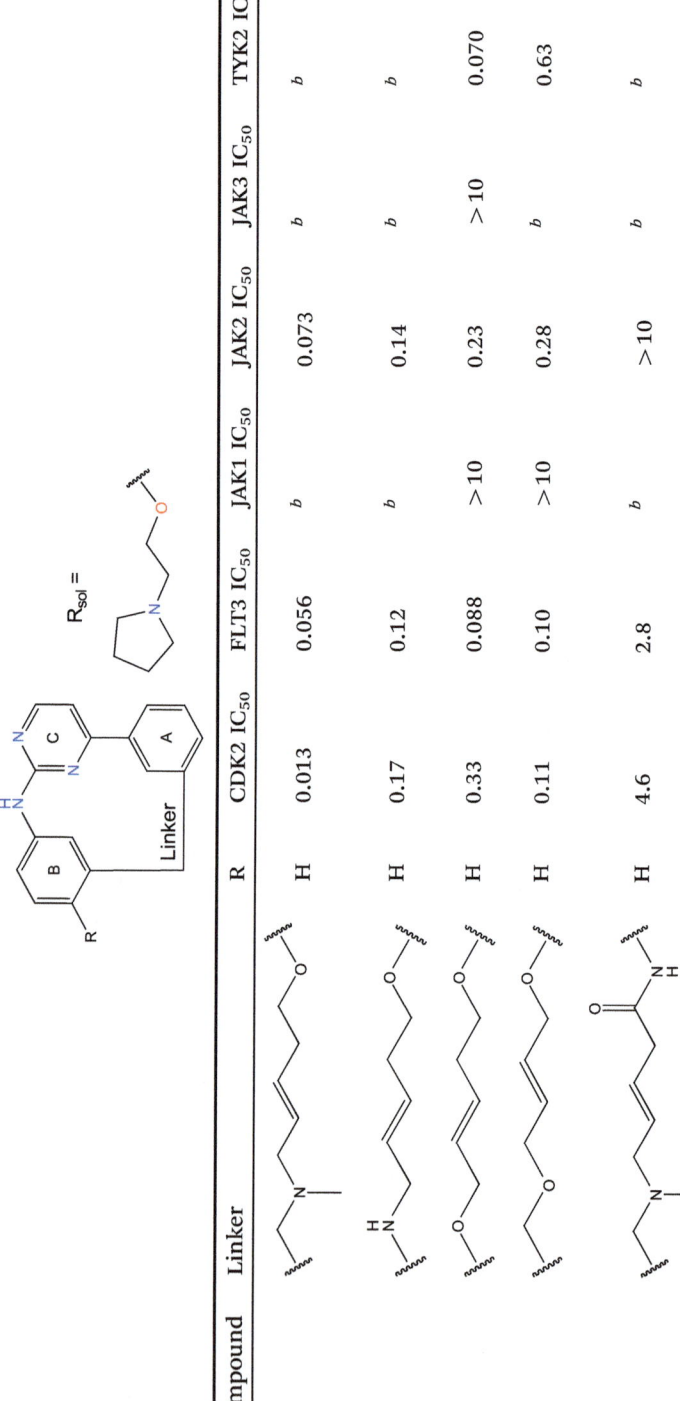

Compound	Linker	R	CDK2 IC$_{50}$	FLT3 IC$_{50}$	JAK1 IC$_{50}$	JAK2 IC$_{50}$	JAK3 IC$_{50}$	TYK2 IC$_{50}$
3		H	0.013	0.056	b	0.073	b	b
42		H	0.17	0.12	b	0.14	b	b
43		H	0.33	0.088	>10	0.23	>10	0.070
44		H	0.11	0.10	>10	0.28	b	0.63
45		H	4.6	2.8	b	>10	b	b

No.	Linker	R						
46		H	>10	>10	b	>10	b	b
47		H	0.099	0.31	3.2	0.23	b	0.83
1		R_{sol}	3.9	0.022	1.28	0.023	0.52	0.050
48		R_{sol}	3.9	0.080	2.2	0.065	1.1	0.23
49		R_{sol}	1.3	0.027	1.1	0.076	1.6	0.11
50		R_{sol}	3.5	0.037	2.8	0.073	0.57	0.22

[a]See Figure 5.10c for a definition of the linker. IC_{50} values are in micromolar and are the mean of at least two individual determinations.[9,10]
[b]Not available.

the isomers were weakly active but equipotent. The double bond in the linker resulting from the ring closing metathesis was originally envisaged to be reduced or functionalized as it was expected to be a metabolic liability. In fact, this turned out not to be the case and the olefin was retained in most compounds. In analog **49** the double bond was reduced resulting in 3-fold increased CDK2 activity and similar JAK2 activity. Compound **50** in which the double bond of **1** has been converted into a cyclopropyl group was less potent compared to **1** against JAK2 (3-fold) and TYK2 (4-fold). No further derivatization of the linker double bond was attempted.

The observation that macrocycles with a basic nitrogen in the linker, such as **3**, are potent CDK2 and FLT3 inhibitors is consistent with the formation of a salt bridge between this basic nitrogen and Asp86 in CDK2 and Asp698 in FLT3. This residue is highlighted in green in the alignment in Figure 5.12.[7] When the basic nitrogen is exchanged for an oxygen the FLT3 and CDK2 activity was expected to drop significantly but this was only observed for CDK2 while FLT3 activity remained as for **1**. When docked into CDK2, poses of **1** were either high energy conformations or had repulsive electrostatic interactions with the Asp86 side chain (Figure 5.13a). This was not the case for FLT3 where poses of **1** were found to form a hydrogen bond to the backbone NH of Asp698 (Figure 5.13b). In CDK2 there is a deletion of one residue between the kinase hinge and Asp86 as compared to the other kinases studied. Due to the shorter distance between the kinase hinge and the backbone NH of Asp86 the ether oxygen of **1** may not form the hydrogen bond to CDK2 that was observed in the FLT3 pose. The equivalent residue in JAK1, JAK2, and TYK2 is a serine and in poses docked into JAK2 the hydroxyl of Ser936 forms a hydrogen bond with both the oxygen- and nitrogen-linked macrocycles. This is shown in Figure 5.13c for **1**. This also explains the good TYK2 activity, but not the poor JAK1 activity of compound **1**. This remained unexplained until a JAK1 X-ray structure was published wherein the serine hydroxyl group forms two hydrogen bonds with Glu966 and Lys965, thus preventing the hydroxyl from hydrogen bonding with the inhibitor.[86] The equivalent residue to Ser936 in JAK3 is the much more hydrophobic Ser909, the side chain of which does not interact well with either the basic nitrogen or the ether oxygen in the macrocyclic linker. Thus the nature of the residue highlighted in green in Figure 5.12 explains the overall selectivity profile of both the nitrogen and the oxygen linked macrocycles.[7]

Amine-linked compounds also tolerated substitution larger than a methyl group on the basic nitrogen. Comparing analogs **51–54** to **3** (Table 5.6) it is apparent that the optimal substituent for CDK2 activity is a methyl group as in **3**. Macrocycle **51**, without any substituent, is approximately half as potent as **3** against CDK2, FLT3 and JAK2. Increasing the bulk of the R_3 substituent gradually decreases activity and compound **54** with a *neo*-pentyl substituent has no measurable activity. These observations were consistent with docked poses of compounds **53** and **54** where the larger substituents either clashed with the kinase or prevented salt bridge formation to Asp86 in CDK2. The slightly decreased activity of **51** compared to **3** may be due to a

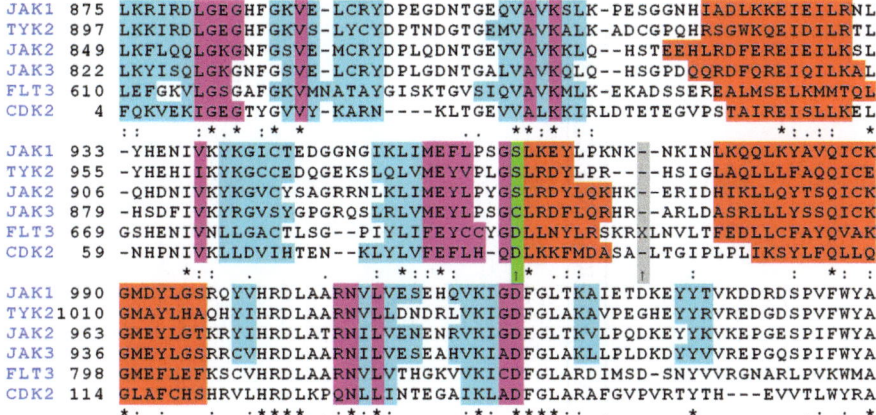

```
JAK1  875 LKRIRDLGEGHFGKVE-LCRYDPEGDNTGEQVAVKSLK-PESGGNHIADLKKEIEILRNL
TYK2  897 LKKIRDLGEGHFGKVS-LYCYDPTNDGTGEMVAVKALK-ADCGPQHRSGWKQEIDILRTL
JAK2  849 LKFLQQLGKGNFGSVE-MCRYDPLQDNTGEVVAVKKLQ--HSTEEHLRDFEREIEILKSL
JAK3  822 LKYISQLGKGNFGSVE-LCRYDPLGDNTGALVAVKQLQ--HSGPDQQRDFQREIQILKAL
FLT3  610 LEFGKVLGSGAFGKVMNATAYGISKTGVSIQVAVKMLK-EKADSSEREALMSELKMMTQL
CDK2    4 FQKVEKIGEGTYGVVY-KARN----KLTGEVVALKKIRLDTETEGVPSTAIREISLLKEL
            ::      :*.* :*  *          .. **:* ::           *:.:: *

JAK1  933 -YHENIVKYKGICTEDGGNGIKLIMEFLPSGSLKEYLPKNK--NKINLKQQLKYAVQICK
TYK2  955 -YHEHIIKYKGCCEDQGEKSLQLVMEYVPLGSLRDYLPR----HSIGLAQLLLFAQQICE
JAK2  906 -QHDNIVKYKGVCYSAGRRNLKLIMEYLPYGSLRDYLQKHK--ERIDHIKLLQYTSQICK
JAK3  879 -HSDFIVKYRGVSYGPGRQSLRLVMEYLPSGCLRDFLQRHR--ARLDASRLLLYSSQICK
FLT3  669 GSHENIVNLLGACTLSG--PIYLIFEYCCYGDLLNYLRSKRXLNVLTFEDLLCFAYQVAK
CDK2   59 -NHPNIVKLLDVIHTEN--KLYLVFEFLH-QDLKKFMDASA-LTGIPLPLIKSYLFQLLQ
            *::    .      .   *::*:    *  .::         :      : *: :

JAK1  990 GMDYLGSRQYVHRDLAARNVLVESEHQVKIGDFGLTKAIETDKEYYTVKDDRDSPVFWYA
TYK2 1010 GMAYLHAQHYIHRDLAARNVLLDNDRLVKIGDFGLAKAVPEGHEYYRVREDGDSPVFWYA
JAK2  963 GMEYLGTKRYIHRDLATRNILVENENRVKIGDFGLTKVLPQDKEYYKVKEPGESPIFWYA
JAK3  936 GMEYLGSRRCVHRDLAARNILVESEAHVKIADFGLAKLLPLDKDYYVVREPGQSPIFWYA
FLT3  798 GMEFLEFKSCVHRDLAARNVLVTHGKVVKICDFGLARDIMSD-SNYVVRGNARLPVKWMA
CDK2  114 GLAFCHSHRVLHRDLKPQNLLINTEGAIKLADFGLARAFGVPVRTYTH---EVVTLWYRA
            *: :   :   :**** .:*:*:    :*: ****::   .      *     .: : *
```

Figure 5.12 Clustal W alignment of the protein kinase targets. Cyan: Beta strand; Red: Alpha helix; Magenta: Binding site residues. Secondary structure information is taken from X-ray structures. The X highlighted in grey denotes the FLT3 insertion residues 708–779. The arrow highlighted with green indicates a residue essential for the selectivity of the described macrocycles (Ser936 in JAK2, Asp689 in FLT3 and Asp86 in CDK2). There is a deletion in CDK2 of one residue just before Asp86. Figure 5.12 reproduced with kind permission from Springer Science + Business Media, *J. Comput. Aided Mol Des.*, 2012, **26**, 437, Figure 1.

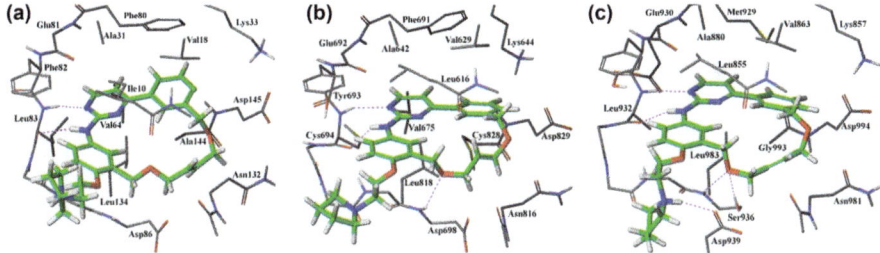

Figure 5.13 Selectivity of O-linked macrocycles. Compound **1** docked into (a) CDK2, (b) FLT3, and (c) JAK2. The interaction of the ether oxygen linker with Ser936 in JAK2 and Asp698 in FLT3 explain the observed selectivity profile. The macrocycle cannot hydrogen bond to the backbone NH of the homologous residue in CDK2 (Asp86) due to the deletion before this residue (see alignment in Figure 5.12).

conformational or solvation effect as a result of a lack of a substituent on the basic amine. As methyl was found to be the optimal nitrogen substituent most N-linked macrocycles were synthesized with this group.

We next turned our attention to the exploration of substitutions on the B-ring (R_1 and R_2). Docked poses of the macrocycles indicated that the 4- and 5-positions of the B-ring point out of the ATP-binding site toward solvent and therefore these positions were proposed to be substituted with solubilizing groups. Compound **55** with a pyrrolidine connected to the 4-position

Table 5.6 SAR of substituents in the B-ring, solubility tags and N-substituents.[a]

Compound	R₁	R₂	R₃	CDK2 IC₅₀	FLT3 IC₅₀	JAK1 IC₅₀	JAK2 IC₅₀	JAK3 IC₅₀	TYK2 IC₅₀
51	H	H	H	0.021	0.11	0.18	0.15	b	0.081
3	H	H	Me	0.013	0.056	b	0.073	b	b
52	H	H	cPr	0.036	0.042	b	0.090	b	b
53	H	H	iBu	0.2	0.19	b	1.5	b	b
54	H	H	CH₂tBu	>10	>10	b	>10	b	b
55	2-(pyrrolidin-1-yl)ethoxy	H	Me	0.25	0.035	b	0.056	b	b
56	OMe	H	Me	0.077	0.066	b	0.28	b	b
57	SO₂Et	H	Me	0.022	0.44	b	0.10	b	b
58	Morpholino	H	Me	0.074	0.071	b	0.049	b	b
59	H	NH₂	Me	0.0065	0.019	b	0.050	b	b
60	H	NHSO₂Et	Me	0.0080	0.14	b	0.018	b	b
61	H	NHCO-morpholine	Me	0.087	0.037	b	0.044	b	b
1	2-(pyrrolidin-1-yl)ethoxy	H		3.9	0.022	1.28	0.023	0.52	0.050
62	2-(NEt₂)ethoxy	H		4.7	0.029	3.5	0.024	0.62	0.079
63	4-Me-piperazine	H		>10	0.030	3.6	0.041	b	0.19
64	Morpholine	H		>10	0.032	8.7	0.060	b	0.16
65	EtSO₂-piperazine	H		>10	0.15	>10	0.15	>10	0.14
66	H	NH₂		0.24	0.052	b	0.035	1.75	b
67	H	NH₂COCH₂CH₂N(Et)₂		0.4	0.078	1.9	0.044	0.39	0.018

[a]See Figure 5.10c for a definition of the rings. IC₅₀ values are in micromolar and are the mean of at least two individual determinations.[9,10] R=H unless stated.
[b]Not available.

(R$_1$) by an ethoxy linker, as for compound **1**, was found to be equipotent with **3** against FLT3 and JAK2 but lost 20-fold CDK2 activity. The smaller methoxy substituent of **56** resulted in a reduction of CDK2 activity of 6-fold, whereas the ethyl sulfone substituent of **57** decreased FLT3 activity 8-fold without altering JAK2 and CDK2 activity significantly. The more bulky morpholine substituent of **58** did not change JAK2 and FLT3 activity but decreased CDK2 activity 6-fold as compared to **3**. Conformational analysis of **56** and **57** indicated that N-linked macrocycles with an acceptor atom in the 4-position of the B-ring may form an internal hydrogen bond to the protonated basic nitrogen that increased the conformational energy of the bioactive conformation. Where this is not offset by favorable interactions of the substituent with the kinase, the increased conformational energy may explain the general trend of 4-substituents lowering inhibitory activity.

The 5-position (R$_2$) of the B-ring was found to be close to the carbonyl backbone of His84 when macrocycles were docked into CDK2. Poses of compounds with a solubilizing group attached to the 5-position *via* a nitrogen formed an additional hydrogen bond to His84 of the CDK2 kinase hinge (Figure 5.14a). Compound **59** with an aniline at the 5-position had 2- and 3-fold increased CDK2 and FLT3 potency, respectively, compared to **3**, but JAK2 activity remained unchanged. These observations are consistent with an extra hydrogen bond being formed to the kinase hinge of CDK2 and possibly FLT3 but not for JAK2. However, when the aniline was further substituted, as in the ethyl-sulfonamide **60** or the morpholine-urea **61**, either FLT3 or CDK2 activity was decreased compared to **59**.

N-Linked macrocycles without B-ring substituents, such as **3**, had reasonable aqueous solubility (Table 5.11) and, given the aforementioned SAR, it was decided not to pursue addition of solubilizing groups to this series. However, this was not the case for the *O*-linked series where a solubilizing

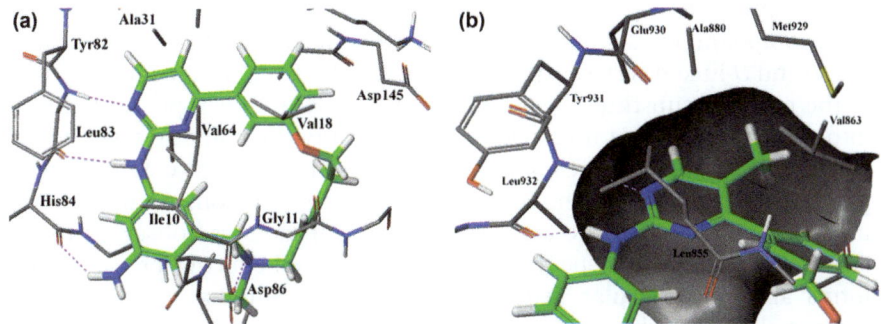

Figure 5.14 Compounds with substituents in the B and C-ring. (a) Compound **59** docked into CDK2. The aniline nitrogen in the 5-position of the B-ring may form an additional hydrogen bond to the end of the kinase hinge. (b) Compound **78** docked into JAK2. The 5-Me substituent has hydrophobic interactions with the gatekeeper residue Met929. Notice that the 6-position hydrogen is pointing towards the backbone carbonyl of Glu930.

group was required to achieve good solubility. The internal hydrogen bond formation found in the *N*-linked series is not possible for the *O*-linked series as long as the 4-substituent linker is not attached *via* a hydrogen bond donor. Compounds in the *O*-linked series with a solubilizing group attached by an ethoxy linker to the 4-position, such as **1** and **62**, showed low nanomolar JAK2 and FLT3 activity while their CDK2 activity was in the micromolar range. When docked into JAK2, the pyrrolidine of **1** forms a salt bridge to Asp939, consistent with the high JAK2 activity. More bulky solubilizing groups were also accommodated in the 4-position although this generally resulted in a slight decrease in activity compared to **1**. Methyl-piperazine **63** and morpholine substituted analog **64** had a similar profile while the JAK2 and FLT3 activity dropped significantly for the sulfonyl-piperazine **65**.

Substitution at the 5-position to form an aniline in the *O*-linked series, as in compound **66** and the further substituted **67**, resulted in a large improvement in CDK2 activity while JAK2 and FLT3 activity decreased slightly. This was consistent with SAR for the *N*-linked series, but detrimental to the desired selectivity profile. When a compound with a 6-methyl group was docked into any of the kinases investigated, the hydrogen bonds with the kinase hinge were clearly disrupted, so substitution at the 6-position was judged to be detrimental to kinase activity. The 2-position is facing the center of the macrocycle. Conformational analysis of compounds with substitution at this position indicated that the macrocycle cannot adopt the putative bioactive conformation. Consequently substitution of the 2- and 6-positions were not investigated. It was decided that in the *O*-linked series the 4-position ethoxy–pyrrolidine solubilizing moiety, as in compound **1**, had the most preferred kinase inhibition profile and therefore most compounds in the *O*-linked series were subsequently synthesized with this group in the 4-position of the B-ring.

Limited availability of appropriate starting materials limited the exploration of A-ring SAR (Table 5.7). Substitution of the 4-position by methoxy, as in compound **68**, significantly decreased CDK2 and FLT3 activity in both the *N*- and *O*-linked series. When **68** was docked into CDK2 the methyl group of the methoxy substituent clashed with the kinase. In compounds docked into any of the kinases investigated, the 4-position is pointing towards the side chain of an acidic residue (see docking of **1** in Figure 5.13). It was postulated that a hydrogen bond donor in this position, as in **69**, may interact favorably with the acid, but this substitution was observed to decrease activity. This may be due to a conformational effect where the donor forms an intramolecular hydrogen bond to the adjacent oxygen in the macrocyclic linker thus increasing the conformational energy of the kinase bound conformation. Compound **70** with a fluorine in the 5-position had 2-fold increased FLT3 and CDK activity albeit with a loss of JAK2 activity, as compared to **3**.

In the *O*-linked series substitution of the 4-position by methoxy, as in compound **71**, significantly decreased CDK2 activity. Compared to **1**, the JAK1 activity of **71**, and to a lesser extent JAK3 activity, was decreased while

Table 5.7 SAR of substituents in the A-ring.[a]

Compound	R_1	R_2	R_3	CDK2 IC_{50}	FLT3 IC_{50}	JAK1 IC_{50}	JAK2 IC_{50}	JAK3 IC_{50}	TYK2 IC_{50}
3	H	H	H	0.013	0.056	b	0.073	b	b
68	OMe	H	H	2.3	0.31	b	0.51	b	b
69	NH$_2$	H	H	0.10	0.16	b	0.16	b	b
70	H	F	H	0.0089	0.030	b	0.16	b	b
1	H	H	H	3.9	0.022	1.28	0.023	0.52	0.050
71	OMe	H	H	>10	0.092	>10	0.019	0.89	0.18
72	F	H	H	3.3	0.040	4.6	0.025	0.72	b
73	H	F	H	2.0	0.0077	0.38	0.024	0.50	
74	H	H	OMe	>10	0.012	4.9	0.33	7.2	0.62

[a]See Figure 5.10c for a definition of the rings. IC_{50} values are in micromolar and are the mean of at least two individual determinations.[9,10] R=H unless stated.
[b]Not available.

maintaining JAK2 activity, consistent with our desired target profile. Unfortunately, both FLT3 activity and solubility decreased relative to **1**. The 5-F substituent increased FLT3 activity 3-fold for the *O*-linked analog **73** without compromising JAK2 activity, compared to **1**, but CDK2 activity was also increased 2-fold detrimental to the target product profile of the *O*-linked series. Fluoro substitution of the 4-position, as in **72**, did not change the kinase selectivity profile compared to **1**. The 6-methoxy compound, **74**, had slightly improved FLT3 inhibitory potency but activity towards the JAK family decreased by at least 10-fold, except for the 4-fold decrease in JAK1 activity. Substitution of the 2-position of the A-ring was not investigated as conformational analysis indicated that this would prevent the *O*-linked macrocycles from adopting the putative bioactive conformation.

The effect of substitution on the C-ring on the *N*- and *O*-linked macrocycles was explored through variations at the 5- and 6-positions, R_2 and R_1, respectively (Table 5.8). However, docking indicated that a 6-position substituent would clash with the kinase and/or prevent formation of hydrogen bonds to the hinge. Compounds **75** and **76** in the *N*-linked series were synthesized to challenge the modeling. While **75**, with a 6-methyl substituent, retained micromolar CDK2 and FLT3 activity, **76**, with a larger pyrrolidine substituent, was devoid of any kinase activity. Docking into JAK2 indicated there was room for a small hydrophobic substituent in the 5-position that may interact with the gatekeeper residue Met929. However, JAK2 activity decreased 2-fold for the *N*-linked 5-methylpyrimidine, **77** compared to **3**. In the *O*-linked series, CDK2 activity for the 5-methyl

Table 5.8 SAR of substituents in the C-ring.[a]

Compound	R$_1$	R$_2$	CDK2 IC$_{50}$	FLT3 IC$_{50}$	JAK1 IC$_{50}$	JAK2 IC$_{50}$	JAK3 IC$_{50}$	TYK2 IC$_{50}$
3	H	H	0.013	0.056	*b*	0.073	*b*	*b*
75	Me	H	4.7	1.7	*b*	>10	*b*	*b*
76	pyrrolidin-1-yl	H	>10	>10	*b*	>10	*b*	*b*
77	H	Me	0.15	0.022	*b*	0.18	*b*	*b*
1	H	H	3.9	0.022	1.28	0.023	0.52	0.050
78	H	Me	>10	0.019	1.0	0.0066	0.089	0.057
79	H	F	1.6	0.015	0.83	0.017	1.0	0.14

[a]See Figure 5.10c for a definition of the rings. IC$_{50}$ values are in micromolar and are the mean of at least two individual determinations.[9,10] R=H unless stated.
[b]Not available.

substituted compounds decreased while, as indicated by modelling studies (see Figure 5.14b), JAK2 activity was found to increase 3-fold for compound **78**. Unfortunately the JAK3 activity of **78** increased 6-fold, detrimental to the desired target profile. Compound **79**, with the smaller more polar fluorine substituent, had a profile closer to the unsubstituted analog **1**, but was 2-fold less selective against CDK2 and 2-fold more selective for JAK1.

Aiming to explore compounds with reduced cLogP, a number of heterocycles were explored as A-ring replacements (Table 5.9). Changing the A-ring from a phenyl to a pyridine or a 5-membered heterocycle lowered the cLogP except when the replacement ring was a thiophene. The 4-position of macrocycles with a phenyl A-ring points toward Lys33 and Asp145 when docked into CDK2 (Figure 5.13a). Introducing a pyridine A-ring as in the *N*-linked derivative **80** was expected to increase electrostatic interactions with the kinase, but this did not lead to increased CDK2 activity.

By introducing a more polar A-ring it was expected that solubility would increase, which was one of the principal objectives for the high cLogP *O*-linked series. Pyridine **81** had a disappointing JAK2 IC$_{50}$, 12-fold higher than the phenyl analog **1**. The furans **82** and **2** had 5- and 2-fold increased IC$_{50}$ values for JAK2, respectively, compared to **1**. Even though **2** had decreased JAK2 activity, its selectivity profile was improved over **1** as both CDK2 and JAK1 inhibitory activity decreased 2-fold and JAK3 activity decreased 8-fold. Compound **2** was found to dock into JAK2 with a similar conformation and orientation as **1** (compare Figure 5.15a with Figure 5.13c). This was generally the case for all macrocycles with pyridine or 5-membered A-rings. Compound **83**, the thiophene analog of **2**, had a 7 nM JAK2 IC$_{50}$ and improved selectivity profile compared to **1**, but this came at the cost of decreased

Table 5.9 SAR of heterocyclic A-rings.[a]

Compound	A-Ring	CDK2 IC_{50}	FLT3 IC_{50}	JAK1 IC_{50}	JAK2 IC_{50}	JAK3 IC_{50}	TYK2 IC_{50}
3	Phenyl	0.013	0.056	[b]	0.073	[b]	[b]
80		0.022	0.31	0.17	0.26	>10	0.065
1	Phenyl	3.9	0.022	1.28	0.023	0.52	0.050
81		3.2	0.063	>10	0.29	1.0	0.63
82		>10	0.18	1.9	0.11	9.2	0.31
2		6.7	0.060	2.7	0.046	4.3	0.23
83		2.9	0.024	0.42	0.0073	0.65	0.032
84		>10	0.048	3.0	0.067	8.8	0.12
85		6.8	0.045	1.5	0.017	0.68	0.047

Table 5.9   *(Continued)*

Compound	A-Ring	CDK2 IC$_{50}$	FLT3 IC$_{50}$	JAK1 IC$_{50}$	JAK2 IC$_{50}$	JAK3 IC$_{50}$	TYK2 IC$_{50}$
86		>10	0.046	>10	0.88	*b*	3.4
87		>10	0.092	>10	0.46	5.7	4.3

^{a}See Figure 5.10c for a definition of the rings. IC$_{50}$ values are in micromolar and are the mean of at least two individual determinations.[11]
^{b}Not available.

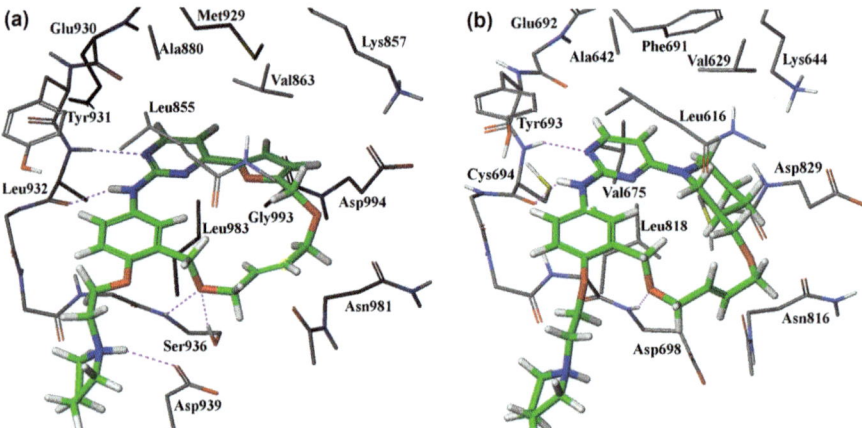

Figure 5.15   Macrocycles with heterocyclic A-rings. (a) Compound 2 (SB1578) docked into JAK2. The putative bioactive conformation and orientation in the JAK2 binding site is similar to that of phenyl analogue **1** (Figure 5.13c). (b) Compound **86** docked into FLT3. There is room for the extra bulk of the aliphatic A-ring in the FLT3 binding site. The putative bioactive conformation and orientation in the FLT3 binding site is similar to that of phenyl analogue **1** (Figure 5.13a).

solubility. Furan **84** had a profile similar to **2** and was more than 100-fold selective for JAK2 over JAK3. The thiophene analog **85** was 3-fold more active against JAK2 than the furan analog **84**, but less selective.

Compounds **86** and **87** have an aliphatic piperidine A-ring. These less potent compounds had the desired selectivity profile for FLT3 and JAK2 while having reduced JAK3 activity and being devoid of CDK2 and JAK1 activity. Docking into JAK2 and FLT3 indicated that there was room for the aliphatic ring and the 1,3-linked and 1,4-linked piperidine were explored

(Figure 5.15b). Compounds **86** and **87** had a rather disappointing JAK2 activity, probably due to the macrocyclic linker, as analogs with different linkers had much improved JAK2 activity (unpublished results).

Two alternate C-rings were also explored. In compounds with a pyrimidine C-ring the 6-position hydrogen is pointing towards the residue after the gatekeeper (Glu930 in JAK2) and is in van der Waals contact with its backbone carbonyl (Figure 5.14b). Some authors have described this interaction as a hydrogen bond with the pyrimidine C6 as the donor.[87] This observation prompted the introduction of a stronger hydrogen bond donor to potentially interact with the kinase hinge. Docking of macrocycles with an -NH$_2$ substituent in the 6-position into JAK2 indicated that the hydrogen bond to the Glu930 backbone carbonyl may be formed but this was at the expense of the hydrogen bond to the Leu932 backbone NH. However, if the pyrimidine were replaced with an -NH$_2$ substituted 5-membered ring, the slightly altered geometry of the C-ring allowed poses of docked compounds to form three hydrogen bonds to the hinge. Compound **88**, with a triazole C-ring, was a potent inhibitor of FLT3 with an IC$_{50}$ of 0.023 μM, but with 10-fold decreased JAK2 activity compared to **1** (Figure 5.16). Except for the disappointing JAK2 activity, the selectivity profile of **88** was desirable with CDK2 and JAK1 activity >10 μM and a JAK3 IC$_{50}$ of 4.5 μM. Unfortunately the heteroatoms of the pyrimidine (A-ring) of **88** were expected to decrease JAK2 affinity (compare **2**, **82** and **88** to **1**). It proved synthetically challenging to replace the pyrimidine of **88** with a phenyl, and for this reason this series was not pursued further. Another way of introducing an additional hydrogen bond donor at the 6-position of the C-ring was by replacing the C-ring with a purine, as in the *N*-linked analog, compound **89** (Figure 5.16). This compound was also potent against FLT3 with an IC$_{50}$ of 0.058 μM but an 8-fold higher JAK2 IC$_{50}$ of 0.45 μM. Interestingly, the *N*-linked purine **89** had poor

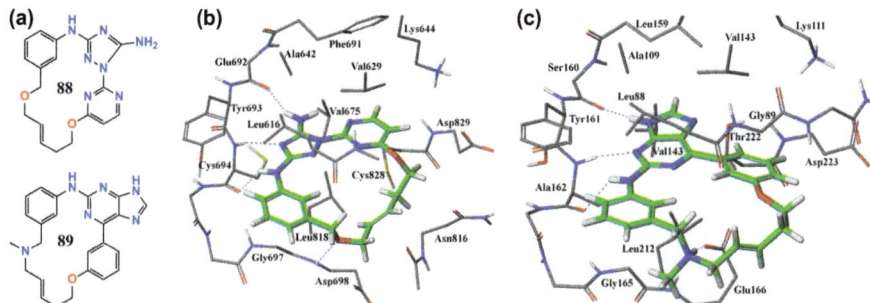

Figure 5.16 (a) Macrocycles with alternative C-rings. **88** was selective for FLT3 with an IC$_{50}$ of 0.023 μM. IC$_{50}$ values for CDK2, JAK1, JAK2, JAK3, and TYK2 were >10, >10, 0.27, 4.5 and 0.67 μM. Compound **89** had JAK2, CDK2, FLT3, and PDK1 IC$_{50}$ of 0.45 μM, 4.1 μM, 0.058 μM and 0.39μM. **89** was used as a lead in our PDK1 project. (b) Compound **88** docked into FLT3 and (c) **89** docked into PDK1. In both compounds the C-ring forms an additional hydrogen bond with the backbone carbonyl of the residue immediately after the gatekeeper.

CDK2 activity of 4.1 μM consistent with the reduced CDK2 activity of 5-substituted pyrimidines like 77. Compound **89** had a PDK1 IC_{50} of 0.39 μM and later became a lead for a PDK1 inhibitor program.[88,89]

5.3.3 *In Vitro* Biology

Cell-based activity for the kinase inhibitors was obtained in cell lines sensitive to inhibition of the target enzymes (Table 5.10). *N*-Linked macrocycles were profiled in a range of solid tumor and hematological cancer cell lines. HL-60 is a FLT3-driven acute myeloid leukemia cell line that is also known to be sensitive to CDK inhibitors. Compounds **3** and **51** were highly potent, inhibiting proliferation in this cell line with IC_{50}s of 0.059 and 0.089 μM, respectively. The more potent CDK2 inhibitor **60** was a less potent antiproliferative agent with an IC_{50} of 0.13 μM, possibly due to the 3-fold decreased FLT3 activity compared to **3**. Compound **52** had a similar FLT3 potency and slightly lower CDK2 activity than **3**, but cellular activities were much reduced as compared to **3**. Similar proliferation inhibitory profiles were observed for the three solid tumor cell lines HCT-116 (colon), COLO205 (colon) and DU145 (prostate). Macrocycle **3** was also potent in the Ramos lymphoma cell line with an IC_{50} of 0.033 μM.

For the *O*-linked macrocycles, profiling of cell proliferation focused initially on a Ba/F3 cell line harboring the JAK2 V617F mutation and MV4-11 cells expressing the FLT3-ITD mutation. Compounds **1**, **62**, and **71** with JAK2 activities in the 0.02 μM range all had similar Ba/F3 IC_{50}s of around 0.1 μM. The 3-fold more potent JAK2 inhibitors, **78** and **83**, were expected to have increased proliferation inhibition. This was the case for thiophene **83**, inhibiting Ba/F3 cell proliferation with an IC_{50} of 0.055 μM, but **78** was found

Table 5.10 Cell-based activities for selected compounds in relevant cell lines.[a]

Compound	Ba/F3 GI_{50}[b]	MV4-11 IC_{50}[c]	HL-60 IC_{50}	HTC116 IC_{50}	Ramos IC_{50}	Colo205 IC_{50}	Du145 IC_{50}
3 (SB1317)	d	d	0.059	0.079	0.033	0.072	0.14
51	d	d	0.089	0.135	d	0.12	0.71
52	d	d	1.38	1.6	d	3.6	3.0
60	d	d	0.13	d	d	d	d
1 (SB1518)	0.16	0.047	d	d	d	d	d
62	0.15	0.037	d	d	d	d	d
71	0.10	0.085	d	d	d	d	d
78	0.18	0.051	d	d	d	d	d
2 (SB1578)	0.25	d	0.85	d	d	d	d
83	0.055	d	0.2	d	d	d	d
84	d	d	0.71	d	d	d	d
85	0.080	d	0.64	d	d	d	d

[a]Activities are in micromolar. Compounds **3**, **51**, **52** and **60** are *N*-linked while the remaining compounds are *O*-linked.
[b]JAK2 V617F mutant cell line.
[c]FLT3-ITD mutant cell line.
[d]Not available.

to be equipotent with **1**. Compounds **1, 62**, and **78** had similar FLT3 activities in the 0.02 µM range and were found to inhibit MV4-11 cell proliferation with IC$_{50}$ values of approximately 0.04 µM. With a 4-fold lower FLT3 activity, compound **71** was half as potent in this assay.

Although the A-ring heterocyclic O-linked macrocycles were intended as potential therapeutics for RA, they were also tested in the HL-60 cell line (AML). Compounds **2** and **83–85** had FLT3 activities around 0.05 µM, except analog **83**, which was twice as potent. These compounds inhibited HL-60 cell proliferation with IC$_{50}$ values in the range of 0.6–0.8 µM, apart from thiophene **83**, which was found to be 3-fold more potent. Additional CDK activity in the N-linked macrocycles was clearly much more effective in inhibition of HL-60 proliferation. Further detailed information on the biological profiles, including cellular pharmacodynamic studies demonstrating intracellular inhibition of the kinases, of compounds **1, 2**, and **3** are available.[77,90,91]

5.3.4 Physical Properties and *In Vitro* ADME

In vitro ADME data was generated for advanced compounds (Table 5.11).[9–11] Cell permeability was not a concern as most compounds had polar surface areas well below 100 Å^2 and were found to have good activity in cellular assays. Kinetic aqueous solubility was generally acceptable for the N-linked compounds, such as **3**, with an N-methyl substituent, which had a solubility of 72 µg mL^{-1}. However, both **51**, without an NH-linker, and **52** with an N-cyclopropyl group, had 5-fold reduced solubility. These observations, together with the favorable kinase activity of **3**, prompted the early selection of methyl as the optimal N-substituent. The O-linked macrocycles had much lower solubility, which led to the incorporation of a solubilizing group. Compounds incorporating a basic amine connected by an ethoxy linker to

Table 5.11 *In vitro* ADME for selected compounds. Compounds **3, 51, 52** and **60** are N-linked while the remaining compounds are O-linked.

Compound	Solubility (µg/mL)[a]	CYP3A4 IC$_{50}$ (µM)	CYP2D6 IC$_{50}$ (µM)	HLM t$_{1/2}$ (min)	MLM t$_{1/2}$ (min)	PPB (%)[b]
3 (SB1317)	71.8	> 25	0.95	45	12	99.4
51	14.7	c	c	48	10	c
52	16.6	c	c	> 60	> 60	c
60	82.4	c	c	30	7	c
1 (SB1518)	> 150	> 5	> 5	> 60	22	99.41
62	147	2.8	> 10	44	16	c
71	60.83	> 10	> 10	> 60	29	c
78	> 150	2.5	> 10	> 60	40	c
2 (SB1578)	> 250	> 10	> 10	> 60	27	87.3
83	154	> 10	> 10	> 60	27	c
84	> 250	> 10	> 10	> 60	18	c
85	218	ND	ND	> 60	25	c

[a]Kinetic slubility, pH 7.
[b]Plasma Protein Binding in mice.
[c]Not vailable.

the 4-position of the B-ring also had increased JAK2 activity, probably due to the formation of a salt bridge to Asp939 (Figure 5.13c). Most *O*-linked macrocycles were synthesized with an ethoxy–pyrrolidine solubility tag that generally increased solubility to >150 µg mL^{-1}. Compounds with additional hydrophobic substituents, such as **71**, with a methoxy in the 4-position of the A-ring, had decreased solubility. Substitution of the A-ring with a more polar heterocycle, such as a furan, for example compounds **2** and **84**, substantially increased solubility to >250 µg mL^{-1}.

Potential for drug-drug interactions was assessed by recombinant enzyme inhibition assays for the major drug metabolizing human cytochrome P450s. Significant CYP3A4 inhibition was not observed for most compounds. Compounds **62** and **78**, both incorporating exposed aliphatic substituents, had CYP3A4 inhibition in the low micromolar range. Inhibition of CYP2D6 was not an issue for *O*-linked macrocycles. However, the *N*-linked macrocycle **3** was a moderate inhibitor of CYP2D6 with an IC$_{50}$ of 1 µM, approximately similar to the plasma C$_{max}$ observed at the maximum tolerated dose in mice. Compounds **1**, **2**, and **3** were found to be devoid of CYP1A2, 2C9, and 2C19 inhibition except for **1** which inhibited CYP2C19 with an IC$_{50}$ of 1.4 µM.

Metabolic stability was measured in mouse (MLM) and human liver microsomal (HLM) assays. Stability in HLM was good for the *O*-linked macrocycles and moderate for the *N*-linked analogs. The *O*-linked compound **62**, with two exposed *N*-ethyl groups, was found to have reduced stability whereas the *N*-linked derivative **52**, with an *N*-cyclopropyl substituent, had increased stability. Stability in MLMs was poor to moderate for all compounds except **52**. This was expected to be an issue for the study of these compounds in mouse xenograft models, however good efficacy was demonstrated in these models (Figures 5.17 and 5.18). This may be due to high plasma protein binding (PPB) *in vivo* as only the non-bound fraction is free to be metabolized.[92] Human mouse and dog PPB was found to be >99% for **1**, **2**, and **3**.

5.3.5   Animal Models and Preclinical DMPK

Based on their desirable kinase inhibition profiles and attractive *in vitro* ADME properties **1**, **2**, and **3** were selected for preclinical DMPK studies (Table 5.12).[9–11] Macrocycle **3** showed high systemic clearance compared to liver blood flow in mice (Cl = 6.6 L h^{-1} kg^{-1} after 5 mg kg^{-1} iv administration) and high volume of distribution at steady state. Following a single oral dose of 75 mg kg^{-1}, **3** had a mean terminal half-life of 6.1 h. At this high dose it was rapidly absorbed (t$_{max}$ = 0.5 h) and had a mean C$_{max}$ and AUC of 1029 ng mL^{-1} and 2523 ng·h mL^{-1}, respectively. The oral bioavailability was moderate at 24%. Exposures of the free drug achieved in mice at the 75 mg kg^{-1} dose (Free C$_{max}$ = 0.017 µM) equaled the CDK2 enzyme inhibition concentration, correlating with the observed efficacy in xenograft models at similar doses (Figure 5.17).

Compound **1** also showed rapid absorption in mice (t$_{max}$ = 1.0 h), with a mean C$_{max}$ and AUC of 292 ng mL^{-1} and 399 ng·h mL^{-1}, respectively, and

Table 5.12 Preclinical Pharmacokinetics for oral dosing of development candidates.

Compound	Species	Dose (mg/kg)	T_{max} (h)	C_{max} (ng/mL)	$t_{1/2}$ (h)	$AUC_{0-\infty}$ (ng·h/mL)	F (%)
1 (SB1518)	Mouse	30	1.0	292	0.84	399	39
1 (SB1518)	Rat	10	4.0	114	5.7	599	24
1 (SB1518)	Dog	3	2.0	11.5	3.4	53	10
2 (SB1578)	Mouse	50	0.5	1227	0.8	2020	34
2 (SB1578)	Rat	50	2.3	231	3.6	1499	6
2 (SB1578)	Dog	5	3.0	27	1.5	96	6
2 (SB1578)	Monkey	20	2.0	1976	1.1	7590	32
3 (SB1317)	Mouse	75	0.5	1029	6.1	2523	24

a mean terminal half-life of 0.8 h following a single oral dose of 30 mg kg^{-1}. The promising efficacy of **1** in pre-clinical pharmacology models (Figure 5.17) was consistent with this exposure. In rats, **1** showed moderately slow absorption ($t_{max} = 4$ h), with a peak concentration of 114 ng mL^{-1}, an AUC of 599 ng·h mL^{-1}, and a terminal half-life of nearly 6 h following a single oral dose of 10 mg kg^{-1}. In dogs, **1** was rapidly absorbed ($t_{max} = 2.0$ h), with a peak concentration of nearly 12 ng mL^{-1}, an AUC of 53 ng·h mL^{-1}, and a terminal half-life of 3.4 h following a single oral dose of 3 mg kg^{-1}.

Compound **2** showed rapid to moderately fast absorption. The t_{max} ranged between 0.5 to 3 h in mice, rats, monkeys and dogs. The terminal $t_{1/2}$ was moderate in mice, dogs, and monkeys (0.8–1.5 h) and longer in rats (3.6 h). The oral bioavailability was moderate in mice and monkeys (32–34%) and poor in rats and dogs (6%). Exposures of free compound achieved in mice at 50 mg kg^{-1} (Free $C_{max} = 0.34$ μM) exceeded the enzyme inhibition concentrations of JAK2 and FLT3 and the GI$_{50}$ of Ba/F3.

Efficacy of **1**, **2**, and **3** was assessed in a range of mouse models of cancer (Figure 5.17 and Figure 5.18).[77,90,91] Prior to conducting these experiments, dosing regimens for the compounds were explored and optimal schedules selected for each model for the duration of the experiment. The CDK2/FLT3/JAK2 inhibitor **3** was evaluated in two human tumor xenograft mouse models.[10] In a colon cancer model, HCT-116 cells were injected subcutaneously and tumors were established with mean group sizes of approximately 100 mm^3. Treatment with **3** at doses of 50 and 75 mg kg^{-1} po 3 times per week was started 8 days after cell inoculation and continued for 15 days. Treatment with **3** significantly inhibited the growth of tumors in a dose dependent manner with the 75 mg kg^{-1} cohort showing a mean tumor growth inhibition (TGI) of 82% (Figure 5.17a and b).

In the Ramos lymphoma model cells were injected subcutaneously and tumors were established with mean group sizes of approximately 200 mm^3. Two different dosing regimens of **3** were explored in this model: 75 mg kg^{-1} po qd on a 2 days on and 5 days off schedule and 15 mg kg^{-1} ip qd on a 5 days on, 5 days off, schedule. First doses were given 12 days after cell inoculation and continued for 15 days. Treatment with **3** using either regimen

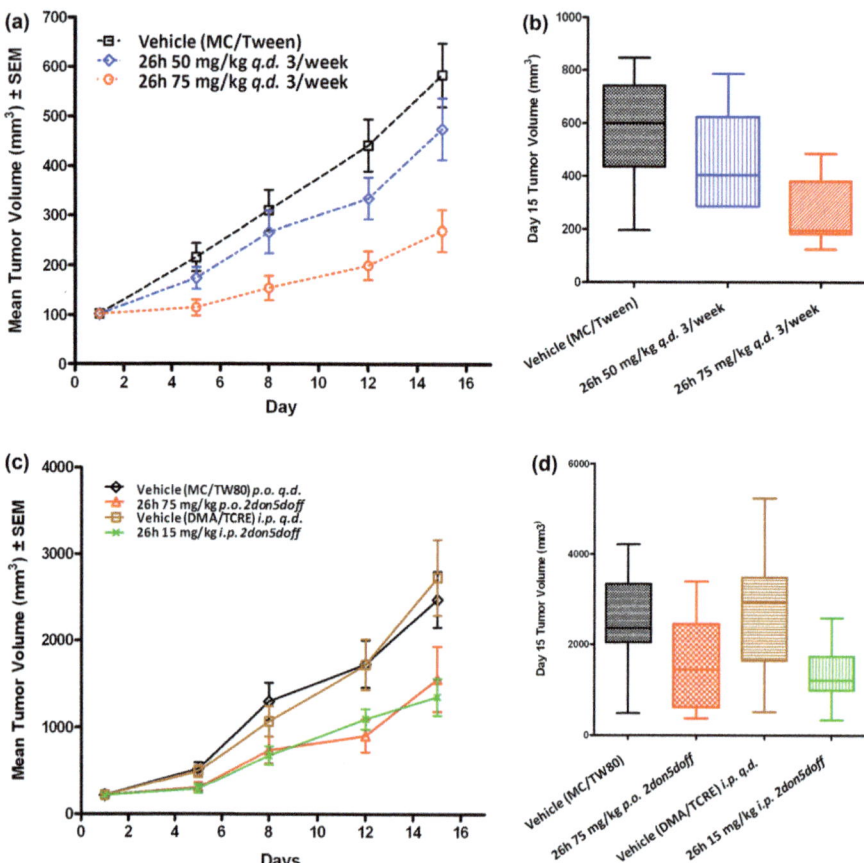

Figure 5.17 Animal models for the clinical candidate **3** (SB1317 – indicated as **26h** in this figure).[10] Mean tumor volumes in (a+b) HCT-116 colon cancer and (c+d) Ramos lymphoma Xenograft models for SB1317 treated mice.
Reprinted with permission from *J. Med. Chem.*, 2012, **55**, 169. Copyright (2012) American Chemical Society.

significantly inhibited the growth of tumors with mean TGIs of 42% for the oral and 63% for the ip route of administration (Figure 5.17c and d). Given the encouraging TGIs observed in both animal models, **3** (SB1317) was selected for further preclinical development. It is ironic that the first macrocycle synthesized for an aurora kinase inhibitor project was selected for development as a multikinase CDK/FLT/JAK2 inhibitor for advanced leukemias and multiple myeloma.[10,90]

Compound **1** was tested in two models that were selected on the basis of their relevance to the molecular targets: Ba/F3-JAK2^{V617F} and MV4-11 mouse allograft and xenograft studies representing cell lines dependent on mutant JAK2 and FLT3 signaling, respectively.[9] The Ba/F3-JAK2^{V617F} allograft is a model for JAK2-driven disease exhibiting hallmark symptoms of myeloproliferative diseases such as splenomegaly and hepatomegaly. Treatment with **1** at doses of 75 and 150 mg kg^{-1} p.o. b.i.d. was started 4 days after cell inoculation and continued for 13 consecutive days. At study termination, vehicle control mice exhibited splenomegaly and hepatomegaly (7-fold and 1.6-fold respectively). Treatment with **1** significantly ameliorated the disease symptoms in a dose dependent manner, with 42% normalization of spleen weight and 99% normalization of liver weight for the 150 mg kg^{-1} dosing regimen with no body weight loss (Figure 5.18a and b).

MV4-11 xenografts were established in nude mice to evaluate *in vivo* efficacy of **1** against FLT3-ITD driven tumors. MV4-11 tumor bearing mice with an average starting tumor size of 130 mm^3 were treated orally once daily at doses of 25, 50, or 100 mg kg^{-1} for 21 consecutive days to identify effects on tumor growth delay. After termination of the treatment, tumor growth was measured for another 34 days, and median survival was

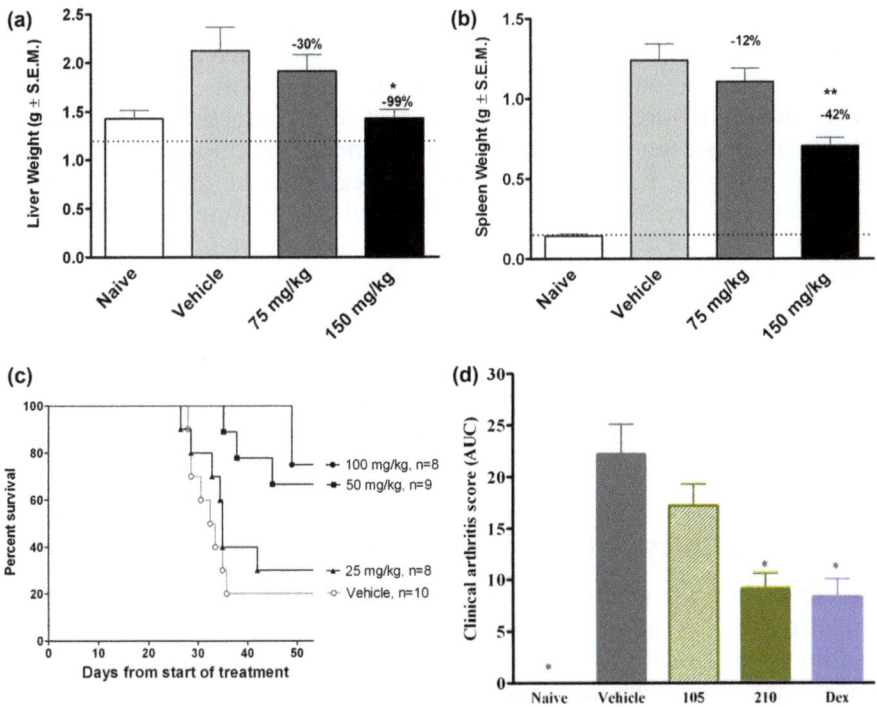

Figure 5.18 Animal models for the clinical candidates **1** (SB1518)[9] and **2** (SB1578).[11] (a+b) Reduction of hepato- and spleno- megaly in a Ba/F3-JAK2^{V617F} allograft model for SB1518 treated mice. (c) Median survival of SB1518 treated mice in a MV4-11 xenograft model. (d) Reduction of collagen Induced arthritis in mice treated with SB1578, at 105 or 210 mg kg^{-1}, or the anti-inflammatory steroid dexamethasone. Figure 5.18a–c
Reprinted with permission from *J. Med. Chem.*, 2011, **54**, 4638. Copyright (2011) American Chemical Society. Figure 5.18d Reprinted with permission from *J. Med. Chem.*, 2012, **55**, 2623. Copyright (2012) American Chemical Society.

calculated. The end point of the experiment for an individual mouse was reached on day 55 or when the tumor reached a size of 1000 mm³, whichever occurred earlier. Figure 5.18c shows the Kaplan-Meier survival curves for the different groups. The median survival was 33 days for the vehicle group. The treatment groups showed a significantly dose dependent increased median survival with no significant body weight loss. Given the encouraging efficacy in these animal models, showing reduction of symptoms (decrease of spleen and liver size) and increased survival, **1** (SB1518, pacritinib) was selected for further clinical development initially as a myelofibrosis and lymphoma agent.[9,91]

Compound **2** was tested for efficacy in a model of RA. Thus, the murine collagen induced arthritis (CIA) model recapitulates the clinical and histological development of human rheumatoid arthritis. Arthritis was induced in mice by immunization with emulsified type II collagen. After arthritis onset, mice were administered twice daily po with doses of 105 mg kg^{-1} or 210 mg kg^{-1} of **2**, and the treatment was continued for 10 days.[11] In the vehicle group, the clinical arthritic score of the mice increased rapidly from day 0 to disease day 11 (Figure 5.18d). Treatment with **2** led to a dose-dependent inhibition of arthritis with a 59% mean reduction in the AUC for the mice administered the higher dose. Treatment effects at the higher dose were comparable to efficacy in mice treated with the anti-inflammatory glucocorticoid steroid dexamethasone. A substantial improvement in the histopathology of the mice treated with **2** shows that inhibition of JAK2 signaling, which is involved in the pathological responses of inflammatory and autoimmune diseases, could be an effective treatment of rheumatoid arthritis. Compound **2** is a slightly weaker inhibitor of JAK2 and FLT3, but a more selective inhibitor compared to **1**, which makes it ideal for a non-oncology indication such as RA where safety is paramount. Macrocycle **2** (SB1578) was therefore selected for further development for the treatment of autoimmune diseases such as arthritis and psoriasis.[11,77]

5.3.6 Summary of Preclinical Development

By constraining an aminopyrimidine scaffold through macrocycle formation mediated by ring closing metathesis a series of small molecule kinase inhibitors were developed in two parallel projects. Selectivity towards the target kinases was achieved mainly by modification to the macrocyclic linker. In total 275 macrocycles were synthesized for these projects, delivering 3 clinical candidates with good PK-PD properties. From the multi-kinase CDK inhibitor project, SB1317 (later renamed TG02), a potent pan-CDK, FLT3 and JAK2 inhibitor with dose-dependent efficacy in the HCT-116 model of colon cancer and a Ramos model of lymphoma was progressed into development for advanced hematological malignancies. The selective JAK2/FLT3 project delivered two candidates SB1518 and SB1578 for oncology and autoimmune indications, respectively. SB1518 demonstrated efficacy in a model of JAK2^{V617F}-driven disease with dose-dependent tumor growth inhibition and normalization of splenomegaly and hepatomegaly at well-tolerated doses. In a second study SB1518 demonstrated significant survival benefits at very well-tolerated doses in a model of FLT3-ITD driven leukemia. SB1578 was highly efficacious in the mouse CIA model and was progressed into development for RA.

5.4   Synthesis

This following sections describe the synthesis of SB1518 (**1**), SB1578 (**2**), and SB1317 (**3**) exploiting the powerful ring-closing metathesis (RCM) reaction as a synthetic tool.

5.4.1   Synthesis of SB1518 (Pacritinib, 1)

Synthesis of SB1518 was conceived by breaking the molecule into two halves that could be convergently joined to provide a diene that underwent macrocyclization using the RCM protocol (Schemes 5.1 and 5.2). The right-hand intermediate **98** was prepared starting from phenol **90** (Scheme 5.1).

Alkylation of **90** with 1,2-dichloroethane (**91**) proceeded smoothly at 100 °C to afford aldehyde **92** in moderate yield.[93] Reduction of **92** with sodium borohydride furnished benzyl alcohol **93** in high yield followed by alkylation with allyl bromide **94** under phase transfer conditions to provide allyl ether **95** in good yield.[94,95] Next, displacement of the terminal chloride of **95** with pyrrolidine proceeded efficiently in the presence of *N,N*-dimethyl acetamide to give pyrrolidinylethoxy **97** in 76% yield.[96] Finally, key aniline intermediate **98** was obtained from **97** by iron assisted reduction of the nitro group.

The left-hand allyl-benzyl ether intermediate **102** was prepared from 2,4-dichloropyrimidine (**99**) (Scheme 5.2). Thus, Suzuki coupling of **99** with boronic acid **100** proceeded smoothly to yield biaryl **101** in moderate yield.[97,98] Alkylation of benzyl alcohol **101** with allyl bromide **94** under phase transfer conditions then provided the key left-hand fragment **102**.

The stage was thus set for the coupling of the two halves to give the key diene intermediate (Scheme 5.2). Intermediates **98** and **102** underwent acid catalysed chloride displacement in *n*-butanol to afford diene **103** in high yield.[99]

Cyclization of **103** *via* RCM was achieved with various catalysts depicted in Figure 5.19. Grubbs 1st and 2nd generation catalysts without additives under normal conditions did not proceed to completion, even after 36 hours. However, with Hoveyda-Grubbs 2nd generation catalyst and/or Zhan-1B catalyst in the presence of additives such as trifluoroacetic acid (TFA) or HCl, the RCM proceeded smoothly with high conversion furnishing the desired macrocycle in 68% yield.[100,101] The final product had *trans : cis* ratios in the range of 85 : 15. Reactions were scaled up to a 50 g scale to obtain material for pre-clinical studies. The *trans/cis* isomers of SB1518 had similar biological activities towards JAK2 kinases and FLT3, hence pre-clinical

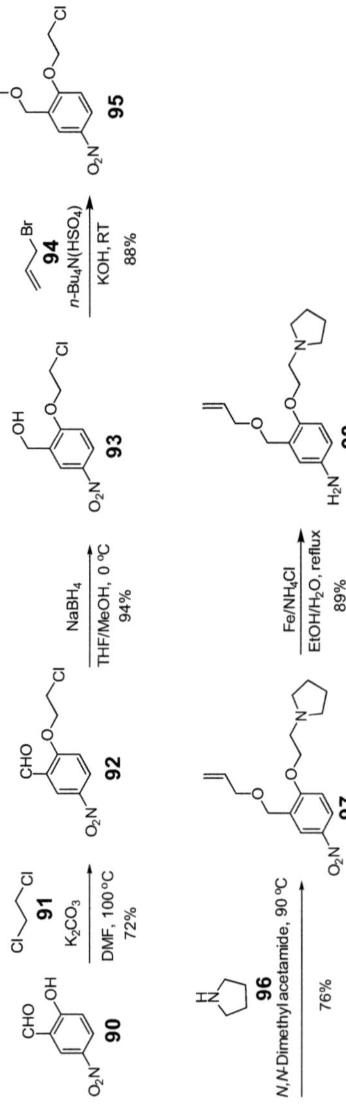

Scheme 5.1 Synthesis of SB1518 (**1**) right-hand fragment **98**.

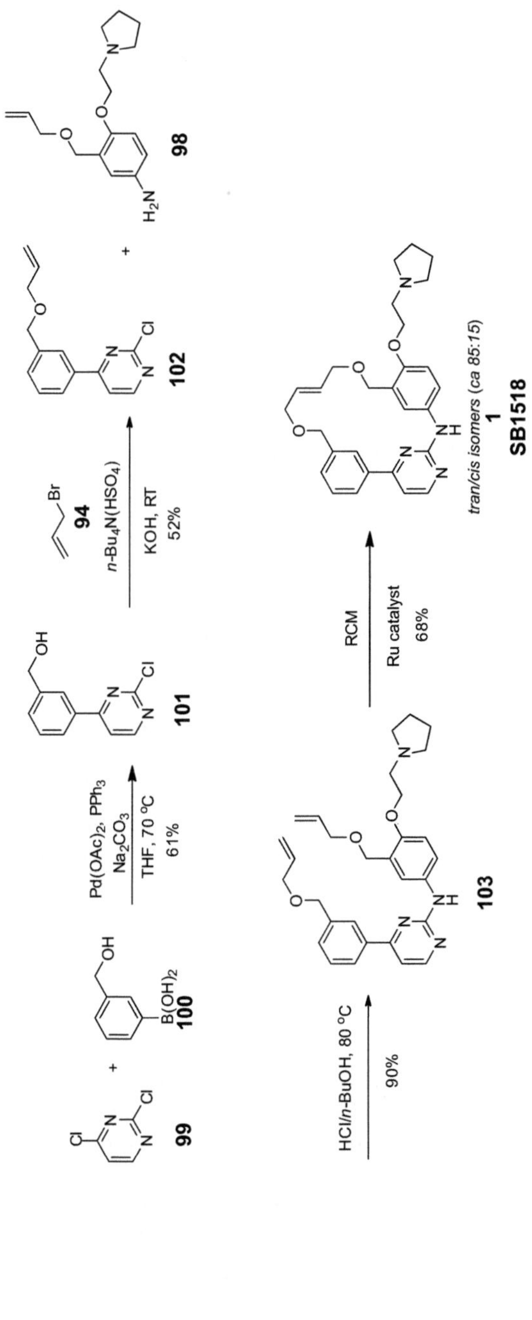

Scheme 5.2 Synthesis of SB1518 (**1**).

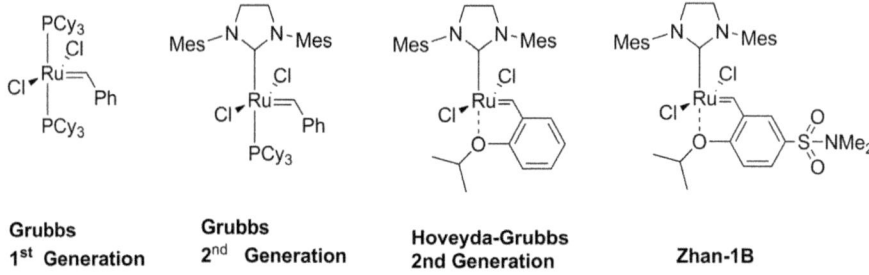

Figure 5.19 Ru catalysts employed for RCM.

activities, including animal models, were performed on mixtures of *tran/cis* isomers (*ca.* 85:15). The *trans* isomer of SB1518 has a JAK2 IC_{50} of 22 nM while the *cis* isomer is slightly less potent with a JAK2 IC_{50} of 50 nM. However, material manufactured for clinical trials was obtained *via* a non-RCM route that provided >99% *trans* isomer (unpublished).

5.4.2 Synthesis of SB1317 (3, TG02)

In a similar strategy to **1**, synthesis of the left-hand side of SB1317 was initiated from 2,4-dichloropyrimidine (**99**) as shown in Scheme 5.3. Suzuki coupling of **99** with boronic acid **104** afforded the biaryl **105** in 80% yield, which was further reacted under phase transfer conditions in the presence of bromide **106** to give alkene **107** in 75% yield.

Preparation of the right-hand half of SB1317 was constructed from 3-nitrobenzaldehyde (**108**). Under reductive amination conditions with *N*-methylallylamine (**109**), allylbenzylamine **110** was obtained in high yield.[102,103] Aniline **111** was then obtained in near quantitative yield by employing $SnCl_2$ reduction conditions (Scheme 5.4).[104]

Coupling of the two halves, **107** and **111**, proceeded efficiently in the presence of HCl to afford **112** in excellent yield. However, RCM on **112** using Grubbs 1st and 2nd generation catalysts failed to afford any product under normal conditions (Scheme 5.5).

As discussed earlier, RCM on compounds with basic centers proceeds best in the presence of an acid as an additive.[105,106] Hence, the reaction was attempted with HCl and under these conditions the desired product formed with >90:<10 *trans: cis* ratios, albeit in low yield, with the 1st generation catalyst. Further improvement was realized with the 2nd generation catalyst affording a moderate yield. However, with TFA as an additive the RCM proceeded most smoothly, with full conversion occurring in just 4 hours to furnish SB1317 in 89% yield with a 94:6 *trans:cis* ratio, after chromatographic purification. Isomeric purity was increased to >98% *trans* by simply washing the solid with cold ethyl acetate, with 90% recovery. Reactions were carried out on 20 g scale to obtain material for pre-clinical studies. Material manufactured for clinical studies was initially prepared as a mixture of

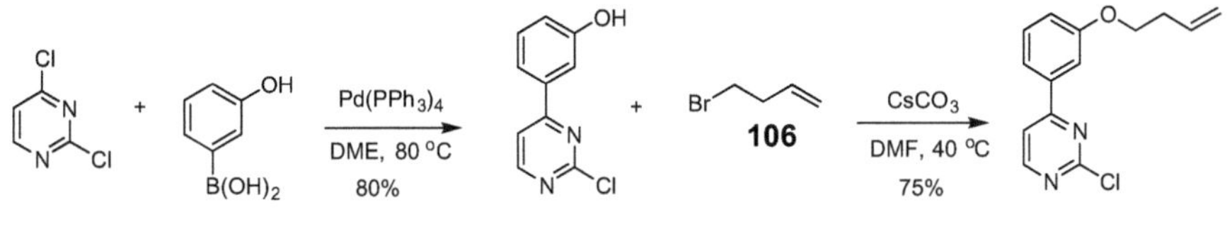

99 104 105 107

Scheme 5.3 Synthesis of SB1317 (3) left-hand fragment.

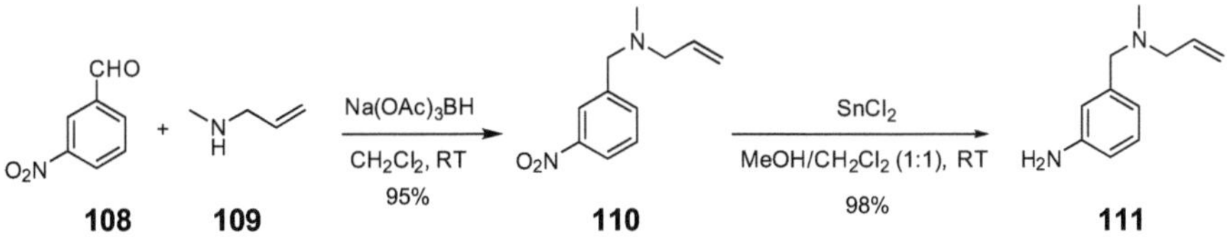

108 109 110 111

Scheme 5.4 Synthesis of SB1317 (3) right-hand fragment 111.

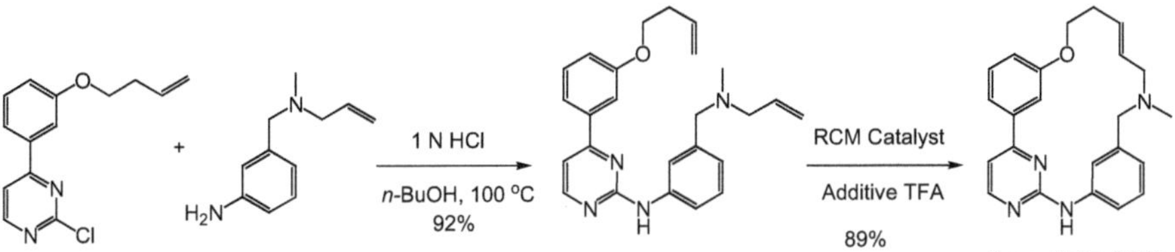

107 111 112

trans: cis (ca 94:6)
3
SB1317 (TG02)

Scheme 5.5 Synthesis of SB1317 (3) *via* RCM.

trans : *cis* isomers (*ca.* 97 : 3). The *cis* isomer was not isolated and was treated as an impurity. Its biological activity has not been determined.

5.4.3 Synthesis of SB1578 (2)

Macrocyclic furanyl pyrimidine SB1578 (2) was also synthesized *via* a convergent route using a RCM as the key step, starting from 2,4-dichloropyrimidine (**99**) as shown in Scheme 5.6. Suzuki coupling of **99** with boronic acid **113** proceeded smoothly to furnish biaryl aldehyde **114** in moderate yield followed by reduction in the presence of sodium borohydride to furnish an almost quantitative yield of alcohol **115.** Alkylation of benzyl alcohol **115** with allyl bromide **94** under phase transfer conditions provided the key left-hand fragment **116.**

Coupling of the two halves, **116** and **98,** proceeded efficiently in the presence of HCl to afford **117** in 90% yield. RCM on diallyl ether **117** using Grubbs 2nd generation catalyst with added TFA then furnished **2** (SB1578) in moderate yield. The final product had a *trans*: *cis* ratio in the range of 70 : 30. Reactions were carried out on a 50 g scale to obtain material for pre-clinical

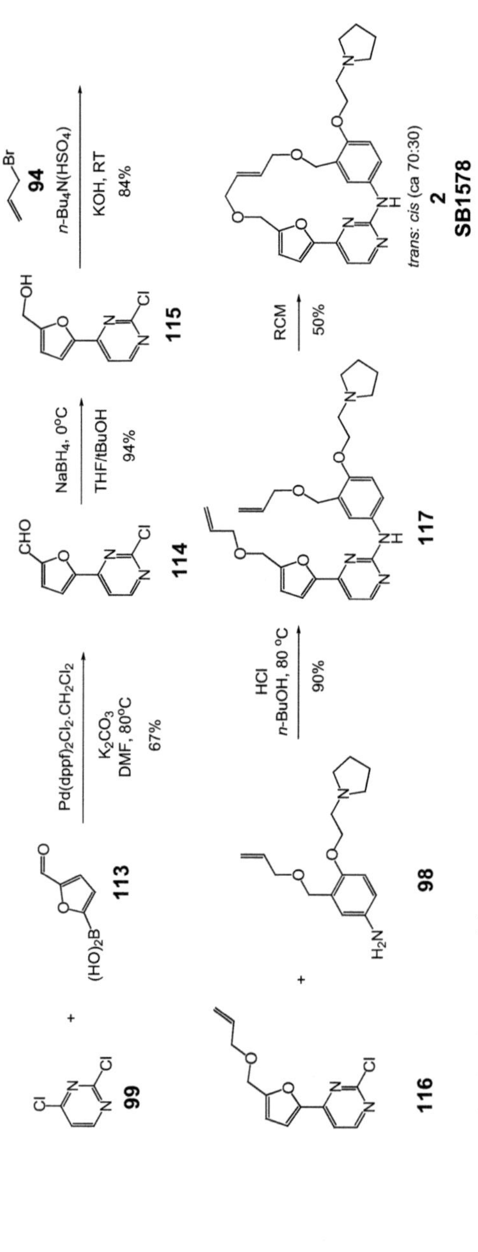

Scheme 5.6 Synthesis of SB1578 (**2**) *via* RCM.

studies. Material manufactured for Phase I clinical trials was obtained as >99% *trans* isomer *via* a non-RCM synthetic route (unpublished).

These efficient synthetic routes show that RCM is a powerful tool for the preparation of novel small molecule macrocycles made for SAR purposes as well as for scale-up for pre-clinical studies. All were prepared with atom efficient syntheses, devoid of protecting groups and with an acceptable overall yield.

5.5 Clinical Trials

5.5.1 Overview

Three macrocyclic kinase inhibitors have entered the clinic: pacritinib (SB1518, **1**), SB1317 (**3**, renamed 'TG02' upon licensing to Tragara Pharmaceuticals), and SB1578 (**2**, Table 5.13). Pacritinib, a JAK2/FLT3 selective inhibitor, is the most advanced having entered Phase III clinical trials December 2012 for the treatment of myelofibrosis.[107] A second Phase III trial was initiated February 2014 to treat myelofibrosis with thrombocytopenia (ClinicalTrials.gov Identifier: NCT02055781). Prior to this, pacritinib had been studied in four other trials in patients with myeloid and lymphoid malignancies seeking to establish safety and a recommended dose for Phase II.[108–111] More recently, pacritinib has been studied in a trial for myelodysplastic syndrome (MDS), sponsored by the MD Anderson Cancer Centre.[112] TG02 (SB1317) has been in phase 1 trials since 2010 focusing on hematological malignancies.[113,114] SB1578 is also a JAK2/FLT3 selective compound but additionally inhibits c-FMS.[77] With a differentiated profile from pacritinib, SB1578 (CT-1578, following licensing to CTI Biopharma Corp. Inc.) is focused on non-oncological indications, hence its overall profile is differentiated from pacritinib. SB1578 entered Phase I clinical trials in 2010 in healthy volunteers in preparation for later studies in rheumatoid arthritis patients and other inflammatory indications.[115]

5.5.2 Pacritinib Clinical Trials

5.5.2.1 Selection of Human Dose

Pacritinib displayed acceptable oral bioavailability in mouse and dog (Table 5.12) hence these species were selected for 28-day, 6 and 9 months pre-clinical toxicology studies (unpublished). Following the 28-day toxicology studies, based on acceptable safety margins and species allometry, the approved first-in-human dose was 100 mg once per day (Table 5.14).

5.5.2.2 Clinical Trial Design

Pacritinib Phase I and II studies were carried out on eligible patients on an open-label escalating dose basis with a continuous oral, daily schedule.

Table 5.13 Summary of clinical studies carried out with macrocyclic kinase inhibitors from clinicaltrials.gov.

Entry	Drug	Sponsor	Study type	Study start date	Study completion date (Est.)	Official title	Number of patients	ClinicalTrials.gov identifier	Ref.
1	Pacritinib (SB1518)	CTI Biopharma Corp.	Phase 3	Dec 2012	(Aug 2017)	A Randomized Controlled Phase 3 Study of Oral Pacritinib Versus Best Available Therapy in Patients With Primary Myelofibrosis, Post-Polycythemia Vera Myelofibrosis, or Post-Essential Thrombocythemia Myelofibrosis	270 (Est.)	NCT01773187	107
2		M.D. Anderson Cancer Center (Collaborator; S*BIO)	Phase 2	Dec 2011	(Dec 2015)	Phase II Study of SB1518 for Patients With Myelodysplastic Syndrome (MDS)	40 (Est.)	NCT01436084	112
3		S*BIO	Phase 2	Dec 2010	Feb 2012	A Phase 2 Safety and Efficacy Study of SB1518 for the Treatment of Advanced Lymphoid Malignancies	28	NCT01263899	110
4		S*BIO	Phase 1/2	Aug 2008	Jan 2012	A Phase 1/2 Study of SB1518 for the Treatment of Advanced Myeloid Malignancies	76	NCT00719836	109
5		S*BIO	Phase 1/2	Aug 2008	Jan 2012	A Phase 1/2 Study of Oral SB1518 in Subjects With Chronic Idiopathic Myelofibrosis	55	NCT00745550	108

No.	Compound	Company	Phase	Start	Completion	Title	Enrollment	NCT number	Ref.
6		S*BIO	Phase 1	Jul 2008	Oct 2011	A Phase 1 Study of SB1518 for the Treatment of Advanced Lymphoid Malignancies	35	NCT00741871	111
7	TG02 (SB1317)	Tragara Pharmaceuticals	Phase 1	Sep 2012	(Aug 2014)	Phase 1 Dose-Escalation and Pharmacokinetic Study of TG02 Citrate in Patients With Relapsed or Refractory Chronic Lymphocytic Leukemia and Small Lymphocytic Lymphoma	30	NCT01699152	114
8		Tragara Pharmaceuticals	Phase 1	Aug 2010	Oct 2013	A Phase 1 Dose-Escalation and Pharmacokinetic Study of TG02 Citrate in Patients With Advanced Hematological Malignancies	120	NCT01204164	113
9	SB1578 (CT-1578)	S*BIO	Phase 1	Aug 2010	Mar 2011	A Phase 1, Randomized, Double-Blind, Placebo-Controlled, Ascending Single and Multiple-Dose Study of the Safety, Tolerability, Pharmacokinetics and Pharmacodynamics of SB1578 When Administered Orally to Healthy Adult Subjects With One Single-Dose Group Crossing Over to Assess Food Effect	40	NCT01235871	115

Table 5.14 Summary of toxicology species used and initial human doses for macrocyclic kinase inhibitors.

Compound	Toxicology species	First-in-human dose
Pacritinib (SB1518)	Mouse, dog	100 mg once per day
TG02 (SB1317)	Mouse, dog	10 mg once per day
SB1578	Mouse, monkey	10 mg once per day

Doses were usually administered once per day as a single agent and taken without food. Later studies in Phase II showed no food effect. One cycle was defined as 28 days of continuous daily treatment. Regular physician safety evaluations determined dose continuation or escalation.

5.5.2.3 Clinical Trial Results

Published data in human studies covers Phase I through to Phase II studies in MF, leukemia and lymphoma patients for pacritinib (see Table 5.13 for details and references). Data from the Phase III study of pacritinib in MF and Phase II study in MDS had not yet been reported at the time of writing.

5.5.2.3.1 Pacritinib Myelofibrosis Trials. Promising clinical activity has been reported in Phase I and II trials for pacritinib in the treatment of myelofibrosis, both primary, post-Polycythemia Vera (post-PV) and post-Essential Thrombocythemia (Post-ET) (Table 5.15). In the Phase I studies doses of 100 to 600 mg d^{-1} were investigated without reaching the maximum tolerated dose (MTD). Biomarker effects were evident from the lowest dose and exposures were dose proportional up to 400 mg. No increase in exposures or pharmacodymamic effects above 400 mg were demonstrated. Furthermore, a higher incidence of toxicities at the higher doses of 500 and 600 mg/d led investigators to recommend a dose of 400 mg d^{-1} for Phase II.

Durable responses have been recorded, particularly for the reduction of splenomegaly, and considerable improvement seen for constitutional symptoms including bone pain, night sweats, pruritus, fatigue, and abdominal pain. Splenomegaly is a particular symptom of MF where the spleen becomes very enlarged in response to impaired hematopoiesis. Spleen measurements by magnetic resonance imaging (MRI) or physical exam (PE) were conducted in these trials with a ratio of 25% spleen volume reduction by MRI equating to above 50% by PE. In a Phase II trial in PMF patients (Study 3, Table 5.15) nearly all evaluable patients (29/30, 97%) experienced a spleen reduction by MRI with 57% having a reduction of 25% or more (Figure 5.20). In the same study, 40–65% reduction in constitutional symptoms was recorded through questionnaires. In another Phase II trial in all MF populations (Study 4, Table 5.15) pacritinib treatment led to a spleen

Table 5.15 Published clinical trial results for pacritinib (SB1518, **1**) in myelofibrosis patients.

Study #	Clinical phase	Indication	Doses (po qd)[b]	Number of patients[a]	Duration	Responses[h]	Toxicity[f]	Ref.
1	Phase 1	MF,[a] AML	100–600 mg d^{-1}	36 (31 MF and 5 AML)	>3 months	Spleen volume reduction,[d]: 7 (41%) ≥35%; 4 (24%) ≥50%	4% Thrombocytopenia (Grade 3/4); 33% diarrhea (4% grade 3); 13% nausea	122
2	Phase 1	MF[a]	100–600 mg d^{-1}	20	>3 months	Clinical improvement in splenomegaly, anemia, platelets	89% diarrhea (11% grade 3 but only at 500 or 600 mg d^{-1}); 39% nausea (6% grade 3 @600 mg d^{-1}); 39% vomiting; 22% abdominal pain, 22% fatigue (11% grade 3 @600 mg d^{-1}); 17% dysgeusia[g]; 17% rash	123
3	Phase 1	PMF	100–600 mg d^{-1}	33	>6 months			124
	Phase 2	PMF	400 mg d^{-1}			Spleen volume reductions in 29 (97%) of these 17 (57%) ≥25%; symptomse improved in 40–65%	81% diarrhea (6% grade 3); 41% nausea; 22% vomiting; 9% fatigue; no grade 3/4 neutropenia or thrombocytopenia	
4	Phase 2	MF[a]	400 mg d^{-1}	34	>6 months	Spleen volume reductionc: 11 (32%) ≥35%; 14 (41%) ≥25%; 2 (6%) anemia improved, of these 1 (3%) transfusion indep.; signif redn in symptoms[e]	Low grade GI effects, easily managed. 24% discontinued due to adverse events	125

[a]Primary MF, post-PV MF and post-ET MF.
[b]Doses were oral once per day.
[c]Spleen volume assessed by MRI.
[d]Spleen assessed by physical exam (PE): 12 (39%) ≥50% and 7 (23%) 100%; reduction by MRI of 25% equated to 50% by PE ($p = 0.043$).
[e]Bone pain, night sweats, pruritus, fatigue, abdominal pain, evaluated each cycle of therapy using the Myelofibrosis Symptom Assessment Form (MFSAF).
[f]Adverse events are all grade 1 or 2 unless otherwise mentioned.
[g]A distortion of the sense of taste.
[h]Evaluable patients only.

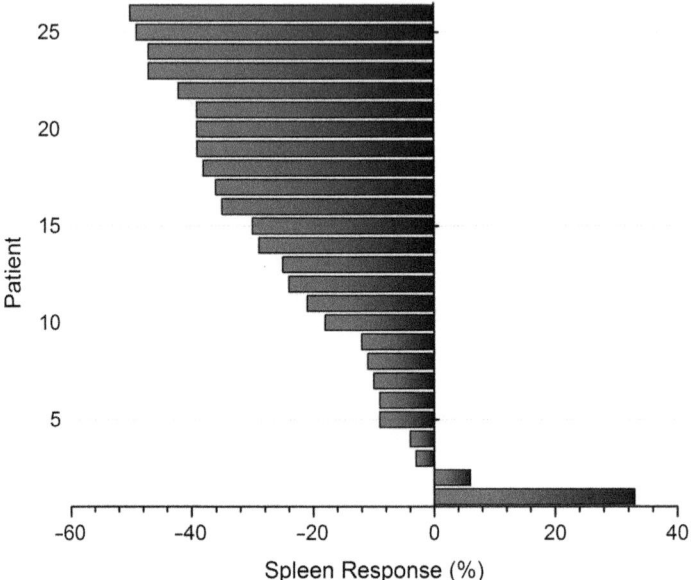

Figure 5.20 Waterfall plot showing the majority of patients treated with pacritinib experience a reduction in spleen volume as measured by MRI. 17 of 30 (57%) patients had response of $\geq 25\%$.
Figure replotted from published data.[125]

volume decrease at or above 25% for 73% of patients with 2 patients (6%) having improvement in anemia and one of those patients becoming transfusion independent. Toxicities suffered by patients on pacritinib therapy were generally gastrointestinal (GI) in nature and well managed with no significant myelosuppression. Sporadic grade 3 and 4 toxicities were seen but were always <10% of patients and usually only at the higher doses of 500 or 600 mg d^{-1}. Typical GI effects were diarrhea (>80%), nausea (40%), vomiting (20–40%) and fatigue (10–20%) among others, but these usually improved after a few cycles, a dose holiday or small dose reduction from 400 to 300 mg d^{-1}.

An analysis of the two Phase I trials (Studies 1 and 2, Table 5.15) in MF and AML (51 and 5 patients, respectively, at the time of reporting) concluded that 70% of MF patients with splenomegaly had a response or stable disease with a progression free survival rate of 67% at 12 months (duration median 20 months) and median time on study of 29 months.[116]

Both response and toxicity were unrelated to platelet levels giving pacritinib access to a significant proportion of MF patients with low platelet counts, a population not currently treated with full dose ruxolitinib.[117]

Pacritinib was orally absorbed slowly with a t$_{max}$ of 3–6 hours and mean elimination half life of 2–3 days in this patient population. At all doses target inhibition was achieved as evidenced by inhibition of phosphorylation of STAT3/5 (also see later discussion in lymphoma trial).

These very encouraging responses and good tolerability prompted initiation of a Phase III trial, PERSIST-1, in MF patients which started recruitment at the end of 2012.[107] Furthermore, the PERSIST-2 Phase III trial focusing on MF patients with low platelet levels (thrombocytopenia), a population that can be treated with full dose pacritinib, was initiated by CTI Biopharma Corp. February 2014 (see http://www.ctibiopharma.com/ and ClinicalTrials.gov Identifier: NCT02055781).

5.5.2.3.2 Pacritinib Lymphoma Trials. Proof of concept has been reported for the first time for a JAK inhibitor in relapsed lymphoma in a Phase I trial of pacritinib.[118] This trial involved any type of relapsed or refractory lymphoma patient, Hodgkin's or non-Hodgkin's, with the exception of Burkitt's and CNS lymphoma (Entry 6, Table 5.13 and Table 5.16). Oral doses ranged from 100 mg to 600 mg d^{-1}. In the 34 patients who received at least one dose, 31 were evaluable for tumor mass assessments by CT or PET scan. Patients were also evaluated for performance status, vital signs, ECG, CBC and blood chemistry and samples analysed for pharmacokinetics and pharmacodynamics (JAK–STAT pathway and FLT3 ligand).

Treatment duration ranged from 1 to 574 days (median 88 days) with 17 patients on study for more than 3 months and 6 patients for more than 6 months. Patients remained on study until disease progression or intolerance. Of the evaluable patients, 55% had a tumor mass reduction of 4–70%, inclusive of 3 partial responses (PRs) and 15 patients achieving stable disease. Of the PRs, two were mantle cell and one follicular all at different doses (Figure 5.21). Responses appeared to be favorable in patients previously treated with rituximab, potentially suggesting that a combination therapy may have value. Further support for combinations with pacritinib can be found in the tolerability data. In general there were few grade 3/4 toxicities, with the majority being gastrointestinal grade 1/2, and infrequent cytopenias. Overall pacritinib was found to be well tolerated in patients with relapsed lymphoma.

Pacritinib was quite slowly absorbed in this population reaching peak concentrations in 5–9 hours then having sustained and high exposure with a mean terminal half life of 1 to 4 days. However AUCs were less than 2-fold increased at day 15 indicating no significant accumulation. With high and sustained total plasma concentrations pacritinib significantly exceeded its IC$_{50}$ concentrations in cell lines.[118]

At all dose levels tested pacritinib inhibited JAK2 signaling. Phospho-STAT5 was quantified in peripheral blood mononuclear cells (PBMCs) by western blot and pSTAT3/5 in whole blood by flow cytometry although in small numbers of patients at each dose level (range 2 to 9). The inhibition was not dose related. Plasma levels of FLT3L increased very significantly (approximately 3-fold) between days 1 and 29 indicating that the inhibition of FLT3 by pacritinib was triggering a negative feedback loop.

Table 5.16 Phase 1 clinical trial of pacritinib in lymphoma patients.

Study	Clinical phase	Indication[a]	Doses (po qd)	Number of patients	Duration (n)[b]	Responses	Toxicity[e]
1	Phase 1	Relapsed lymphoma: Hodgkin or non-Hodgkin	100–600 mg d^{-1}	34 (24M, 10F)	Median 88 days; 3 months (17); 6 months[e]	Reductions in tumor mass in 17 pts (55%[c]; PRs in 3 patients[d]	Mostly grade 1/2 GI effects: 32% diarrhea, 29% nausea, 26% constipation; 18% fatigue, 18% pyrexia

[a]Lymphoma types: Hodgkin's (14), non-Hodgkin's (20), follicular (10), mantle cell (5), B-cell (4), small lymphocytic (1); excluded: Burkitt's and CNS lymphoma.
[b]Range 1–574 days.
[c]Range 4–70% tumor mass reduction, measured by CT or PET scan every 2 cycles.
[d]PR defined as >50% tumor mass reduction; PRs were in mantle cell (2300 mg and 400 mg dose) and follicular (1600 mg dose).
[e]Other side effects above 10%: neutropenia (12–6% grade 3/4), anemia (12–3% grade 3/4), thrombocytopenia (12–3% grade 3/4).

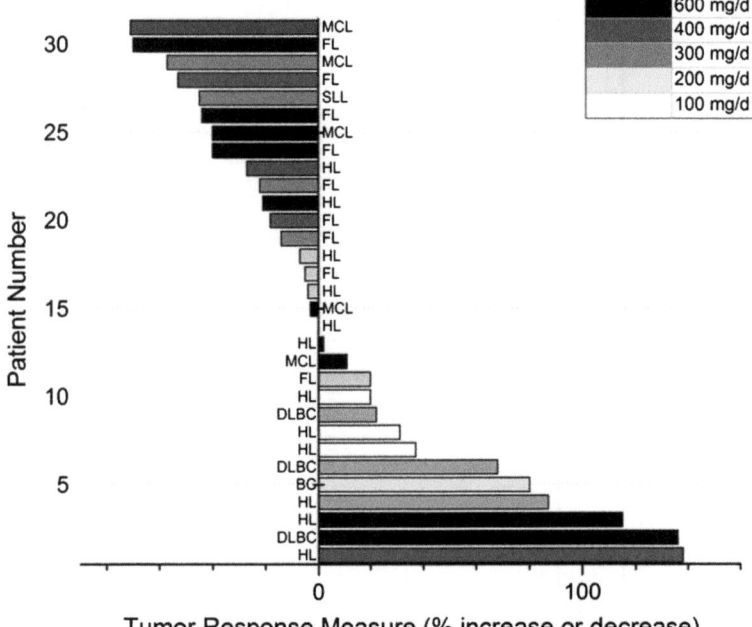

Figure 5.21 Waterfall plot demonstrating percentage change from baseline in target tumor dimensions (best responses by dose level) among evaluable patients (n = 31). Labels in the y-axis identify the histologic subtypes. BC, unclassified B-cell lymphoma; FL, follicular lymphoma; DLBC, diffuse large B-cell lymphoma; MCL, mantle cell lymphoma; SLL, small lymphocytic lymphoma/chronic lymphocytic leukemia; HL, Hodgkin lymphoma. Figure replotted from published data.[118]

These promising responses and tolerability pave the way for further studies of pacritinib in lymphomas.

5.5.3 TG02 (SB1317, 3) Clinical Trials

5.5.3.1 Selection of Human Dose and Clinical Trial Design

Given the likely intervention required to manage the expected toxicities with a potent inhibitor of cell cycle kinases such as TG02 (SB1317, 3), the Phase I plan in patients with hematological malignancies incorporated two schedules: a continuous daily dose and a schedule of 5 days on and 2 days off for 2 weeks (28 day cycles). Pre-clinical pharmacokinetics and metabolism studies determined oral bioavailability in mouse and dog of 24 and 37%, respectively, with rat bioavailability estimated at 3.8%.[119] Similar metabolic profiles between human and pre-clinical species supported the appropriate choice of toxicology species. Pre-clinical toxicology studies (Table 5.14) determined the first-in-human starting dose of TG02 to be 10 mg d^{-1} on a continuous daily basis, with the intermittent schedule supporting a starting human dose of 30 mg d^{-1}.

Table 5.17 Phase 1 first-in-human clinical trial of TG02 (3) in patients with advanced hematological malignancies.

Study	Clinical phase	Indications[a]	Schedule	Doses (po)	Number of patients	Responses	Toxicity
1 – Arm A	Phase 1	AML, CML, MDS	Daily	10–70 mg d^{-1}	26	Not reported	Nausea (46%); vomiting (23%); decreased appetite (19%); neutropenia (19%); diarrhea (15%); fatigue (15%); <15%: constipation, dyspepsia, headache (n = 26)
1 – Arm B	Phase 1	AML, MDS	Intermittent	30–150 mg d^{-1} days 1–5 and 8–12, ×2 weeks	15	One patient had a sustained anti-leukemic response for at least 3 cycles (>80%, >65% reduction in PBMC, bone marrow blasts, respectively)	Nausea (60%); vomiting (46%); fatigue (40%); decreased appetite (27%); diarrhea (27%); neutropenia (20%); 20%: constipation, dyspepsia, headache (n = 15)

[a]AML = Acute Myeloid Leukemia; CML = Chronic Myeloid Leukemia (blast phase); MDS = Myelodysplastic Syndrome.

5.5.3.2 Clinical Trial Results in Advanced Hematological Malignancies

A first in man trial of TG02 in patients with advanced hematological malignancies has been reported.[120] In the Phase I trial arm A dosed daily starting at 10 mg d^{-1} and escalating to 70 mg d^{-1}, and the intermittent regimen, arm B, started at 30 mg d^{-1}, 5 days on with 2 days off, and reached 150 mg d^{-1} (Table 5.17). Safety and PK were determined and MTD was reached in both schedules.

Supported by pre-clinical studies in primary AML cells[90,121] a sustained response was achieved by one patient on the intermittent schedule over >2 cycles starting at 150 mg and reducing to 100 mg. This heavily pre-treated AML patient had considerable reductions in PBMC blasts (>80%) and bone marrow blasts (>65%).

Most toxicities in arm B were GI in nature and manageable: nausea, vomiting, fatigue, decreased appetite, and diarrhea at grade 1/2, among others (see Table 5.17 and Figure 5.22).

Exposures were dose-related but non-proportional reaching pharmacologically active levels (above the IC$_{50}$ for inhibition of cell proliferation) at or above 50 mg (Figure 5.23).

Other studies in multiple myeloma and CLL are on-going with different schedules being investigated. Given its broad and potent suppression of key kinases TG02 is a promising agent for both hematological malignancies and solid tumors.

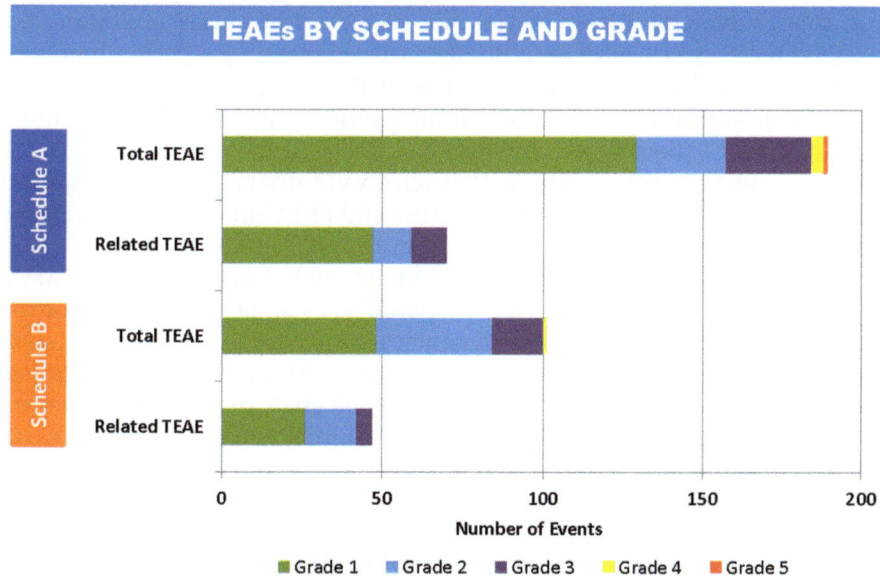

Figure 5.22 TG02 Treatment emergent adverse events by schedule and grade. Figure 5.22 reproduced with kind permission from Tragara Pharmaceuticals Inc.

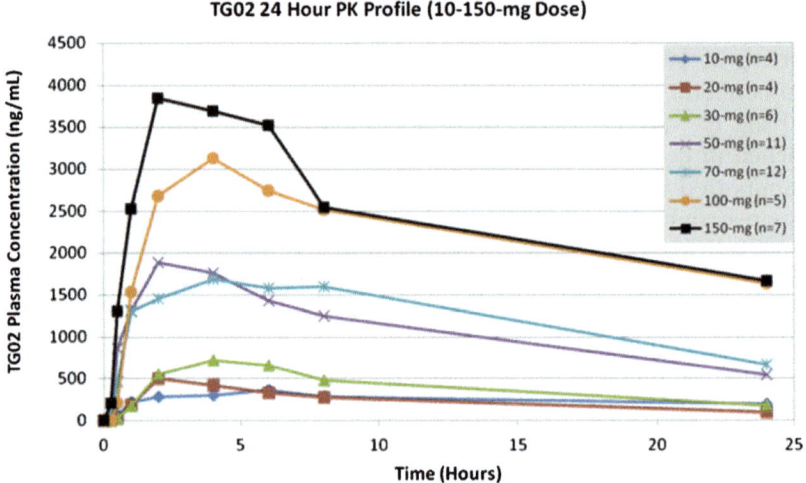

Figure 5.23 TG02 (3) dose response PK profile.
Reproduced with kind permission from Tragara Pharmaceuticals Inc.

5.6   Conclusion

In this chapter the history of an emerging class of kinase inhibitors, designed macrocycles, have been briefly reviewed revealing a small number of
novel chemical entities that have entered the clinic. Macrocycles with reported clinical results are derived from a series of aryl-substituted anilino-
pyrimidines. Following a computational docking analysis of an aurora A
kinase screening hit specific macrocycles were designed and synthesized
and found to have activity for JAK2, CDK2 and FLT3 kinases. These enzymes
are implicated in important pathways in carcinogenesis affecting the JAK-
STAT signaling pathway, cell cycle and mutated FLT3-ITD prevalent in AML.
Combination of those targets was proposed as a compelling strategy for the
treatment of hematological malignancies with later expansion into solid
tumors. Following an extensive medicinal chemistry program three clinical
candidates were identified that met desirable goals of JAK2/FLT3 dual inhibitory activity (without CDK), SB1518 (pacritinib) and SB1578, and a CDK/
JAK2/FLT3 inhibitor, TG02, which was later found to have additional desirable ERK5 activity. Of these three clinical stage compounds the most advanced is pacritinib, having entered Phase III clinical trials for the treatment
of myelofibrosis. At the time of writing TG02 (SB1317), is poised to move into
Phase II clinical trials while SB1578 (CT-1578), also a dual JAK2/FLT3 inhibitor, has been studied in an unpublished Phase I trial in healthy volunteers only. We believe the clinical success of these compounds will spur

growth in the development of synthetic small molecule macrocycles in the coming years.

References

1. P. Boyle and B. Levin, *World Cancer Report*, WHO, ISBN 9789283204237, 2008.
2. J. Baselga, *Science*, 2006, **312**, 1175.
3. P. Cohen, *Nat. Rev. Drug Discovery*, 2002, **1**, 309.
4. J. Chen, X. Zhang and A. Fernandez, *Bioinformatics*, 2007, **23**, 563.
5. Z. A. Knight and K. M. Shokat, *Chem. Biol. (Oxford, U. K.)*, 2005, **12**, 621.
6. M. A. Fabian, W. H. Biggs, 3rd, D. K. Treiber, C. E. Atteridge, M. D. Azimioara, M. G. Benedetti, T. A. Carter, P. Ciceri, P. T. Edeen, M. Floyd, J. M. Ford, M. Galvin, J. L. Gerlach, R. M. Grotzfeld, S. Herrgard, D. E. Insko, M. A. Insko, A. G. Lai, J. M. Lelias, S. A. Mehta, Z. V. Milanov, A. M. Velasco, L. M. Wodicka, H. K. Patel, P. P. Zarrinkar and D. J. Lockhart, *Nat. Biotechnol.*, 2005, **23**, 329.
7. A. Poulsen, A. William, S. Blanchard, A. Lee, H. Nagaraj, H. Wang, E. Teo, E. Tan, K. C. Goh and B. Dymock, *J. Comput.-Aided Mol. Des.*, 2012, **26**, 437.
8. A. Poulsen, A. William, S. Blanchard, H. Nagaraj, M. Williams, H. Wang, A. Lee, E. Sun, E. L. Teo, E. Tan, K. C. Goh and B. Dymock, *J. Mol. Model.*, 2013, **19**, 119.
9. A. D. William, A. C. Lee, S. Blanchard, A. Poulsen, E. L. Teo, H. Nagaraj, E. Tan, D. Chen, M. Williams, E. T. Sun, K. C. Goh, W. C. Ong, S. K. Goh, S. Hart, R. Jayaraman, M. K. Pasha, K. Ethirajulu, J. M. Wood and B. W. Dymock, *J. Med. Chem.*, 2011, **54**, 4638.
10. A. D. William, A. C. Lee, K. C. Goh, S. Blanchard, A. Poulsen, E. L. Teo, H. Nagaraj, C. P. Lee, H. Wang, M. Williams, E. T. Sun, C. Hu, R. Jayaraman, M. K. Pasha, K. Ethirajulu, J. M. Wood and B. W. Dymock, *J. Med. Chem.*, 2012, **55**, 169.
11. A. D. William, A. C. Lee, A. Poulsen, K. C. Goh, B. Madan, S. Hart, E. Tan, H. Wang, H. Nagaraj, D. Chen, C. P. Lee, E. T. Sun, R. Jayaraman, M. K. Pasha, K. Ethirajulu, J. M. Wood and B. W. Dymock, *J. Med. Chem.*, 2012, **55**, 2623.
12. R. U. Vallente, *Genet. Eng. Biotechnol. News*, 2013, **33**, 16.
13. E. M. Driggers, S. P. Hale, J. Lee and N. K. Terrett, *Nat. Rev. Drug Discovery*, 2008, **7**, 608.
14. W. Brandt, V. J. Haupt and L. A. Wessjohann, *Curr. Top. Med. Chem. (Sharjah, United Arab Emirates)*, 2010, **10**, 1361.
15. E. J. Giamarellos-Bourboulis, *Curr. Top. Med. Chem. (Sharjah, United Arab Emirates)*, 2010, **10**, 1470.
16. E. Marsault and M. L. Peterson, *J. Med. Chem.*, 2011, **54**, 1961.
17. A. K. Oyelere, *Curr. Top. Med. Chem. (Sharjah, United Arab Emirates)*, 2010, **10**, 1359.
18. J. Mallinson and I. Collins, *Future Med. Chem.*, 2012, **4**, 1409.

19. M. R. Jirousek, J. R. Gillig, C. M. Gonzalez, W. F. Heath, J. H. McDonald, 3rd, D. A. Neel, C. J. Rito, U. Singh, L. E. Stramm, A. Melikian-Badalian, M. Baevsky, L. M. Ballas, S. E. Hall, L. L. Winneroski and M. M. Faul, *J. Med. Chem.*, 1996, **39**, 2664.

20. S. Hu, G. Xie, D. X. Zhang, C. Davis, W. Long, Y. Hu, F. Wang, X. Kang, F. Tan, L. Ding and Y. Wang, *Bioorg. Med. Chem. Lett.*, 2012, **22**, 6301.

21. Y. Shi, L. Zhang, X. Liu, C. Zhou, S. Zhang, D. Wang, Q. Li, S. Qin, C. Hu, Y. Zhang, J. Chen, Y. Cheng, J. Feng, H. Zhang, Y. Song, Y. L. Wu, N. Xu, J. Zhou, R. Luo, C. Bai, Y. Jin, W. Liu, Z. Wei, F. Tan, Y. Wang, L. Ding, H. Dai, S. Jiao, J. Wang, L. Liang, W. Zhang and Y. Sun, *Lancet Oncol.*, 2013, **14**, 953.

22. G. Georghiou, R. E. Kleiner, M. Pulkoski-Gross, D. R. Liu and M. A. Seeliger, *Nat. Chem. Biol.*, 2012, **8**, 366.

23. Y. Hayashi, J. Morimoto and H. Suga, *ACS Chem. Biol.*, 2012, 7, 607.

24. H. Hirai, I. Takahashi-Suziki, T. Shimomura, K. Fukasawa, T. Machida, T. Takaki, M. Kobayashi, T. Eguchi, H. Oki, T. Arai, K. Ichikawa, S. Hasako, T. Kodera, N. Kawanishi, Y. Nakatsuru, H. Kotani and Y. Iwasawa, *Invest. New Drugs*, 2011, **29**, 534.

25. Z. F. Tao, L. Wang, K. D. Stewart, Z. Chen, W. Gu, M. H. Bui, P. Merta, H. Zhang, P. Kovar, E. Johnson, C. Park, R. Judge, S. Rosenberg, T. Sowin and N. H. Lin, *J. Med. Chem.*, 2007, **50**, 1514.

26. U. Lucking, G. Siemeister, M. Schafer, H. Briem, M. Kruger, P. Lienau and R. Jautelat, *ChemMedChem*, 2007, **2**, 63.

27. Z. Nie, C. Perretta, P. Erickson, S. Margosiak, J. Lu, A. Averill, R. Almassy and S. Chu, *Bioorg. Med. Chem. Lett.*, 2008, **18**, 619.

28. H. C. Zhang, L. V. Bonaga, H. Ye, C. K. Derian, B. P. Damiano and B. E. Maryanoff, *Bioorg. Med. Chem. Lett.*, 2007, **17**, 2863.

29. H. J. Breslin, B. M. Lane, G. R. Ott, A. K. Ghose, T. S. Angeles, M. S. Albom, M. Cheng, W. Wan, R. C. Haltiwanger, K. J. Wells-Knecht and B. D. Dorsey, *J. Med. Chem.*, 2012, **55**, 449.

30. J. Zhang, P. L. Yang and N. S. Gray, *Nat. Rev. Cancer.*, 2009, **9**, 28.

31. P. Y. Dakas, S. Barluenga, F. Totzke, U. Zirrgiebel and N. Winssinger, *Angew. Chem. Int. Ed.*, 2007, **46**, 6899.

32. E. Vakil and A. Tefferi, *Clin. Lymphoma, Myeloma Leuk.*, 2011, 11 Suppl 1, S37.

33. H. Kiu and S. E. Nicholson, *Growth Factors*, 2012, **30**, 88.

34. E. J. Baxter, L. M. Scott, P. J. Campbell, C. East, N. Fourouclas, S. Swanton, G. S. Vassiliou, A. J. Bench, E. M. Boyd, N. Curtin, M. A. Scott, W. N. Erber, A. R. Green and P. Cancer Genome, *Lancet*, 2005, **365**, 1054.

35. C. James, V. Ugo, J. P. Le Couedic, J. Staerk, F. Delhommeau, C. Lacout, L. Garcon, H. Raslova, R. Berger, A. Bennaceur-Griscelli, J. L. Villeval, S. N. Constantinescu, N. Casadevall and W. Vainchenker, *Nature*, 2005, **434**, 1144.

36. R. Kralovics, F. Passamonti, A. S. Buser, S. S. Teo, R. Tiedt, J. R. Passweg, A. Tichelli, M. Cazzola and R. C. Skoda, *N. Engl. J. Med.*, 2005, **352**, 1779.

37. R. L. Levine, M. Wadleigh, J. Cools, B. L. Ebert, G. Wernig, B. J. Huntly, T. J. Boggon, I. Wlodarska, J. J. Clark, S. Moore, J. Adelsperger, S. Koo, J. C. Lee, S. Gabriel, T. Mercher, A. D'Andrea, S. Frohling, K. Dohner, P. Marynen, P. Vandenberghe, R. A. Mesa, A. Tefferi, J. D. Griffin, M. J. Eck, W. R. Sellers, M. Meyerson, T. R. Golub, S. J. Lee and D. G. Gilliland, *Cancer Cell*, 2005, **7**, 387.
38. Novartis/Incyte, www.jakafi.com.
39. S. Verstovsek, R. A. Mesa, J. Gotlib, R. S. Levy, V. Gupta, J. F. DiPersio, J. V. Catalano, M. Deininger, C. Miller, R. T. Silver, M. Talpaz, E. F. Winton, J. H. Harvey Jr., M. O. Arcasoy, E. Hexner, R. M. Lyons, R. Paquette, A. Raza, K. Vaddi, S. Erickson-Viitanen, I. L. Koumenis, W. Sun, V. Sandor and H. M. Kantarjian, *N. Engl. J. Med.*, 2012, **366**, 799.
40. C. Harrison, J. J. Kiladjian, H. K. Al-Ali, H. Gisslinger, R. Waltzman, V. Stalbovskaya, M. McQuitty, D. S. Hunter, R. Levy, L. Knoops, F. Cervantes, A. M. Vannucchi, T. Barbui and G. Barosi, *N. Engl. J. Med.*, 2012, **366**, 787.
41. Pfizer: http://www.xeljanz.com [accessed Feb. 2014].
42. E. Leah, *Nat. Rev. Rheumatol.*, 2012, **8**, 561.
43. K. Garber, *Nat. Biotechnol.*, 2011, **29**, 467.
44. FDA approves Xeljanz for rheumatoid arthritis. http://www.fda.gov/NewsEvents/Newsroom/PressAnnouncements/ucm327152.htm (Nov. 2012) [accessed Feb. 2014].
45. G. R. Stark and J. E. Darnell Jr, *Immunity*, 2012, **36**, 503.
46. B. A. Croker, H. Kiu and S. E. Nicholson, *Semin. Cell Dev. Biol.*, 2008, **19**, 414.
47. S. J. Rodig, M. A. Meraz, J. M. White, P. A. Lampe, J. K. Riley, C. D. Arthur, K. L. King, K. C. Sheehan, L. Yin, D. Pennica, E. M. Johnson Jr and R. D. Schreiber, *Cell*, 1998, **93**, 373.
48. H. Neubauer, A. Cumano, M. Muller, H. Wu, U. Huffstadt and K. Pfeffer, *Cell*, 1998, **93**, 397.
49. E. Parganas, D. Wang, D. Stravopodis, D. J. Topham, J. C. Marine, S. Teglund, E. F. Vanin, S. Bodner, O. R. Colamonici, J. M. van Deursen, G. Grosveld and J. N. Ihle, *Cell*, 1998, **93**, 385.
50. E. Derenzini and A. Younes, *Expert Opin. Invest. Drugs*, 2013, **22**, 775.
51. M. A. Weniger, I. Melzner, C. K. Menz, S. Wegener, A. J. Bucur, K. Dorsch, T. Mattfeldt, T. F. Barth and P. Moller, *Oncogene*, 2006, **25**, 2679.
52. A. Navarro, T. Diaz, A. Martinez, A. Gaya, A. Pons, B. Gel, C. Codony, G. Ferrer, C. Martinez, E. Montserrat and M. Monzo, *Blood*, 2009, **114**, 2945.
53. A. Mottok, C. Renne, K. Willenbrock, M. L. Hansmann and A. Brauninger, *Blood*, 2007, **110**, 3387.
54. I. Melzner, M. A. Weniger, A. J. Bucur, S. Bruderlein, K. Dorsch, C. Hasel, F. Leithauser, O. Ritz, M. J. Dyer, T. F. Barth and P. Moller, *Int. J. Cancer*, 2006, **118**, 1941.

55. I. Melzner, A. J. Bucur, S. Bruderlein, K. Dorsch, C. Hasel, T. F. Barth, F. Leithauser and P. Moller, *Blood*, 2005, **105**, 2535.
56. P. Macchi, A. Villa, S. Giliani, M. G. Sacco, A. Frattini, F. Porta, A. G. Ugazio, J. A. Johnston, F. Candotti, J. J. O'Shea, P. Vezzoni and L. D. Notarangelo, *Nature*, 1995, **377**, 65.
57. S. M. Russell, N. Tayebi, H. Nakajima, M. C. Riedy, J. L. Roberts, M. J. Aman, T. S. Migone, M. Noguchi, M. L. Markert, R. H. Buckley, J. J. O'Shea and W. J. Leonard, *Science*, 1995, **270**, 797.
58. K. Suzuki, H. Nakajima, Y. Saito, T. Saito, W. J. Leonard and I. Iwamoto, *Int. Immunol.*, 2000, **12**, 123.
59. Lilly/Incyte, Lilly and Incyte Announce Baricitinib Efficacy and Safety Data from the Open-Label, Long-Term Extension of the Phase 2b JADA Study in Patients with Rheumatoid Arthritis - Results from 52-week study presented at EULAR 2013, 13 June 2013.
60. Pfizer, Pfizer Receives CHMP Negative Opinion Regarding Marketing Authorization In Europe For Rheumatoid Arthritis Treatment XEL-JANZ® (tofacitinib citrate), 25 April, 2013, http://press.pfizer.com/press-release/pfizer-receives-chmp-negative-opinion-regarding-marketing-authorization-europe-rheumat [accessed Feb. 2014].
61. K. Migita, A. Komori, T. Torigoshi, Y. Maeda, Y. Izumi, Y. Jiuchi, T. Miyashita, M. Nakamura, S. Motokawa and H. Ishibashi, *Arthritis Res. Ther.*, 2011, **13**, R72.
62. M. H. Shaw, V. Boyartchuk, S. Wong, M. Karaghiosoff, J. Ragimbeau, S. Pellegrini, M. Muller, W. F. Dietrich and G. S. Yap, *Proc. Natl. Acad. Sci. U. S. A.*, 2003, **100**, 11594.
63. M. Ishizaki, T. Akimoto, R. Muromoto, M. Yokoyama, Y. Ohshiro, Y. Sekine, H. Maeda, K. Shimoda, K. Oritani and T. Matsuda, *J. Immunol.*, 2011, **187**, 181.
64. V. Paunovic, H. P. Carroll, K. Vandenbroeck and M. Gadina, *Rheumatology*, 2008, **47**, 771.
65. M. Prchal-Murphy, C. Semper, C. Lassnig, B. Wallner, C. Gausterer, I. Teppner-Klymiuk, J. Kobolak, S. Muller, T. Kolbe, M. Karaghiosoff, A. Dinnyes, T. Rulicke, N. R. Leitner, B. Strobl and M. Muller, *PloS One*, 2012, 7, e39141.
66. M. Ishizaki, R. Muromoto, T. Akimoto, Y. Ohshiro, M. Takahashi, Y. Sekine, H. Maeda, K. Shimoda, K. Oritani and T. Matsuda, *Int. Immunol.*, 2011, **23**, 575.
67. J. T. Reilly and Leuk, *Lymphoma*, 2003, **44**, 1.
68. H. Kiyoi and T. Naoe, *Int. J. Hematol.*, 2006, **83**, 301.
69. A. Y. Leung, C. H. Man and Y. L. Kwong, *Leukemia*, 2013, **27**, 260.
70. M. Knockaert, P. Greengard and L. Meijer, *Trends Pharmacol. Sci.*, 2002, **23**, 417.
71. D. O. Morgan, *Annu. Rev. Cell Dev. Biol.*, 1997, **13**, 261.
72. D. Cai, V. M. Latham Jr., X. Zhang and G. I. Shapiro, *Cancer Res.*, 2006, **66**, 9270.
73. R. Jorda, K. Paruch and V. Krystof, *Curr. Pharm. Des.*, 2012, **18**, 2974.

74. R. T. Paniagua, A. Chang, M. M. Mariano, E. A. Stein, Q. Wang, T. M. Lindstrom, O. Sharpe, C. Roscow, P. P. Ho, D. M. Lee and W. H. Robinson, *Arthritis Res. Ther.*, 2010, **12**, R32.
75. H. Ohno, Y. Uemura, H. Murooka, H. Takanashi, T. Tokieda, Y. Ohzeki, K. Kubo and I. Serizawa, *Eur. J. Immunol.*, 2008, **38**, 283.
76. J. G. Conway, H. Pink, M. L. Bergquist, B. Han, S. Depee, S. Tadepalli, P. Lin, R. C. Crumrine, J. Binz, R. L. Clark, J. L. Selph, S. A. Stimpson, J. T. Hutchins, S. D. Chamberlain, T. A. Brodie and J. Pharmacol, *Exp. Ther.*, 2008, **326**, 41.
77. B. Madan, K. C. Goh, S. Hart, A. D. William, R. Jayaraman, K. Ethirajulu, B. W. Dymock and J. M. Wood, *J. Immunol.*, 2012, **189**, 4123.
78. P. A. Lochhead, R. Gilley and S. J. Cook, *Biochem. Soc. Trans.*, 2012, **40**, 251.
79. H. Song, X. Jin and J. Lin, *Oncogene*, 2004, **23**, 8301.
80. J. C. Montero, A. Ocana, M. Abad, M. J. Ortiz-Ruiz, A. Pandiella and A. Esparis-Ogando, *PloS One*, 2009, **4**, e5565.
81. Q. Yang, X. Deng, B. Lu, M. Cameron, C. Fearns, M. P. Patricelli, J. R. Yates, 3rd, N. S. Gray and J. D. Lee, *Cancer Cell*, 2010, **18**, 258.
82. M. J. Ortiz-Ruiz, L. A. Cheatham, K. R. Meshaw, F. J. Burrows, A. Pandiella and A. Esparís-Ogando, ASCO, Berlin, 2011.
83. S. Alvarez-Fernandez, M. J. Ortiz-Ruiz, T. Parrott, S. Zaknoen, E. M. Ocio, J. San Miguel, F. J. Burrows, A. Esparis-Ogando and A. Pandiella, *Clin. Cancer Res.*, 2013, **19**, 2677.
84. A. Poulsen, A. William, A. Lee, S. Blanchard, E. Teo, W. Deng, N. Tu, E. Tan, E. Sun, K. L. Goh, W. C. Ong, C. P. Ng, K. C. Goh and Z. Bonday, *J. Comput.-Aided Mol. Des*, 2008, **22**, 897.
85. D. J. G. Matthews, M. E., *Targeting Protein Kinases for Cancer Therapy*, Wiley, Hoboken, New Jersey, 2010.
86. N. K. Williams, R. S. Bamert, O. Patel, C. Wang, P. M. Walden, A. F. Wilks, E. Fantino, J. Rossjohn and I. S. Lucet, *J. Mol. Biol.*, 2009, **387**, 219.
87. G. R. S. Desiraju, T., *The Weak Hydrogen Bond In Structural Chemistry and Biology*, Oxford University Press, New York, 1999.
88. S. Blanchard, C. K. Soh, C. P. Lee, A. Poulsen, Z. Bonday, K. L. Goh, K. C. Goh, M. K. Goh, M. K. Pasha, H. Wang, M. Williams, J. M. Wood, K. Ethirajulu and B. W. Dymock, *Bioorg. Med. Chem. Lett.*, 2012, **22**, 2880.
89. A. Poulsen, S. Blanchard, C. K. Soh, C. Lee, M. Williams, H. Wang and B. Dymock, *Bioorg. Med. Chem. Lett.*, 2012, **22**, 305.
90. K. C. Goh, V. Novotny-Diermayr, S. Hart, L. C. Ong, Y. K. Loh, A. Cheong, Y. C. Tan, C. Hu, R. Jayaraman, A. D. William, E. T. Sun, B. W. Dymock, K. H. Ong, K. Ethirajulu, F. Burrows and J. M. Wood, *Leukemia*, 2012, **26**, 236.
91. S. Hart, K. C. Goh, V. Novotny-Diermayr, C. Y. Hu, H. Hentze, Y. C. Tan, B. Madan, C. Amalini, Y. K. Loh, L. C. Ong, A. D. William, A. Lee, A. Poulsen, R. Jayaraman, K. H. Ong, K. Ethirajulu, B. W. Dymock and J. W. Wood, *Leukemia*, 2011, **25**, 1751.
92. D. A. Smith, L. Di and E. H. Kerns, *Nat. Rev. Drug Discovery*, 2010, **9**, 929.

93. I. R. Hardcastle, M. G. Rowlands, J. Houghton, I. B. Parr, G. A. Potter, M. Jarman, K. J. Edwards, C. A. Laughton, J. O. Trent and S. Neidle, *J. Med. Chem.*, 1995, **38**, 241.

94. P. Köhling, A. M. Schmidt and P. Eilbracht, *Org. Lett.*, 2003, **5**, 3213.

95. H. S. P. Rao and S. P. Senthilkumar, *Proc. Indian Acad. Sci.*, 2001, **113**, 191.

96. C. Niu, D. H. Boschelli, L. N. Tumey, N. Bhagirath, J. Subrath, J. Shim, Y. Wang, B. Wu, C. Eid, J. Lee, X. Yang, A. Brennan and D. Chaudhary, *Bioorg. Med. Chem. Lett.*, 2009, **19**, 5829.

97. N. Miyaura and A. Suzuki, *Chem. Rev. (Washington, DC, U. S.)*, 1995, **95**, 2457.

98. A. Suzuki, *Pure Appl. Chem.*, 1991, **63**, 419.

99. S. Joshi, G. C. Maikap, S. Titirmare, A. Chaudhari and M. K. Gurjar, *Org. Proc. Res. Devel.*, 2010, **14**, 657.

100. Q. Cai, Z. A. Zhao and S. L. You, *Angew. Chem. Int. Ed.*, 2009, **48**, 7428.

101. B. Schmidt, *Angew. Chem. Int. Ed.*, 2003, **42**, 4996.

102. A. F. Abdel-Magid, K. D. Carson, B. D. Harris, C. A. Maryanoff and R. D. Shah, *J. Org. Chem.*, 1996, **61**, 3849.

103. E. W. Baxter and A. B. Reitz, *Reductive Aminations of Carbonyl Compounds with Borohydride and Borane Reducing Agents, Org. React.*, **59**, Wiley, 2002.

104. F. D. Bellamy and K. Ou, *Tetrahedron Lett.*, 1984, **25**, 839.

105. A. Deiters and S. F. Martin, *Chem. Rev. (Washington, DC, U. S.)*, 2004, **104**, 2199.

106. S. Kim, W. Hwang, I. S. Lim, S. H. Kim, S.-g. Lee and B. M. Kim, *Tetrahedron Lett.*, 2010, **51**, 709.

107. CTI Biopharma Corp.: Oral Pacritinib Versus Best Available Therapy to Treat Myelofibrosis (Phase 3 trial), http://www.clinicaltrials.gov/ct2/show/NCT01773187 [accessed Feb. 2014].

108. S*BIO PTE LTD: A Phase 1/2 Study of Oral SB1518 in Subjects With Chronic Idiopathic Myelofibrosis, http://www.clinicaltrials.gov/ct2/show/NCT00745550 [accessed Feb. 2014].

109. S*BIO PTE LTD: A Phase 1/2 Study of SB1518 for the Treatment of Advanced Myeloid Malignancies, http://www.clinicaltrials.gov/ct2/show/NCT00719836 [accessed Feb. 2014].

110. S*BIO PTE LTD: A Safety and Efficacy Study of SB1518 for the Treatment of Advanced Lymphoid Malignancies, http://www.clinicaltrials.gov/ct2/show/NCT01263899 [accessed Feb. 2014].

111. S*BIO PTE LTD: A Phase 1 Study of SB1518 for the Treatment of Advanced Lymphoid Malignancies, http://www.clinicaltrials.gov/ct2/show/NCT00741871 [accessed Feb. 2014].

112. M.D. Anderson Cancer Center, S*BIO PTE LTD: SB1518 for Patients With Myelodysplastic Syndrome (MDS), http://www.clinicaltrials.gov/ct2/show/NCT01436084 [accessed Feb 2014].

113. Tragara Pharmaceuticals, Inc.: A Phase I Dose-Escalation and PK Study of TG02 Citrate in Patients with Advanced Hematological Malignancies, http://www.clinicaltrials.gov/ct2/show/NCT01204164 [accessed Feb. 2014].

114. Tragara Pharmaceuticals, Inc.: Phase 1 Study of TG02 Citrate in Patients With Chronic Lymphocytic Leukemia and Small Lymphocytic Lymphoma, http://www.clinicaltrials.gov/ct2/show/NCT01699152 [accessed Feb. 2014].

115. S*BIO PTE LTD: A Single and Multiple-Dose Study of SB1578, http://www.clinicaltrials.gov/ct2/show/NCT01235871 [accessed Feb. 2014].

116. J. Seymour, B. Scott, A. Roberts, B. To, O. Odenike, Z. Estrov, J. Cortes, D. Thomas, J. Zhu, A. Dorr, H. Kantarjian, H. Deeg and S. Verstovsek, 16th EHA Congress, 2011, Abstr. 0907.

117. Incyte-Corporation. Jakafi® (ruxolitinib) Prescribing Information Updated with Expanded Dosing Guidance and New Safety Information, http://investor.incyte.com/phoenix.zhtml?c=69764&p=irol-news&nyo=0 [accessed Feb. 2014].

118. A. Younes, J. Romaguera, M. Fanale, P. McLaughlin, F. Hagemeister, A. Copeland, S. Neelapu, L. Kwak, J. Shah, S. de Castro Faria, S. Hart, J. Wood, R. Jayaraman, K. Ethirajulu and J. Zhu, *J. Clin. Oncol.*, 2012, **30**, 4161.

119. M. K. Pasha, R. Jayaraman, V. P. Reddy, P. Yeo, E. Goh, A. Williams, K. C. Goh and E. Kantharaj, *Drug Metab. Lett.*, 2012, **6**, 33.

120. G. J. Roboz, J. Khoury, J. Shammo, M. Syto, F. Burrows, T. L. Parrott and E. Jabbour, *ASCO Annual Meeting 2012*, 2012, Abstr. 6577.

121. M. Pallis, A. Abdul-Aziz, F. Burrows, C. Seedhouse, M. Grundy and N. Russell, *Br. J. Haematol.*, 2012, **159**, 191.

122. S. Verstovsek, O. Odenike, B. Scott, Z. Estrov, J. Cortes, D. A. Thomas, J. Wood, K. Ethirajulu, A. Lowe, H. J. Zhu, H. Kantarjian and H. J. Deeg, *51st ASH Annual Meeting and Exposition*, New Orleans, LA, 2009, Abstr. 3905.

123. F. Seymour, B. To, A. Goh, L. Meadows, A. Ethirajulu, A. Wood, A. Zhu and W. Roberts, *Haematologica*, 2010, 95 (suppl 2), 472, Abstr. 1144.

124. H. J. Deeg, O. Odenike, B. L. Scott, Z. Estrov, J. E. Cortes, D. A. Thomas, H. J. Zhu, H. Kantarjian and S. Verstovsek, *J. Clin. Oncol.*, 2011, **29**, Suppl. Abstr. 6515.

125. R. S. Komrokji, M. Wadleigh, J. F. Seymour, A. W. Roberts, L. Bik, H. J. Zhu and R. A. Mesa, *53rd ASH Annual Meeting and Exposition*, New Orleans, LA, 2011, Abstr. 282.

CHAPTER 6

Anti-Inflammatory Macrolides to Manage Chronic Neutrophilic Inflammation

MICHAEL BURNET,*[a] JAN-HINRICH GUSE,[a]
HANS-JÜRGEN GUTKE,[a] LOIC GUILLOT,[b] STEFAN LAUFER,[c]
ULRIKE HAHN,[a] MICHAEL P. SEED,[d] ENRIQUETA VALLEJO,[a]
MARY EGGERS,[a] DOUG McKENZIE,[e] WOLFGANG ALBRECHT[f]
AND MICHAEL J. PARNHAM[g]

[a] Synovo GmbH, Tübingen, Germany; [b] INSERM, UMR_S 938, CDR
Saint-Antoine, Paris, France; [c] The University of Tübingen, Germany;
[d] University of East London, London, UK; [e] Stressor Therapeutics Ltd,
10782 Spur Point, San Diego, CA 92130, USA; [f] c-a-i-r biosciences GmbH,
Tübingen, Germany; [g] Fraunhofer Institute for Molecular Biology and
Applied Ecology IME-TMP, Frankfurt am Main, Germany
*Email: michael.burnet@synovo.com

6.1 Introduction

"Inflammation" broadly describes a tissue response to insult. It may be
pathological, or it may be healthy and regenerative.[1] Therapeutic approaches
to inflammation have tended to centre on the inhibition or neutralisation
of pro-inflammatory signals or cascades. While preventing the onset of
inflammation is attractive, experience suggests that there may also be
unintended consequences to this approach, namely inhibition of resolution

RSC Drug Discovery Series No. 40
Macrocycles in Drug Discovery
Edited by Jeremy Levin
© The Royal Society of Chemistry 2015
Published by the Royal Society of Chemistry, www.rsc.org

processes (*e.g.* with COX2 inhibitors),[2] or, upon discontinuation of therapy, a resurgence of pro-inflammatory processes (*e.g.* with glucocorticoids).[3]

An alternative is to attempt to find means to support the resolution of inflammation or the maintenance of a non-inflamed or non-inflammation prone state. The antibacterial macrolides are a class of compounds that appear to exert such an effect. Clinical studies of chronic macrolide therapy suggest that a general effect of the class is to reduce apparent inflammation in a way that is not easily explained by antibacterial effects alone. Rather, it appears that the macrolides modify the responsiveness of myeloid derived immune cells, notably neutrophils and macrophages, with the effect of promoting a pro-resolution state that may be observed in the balance of anti- and pro-inflammatory cytokines that these cells produce.[4,5]

The particular effect of macrolides on neutrophils is enhanced not least in part through their very high partitioning into the phagosomes. Depending on the structure of specific macrolides, and the activation state of the immune cells, the concentration in neutrophils can be up to 1000-fold that of plasma. This accumulation in neutrophils and other phagocytes leads to an important beneficial effect in use, namely the transport to, and accumulation of drug in, zones of active inflammation. Macrolide pharmacokinetics are characterised by accumulation in acidic compartments. Thus, the amphiphilic macrolide ring system passes readily through membranes while the amine of the desosamine ring is subject to protonation in the phagosomes leading to acid trapping. For an anti-bacterial compound this means that, in so far as the site of infection attracts neutrophils and monocytes, the macrolide will be transported to the site of infection and accumulated there. The same process functions in non-infective inflammations. Thus, despite their relatively low potency, macrolides exert clinically useful anti-inflammatory effects in chronic use by virtue of their very high and stable concentrations at sites of disease. A similar conclusion can be made in the context of their antibacterial effects where again relatively low *in vitro* potency is associated with an adequate *in vivo* effect.

6.2 Efforts Toward the Discovery of Anti-Inflammatory Macrolides

The clinical observations of generalised anti-inflammatory effects led a range of researchers to use the macrolides as a scaffold for new agents, or to deliver other pharmacological agents. In one approach, simple variation of the macrolide ring and pendant groups leads to compounds that can be screened directly for suitable anti-inflammatory activity.[6] In another approach, stable conjugates of small molecules to macrolides adopt many of the positive pharmacological characteristics of the parent macrolide while usually retaining the binding activity of the conjugated compound to its target.[7,8] Thus, macrolide conjugation also provides a means to improve the pharmacokinetics and distribution of compounds that may be otherwise insufficiently stable or soluble.

Objections to the use of the macrolides as anti-inflammatory therapies are usually made in the following order:

1. The antibacterial effect selects for resistance, and often multiple re-sistance, in a range of potentially pathogenic bacteria.
2. The macrolides have been associated with cardiotoxicity related to long QT syndrome (The QT wave interval is a measure of normal cardiac function).
3. The macrolides have been associated with ototoxicity, albeit to a far lesser extent than is known for aminoglycosides.
4. The accumulation of macrolides in lysosomes is associated with phospholipidosis.

The concerns over selection for resistance in commensal bacteria have been borne out in clinical studies where the majority of patients carry re-sistant organisms after treatment over a period of months.[9] While macrolide resistance has become so common that this in itself is tolerable in certain settings, the fact that macrolide resistance is often carried on multi-resist-ance plasmids makes it more problematic. The official consensus has, therefore, been to avoid the promotion of macrolides for inflammation. However, in certain indications their use is so beneficial that concerns over resistance have been put aside by individual practitioners.

Nonetheless, the promotion of resistance has led most regulators to oppose the wider use of macrolides. The resulting issue has not been lost on researchers in the field and a number of groups are working towards the clinical development of "non-antibacterial, anti-inflammatory macrolides" (NAMs). The development of this class of compounds has been hindered in part by the fact that macrolides are so inherently antibacterial that complete elimination of antibacterial effect is rather difficult, and by the issues of mode of action and safety.

6.3   Issues in Development of Anti-Inflammatory Macrolides

Starting with safety, the absence of a single, easily defined mode of action leads to concerns over what toxicity models will be relevant and what biomarkers or genotypes to use for the selection of potentially responsive patients. These concerns may be relatively easily approached with practical pharmacology.

For example, potential cardiotoxicity is associated with an abnormal ECG at baseline.[10] In studies where ECGs are taken at the outset and used to exclude patients with abnormal signals or QT intervals, there is no evidence of macrolide-associated adverse cardiac events. These reports suggest that the now standard practice of conducting ECG prior to commencing chronic macrolides[1] is not associated with cardiac events beyond those observed in placebo or control arms. In contrast to their use in chronic settings, the use of macrolides as antibacterials is considered so ordinary and low cost that ECG is rarely performed prior to their prescription. Thus, in meta-analyses of cardiac events, the few events that are noted are mainly associated with short-term use as antibacterials. These data suggest that while the issue is a real one, it can be managed more satisfactorily than at present.

Phospholipidosis presents an alternative but rather benign effect of macrolides. Although it is reported in chronic macrolide therapy, there are no obvious negative effects and there is a possibility that it contributes to beneficial effects, notably in inflammatory bowel and eye diseases[11] where additional phospholipids correct surfactant deficiencies.[12] Various studies show that phospholipidosis resolves on discontinuation of macrolide therapy and there are no clinical reports of negative outcomes associated with it. Thus phospholipidosis is probably mechanistically linked to effects in immune cells and it seems to present therapeutic opportunities in phospholipid deficiencies rather than any obvious adverse effects in clinical practice.

The last well known safety issue in macrolide use is hearing loss. Reversible effects on hearing are reported in conventional oral dosing regimens while exposure to high doses such as in hospital intravenous administration may be associated with permanent hearing loss.[13] Where studied, reversible hearing loss appears to be more frequent with co-medication (*e.g.* ketoconazole) and appears to recover in the range of 4 to 11 weeks after discontinuing the macrolide.[14] In the most recent study of long-term macrolide therapy in chronic disease, Albert *et al.*,[15] reported hearing decrements in 25% of subjects taking azithromycin and 20% of subjects allocated to placebo ($p = 0.04$). Discontinuation of treatment led to improvements in audiogram results in 34% of patients taking azithromycin *vs.* 38% of patients taking placebo. Of the patients who remained on treatment, 32% of azithromycin treated patients and 25% of placebo patients also showed improvements in audiogram scores. These data suggest that while hearing effects may be present, the effect is not easily measured.

6.4 Is the Anti-Inflammatory Activity of Macrolides Related to their Effects on Normal Flora or Colonisation by Pathogens?

A wide variety of clinical studies report beneficial effects from macrolide therapy in many inflammatory diseases and notably lung diseases. In many instances, these effects are obtained in the absence of clear infections. This had led to considerable debate as to whether the main mode of action in these settings is one of anti-inflammatory activity or whether subtle modulation of bacterial vigour leads to greater benefits than might be expected. Effects on bacteria may also include interference in quorum sensing or biofilm formation that may not be associated with effects on growth rate of planktonic forms in culture.

The possible mechanisms of immune modulation by macrolides have been reviewed recently.[5,16] Their conclusions can be summarised briefly as follows using azithromycin as a model macrolide. Over short periods of exposure, azithromycin modulates the function of the plasma and lysosomal membranes to cause initial immune stimulation manifested, for example, in increased phagocytic activity, or increased IL-17 production following stimulus. Over longer exposure, and at higher concentrations, the membranes and the lysosome become so highly loaded that general membrane and protein maturation functions are inhibited leading to reduced synthesis of arachidonic acid and reductions in signalling *via* the well-known transcription systems (*e.g.* NfκB and AP-1).

While immune-modulatory concepts for macrolide action are repeatedly observed, there is also the possibility that a combination of both anti-bacterial and immune modulatory actions is important for clinical benefit. For the bacterial modulation hypothesis, there are reports that indicate that in certain studies, slightly greater effect is obtained in patients carrying pathogenic strains of *Pseudomonas aeruginosa*, or that the frequency of culturable *Staphylococcus aureus* declines during therapy (Table 6.1).[1,17] Similarly, the fact that high levels of macrolide resistance are evident after 3 to 12 months of continuous therapy suggests that even though treatment is not grossly altering the culturable flora in nasopharyngeal swabs, there must be some degree of selection for tolerance to the compound that may involve a period of decreased bacterial activity.

More recently, it has been possible to study bacterial population dynamics by sequencing bacterial DNA harvested from bronchoalveolar lavage samples from asthma patients.[19] By analysing the frequency of sequences, an impression of the relative abundance of different genera can be obtained. Initial data from patients suggest that after six weeks of daily azithromycin (250 mg), changes in flora included reductions in *Pseudomonas* and *Staphylococcus sp.* and increases in *Anaerococcus*. Changes in flora disfavouring pathogens while maintaining other genera suggests a selective antibacterial effect that is consistent with reports of clinical benefit. These studies are, however, too short to suggest the basis for benefit in longer term

Table 6.1   Observations of cystic fibrosis patients treated with azithromycin for 168 days and selected according to the presence of *Pseudomonas aeruginosa*.

Parameter	Effect of daily azithromycin	
P. aeruginosa status	Negative[b]	Positive[c]
N	130	100
FEV1[a] (L) – *p* value	0.02	0.09
Weight (kg) increase – *p* value	0.58	0.70
Exacerbation reduction (%)	50	50

[a]FEV1, Forced Expiratory Volume in the first second of exhalation.
[b]For data on patients negative for *Pseudomonas aeruginosa* infection, see ref. 18.
[c]For data on patients negative for *Pseudomonas aeruginosa* infection, see ref. 17 (no effect on colonisation observed).

studies. These data are also consistent with observations of selection for resistance that, by definition, requires a selective disadvantage for sensitive strains. That genera associated with pathogens were among the most responsive to azithromycin perhaps serves to indicate that very successful antibacterials have nuanced *in vivo* actions as opposed to broad spectrum bacterial suppression.

Against the bacterial modulation concept are a range of arguments that involve both mechanistic studies on inflammatory processes reported here and more circumstantial evidence derived from clinical studies. For example, in lung transplant, one phenomenon of chronic rejection of the graft is known as bronchiolitis obliterans. Around 40% of patients with this condition respond to treatment with azithromycin and detailed studies suggest that these are the sub-set of patients in which neutrophilia in the airway contributes to the apparent disease. Administration of azithromycin leads to fewer neutrophils in the airway and recovery of airway function. Other forms of bronchiolitis obliterans appear not to respond to azithromycin. Responses are obtained in the absence of clear infection and so in this example it is reasoned that the macrolide effect is an immunomodulatory one.[20,21]

Similarly, there is a very clear systemic response of plasma inflammatory markers to azithromycin soon after commencement of therapy in cystic fibrosis patients that is sustained for 3 to 6 months.[22] The most notable feature of this response is a decline in circulating neutrophils that may correspond to changes in neutrophil infiltration in airways.

Although various studies demonstrate these benefits, each example can be countered. For example, reductions in circulating neutrophils can also simply indicate the reduction of an infection. Similarly, cryptic infection may underlie many inflammatory conditions and these cryptic infections are by definition difficult to demonstrate. In both COPD and cystic fibrosis there is a plateau in response to azithromycin after one to three years that may relate to either some change in flora that has not yet been observed or accommodation by the immune system.

To investigate the question of whether macrolide action is due to direct immune modulatory effects or antibacterial effects more deeply, screens were executed to discover macrolides that are both non-antibacterial and anti-inflammatory. The compound on the left in Figure 6.1, CSY0073, is one example of the structures identified through those efforts, as compared to azithromycin shown on the right.

CSY0073 applied in the range of 5 to 30 mg kg^{-1} day^{-1} to mice with dextran sulfate-induced colitis exerts anti-inflammatory effects that both reduce signs of acute inflammation and also preserve intestinal wall structure. That this effect is not due to effects on intestinal bacteria has been demonstrated by comparison of fecal flora of healthy mice treated with either azithromycin or CSY0073. Thus, CSY0073 has no obvious effect on the composition of intestinal flora while azithromycin causes Gram positive organisms in particular to be reduced to less than 10% of the culturable

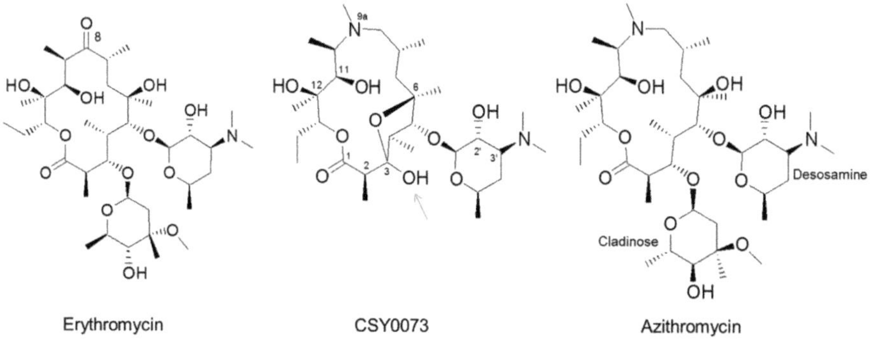

Figure 6.1   Structures of non-antibacterial macrolide CSY0073 and azithromycin. Standard macrolide ring numbering is shown for CSY0073. The blue arrow indicates the position at which CSY0073 is modified relative to azithromycin, namely loss of cladinose and oxidation of the resulting hydroxyl group to a ketone that cyclises to the hemiketal.

organisms *vs. ca.* 50% in untreated animals.[23] Both CSY0073 and azithromycin have similar potency in assays on the response of cultured cells, airways, the gut lining or lamina propria cells to stimulation with LPS. Given that this effect occurs on a time-scale of minutes to hours and that it is not dependent on the presence of bacteria, there is a reasonable possibility that both compounds are acting on independent pathways of macrolide effect that include direct anti-inflammatory action.

6.5   General Properties of Macrolides

Shown in Figure 6.1 are three macrolides, one of which, CSY0073, has been stripped of antibacterial activity. The macrolactone ring of each of these is decorated with a range of hydroxyl groups and sugars. It appears that in an aqueous environment, these generally hydrophilic groups are displayed to solvent and the amines are protonated. This appears to confer macrolides with high solubility in acid environments.

Given the abundance of hydrophilic groups, and their overall size, the apparent high uptake of macrolides by cells would be unexpected. It appears that cellular uptake of macrolides is a process that is favoured in living cells that are able to generate proton gradients across outer and inner membranes. The current hypothesis on the mechanism by which uptake occurs in living cells can be summarised for brevity as follows: the macrolides are attracted to the membrane surface *via* the interaction of their amines with surface phospholipids and that, once in contact with a hydrophobic environment, they effectively invert to direct their hydroxy groups to the ring interior becoming hydrophobic in the process. Exit of the macrolide from the membrane is supposed to be favoured by the protonation of the amines at the lower intracellular pH, most notably in lysosomes and phagosomes.

It is nonetheless, thought that the macrolides remain associated with the membranes *via* their amines even in the lysosome.

The desosamine sugar is the main determinant of the pK_a of the macrolide and also confers binding to the prokaryotic ribosome. The hydroxy group next to the dimethylamine is activated by the amine and is the most reactive hydroxy group in the molecule. Bulky alterations at this position and the amine have the most dramatic effect on antibacterial potency.

The cladinose sugar is not known to confer particular pharmacological effects and it is easily hydrolysed under acidic conditions such as that of the stomach. This cleavage product is one of the main metabolites of erythromycin and its lability is one of its main limits to activity. A range of anti-inflammatory and antibacterial (ketolide) macrolides lack the cladinose.

The 8-position of the macrolide is the position where erythromycin is opened *via* its oxime derivative to generate azithromycin (see position 9a of CSY0073, Figure 6.1). This position is also amenable to chemistry to link compounds to erythromycin, with the oxime a useful starting point. The 11-position of the macrolide (*e.g.* azithromycin, Figure 6.1) offers the potential for direct coupling and for diol chemistry. Various antibacterial compounds are based on addition of extended groups *via* the 11 position.

6.6 Reducing Antibacterial Effects of 14- and 15-Membered Macrolactone Macrolides

There are two main means of modulating the antibacterial effect of the macrolactones derived from erythromycin. The first involves direct interruption of the interactions between the desosamine sugar and its main target in the bacterial ribosome. The hydroxyl and secondary amine functions of desosamine interact directly with the ribosome. Substitution of the methyl groups on the amine for bulkier groups, combined with an *O*-substitution results in a general reduction in antibacterial effect in the macrolide analogs in which this has been tested. In a general sense, the bulkier the groups, the larger the reduction in antibacterial effect that is observed. While this rule is broadly useful, substitution of long alkyl chains onto the amine group (*e.g.* stearic acid) have greater antibacterial activity than may have been predicted from ribosome binding models. While broadly effective, this approach has the main disadvantage that it increases molecular weight and thereby increases the probability of undesirable effects.

The alternative means to modulate antibacterial effects is to change the rigidity and properties of the macrolactone ring. This is illustrated in Figure 6.2a where a series of analogs derived from azithromycin is described. The first modification is the removal of the cladinose sugar by acid hydrolysis to yield CSY1239, with an additional hydroxyl group. This metabolite is produced *in vivo* in gastric secretions and it is notably less antibacterial than the parent azithromycin. Acetylation of the 2-OH of desosamine of CSY1239 to give CSY0072 further reduces antibacterial effect.

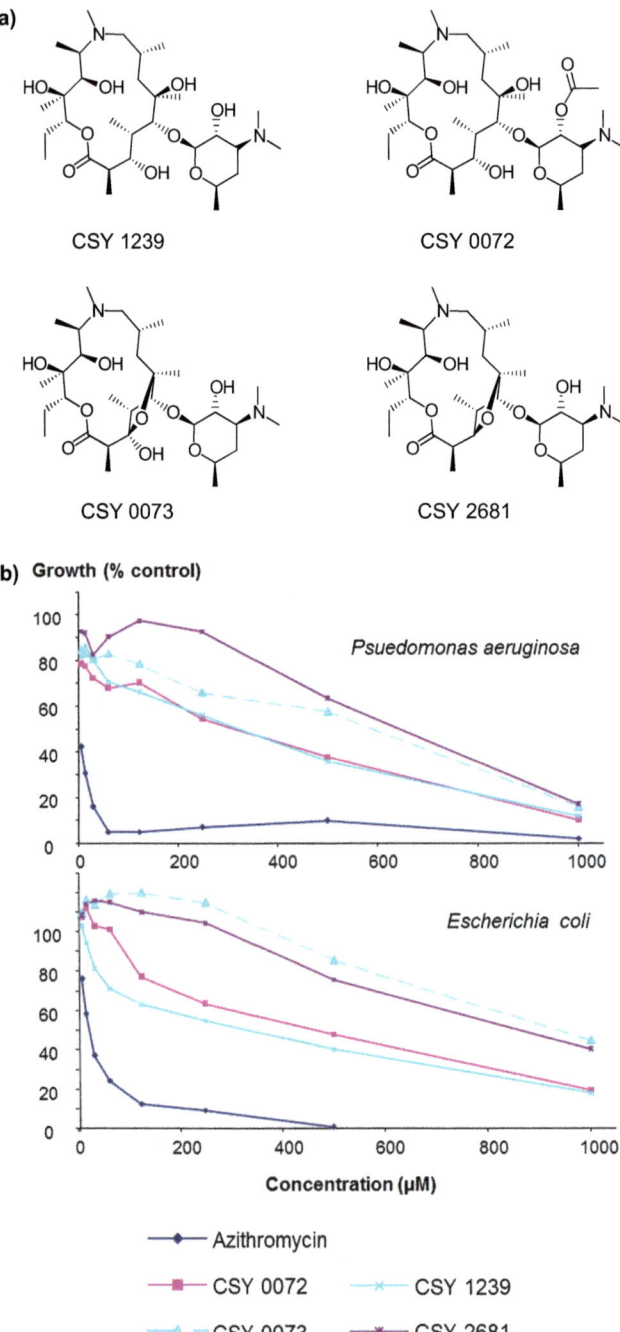

Figure 6.2 (a) Structures of non-antibacterial macrolides based on descladinosyl azithromycin. (b) Antibacterial effects of compounds in (a) for two example strains in comparison with azithromycin.

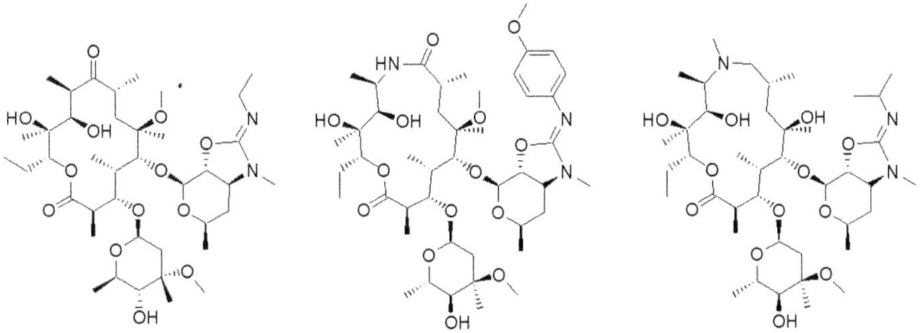

Figure 6.3 Non-antibacterial macrolides reported in ref. 10 with an IC_{50} against *Streptococcus pyogenes* of greater than 64 µg mL^{-1}. These structures have a blocking group preventing the interaction of the ribosome with the desosamine OH and amine groups.

Oxidation of CSY1239 to the ketone, to yield CSY0073, results in a molecule that can also form an intramolecular anomeric bridge to one of the existing ring hydroxyl groups. This hemiketal, changes the ring properties such that the compound is significantly less antibacterial than the unoxidised form. The removal of the hydroxy group completely from CSY1239 to yield CSY2681 provides a similarly non-antibacterial compound.

The differential activity observed in this series is most apparent in Gram negative test organisms (Figure 6.2b). In both *Ps. aeruginosa* and *E. coli*, the descladinosyl analogs CSY1239 and CSY0072 have an intermediate effect on growth reduction relative to azithromycin. The ring oxidised forms, in contrast, are significantly less antimicrobial in both test strains. Gram positive species such as *Staphylococcus carnosus* respond more uniformly to the series, suggesting that a part of the variation in activity observed may be attributed to differential penetration of the cell wall.

The main advantage of ring structure changes is that the molecular weight of the compounds is reduced relative to the parent compounds, and this in turn can reduce their potential for new interactions with off-target sites. In the series of analogs shown in Figure 6.2a molecular weights are in the range of 580 daltons, in comparison to 749 for azithromycin. In compounds where the desosamine interactions are blocked, such as those shown in Figure 6.3, molecular weights are typically in the range of 800 to 1100.[24]

6.7 Appropriate Doses for Anti-Inflammatory Effects

If NAMs are to be successful in the clinic, they will need to preserve the clinical anti-inflammatory efficacy of the antibacterial macrolides while also improving on the already good safety of the class. What stands in their favour is that after nearly 50 years of clinical experience with macrolides, their pharmacology is very well understood and key aspects of safety can be easily addressed. However, there is still much to learn about the clinical use of macrolides and in particular, the potential to reduce doses. In the past, doses have been calculated largely based on those useful for treating infection. More studies are now emerging demonstrating that doses in the chronic setting can be reduced without the loss of anti-inflammatory effect. These data are supported by the fact that macrolides, notably azithromycin, have very long terminal half-lives (50–70 hours, see ref. 5) and that their anti-inflammatory effects are obtained over the long (weeks) rather than the short term.

The other key issue to solve in the clinical use of NAMs is the question over whether an antibacterial effect, however weak, is required to produce the observed clinical effect of the known macrolides. To date, most studies, either pre-clinical or clinical, suggest that this is not the case.

In the following sections, the various structure classes of the NAMs that are either candidates themselves, or candidate carriers for conjugated drugs are reviewed. What is known about the anti-inflammatory mode of action of the compounds and their effects *in vivo* will also be discussed. Finally, the clinical experience to date and likely fields of early application is summarised.

6.8 NAM Mode of Action – Multiple Effects with a Common Element, or a Fortunate Collection of Mutually Supportive Actions?

To illustrate the complexity of the anti-inflammatory mode of action of macrolides, azithromycin (AZI) will serve as a model compound. Azithromycin is also the most widely used macrolide for clinical anti-inflammatory purposes. Its known effects are many, and need to be understood in the context of whole organism physiology and pharmacology. In Table 6.2, are listed some of the best established aspects of AZI pharmacology. In reviewing these data it is important to bear in mind that AZI is highly concentrated in cells *in vitro* and *in vivo*. Thus, in a cell culture system, the effective cell concentration may be many times the assumed concentration in medium. Addition of high levels of serum may modulate this accumulation. However, one must assume that cell and membrane concentrations of azithromycin are likely to be in the hundreds of micromolar even when medium concentration is in the range of 1 to 10 µM.

6.9 Molecular Mechanisms of Macrolide Modulation of Inflammation

Azithromycin inhibits arachidonic acid release and prostaglandin E2 synthesis in LPS-stimulated J774A macrophages.[23,28] Downstream effects include interference with the nuclear expression of activator protein-1 (AP-1)[4] and NFκB.[29] Azithromycin reduces IL-12p40 transcriptional activity by inhibiting the binding of AP-1 to the promoter site.[30] The p40 subunit is a

Table 6.2 Summary of pharmacological targets or processes influenced by macrolides.

Target or process	Pharmacological consequence or effect	Example ref.
Motilin receptor	Induction of GI motility, GI cramps, diarrhea in some patients. This is difficult to distinguish from effects on GI flora. Stimulation of motilin receptor is also thought to be associated with increased downward peristalsis leading to a reduction in gastroesophageal reflux and reductions in aspiration of GI fluids into the bronchi.	25
hERG	Macrolides are associated with QT prolongation, generally in the context of a pre-existing long-QT condition. It is not, however, clear what the target is in this context. WT hERG is not sensitive to macrolides below the mM range.	10, 26
Membrane and tight junction modulation	Macrolides influence membrane properties, most likely *via* insertion and thereby function in both ion permeability and the interaction with membrane proteins.	27
Immune cell reactivity	Levels of various inflammatory mediators are moderated in the presence of macrolides. Inhibition of phospholipases, mobility of NFκB and elevation of lysosomal pH are thought to partly explain these effects.	5, 16

Table 6.3 Macrophage T cell combinations in inflammation and immunity.

Name	M17	M1	M2
Macrophage Function	Pro-inflammatory	Pro-inflammatory	Anti-inflammatory, Reparative
Principal lymphokine(s) driving T cell deviation	IL1B, IL23 (p40/p19)	IL12 (p40/p35)	IL10
T cell deviation state	Th17	Th1	Treg, Th2
T cell role	Active immune response	Active immune response	Tolerance
Principal lymphokine produced by T cell	IFNgamma, IL17	IFNgamma, IL2	IL10

common to both interleukin-12 family members IL-12 and IL-23. Azithromycin also blocks interleukin-1β (IL-1β) synthesis by macrophages through its effect on AP-1.[4] These three lymphokines, IL-1β, IL12, and IL23, represent the primary macrophage and dendritic cell lymphokines responsible for the "deviation" of T helper cells towards potentially pathogenic phenotypes (see Table 6.3).

The non-antimicrobial macrolide CSY0073 (Figure 6.2b) polarises macrophages towards the anti-inflammatory reparative phenotype referred to as M2, alternatively called the alternate activation state,[31] distinguishing them from pro-inflammatory M1 macrophages and from pro-inflammatory "M17" macrophages, a new phenotype that is introduced and discussed later in this chapter. The M1, M2, and M17 macrophages produce different sets of factors consistent with their function; IL-12 and IL23 are the proto-typic pro-inflammatory lymphokines produced by M1 and M17, respectively, while IL-10 is the prototypic anti-inflammatory lymphokine made by M2. Macrophage-derived lymphokines coordinate system-wide immunity through their effects on effector T cells (*vide infra* and Table 6.3). The same polarisation of macrophage phenotype towards the M2 state is obtained through gene deletion of the NADPH oxidase functional p47(phox) subunit or disruption of TLR4 signaling.[32,33]

Azithromycin creates a phenotype state in macrophages and dendritic cells in which pro-inflammatory IL1 β, IL12, and IL23 lymphokine pro-duction is blocked, but where M2 anti-inflammatory lymphokine production remains intact. This property has considerable therapeutic utility.

6.10 Pulmonary Disease, Azithromycin, and Underlying Polarisation of Immune Responses

Azithromycin is a widely used antibacterial agent whose immunomodulatory activity is well known. The activity of AZI in pulmonary disease provides substantial insight into the drug's biological activity for modulating immune responses. These uses are summarized in Table 6.4 along with the number of patients in studies and the outcomes observed.

Thus, AZI ameliorated LPS-induced pulmonary neutrophilia through AP-1 mediated inhibition of IL-1β synthesis by alveolar macrophage.[4] In a mouse pseudomonas lung infection model, AZI reduced the influx of neutrophils into the interstitial and alveolar compartments while promoting a pheno-typic conversion of macrophages to the M2 state.[34] In this model, early neutrophil recruitment has been shown to be induced by IL-1β acting in synergy with IL-23, another product of activated macrophages. At later time points, IL-23 acted on lung γδ T cells to induce expression of IL-17, consistent with its known role in derivation of Th17 cells.[35]

Azithromycin also reduced broncholaveolar lavage (BAL) neutrophilia and lymphocytic bronchiolitis (LB) after lung transplantation. LB subjects showed a significant presence of IL-17 + cells in lamina propria compared with stable rejection and infection groups, the levels of which correlated with broncholaveolar lavage neutrophilia. AZI significantly reduced both the neutrophilia and IL-17 + cells, the majority of which were CD8 + .[36] Vanaudenaerde *et al.*, analyzed 132 BAL samples from lung transplant recipients and found a >10-fold increase in IL17 and IL23 mRNA expression consistent with activation of the IL17/IL23 signalling pathway.[37] In patients

Table 6.4 Summary of clinical studies conducted with macrolides in pulmonary diseases.

Disease	End-point or outcome	Patients in trial (total)	Duration (months)	Conclusions	Ref.
Asthma	Exacerbations, Asthma Control Questionnaire (ACQ), Asthma Quality of Life Questionnaire (AQLQ) and lower respiratory tract infections	99	6	Exacerbations only significantly reduced in non-eosinophilic severe asthma (blood eosinophilia $\leq$200/μl). Azithromycin significantly improved the AQLQ score, but also increased macrolide-resistant streptococci	59
COPD	Exacerbations and SGRQ[a]	1577	12	Significant reduction in exacerbations in azithromycin group	1, 60, 61
Cystic Fibrosis CF	FEV1[b] change	185	6	FEV1 increased (0.097L). Reduction in exacerbations in azithromycin group	17, 62
CF	FEV1 change	260	6	No effect on FEV1. Reduction in exacerbations and weight increase in azithromycin group.	18, 60, 63, 64, 65
CF	FEV1 change, exacerbation	959	6	Improvement of FEV1 and weight, reduction in exacerbations in azithromycin group	66
Non-CF bronchiectasis with 3 or more lower respiratory tract infections	FEV1 change, exacerbations	83	12	Significant reduction in exacerbations and improvement in FEV1, macrolide resistance rate 88% in azithromycin-treated individuals *vs.* 26% in placebo	2, 67
Severe asthma and/ or bronchiectasis	FEV1 change, symptom score	108	2	Significant increase in FEV1.	35,68
Diffuse panbronchiolitis	Clinical and radiological findings, arterial gas analysis, lung function, and sputum bacteria	51	12	Improvement in 70% of patients	11

Table 6.4 (*Continued*)

Disease	End-point or outcome	Patients in trial (total)	Duration (months)	Conclusions	Ref.
Allograft rejection, Post-transplant BOS[d]	FEV1 increase. BAL[c] neutrophilia and levels of IL-8, 8-isoprostane	62	12	Azithromycin reduced BOS frequency by 44% if given prophylactically	69, 70
Post-transplant BOS	FEV1 change, BAL neutrophils	81	6	Improvements with both therapeutic and prophylactic use, with BAL neutrophilia a predictor of response, and suggestion of interaction with reflux disease	71, 72
Lymphocytic bronchiolitis	Histology, IL-17 + cells, neutrophilia	7	Not given	Reduction in local IL-17 + cells which correlated with reduction in neutrophilia	36

[a]SGRQ: St. George's Respiratory Questionnaire.
[b]FEV1: Forced expiratory volume in 1 second.
[c]BAL: Bronchoalveolar lavage.
[d]BOS: Bronchiolitis obliterans syndrome.

with diffuse panbronchiolitis, the number of CD8+ CD11b-cytotoxic T cells in broncholaveolar lavage fluid (BALF) (26.69 $+/-$ $5.86 \times 10(3)$/ml) was higher than the control (2.02 $+/-$ $0.38 \times 10(3)$ ml^{-1}; $p < 0.001$).[38] The authors noted that macrolide therapy reduced the number of these cells, irrespective of bacterial infection.

Obliterative airway lesions, a correlate of chronic rejection following human lung transplantation, were accompanied by enhanced accumulation of neutrophils along with self-antigen-specific Th17 cells.[39] Patients receiving AZI prophylactically during lung transplantation demonstrated statistically better FEV1 (Forced Expiratory Volume in the first second of expiration), lower airway neutrophilia and systemic C-reactive protein levels over time, as well as better survival rates. Bronchiolitis obliterans syndrome (BOS) occurred less in lung transplant patients receiving AZI: 12.5 *vs.* 44.2% ($p = 0.0017$).[21] Azithromycin significantly reduced airway neutrophilia and IL-8 mRNA in patients with BOS. Plasma CRP concentration correlated positively with BAL total cell count and neutrophilia, suggesting systemic inflammation in BOS.[40] BAL neutrophilia can be used as a predictor for the FEV1 response to azithromycin. Interestingly, Vanaudenaerde *et al.*,[37] has noted that BOS patients with elevated neutrophils had reversible allograft dysfunction which responded to AZI, whereas in other reports, patients with fibroproliferative BOS were resistant.[40] This observation presages a companion diagnostic for identifying potentially treatment-responsive BOS patients, a highly desirable situation given the paucity of treatment options for these patients.

These studies in pulmonary disorders suggest the presence of an underlying active IL23/IL-17 response, and that AZI is impacting it. Azithromycin has distinct effects on polarising macrophages towards the M2 phenotype. These data suggest that azithromycin could be mediating its effects in pulmonary disorders through the beneficial polarisation of a distinct pro-inflammatory pathogenic macrophage/dendritic cell into a non-pathogenic M2 state. To simplify discussion of this point, the potential pathogenic starting macrophages are designated as "M17".

6.11 The "M17" Macrophages/Dendritic State

Extracellular adenosine triphosphate (ATP) released during tissue injury can serve as a trigger of inflammation (see ref. 41). Extracellular ATP has been associated with chronic obstructive pulmonary disease, and COPD is characterised by a strong and persistent up-regulation of extracellular ATP in the airways. Bronchoalveolar lavage fluid ATP concentrations in COPD have been shown to correlate negatively with lung function and positively with BALF neutrophil counts. Patients with COPD exhibit an up-regulation of specific purinergic receptors in blood neutrophils and airway macrophages, and the macrophages respond with an increased secretion of pro-inflammatory and tissue-degrading mediators after ATP stimulation. ATP was shown to induce stronger chemotaxis and a robust elastase release in COPD blood neutrophils. Extracellular ATP appears to contribute to the patho-genesis of COPD by promoting inflammation and tissue degradation.[42] In *Pseudomonas aeruginosa*-induced pneumonia, the massive recruitment and activation of neutrophils is accompanied by the extracellular release of active neutrophil elastase in the lungs[43] which is associated with the induction of inflammatory lymphokine expression that is mediated at least in part through Toll-like receptor (TLR) 4.[44] Clearly, the conditions within the pulmonary compartment favour activation of specific forms of inflammation.

In vitro activation of the alveolar macrophage cell line MH-S, as well as primary alveolar macrophages, with LPS results in the release of IL-23.[45] The ability to mount pathogenic Th17 cell responses is genetically determined and depends on the production of IL-23 and IL-1β by antigen presenting cells.[46] Recently, studies examining dendritic cell polarization have shown that TLR2 ligands in combination with physiologically relevant levels of extracellular ATP induce a distinct activation state favoring IL-23 and IL-1β production and leading to the promotion of a Th17-type response. At the same time that the ATP creates a state favouring IL23 synthesis, it disfavours IL-12 production, showing that the IL-12 family members are reciprocally regulated. The ATP-dependent regulation was mediated by two distinct purinergic (*i.e.* P$_2$) receptors and is similarly induced by prostaglandin E(2). In parallel, the ATP-induced dendritic cells express higher levels of MHC class II, costimulatory molecules, and TLRs and exhibit increased activation of the NFκB-signaling pathway.[47] This differential regulation by nucleotides appears to be an adaptive response used by macrophages and dendritic cells to gear their synthetic responses to specific stages of T-cell responses. That pattern of polarisation may be an underlying player in pulmonary disorders, responding to the conditions within the lung compartment, and it may play a much bigger role in Th17 disorders in general.[48]

6.12   Macrophage Polarization

States of chronic inflammation appear to be conditions in which macrophage polarisation is oriented toward the maintenance of inflammation rather than its resolution. In various settings from cancer to autoimmune diseases, the macrophages appear to adopt pathological polarisation states that can be influenced by macrolides. As with dendritic cells, macrophages switch between phenotypes that are geared towards their role in immunity. In various models of induced tissue injury there is a distinct temporal pattern to immune cell influxes; an early wave of neutrophils precedes a wave of M1 macrophages that eventually gives way to reparative M2 macrophages as the immune response resolves. This pattern presumably reflects the functional roles of cells in staging the inflammation and immune response. In this chapter the possibility that a separate macrophage phenotype, the M17, can be generated during the early neutrophil influx is considered. Thus, the early induction and execution phase of inflammation involves macrophages, be they M17 or M1, which are pro-inflammatory.

M2 macrophages, besides producing anti-inflammatory lymphokines (*e.g.* IL-10) are involved in the removal of cellular debris and tissue repair and regeneration. In CNS injury, M1 macrophage response is rapidly induced and then maintained at sites of traumatic spinal cord injury and this response overwhelms a comparatively smaller and transient M2 macrophage response.[49] The time course of myeloid cell apoptosis following acute injury coincides with the shift in macrophage phenotype towards the M2 state, providing support to the notion that efferocytosis drives their phenotype shift.[31,50,51] Importantly, IL-4 from macrophages contributes to alternative activation of peritoneal exudate macrophages and augments cytokine production to suppress inflammation.[52] Azithromycin appears to recapitulate the signals used in driving the M2 phenotypic shift. Recently, experimental treatments for EAE (experimental autoimmune encephalomyelitis) have validated that the polarisation of M1 to M2 is associated with a therapeutic response in this animal model.[53,54]

6.13   T Cell Polarisation

T helper responses have now grown to include three subsets: Th1, Th2 and Th17. Th1 are traditional helper T cells expressing IL2 and interferon-gamma whose deviation occurs through interaction with IL-12 producing M1 macrophages. The Th17 lineage selectively produces pro-inflammatory cytokines including IL-17, IL-21, and IL-22 while IL-1, IL-6, and IL-23 derived from macrophages or dendritic cells promote their differentiation. Pathogenic IL-23-dependent Th17 cells have been shown to be critical for the development of many diseases, and to play a role in models like EAE. In Th17 EAE, Axtel *et al.*, demonstrated a neutrophilic infiltration in the optic nerve and spinal cord that was not present in Th1 EAE.[55] Blockade of neutrophil elastase blocked Th17 EAE but not Th1 EAE. Gery *et al.*, studied the kinetics of Th1 versus Th17 in ocular inflammation in mice expressing eye-restricted hen egg lysozyme.[56] It was found that Th1 cells initially proliferated considerably faster and invaded the eye more quickly than their Th17 counterparts, but then disappeared rapidly. By contrast, Th17 cells accumulated and remained the majority of the infiltrating CD4 + cells in the eye for as long as 25 days after transfer, mediating more long-lasting pathological changes. Th17-induced ocular inflammation also differed from Th1-induced inflammation by having a neutrophil component.

It has been shown that modulation of macrophage phenotypes can reprogram Th cell populations and terminate disease. For example, in a mouse model of murine lupus nephritis, macrophages possessed pro-inflammatory phenotypes which polarised T cells toward disease-prone Th1 cells and Th17 cells. Agents that reprogrammed the macrophages to make more IL-10 eliminated the induction of Th1/Th17 and alleviated disease.[57] The balance between pathogenic Th17 and disease-resolving Tregs also has prognostic value and is increasingly evaluated in immune disorders. Multiple sclerosis patients in remission, but not during relapse, exhibited increases in Treg cells relative to Th17 cells, suggesting that waning Tregs allow the manifestation of disease. Modulation of M2 macrophages provides one avenue for increasing the levels of Tregs for clinical purposes.[58] The thrust of these data in the context of macrolides is that chronic inflammatory states are the result of an interplay of anti-resolution regulation by myeloid and lymphoid cells. Although there is significant focus on pathological T-cells, there are many examples of drug regulation of myeloid cells that lead to profound changes in T-cell activity. These observations include those in the cancer microenvironment, or airways of transplant patients, where macrophage targeted therapies are responsible for changes in the activity of the bulk of the immune cells present. Macrolides, by exerting a pleiotropic brake on the inflammatory state are able to cause a broad but limited re-polarisation to a pro-resolution state, as much by preventing the metabolic activity necessary for the inflamed state as through specific regulation of pro-inflammatory targets.

6.14   Dendritic Cells

Finally, AZI has also been shown to induce the differentiation of human blood monocytes to a distinctive type of dendritic cells displaying enhanced phagocytic and efferocytic capabilities, as well as decreased surface molecule expression co-stimulatory molecules (CD40 and CD86) required for T cell activation, decreased production of IL-12, increased IL-10 production and reducing allostimulatory capacity MLR-reducing properties.[5] Dendritic cells with these properties are effective at generating Tregs. In general, the effects of AZI on macrophages are recapitulated in its effects on dendritic cells, both driving T cells responses toward quiescence and tolerance.

6.15   Conjugated Anti-Inflammatory Macrolides

The previous sections have focused on the direct effects of the macrolactone/ macrolide backbone on inflammatory process, primarily on immune cells. While the potency of these effects on such processes are sufficient for clinical benefits to be observed, the transport-targeting function of the macrolides provides another opportunity to modulate inflammation. Therefore, by conjugating potent anti-inflammatory compounds to the macrolide backbone, the physical properties of the resultant molecule are dominated by those of the macrolide and are subject to concentration in the immune cell fraction. Examples of such structures are provided in Figure 6.4. When such structures were first contemplated, it was assumed that the pendant anti-inflammatory cargo molecule would require release from its macrolide carrier before becoming fully active. To this end, conjugations were made primarily *via* ester linkages on the desosamine moiety. Other linkage options included the 11-OH and the ring nitrogen at the 9a position (see Figure 6.1 for numbering).

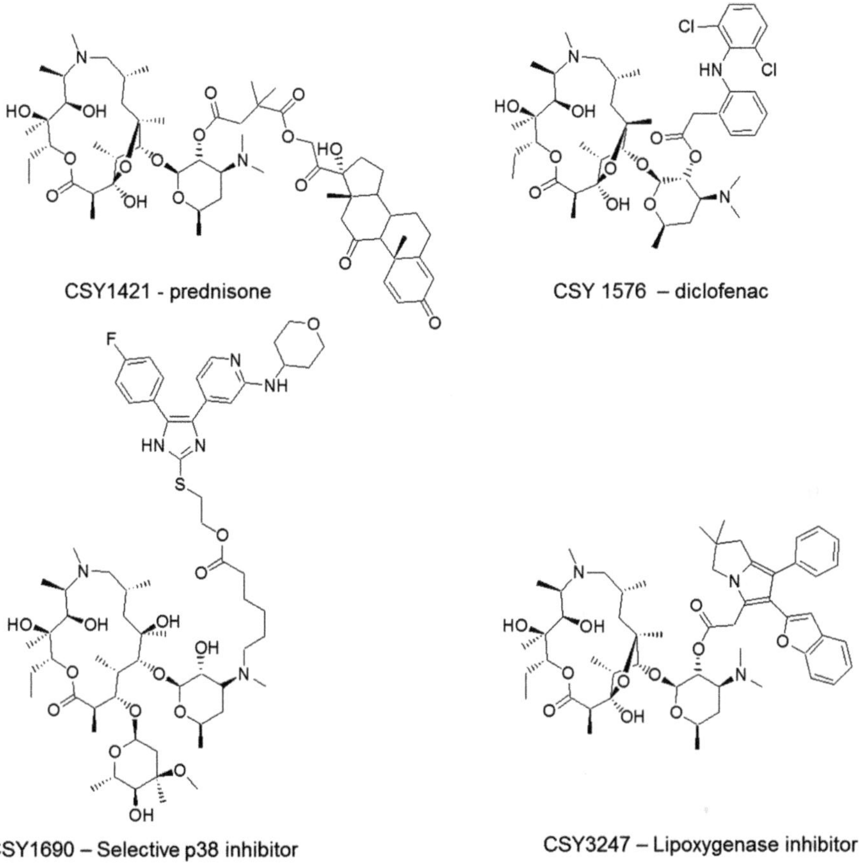

CSY1421 - prednisone

CSY 1576 – diclofenac

CSY1690 – Selective p38 inhibitor

CSY3247 – Lipoxygenase inhibitor

Figure 6.4 Macrolide conjugates of anti-inflammatory compounds. The compound code and its conjugated drug are indicated below the structure.

Compounds of this type exhibited enhanced biological activity relative to their unconjugated parent compounds.[7,8,73,74] However, this was not necessarily due to targeted release of the cargo compound, but rather a combination of factors as described below:

1. the conjugate compounds were partitioned to immune cells;
2. the cargo compounds retained significant affinity for their targets despite conjugation to the macrolide;
3. in many instances, these higher molecular weight macrolides exhibited direct anti-inflammatory effects in a manner analogous to those discussed for azithromycin;
4. the high molecular weight conjugates exhibited higher volumes of distribution and longer half-lives than the unconjugated compounds, which can be attributed to the pharmacokinetic effects of the macrolide and overall increases in lipophilicity.

The first macrolide conjugate discussed is CSY1421 (Figure 6.4), an example of a glucocorticoid, in this case prednisone, connected through an ester linkage to CSY0073, the non-antibacterial analog of azithromycin. The dimethyl succinate linker was used to stabilise the conjugate *in vivo*. Similar conjugates can be made to other glucocorticoids such as triamcinolone, beclamethasone or dexamethasone. In each case, the macrolide conferred a two to 6-fold increase in molar potency in murine collagen induced arthritis (CIA) models versus the unconjugated glucocorticoid alone when administered orally. Contrary to expectations, the conjugated drug was recovered from various organs intact and ester cleavage products were not apparent.

The macrolide conjugate CSY1576 is an ester derivative of the non-steroidal anti-inflammatory agent diclofenac appended directly onto the 2^1-hydroxyl group of the desosamine moiety of CSY0073. This compound was significantly more potent than diclofenac alone in murine and rat CIA as well as in rat experimental autoimmune encephalomyelitis (EAE) *via* the oral route. Depending on the model and the stage of disease at introduction, CSY1576 was between four and 8-fold more active than diclofenac in suppressing signs and onset of inflammation. Toxicity to the gut lining prevents use of diclofenac in mice at doses high enough to abolish signs of arthritis in CIA. In contrast, the toxicity of CSY 1576 was sufficiently moderated that it could be administered at 20 µmol kg^{-1} to obtain full suppression of CIA-associated arthritis without negative effects on animal weight associated with the action of diclofenac on the gut mucosa. At lower doses (*e.g.* 10 µmol kg^{-1} once daily), diclofenac has moderate effects on signs in CIA, but CSY1576 maintains effects nearer to baseline (Figure 6.5).

Diclofenac inhibits COX I and II and *via* these enzymes is implicated in a range of processes including the growth of intestinal polyps and in neovascularisation or angiogenesis that is in turn an aspect of tissue remodelling following insult. Prostaglandins derived from COX II activity play an important role in these processes. Administration of the diclofenac-macrolide conjugate CSY1576 exerts a more pronounced effect on neovascularisation in the cornea than the same dose of diclofenac (see Figure 6.6).

The macrolide CSY1690 is a conjugate of azithromycin and an inhibitor of p38 kinase, a member of a family of mitogen-activated protein kinases that are involved in the regulation of pro-inflammatory cytokines such as TNF-α, IL-1β and IL6. This molecule was synthesised for potential use in both cancer and inflammation. Like the prednisone example above, the compound proved quite stable *in vitro* and *in vivo*. In anti-bacterial assays, it is in active. In assays of direct inhibition of p38 alpha *in vitro*, CSY1690 has an IC$_{50}$ in the range of 24 nM while the unconjugated p38 inhibitor in the same assays has an IC$_{50}$ in the range of 9 nM. Similar results were obtained from other analogs and conjugates from this series suggesting that the carrier macrolide was less of a steric impediment than expected for this target given that the ribose binding site would be near to the linking site on the macrolide. Conjugate CSY1690 is a particularly potent inhibitor of IL-10

Increase in paw thickness (%)

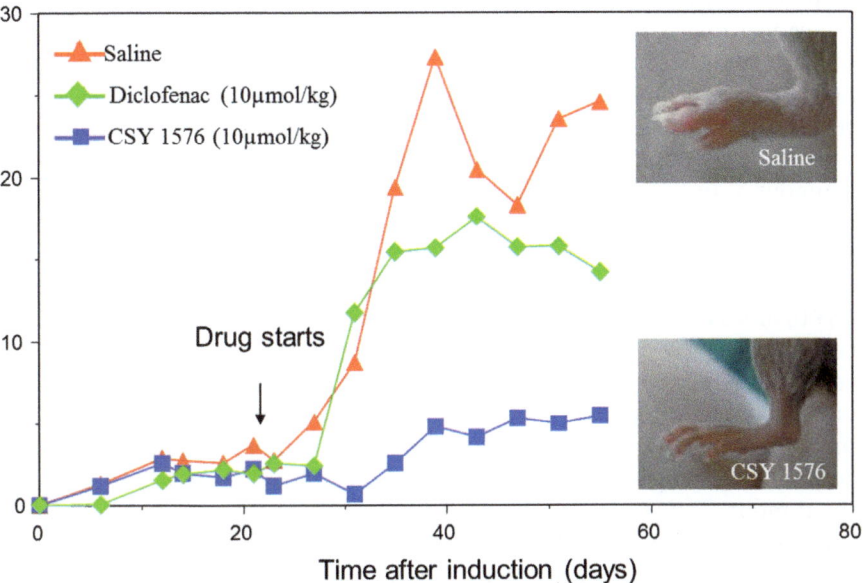

Figure 6.5 The effect of macrolide conjugated diclofenac (CSY1576) *vs.* diclofenac at the equimolar dose of 10 μmol kg^{-1} day^{-1} on development of paw thickness in collagen induced arthritis in the DBA mouse.

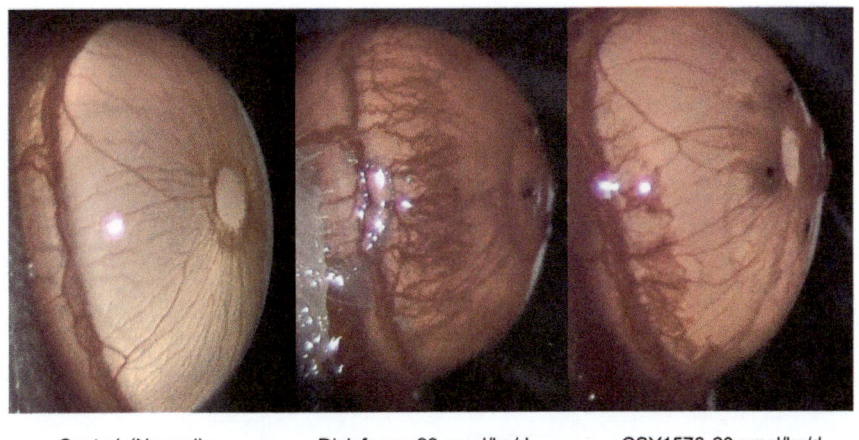

Control (Normal)   Diclofenac 20 μmol/kg/d   CSY1576 20 μmol/kg/d

Figure 6.6 The effect of macrolide-conjugated diclofenac (CSY1576) *vs.* diclofenac at the equimolar dose of 20 μmol kg^{-1} day^{-1} on development of corneal vascular outgrowths following the insertion of sutures into the mouse cornea. In this setting, the macrophage mediated process of vascular outgrowth appears to be more susceptible to the conjugated compound.

production by stimulated macrophages and following this observation it was employed in models of various cancers to explore its potential in modulating the cancer microenvironment. Inhibition of IL-10 and the related stimulus of IL-12 production helps break immune suppression around tumours. Administration of CSY1690, at 10 mg kg^{-1} ip, in models of pancreatic cancer, bladder cancer and lymphoma was associated with reductions in tumour development that were accentuated when combined with a cytotoxic compound. In the data shown in Figure 6.7, significant changes in tumour cytokine expression with CSY1690 alone were sufficient to cause regression and ultimately rejection of the MB49 tumour cells meaning that the remnant tumour was difficult to recover or quantify. On systemic administration, CSY1690 was recovered from tumours at levels 3 to 4-fold over blood concentrations suggesting that it was either being carried by migrating immune cells, or that it is well absorbed by acidic compartments either in the tumour or its infiltrate. These data suggest that a compound like CSY1690 can exert a macrophage driven response at the level of a tumour that results in both activation of lymphocytes and myeloid cells to break immune tolerance of the tumour.

Macrolide CSY3247 is a conjugate to a small molecule lipoxygenase inhibitor.[75] The lipoxygenases are a class of non-heme iron-containing enzymes that catalyse the hydroperoxidation of polyunsaturated fatty acids, ultimately resulting in the generation of leukotrienes that have been implicated in diseases including rheumatoid arthritis, atherosclerosis and psoriasis. In this case, as for diclofenac, improved anti-inflammatory potency was observed for the conjugate versus the unconjugated compound.

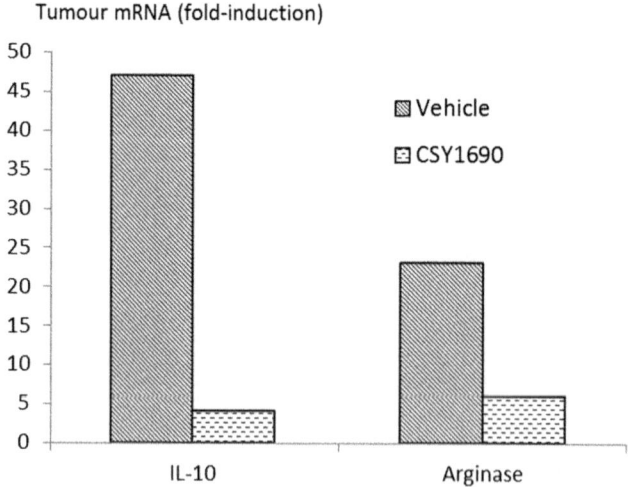

Figure 6.7 The effect of CSY1690 on expression of macrophage secreted cytokines in a tumour extract from a murine MB49 tumour following treatment for 14 days with 10 mg/kg i.p. of CSY1690. These cytokine levels were associated with tumour regression. Arginase is a marker of the M2 phenotype.

Of particular interest for this compound is that it is inherently fluorescent with UV excitation. This allowed the investigation of the question of whether the conjugate mediated targeted transport of the lipoxygenase inhibitor *in vivo* toward immune cells. The conjugate was administered to mice at 10 mg kg^{-1} po and the molar equivalent of the unconjugated inhibitor or vehicle was administered to separate groups of mice. Following ip dosing of LPS blood was drawn at 90 minutes post-stimulation. Whole blood was assessed by cytometry and the neutrophil fraction was identified by side-scatter (Figure 6.8). Fluorescence associated with neutrophils was higher in

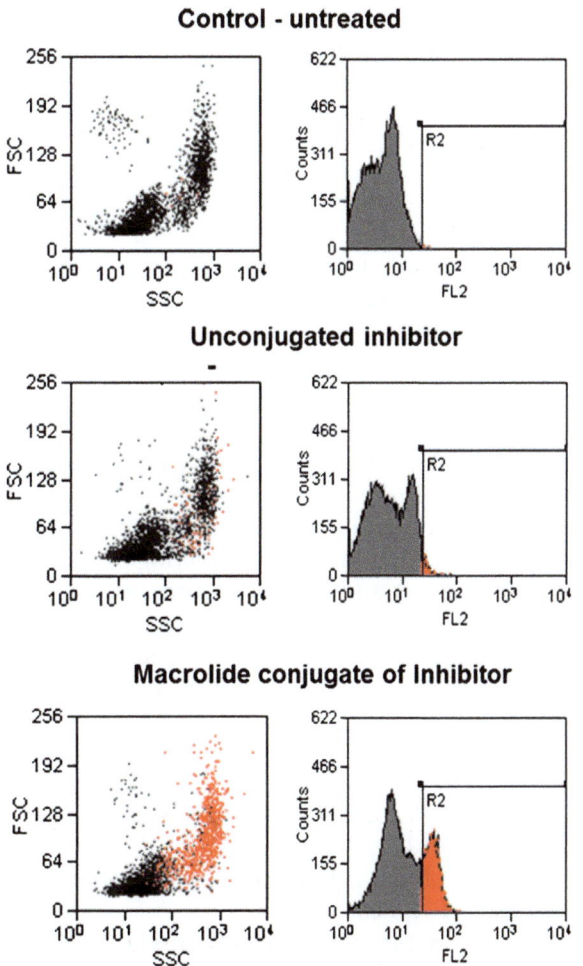

Figure 6.8   Cytometric analysis of drug fluorescence in blood cells following oral administration of CSY3247 and its unconjugated lipoxygenase inhibitor payload. Red coloured cells have fluorescence associated with the anti-inflammatory drug of interest. When the drug is macrolide-conjugated (CSY3247), fluorescence is more intensely associated with the neutrophil fraction.

animals receiving the conjugate, indicating that the conjugated species could indeed direct the compound to the neutrophil compartment *in vivo*. While the blood levels of the two compounds were similar on a molar basis, it is clear that the conjugate has a different cellular distribution. This provided a very clear example of how the partition properties of small molecules can be directed to cell subsets without formulation or packaging but instead relying on inherent properties. It is also relatively rare to be able to influence the distribution of compounds in the body after oral administration.

Finally, the same approach has also been effective in malaria therapy (data not shown) indicative of the broad therapeutic potential of this macrolide conjugation strategy. Various anti-malarial drugs can be conjugated to the macrolide desosamine ring that in turn mediates their uptake into the parasite vacuole leading to improved overall efficacy *in vivo*. Examples using this approach include certain kinase inhibitors, and antimicrobial compounds as the small molecule payloads.

6.16   Conclusion

The macrolides are a highly bioavailable compound class that exert both antibacterial and anti-inflammatory effects *via* a combination of selective uptake, lysosome pH elevation and direct interactions with inflammatory regulators. Their use as anti-inflammatories has been limited in the past because of a reluctance to over-use antibacterial compounds in the community for uses not involving infection. The separation of their antibacterial from their anti-microbial functions now provides an opportunity to test which of these modes of action is dominant in the various diseases which respond to macrolide therapy. The availability of non-antibacterial macrolides also provides a means to take advantage of the targeting potential of macrolides in the context of inflammatory and neoplastic diseases. The observation that a macrolide conjugate can still bind its target suggests that, in certain applications, using a macrolide carrier to mediate ideal pharmacokinetic performance may be a feasible means to enhance specific drug performance.

References

1. S. S. Sohal, C. Ward, W. Danial, R. Wood-Baker and E. H. Walters, *Expert Rev. Respir. Med.*, 2013, 7, 275.
2. K. Fukunaga, P. Kohli, C. Bonnans, L. Fredenburgh and B. D. Levy, *J. Immunol.*, 2005, **174**, 5033.
3. E. Garcia-Planella, M. Mañosa, M. Van Domselaar, J. Gordillo, Y. Zabana, E. Cabré, A. López San Roman and E. Domènech, *Dig. Liver Dis.*, 2012, **44**, 206.
4. M. Bosnar, S. Čužić, B. Bošnjak, K. Nujić, G Ergović, N. Marjanović, I. Pašalić, B. Hrvačić, D. Polančec, I. Glojnarić, V. Eraković and V. Haber, *Int. Immunopharmacol.*, 2011, **11**, 424.

5. M. J. Parnham, V. Haber, E. Giamarellos-Bourboulis, G. Perletti, G. Verleden and R. Vos, *Pharmacol. Ther.*, 2014, DOI: 10.1016/j.pharmthera.2014.03.003.

6. M. Del Tacca, C. Blandizzi and G. Morazzoni, Zambon S. p. A., Italy, *PCT Int. Appl.* WO2006100195, 2006.

7. M. Burnet, J. Guse, C. Bauerlein and U. Hahn, Synovo GmbH, Germany, *U. S. Pat. Appl.* 20130045938, 2013.

8. M. Burnet, J. Guse and H. Gutke, Synovo GmbH, Germany, *U. S. Pat.* 7579324, 2009.

9. G. Tramper, T. Wolfs, A. Fleer, J. Kimpen and C. van der Ent, *Pediatr. Infect. Dis. J.*, 2007, **26**, 8.

10. W. A. Ray, K. T. Murray, K. Hall, P. G. Arbogast and C. M. Stein, *N. Engl. J. Med.*, 2012, **366**, 1881.

11. Y. Liu, W. R. Kam, J. Ding and D. A. Sullivan, *Toxicology*, 2014, **320**, 1.

12. G. Thouvenin, N. Nathan, R. Epaud and A. Clement, *BMJ Case Rep.*, published online 24 June 2013, DOI: 10.1136/bcr-2013-009988.

13. A. L. Tseng, L. Dolovich and I. E. Solit, *Clin. Infect. Dis.*, 1997, **24**, 76.

14. E. D. Bizjak, M. T. Haug, R. J. Schilz, B. D. Sarodia and J. M. Dresing, *Pharmacotherapy*, 1999, **19**, 245.

15. R. K. Albert, J. C. Connett, W. C. Bailey, R. Casaburi, J. A. D. Cooper, G. J. Criner, J. L. Curtis, M. T. Dransfield, M. K. Han, S. C. Lazarus, B. Make, N. Marchetti, F. J. Martinez, N. E. Mandinger, C. McEvoy, D. E. Niewoehner, J. Porsasz, C. S. Price, J. Reilly, P. D. Scanlon, F. C. Sciurba, S. M. Scharf, G. R. Washko, P. G. Woodruff and N. R. Anthonisen, *N. Engl. J. Med.*, 2011, **365**, 689.

16. S. Kanoh and B. K. Rubin, *Clin. Microbiol.*, 2010, **23**, 590.

17. L. Saiman, B. C. Marshall, N. Mayer-Hamblett, J. L. Burns, A. L. Quittner, D. A. Cibene, S. Coquillette, A. Y. Fieberg, F. J. Accurso and P. W. Campbell, *JAMA*, 2003, **290**, 1749.

18. L. Saiman, M. Anstead, N. Mayer-Hamblett, L. C. Lands, M. Kloster, J. Hocevar-Trnka, C. H. Goss, L. M. Rose, J. L. Burns, B. C. Marshall and F. Ratjen, *JAMA*, 2010, **303**, 1707.

19. M. Slater, D. W. Rivett, L. Williams, M. Martin, T. Harrison, I. Sayers, K. D. Bruce and D. Shaw, *Thorax*, 2013, DOI: 10.1136/thoraxjnl-2013-204517.

20. R. Vos, B. M. Vanaudenaerde, A. Ottevaere, S. E. Verleden, S. I. De Vleeschauwer, A. Willems-Widyastuti, S. Wauters, D. E. Van Raemdonck, T. S. Nawrot, L. J. Dupont and G. M. Verleden, *J. Heart Lung Transpl.*, 2010, **29**, 1358.

21. R. Vos, B. M. Vanaudenaerde, S. E. Verleden, D. Ruttens, A. Vaneylen, D. E. Van Raemdonck, L. J. Dupont and G. M. Verleden, *Transplantation*, 2012, **94**, 101.

22. F. Ratjen, L. Saiman, N. Mayer-Hamblett, L. C. Lands, M. Kloster, V. Thompson, P. Emmett, B. Marshall, F. Accurso, S. Sagel and M. Anstead, *Chest*, 2012, **142**, 1259.

23. A. Mencarelli, E. Distrutti, B. Renga, S. Cipriani, G. Palladino, C. Booth, G. Tudor, J. H. Guse, U. Hahn, M. Burnet and S. Fiorucci, *Eur. J. Pharmacol.*, 2011, **665**, 29.

24. M. Bosnar, G. Kragol, S. Kostrun, I. Vujasinovic, B. Bosnjak, V. B. Mihaljevic, Z. M. Istuk, S. Kapic, B. Hrvacic, K. Brajsa, B. Tavcar, D. Jelic, I. Glojnaric, D. Verbanac, O. Culic, J. Padovan, V. E. Haber and R. Spaventi, *J. Med. Chem.*, 2012, **55**, 611.

25. T. Peeters, G. Matthijs, I. Depoortere, T. Cachet, J. Hoogmartens and G. Vantrappen, *Am. J. Physiol.*, 1989, **257**, G470.

26. H. Svanström, B. Pasternak and A. Hviid, *N. Engl. J. Med.*, 2013, **368**, 1704.

27. V. Asgrimsson, T. Gudjonsson, G. H. Gudmundsson and O. Baldursson, *Antimicrob. Agents Chemother.*, 2006, **50**, 1805.

28. K. Nujić, M. Banjanac, V. Munić, D. Polančec and V. E. Haber, *Cell. Immunol.*, 2012, **279**, 78.

29. C. Cigana, B. M. Assael and P. Melotti, *Antimicrob. Agents Chemother.*, 2007, **51**, 975.

30. K. Yamauchi, Y. Shibata, T. Kimura, S. Abe, S. Inoue, D. Osaka, M. Sato, A. Igarashi and I. Kubota, *Int. J. Biol. Sci.*, 2009, **5**, 667.

31. B. S. Murphy, V. Sundareshan, T. J. Cory, D. Hayes, M. I. Anstead and D. J. Feola, *J. Antimicrob. Chemother.*, 2008, **61**, 554.

32. S. H. Choi, S. Aid, H. W. Kim, S. H. Jackson and F. Bosetti, *J. Neurochem.*, 2012, **120**, 292.

33. X. D. Shen, B. Ke, Y. Zhai, F. Gao, S. Tsuchihashi, C. R. Lassman, R. W. Busuttil and J. W. Kupiec-Weglinski, *Liver Transpl.*, 2007, **13**, 1435.

34. D. J. Feola, B. A. Garvy, T. J. Cory, S. E. Birket, H. Hoy, D. Hayes and B. S. Murphy, *Antimicrob. Agents Chemother.*, 2010, **54**, 2437.

35. P. J. Dubin, A. Martz, J. R. Eisenstatt, M. D. Fox, A. Logar and J. K. Kolls, *Infect. Immun.*, 2012, **80**, 398.

36. S. E. Verleden, R. Vos, E. Vandermeulen, D. Ruttens, A. Vaneylen, L. J. Dupont, E. K. Verbeken, G. M. Verleden, D. E. Van Raemdonck and B. M. Vanaudenaerde, *J. Heart Lung Transpl.*, 2013, **32**, 447.

37. B. M. Vanaudenaerde, S. I. De Vleeschauwer, R. Vos, I. Meyts, D. M. Bullens, V. Reynders, W. A. Wuyts, D. E. Van Raemdonck, L. J. Dupont and G. M. Verleden, *Am. J. Transplant.*, 2008, **8**, 1911.

38. K. Kawakami, J. Kadota, K. Iida, T. Fujii, R. Shirai, Y. Matsubara and S. Kohno, *Clin. Exp. Immunol.*, 1997, **107**, 410.

39. V. Tiriveedhi, M. Takenaka, S. Ramachandran, A. E. Gelman, G. A. Patterson and T. Mohanakumar, *Am. J. Transplant.*, 2012, **12**, 2663.

40. G. M. Verleden, B. M. Vanaudenaerde, L. J. Dupont and D. E. Van Raemdonck, *Am J Respir Crit Care Med.*, 2006, **174**, 566.

41. H. K. Eltzschig, M. V. Sitkovsky and S. C. Robson, *N. Engl. J. Med.*, 2012, **367**, 2322.

42. M. Lommatzsch, S. Cicko, T. Müller, M. Lucattelli, K. Bratke, P. Stoll, M. Grimm, T. Dürk, G. Zissel, D. Ferrari, F. Di Virgilio, S. Sorichter, G. Lungarella, J. C. Virchow and M. Idzko, *Am. J. Respir. Crit. Care Med.*, 2010, **181**, 928.

43. J. Altenburg, C. S. de Graaff, Y. Stienstra, J. H. Sloos, E. H. van Haren, R. J. Koppers, T. S. van der Werf and W. G. Boersma, *JAMA*, 2013, **309**, 1251.

44. R. Benabid, J. Wartelle, L. Malleret, N. Guyot, S. Gangloff, F. Lebargy and A. Belaaouaj, *J Biol Chem.*, 2012, **287**, 34883.

45. M. Bosmann, J. J. Grailer, N. F. Russkamp, R. Ruemmler, F. S. Zetoune, J. V. Sarma and P. A. Ward, *Shock*, 2013, **39**, 447.

46. B. M. Larkin, P. M. Smith, H. E. Ponichtera, M. G. Shainheit, L. I. Rutitzky and M. J. Stadecker, *Semin. Immunopathol.*, 2012, **34**, 873.

47. T. Khayrullina, J. H. Yen, H. Jing and D. Ganea, *J. Immunol.*, 2008, **181**, 721.

48. M. Schnurr, T. Toy, A. Shin, M. Wagner, J. Cebon and E. Maraskovsky, *Blood*, 2005, **105**, 1582.

49. K. A. Kigerl, J. C. Gensel, D. P. Ankeny, J. K. Alexander, D. J. Donnelly and P. G. Popovich, *J. Neurosci.*, 2009, **43**, 13435.

50. X. Yan, A. Anzai, Y. Katsumata, T. Matsuhashi, K. Ito, J. Endo, T. Yamamoto, A. Takeshima, K. Shinmura, W. Shen, K. Fukuda and M. Sano, *J. Mol. Cell. Cardiol.*, 2013, **62**, 24.

51. Y. Kharraz, J. Guerra, C. J. Mann, A. L. Serrano and P. Muñoz-Cánoves, *Mediators Inflammation*, 2013, **2013**, 491.

52. M. Y. Zeng, D. Pham, J. Bagaitkar, J. Liu, K. Otero, M. Shan, T. A. Wynn, F. Brombacher, R. R. Brutkiewicz, M. H. Kaplan and M. C. Dinauer, *Blood*, 2013, **121**, 3473.

53. C. Liu, Y. Li, J. Yu, L. Feng, S. Hou, Y. Liu, M. Guo, Y. Xie, J. Meng, H. Zhang, B. Xiao and C. Ma, *PloS One*, 2013, **8**, e54841.

54. H. R. Jiang, M. Milovanović, D. Allan, W. Niedbala, A. G. Besnard, S. Y. Fukada, J. C. Alves-Filho, D. Togbe, C. S. Goodyear, C. Linington, D. Xu, M. L. Lukic and F. Y. Liew, *Eur. J. Immunol.*, 2012, **42**, 1804.

55. K. Herges, B. A. de Jong, I. Kolkowitz, C. Dunn, G. Mandelbaum, R. M. Ko, A. Maini, M. H. Han, J. Killestein, C. Polman, A. L. Goodyear, J. Dunn, L. Steinman and R. C. Axtell, *Mult. Scler.*, 2012, **18**, 398.

56. G. Shi, M. Ramaswamy, B. P. Vistica, C. A. Cox, C. Tan, E. F. Wawrousek, R. M. Siegel and I. Gery, *J. Immunol.*, 2009, **183**, 7547.

57. W. Zhang, W. Xu and S. Xiong, *J Immunol.*, 2011, **187**, 1764.

58. E. Peelen, J. Damoiseaux, J. Smolders, S. Knippenberg, P. Menheere, J. W. Tervaert, R. Hupperts and M. Thewissen, *J. Neuroimmunol.*, 2011, **240–241**, 97.

59. C. Brusselle, R. Deman, H. Slabbynck, V. Ringoet, G. Verleden, K. Demedts, K. Verhamme, B. Demeyere and G. Joos, *Thorax*, 2012, **202**, 698.

60. U. Baumann, M. King, E. M. App, S. Tai, A. König, J. J. Fischer, T. Zimmermann, W. Sextro and H. von der Hardt, *Can. Respir. J.*, 2004, **2**, 151.

61. F. Blasi, D. Bonardi, S. Aliberti, M. Confalonieri, O. Amir, M. Carone, F. Di Marco, S. Centanni and E. Guffanti, *Pulm. Pharmacol. Ther.*, 2010, **23**, 200.

62. J. Wolter, S. Seeney, S. Bell, S. Bowler, P. Masel and J. McCormack, *Thorax*, 2002, **57**, 212.
63. C. R. Hansen, T. Pressler, C. Koch and N. Høiby, *J. Cystic Fibrosis*, 2005, **4**, 35.
64. A. Clement, E. Tamalet, E. Leroux, S. Ravilly, B. Fauroux and J. P. Jais, *Thorax*, 2006, **61**, 895.
65. A. Equi, I. M. Balfour-Lynn, A. Bush and M. Rosenthal, *Lancet*, 2002, **360**, 978.
66. K. W. Southern, *Paediatr. Respir. Rev.*, 2012, **13**, 228.
67. C. Wong, L. Jayaram, N. Karalus, T. Eaton, C. Tong, H. Hockey, D. Milne, W. Fergusson, C. Tuffery, P. Sexton, L. Storey and T. Ashton, *Lancet*, 2012, **380**, 660.
68. M. Coeman, Y. van Durme, F. Bauters, E. Deschepper, I. Demedts, P. Smeets, G. Joos and G. Brusselle, *Ther. Adv. Respir. Dis.*, 2011, **5**, 377.
69. M. Federica, S. Nadia, M. Monica, C. Alessandro, O. Tiberio, B. Francesco, V. Mario and F. Maria, *Clin. Transplant.*, 2011, **25**, E381.
70. J. Gottlieb, J. Szangolies, T. Koehnlein, H. Golpon, A. Simon and T. Welte, *Transplantation*, 2008, **85**, 36.
71. N. Porhownik, W. Batobara, W. Kepron, H. W. Unruh and Z. Bshouty, *Can. Respir. J.*, 2008, **15**, 199.
72. D. Shitrit, D. Bendayan, S. Gidon, M. Saute, I. Bakal and M. R. Kramer, *J. Heart Lung Transpl.*, 2005, **24**, 1440.
73. M. Mercep, M. Mesic, S. Markovic, D. Pesic, I. Landek, M. Komac, O. Stegic, S. Selmani, L. Tomaskovic and M. Banjanac, GlaxoSmithKline, USA, *U. S. Pat. Appl.* 20080096830, 2008.
74. M. Mercep, M. Mesic, L. Tomaskovic, S. Markovic, B. Hrvacic, V. Poljak, and O. Makaruha, GlaxoSmithKline, USA, *PCT Int. Appl.* WO2004/094449.
75. S. Laufer, W. Albrecht, M. Burnet and H. Gutke, Merckle GmbH, Germany, *U. S. Pat. Appl.* 20090221697, 2009.

CHAPTER 7

Linear and Macrocyclic Hepatitis C Virus Protease Inhibitors: Inhibitor Design and Macrocyclization Strategies for HCV Protease and Related Targets

WIESLAW M. KAZMIERSKI,*[a] RICHARD L. JARVEST,[c] JACOB J. PLATTNER[b] AND XIANFENG LI*[b]

[a] GlaxoSmithKline, Five Moore Drive, Research Triangle Park, NC 27709, USA; [b] Anacor Pharmaceuticals, Inc., 1020 E. Meadow Circle, Palo Alto, CA 94303, USA; [c] GlaxoSmithKline, Gunnels Wood Road, Stevenage, Herts, SG1 2NY, UK
*Email: wieslaw.m.kazmierski@gsk.com; xli@anacor.com

7.1 Introduction

Recent years have witnessed extraordinary progress in the discovery and development of agents to combat the hepatitis C virus (HCV), the causative agent of hepatitis C. New treatment paradigms are promising to radically simplify treatment and improve patient outcomes. HCV protease inhibitors (HCV PIs) play a prominent role in these new and promising regimens. This chapter will attempt to summarize key approaches to designing HCV PIs and

RSC Drug Discovery Series No. 40
Macrocycles in Drug Discovery
Edited by Jeremy Levin
© The Royal Society of Chemistry 2015
Published by the Royal Society of Chemistry, www.rsc.org

their structural features, with a particular emphasis on macrocyclization strategies. In part owing to the lack of many suitable small molecule high-throughput hits, HCV PI discovery efforts, similarly to HIV PIs discovered earlier, were based on peptide substrate-peptidomimetic approach and structure-based design. These approaches resulted in a series of major scientific breakthroughs as manifested by a number of FDA-approved and advanced clinical compounds. These efforts took two decades of intensive basic research across many pharmaceutical and biotech industry laboratories and had to overcome a significant amount of skepticism about whether peptide-based approaches could deliver viable oral drugs. High expectations and pent-up demand for this novel oral therapy contributed to telaprevir (Incivek, VX-950, Figure 7.1), the first generation HCV PI on the market, becoming the fastest drug in history to reach the $1 billion mark.[1] After the initial success with linear inhibitors such as telaprevir and boceprevir (Victrelis, Figure 7.1), macrocyclization emerged as a particularly powerful approach to designing compounds with improved potency and pharmacokinetic properties. Key medicinal chemistry and computer-assisted drug design milestones and considerations employed in constructing these macrocycles, arguably among the most elegant and impactful achievements in recent medicinal chemistry, will be described in this review. Mechanistic details of common HCV protease inhibitor C-terminal moieties, such as ketoamides, sulfonamides, phosphinic and carboxylic acids, interacting with the HCV protease catalytic Ser139 and adjacent subsites, will also be discussed. This is followed by a brief presentation of key clinical protease inhibitors, both linear and macrocyclic (Section 7.4). Section 7.5 will describe some of the work done by the authors and their colleagues on boron-containing warheads in the context of both linear and macrocyclic HCV protease inhibitors. Continuing the macrocyclization theme, this chapter will also briefly cover key developments in the related areas of macrocyclic inhibitors of HCV RNA-dependent RNA polymerase NS5B (Section 7.6.1) and non-HCV macrocyclic protease inhibitors (Section 7.6.2). Although slightly outside of the chapter's main topic, these sections will offer additional useful insights into designing macrocyclic drugs, especially since they are not discussed elsewhere in this book. This chapter is dedicated to those who relentlessly pursued scientific and medical progress in this area, pushing the boundaries of science and most of all delivering innovative, life-saving medicines to patients.

7.2   Hepatitis C Virus and Current Treatment Options

Hepatitis C virus (HCV), sometimes termed a 'silent killer', was identified in 1989 as the infectious agent responsible for community-acquired non-A non-B hepatitis.[2] HCV is an asymptomatic disease affecting more than 170 million individuals worldwide (about 3% of the population) and is the major cause of chronic liver disease that can lead to steatosis, cirrhosis, hepatocellular carcinoma and liver failure. Despite many preventive

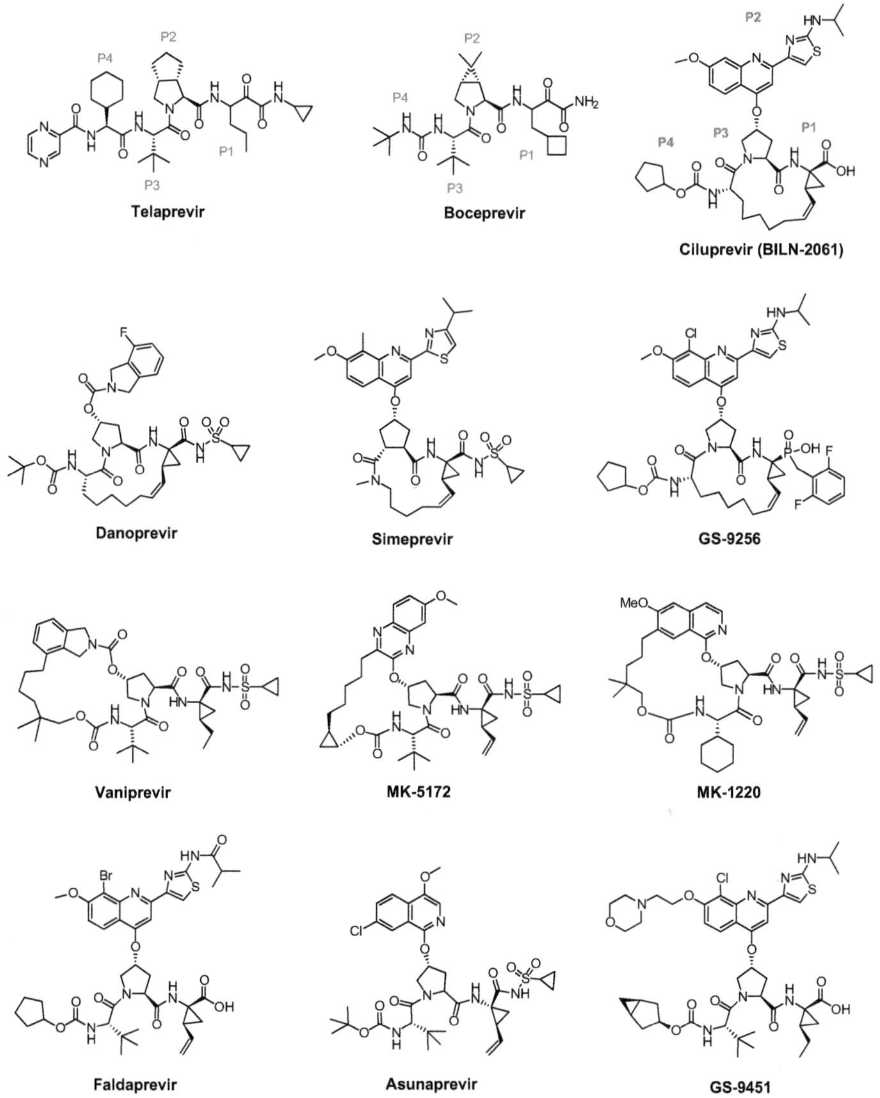

Figure 7.1 Key HCV NS3 protease inhibitors.

measures introduced over the years, it is estimated that up to 4.7 million new infections occur worldwide each year. Based on genetic diversity, HCV is divided into six major genotypes (genotype 1–6) and numerous subtypes in different geographic locations. While genotype 1a (GT1a) is the most abundant in the US, the majority of sequences in Europe, Japan and China are from GT1b. As a result of the recent approval of the first HCV PIs, Vertex's telaprevir[3,4] and Merck's boceprevir[5,6] (Figure 7.1), at the time of writing the current gold standard treatment for HCV infection involves a combination therapy of an oral protease inhibitor, injectable pegylated interferon-α

(PEG-IFN) and the oral drug ribavirin (RBV), and further direct-acting HCV antivirals are progressing through regulatory approval.

While new treatments are more effective in patients with GT1 than the previous PEG-IFN/RBV only regimen, they nonetheless are less than ideal because of side effects associated with PIs and PEG-IFN as well as the three times a day (tid) dosing regimen. Since HCV has a high replication rate and does not have a proof-reading mechanism, numerous resistant HCV variants likely pre-exist and will rapidly outgrow wild type virus (WT) under drug selection pressure. Both telaprevir and boceprevir, when administered as single agents, have a low barrier to resistance and require co-administration with PEG-IFN/RBV to prevent the emergence of resistant mutants.[7] Thus, more effective HCV PIs that can support a once daily (qd) dosing regimen, improve patient compliance, and enable a fixed-dose combination with other oral HCV agents are needed.

7.3   HCV Protease Inhibitors: Structural and Design Considerations

The NS3/4A serine protease is a heterodimer of a catalytic NS3 protein and an activating cofactor NS4A, responsible for cleavage at four sites of the HCV polyprotein (NS3/4A, NS4A/4B, NS4B/5A, and NS5A/5B) to produce functional proteins (Figure 7.2a).[8,9] Viral replication can initiate only after the individual functional proteins are cleaved from the polyprotein. The NS3 protease also appears to contribute to the ability of HCV to attenuate innate antiviral defenses and maintain persistent infection, by proteolytic cleavage of key host proteins in both the TLR3 and RIG-1 signaling pathways.[10,11]

X-ray crystal structures of the HCV NS3 protease have been determined and have provided a wealth of information on inhibitor binding and

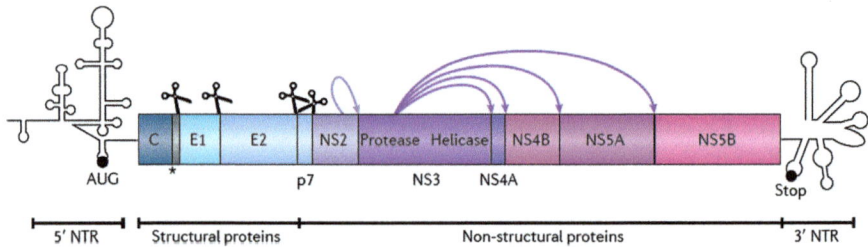

Figure 7.2a   Hepatitis C Virus RNA genome, indicating encoded proteins. The structural core (C) protein, envelope glycoproteins (E1 and E2), p7 and NS2 are required for virus assembly. Remaining non-structural proteins are required for the RNA replication. Arrows indicate cleavage of translated polyprotein by the viral proteases.
Reprinted with permission from R. Bartenschlager, V. Lohmann and F. Penin, *Nat. Rev. Microbiol.*, 2013, **11**, 482.

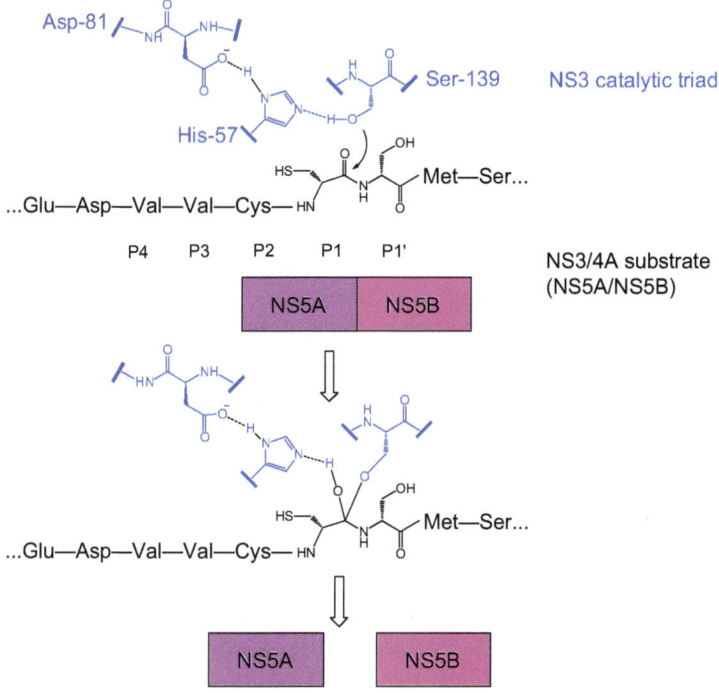

Figure 7.2b Simplified mechanism of NS3/4A protease cleaving NS5A-NS5B junction.

design.[12,13] The NS3 protease is a typical ß-barrel serine protease with a classical Asp-His-Ser catalytic triad that cleaves the Cys (P1)-Ser (P1')[14] amide bond (Figure 7.2b). This is illustrated in an abbreviated way in Figure 7.2b, where the NS5A Cys (P1) carbonyl group in the NS5A-NS5B polypeptide juncture[15] is attacked by the hydroxyl group of Ser139 from NS3 catalytic triad (Asp-81, His-57 and Ser-139). This process proceeds through the formation of an oxyanion hole-stabilized tetrahedral intermediate and its subsequent hydrolysis to NS5A and NS5B-containing polypeptides. The enzyme is characterized by a flat, shallow and solvent-exposed active site, and thus the substrate binding by the NS3 protease requires multiple interactions over a large surface area. Identifying a classic small molecule inhibitor of HCV protease with reasonable binding activity has proven to be a significant challenge, and high throughput screening efforts have been relatively ineffective. Similarly to the success of HIV protease inhibitors, rational, substrate-based inhibitor design has proved the most effective approach to discovering HCV PIs.

An investigation of HCV protease inhibition by substrate cleavage products revealed that hexapeptide SMSYTW-OH, the N-terminal fragment of the cleaved NS5B polyprotein, was inactive. However, hexapeptide DDIVPC-OH, which is closely related to the C-terminal portion of the cleaved NS5A polyprotein, and its acetylated derivative Ac-DDIVPC-OH (**1**, Figure 7.3a), were inhibitory in the enzyme assay with IC_{50}s of 71 µM[16] and 28 µM, respectively.[17] This finding encouraged the Boehringer Ingelheim (BI) group to optimize the sequence of **1**. Initial attempts to replace the chemically and metabolically labile cysteine moiety identified norvaline as a suitable cysteine replacement in Ac-DDIVPNva-OH (**2**, IC_{50} = 150 µM).[17] Subsequent substitution of one of the aspartic acids by its D-enantiomer in Ac-DdIVPNva-OH (**3**) further improved enzymatic potency (IC_{50} = 17 µM).[17] A significant event was the discovery that aromatic substituents at the 4-position of the proline residue of analogs such as **3** occupied additional enzyme–ligand interaction subsites (designated P2*), contributing to significant potency improvement in compounds **4** and **5**. Subsequent use of D-glutamic acid at position P5 and cyclohexyl at position P4 resulted in inhibitor **6** with nanomolar potency.[18]

NMR studies of inhibitor **4** bound to NS3 suggested that it binds in an extended β-strand conformation,[19] similarly to the NS3 binding mode of a simplified inhibitor, tripeptide **7** (Figure 7.3b), which featured an optimized 1-aminocyclopropylcarboxylic acid (ACCA) P1 residue.[20] However, the conformation of the ACCA observed for NS3-free and NS3-bound **7** were found to be distinctly different, with binding of **7** to NS3A resulting in a higher energy conformation of ACCA. This is due to the ϕ angle (defined as the angle between the $C–CO_2^-$ bond and the NHAc carbonyl bond) of ACCA rotating 180° in the bound conformation, allowing its carboxylate to interact with the oxyanion hole of NS3.[21] The BI group then designed a series of macrocyclic scaffolds linking the P1 and P3 residues in order to preorganize the ϕ angle in a way consistent with the enzyme-bound conformation to relieve the entropic penalty inhibitor **7** pays when binding to NS3. This was achieved by subjecting P2-quinoline based tripeptide **8** to ring-closing metathesis (RCM), resulting in the 15-membered macrocycle **9**, a process which yielded about a 30-fold potency gain for **9** (Figure 7.3b). Additional HCV NS3 subsites were explored by probing substitutions on the P2 quinoline. Addition of 7-methoxyquinoline to tetrapeptide **10** as the P2* moiety to give **11** improved potency more than 700-fold compared to **10**. This significantly greater gain compared to the potency boost on derivatization of **2** to provide **4** (21-fold) reflects a bigger P2* group and suggests that further substitutions could benefit potency. While the interactions of the P2* moiety with the shallow S2* enzyme pocket appear mostly hydrophobic in nature, the X-ray structure of the enzyme–inhibitor complex positions P2* close to both the Asp–His catalytic pair and to the Arg155 side chain, suggesting a possibility that the guanidinium moiety of Arg155 and the 7-methoxy substituent in P2* could be stabilizing this complex through electrostatic interactions. Significant potency gain with large P2* groups is clearly observed in both the linear tripeptide **12** and the 15-membered macrocycle **13**, with the latter about 140-fold more potent than **9**.

Additional SAR along these lines led to the discoveries of both the cyclic HCV PI ciluprevir (discontinued) and the linear inhibitor faldaprevir,

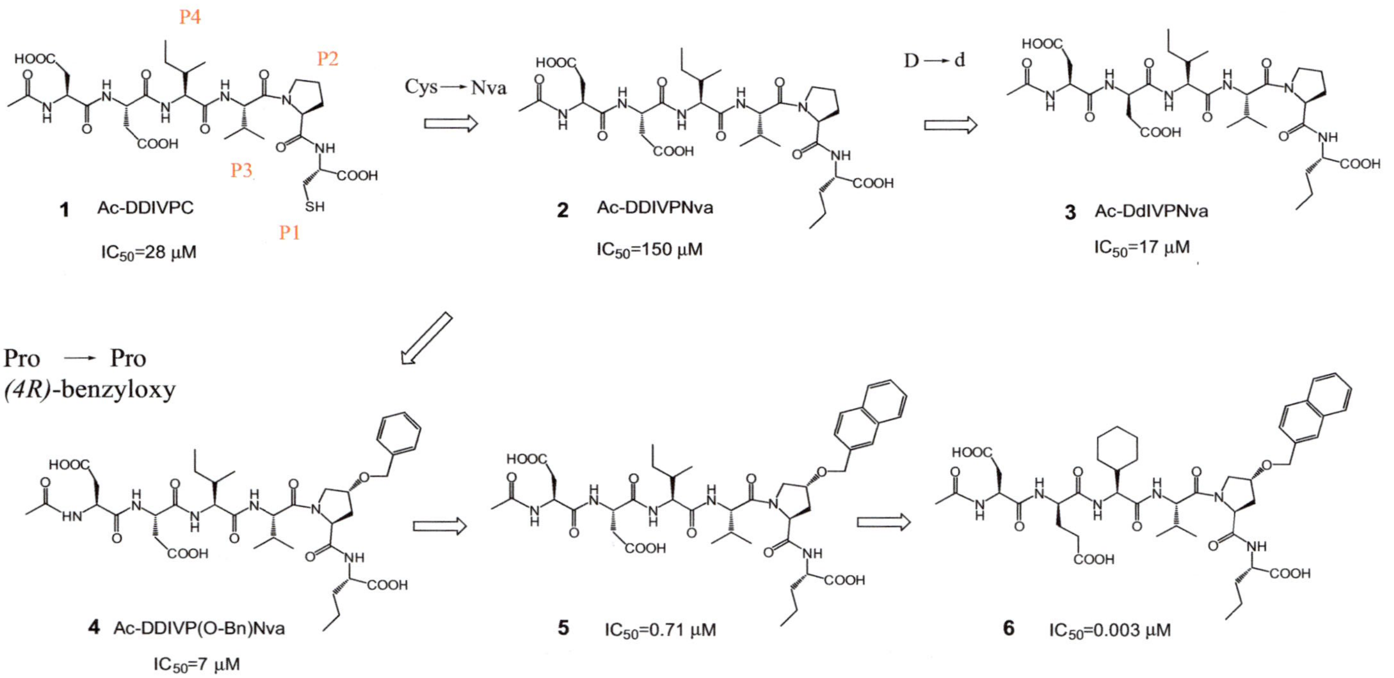

Figure 7.3a Early SAR in the substrate-based approach to HCV PIs discovery: linear analogs with improved potency and role of the P2* moieties.

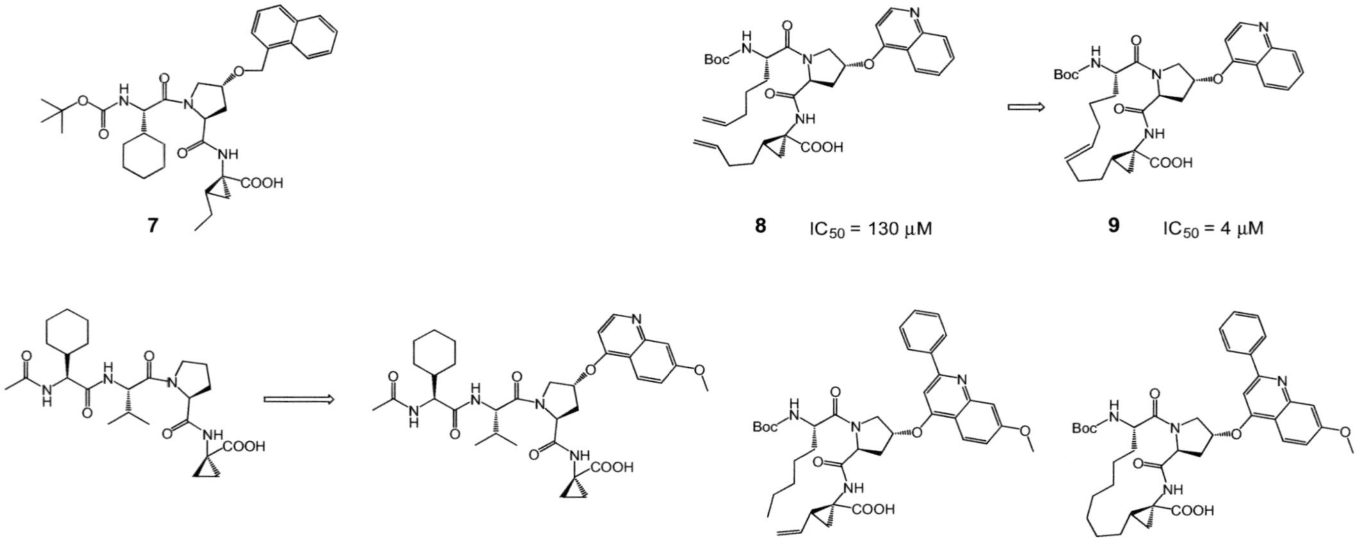

Figure 7.3b Additional P2* SAR and the impact of macrocyclization on potency.

currently in Phase III clinical trials (Figure 7.1). Careful conformational analysis of several enzyme-bound HCV PIs, including ciluprevir and faldaprevir, revealed similar conformations of both inhibitors[22] (Figure 7.4a). Thus, specific substitutions in faldaprevir biased its conformation compared to the starting peptide DDIVPC-OH, in a way similar to that achieved by the macrocyclization in ciluprevir.

The Merck group noticed that the significant potency increase upon incorporation of the P2 aryl moiety (*e.g.* compare compound **2** to **4** and compound **10** to **11**) could not be easily explained by the model of a close analog (unsaturated rather than saturated macrocycle) of compound **13** bound to NS3 protease,[23] in which the P2 quinoline moiety does not appear to interact with many protein surface features.[24] However, analysis of ciluprevir's interactions with full length NS3/4A, containing the large helicase domain, suggested that the latter could provide the needed surface, including a site to accommodate the thiazole substituent of this inhibitor. In addition, this model suggested an alternative macrocyclic connection between the P2 quinoline and P4, rather than between the P1 and P3 moieties.[24] This led to a new, potent macrocyclic P2-P4 series exemplified by **14** (Figure 7.4b). This compound turned out to be quite potent in the genotype 1b enzyme assay ($K_i = 8.5$ nM) compared to ciluprevir ($K_i = 0.3$ nM), and was thus followed up by other P2-P4 macrocycles, such as vaniprevir,[25] MK-1220[26] and MK-5172 (Figure 7.1).[27]

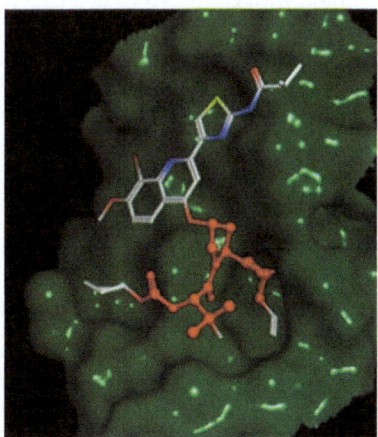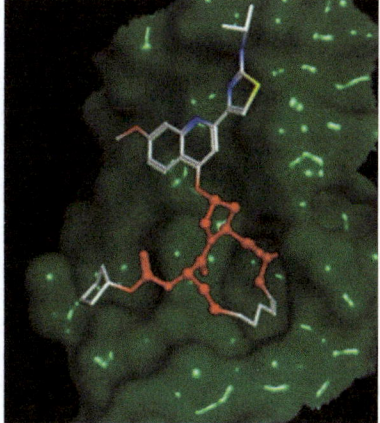

Figure 7.4a (left) Faldaprevir (X-ray structure), (right) ciluprevir (created by modification of an X-ray structure of a related macrocyclic compound and energy minimization). Both are superimposed on the enzyme derived from the X-ray structure of the faldaprevir complex. Common scaffold colored red.

Reprinted with permission from S. R. LaPlante, H. Nar, C. T. Lemke, A. Jakalian, N. Aubry and S. H. Kawai, *J. Med. Chem.*, 2014, **57**, 1777. Copyright (2013) American Chemical Society.

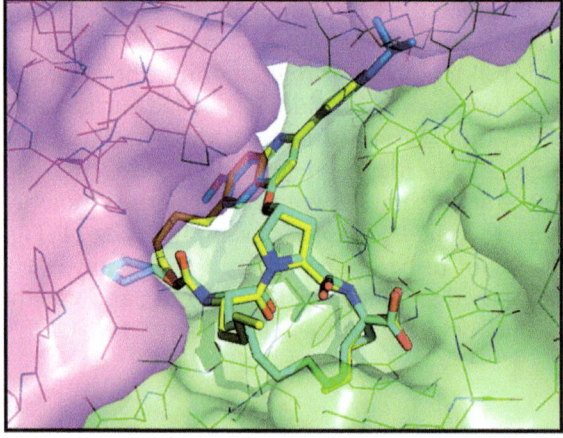

Figure 7.4b   Target macrocycle **14** (yellow) overlaid with ciluprevir (blue). Green: full
length NS3/4A; purple: helicase.
Reprinted with permission from N. J. Liverton, M. K. Holloway, J. A.
McCauley, M. T. Rudd, J. W. Butcher, S. S. Carroll, J. DiMuzio, C.
Fandozzi, K. F. Gilbert, S. S. Mao, C. J. McIntyre, K. T. Nguyen, J. J.
Romano, M. Stahlhut, B. L. Wan, D. B. Olsen and J. P. Vacca, *J. Am.
Chem. Soc.,* 2008, **130**, 4607. Copyright (2008) American Chemical
Society.

A number of C-terminal moieties have been used to increase the inhibitory
potency or optimize other properties of HCV PIs. Telaprevir and boceprevir,
the first HCV PIs to reach the market (Figure 7.1), contain the electrophilic
α-ketoamide P1–P1$'$ 'warhead', which traps the active-site Ser139 to form a
reversible covalent tetrahedral intermediate.[3–6,28] Covalent drugs are considered more risky to develop due to potential irreversible binding to
mechanistically unrelated biomolecules, and thus the potential for idio-
syncratic toxicity. However, the measured reactivation half life ($t_{1/2}$) of the
inhibited enzyme suggests that reversibility of the covalent ketoamide
binding could be a mitigating factor.[6] All of the other clinical HCV PIs in
Figure 7.1 are non-covalent inhibitors. The carboxylate moiety in faldaprevir
analog, compound **1**$'$ (Figure 7.5a),[22] and acyl-sulfonamide moiety in
danoprevir[29] develop prominent stabilizing interactions with the enzyme's

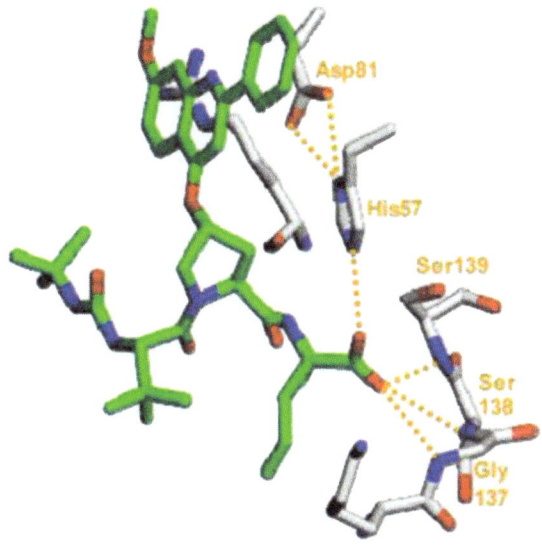

Figure 7.5a Details of the interaction of the C-terminal carboxylate of faldaprevir analog (compound 1', reference 22) with the oxyanion hole and the hydrogen-bonding network from the catalytic triad His57, Asp81 and Ser139.
Reprinted with permission from S. R. LaPlante, H. Nar, C. T. Lemke, A. Jakalian, N. Aubry and S. H. Kawai, *J. Med. Chem.*, 2014, **57**, 1777. Copyright (2013) American Chemical Society.

oxyanion hole and surrounding subsites as shown in Figure 7.5b. Except for the phosphinic acid-based inhibitor GS-9256, all of the clinical macrocyclic inhibitors in Figure 7.1 contain the acyl-sulfonamide moiety, also present in the linear asunaprevir (BMS-650032)[30] and its closely related clinical predecessor BMS-605339 (structure not shown).[31] SAR leading to discovery of BMS-605339 indicated a clear preference for the cyclopropyl substitution in the acyl-sulfonamide moiety among a number of alicyclic, aliphatic, aromatic substituents, as well as over a simple carboxylate.[31] Section 7.5 will detail a family of boron-based HCV protease inhibitor warheads, which has been extensively evaluated by the GSK and Anacor scientists.

The 15-membered, P1-P3 macrocyclic inhibitor, ciluprevir (BILN-2061, Boehringer Ingelheim, Figure 7.1), was the first NS3 protease inhibitor to enter clinical trials and to establish the proof-of-concept in humans.[32] Ciluprevir is a potent and specific inhibitor in both the NS3 protease enzyme assay (GT1b, $IC_{50} = 3.6$ nM) and cell-based replicon assay (GT1b replicon, $EC_{50} = 1.2$ nM).[33] Ciluprevir was well tolerated and efficacious in Phase I and II clinical studies and produced 2–3 log reductions of HCV RNA plasma levels when given to GT1 HCV patients twice daily (bid) as monotherapy. Although its development was discontinued due to concern about cardiac issues in animal studies, ciluprevir validated HCV protease as a drug target and prompted extensive investigation into optimization of the

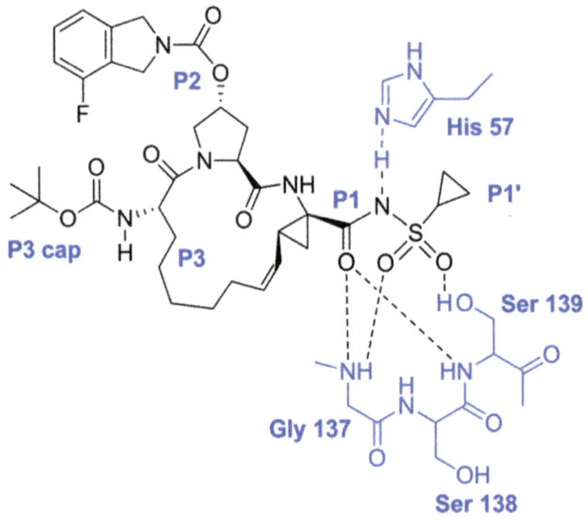

Figure 7.5b   Danoprevir acylsulfonamide moiety interactions with the oxyanion hole and the S1′ HCV protease pocket.
Reprinted with permission from Y. Jiang, S. W. Andrews, K. R. Condroski, B. Buckman, V. Serebryany, S. Wenglowsky, A. L. Kennedy, M. R. Madduru, B. Wang, M. Lyon, G. A. Doherty, B. T. Woodard, C. Lemieux, M. G. Do, H. Zhang, J. Ballard, G. Vigers, B. J. Brandhuber, P. Stengel, J. A. Josey, L. Beigelman, L. Blatt and S. D. Seiwert, *J. Med. Chem.*, 2014, **57**, 1753. Copyright (2013) American Chemical Society.

inhibitor peptide framework and macrocyclization strategies. Section 7.4 will detail other P1-P3 macrocyclic inhibitors that have entered clinical trials, including danoprevir, simeprevir (TMC435) and GS-9256 as well as the P2–P4 macrocyclic inhibitors vaniprevir, MK-1220 and MK-5172, followed by next generation, non-covalent linear inhibitors faldaprevir, asunaprevir and GS-9451. These new linear inhibitors are highly potent and, in addition, the pharmacokinetic properties of faldaprevir and GS-9451 allow their development as qd agents. Nonetheless, a systematic comparative evaluation of linear and cyclic analogs of asunaprevir, danoprevir, vaniprevir, and MK-5172 in enzyme and replicon assays found that the macrocyclization, especially in a P1–P3 fashion, resulted in potency increase and a decreased sensitivity to the effect of HCV PI mutations.[34–36]

7.4   Clinical HCV Protease Inhibitors

The key features of clinical HCV PIs will be briefly described in the following section. The current information about ongoing clinical trials is mainly from the government website found at www.clinicaltrials.gov. Some of these inhibitors were recently extensively reviewed.[37] During the final preparation of this chapter, the macrocyclic simeprevir received approval for the treatment of chronic HCV infection in combination with PEG-IFN/RBV in Japan, Canada and the USA.[38]

7.4.1 Danoprevir (ITMN-191)

Danoprevir (Roche, Figure 7.1) is a 15-membered P1–P3 macrocyclic inhibitor that contains acyl sulfonamide, fluoroisoindoline, and *t*-butyl carbamate moieties at the P1, P2*, and P4 sites of the natural substrate, respectively.[29] This compound contains the same macrocyclic core as ciluprevir. In this series, the replacement of the carboxylic acid group at P1 with an acylsulfonamide as a bioisostere provided over 100-fold potency improvement in the enzyme assay and in the replicon assay. The 15-membered macrocyclic inhibitor was shown to be more active than the corresponding compounds with a 14-membered linker or an oxygen-containing linker. Danoprevir was identified as the clinical candidate based on its favorable potency profile against multiple HCV genotypes 1-6 and key mutants (GT1b, $IC_{50} = 0.2–0.4$ nM; replicon GT1b, $EC_{50} = 1.6$ nM), desirable *in vitro* ADME profile and good *in vivo* liver exposure across multiple animal species (oral bioavailability 15% in rat, liver/plasma ratio ~10 in rat).[29,39] The X-ray crystal structure of danoprevir bound to the HCV NS3 protease revealed molecular details of their interaction, including specific contacts made by the C-terminal acyl-sulfonamide moiety (Figure 7.5b).[29] In early clinical trials, patients given high doses of this agent were observed to have increased levels of aminotransferases. The co-administration of ritonavir (a commonly used HIV protease inhibitor to inhibit the CYP3A enzyme) has allowed it to move forward into advanced trials without the hepatotoxicity concern.[40] Danoprevir is a twice-daily, ritonavir-boosted HCV PI. Currently, it is in Phase III trials both in combination with PEG-IFN/RBV[41] and with other direct-acting antiviral agents including NS5B inhibitor mericitabine.[42]

7.4.2 Simeprevir (TMC435)

Simeprevir (Janssen/Medivir, Figure 7.1) is a 14-membered P1-P3 macrocyclic inhibitor that involves the replacement of the hydroxyproline moiety of ciluprevir by a cyclopentane surrogate as well as modification of the peptidic framework.[38,43] In this new cyclopentane series the macrocycles were optimized by exploring different amide-containing macrocyclic ring sizes and P4 truncations. The 14-membered macrocyclic inhibitor was found to be more potent than the corresponding 13-, 15-, and 16-membered macrocyclic analogs. Further optimization by incorporating a P1 acylsulfonamide moiety led to the discovery of TMC435. This compound inhibited HCV GT1b NS3 protease activity at subnanomolar concentrations ($K_i = 0.36$ nM) and with good replicon potency (GT1b replicon, $EC_{50} = 7.8$ nM). It also exhibited a favorable PK profile with good oral bioavailability (44% in rat) and displayed high liver exposure after oral dosing (liver/plasma ratio of 32).[44] Simeprevir was approved as the first once-daily HCV PI for the treatment of genotype 1 infected patients in combination with PEG-IFN/RBV.[45,46] It is also being developed in clinical trials with other direct-acting antiviral agents such as daclatasvir (an NS5A inhibitor),[47] sofosbuvir (a nucleotide analog inhibitor of HCV polymerase),[48] GSK2336805 (an HCV NS5A inhibitor)[49] and TMC647055 (a non-nucleotide polymerase inhibitor).[50]

7.4.3 GS-9256

GS-9265 (Gilead, Figure 7.1) is a 15-membered P1-P3 macrocyclic inhibitor which conserves the macrocyclic core of ciluprevir, with a modified P2-quinoline heterocycle and a novel phosphinic acid at the carboxyl terminus.[51] The phosphinic acid was employed as a carboxylate bioisostere to mimic the interaction of product-like carboxylate based inhibitors. Two *ortho*-substituted fluorine atoms incorporated on the benzyl group of the phosphinic acid were shown to improve the replicon activity and cell permeability. Further introduction of a chlorine atom at the C-8 position of the quinoline ring was found to result in a significant increase of bioavailability (21% in dog). GS-9256 was selected for clinical development due to its combination of potency (GT1b, $IC_{50} = 4$ nM; GT1b replicon, $EC_{50} = 20$ nM) and PK properties. It is a twice-daily HCV protease inhibitor that is in Phase II trials in combination with PEG-IFN/RBV[52] and with other direct-acting antiviral agents including tegobuvir (an NS5B inhibitor).[53]

7.4.4 Vaniprevir (MK-7009)

Vaniprevir (Merck, Figure 7.1) is a 20-membered P2-P4 macrocyclic inhibitor with a carbamate linkage between the P2-proline and the linked P2-isoindoline substituent.[25] Molecular modeling analysis based on the full crystal structure of the NS3 protease suggested the feasibility of an alternative macrocyclization between the P2 heterocycle and the P4 side chain to generate a structurally distinct series of inhibitor.[24] Subsequently, extensive chemistry exploration of the P2 heterocycle, the P2 to P4 linker, and the P1 side chain led ultimately to the discovery of vaniprevir. Vaniprevir inhibited HCV GT1b NS3 protease at subnanomolar concentrations ($K_i = 0.05$ nM) and with good replicon potency (GT1b replicon, $EC_{50} = 5.0$ nM). It showed good plasma exposure in dog and chimpanzee but low plasma exposure in rat and rhesus monkey (oral bioavailability <15%).[54] Since it demonstrated high liver exposure following oral dosing in multiple species, especially in the chimpanzee model (2400-fold over the GT1b EC_{50}), vaniprevir was selected for clinical evaluation. Vaniprevir is a twice-daily HCV PI that is in Phase II trials in combination with PEG-IFN and RBV.[55,56]

7.4.5 MK-5172

MK-5172 (Merck, Figure 7.1) is an 18-membered P2–P4 macrocyclic inhibitor with an ether linkage between the P2 proline and the linked P2-quinoxaline substituent.[27] To further improve the activity against the NS3A protease as well as key clinically relevant mutants and the poor PK profile observed with

MK-7009, scientists at Merck continued to explore the P2–P4 macrocyclic inhibitor series. Extensive optimization of the P2 heterocycle and linker regions of the series led to the identification of MK-5172. MK-5172 exhibited picomolar binding affinity for genotype 1–3 proteases (GT1b, $K_i = 0.02$ nM; GT3a, $K_i = 0.70$ nM; GT1b replicon, $EC_{50} = 7.4$ nM) and a broad panel of clinically relevant mutants including A156T, A156V, D168A, D168V and R155K.[27] MK-5172 also demonstrated modest oral bioavailability of 13% in rat with improved plasma exposure and excellent liver exposure in rat and dog. MK-5172 proved highly efficacious *in vivo* in the chronic HCV-infected chimpanzee, including greater viral load suppression than vaniprevir at an identical dose and frequency.[57] MK-5172 is a once-daily HCV PI that is currently in Phase II trials in combination with PEG-IFN/RBV[27] and with other direct-acting antiviral agents such as MK-8742 (an NS5A inhibitor).[58]

7.4.6   MK-1220

MK-1220 (Merck, Figure 7.1) is another 18-membered P2-P4 macrocyclic inhibitor with an ether linkage between the proline and the linked P2-isoquinoline substituent.[26] To improve plasma and liver exposure of an initial P2-isoquinoline lead series,[24] a large number of analogs were made and tested to identify those compounds which combined the highest enzyme and replicon potency, rat oral plasma and liver exposure.[26] Further optimization of the P2 heterocycle substitution pattern and the P3 amino acid residue led to MK-1220 in which the macrocycle linker has been attached to the 7-position of the P2-isoquinoline, reminiscent of the macrocyclic motif of vaniprevir. MK-1220 exhibited picomolar potency (GT1b, $K_i = 0.02$ nM; GT1b replicon, $EC_{50} = 4.0$ nM) and improved rat plasma and liver exposure (oral bioavailability of 37% in rat, liver concentration 1000-fold over the GT1b EC_{50}).[26] This compound was reported as a candidate suitable for clinical development, but no patient enrollment information is available.

7.4.7   Faldaprevir (BI 201335)

Faldaprevir (Boehringer Ingelheim, Figure 7.1) is a linear protease inhibitor that contains a large P2 quinoline group and a C-terminal 1-amino-2-vinyl-cyclopropylcarboxylic acid as the P1 residue.[22,59] The initial lead compound in this series was a linear version of ciluprevir,[59] which was 5-fold less active in the enzyme GT1b assay and 20-fold less potent in the GT1b replicon assay compared to ciluprevir. In the optimization process, the introduction of a bromine atom at the C8-position of the P2 quinoline and the modification of the isopropyl group of the aminothiazole moiety significantly improved the potency and PK profile. These studies resulted in the discovery of BI 201335, which showed good HCV protease activity (GT1b, $IC_{50} = 3.0$ nM) and replicon potency (GT1b replicon, $EC_{50} = 3.0$ nM). It also exhibited a good PK profile with oral bioavailability of 40% in rats and a favorable partition ratio into the rat liver with a 40-fold liver *vs.* plasma concentration ratio after oral dosing.[60] Faldaprevir is a once-daily HCV PI that is currently in Phase III trials in combination with PEG-IFN/RBV[61-63] and with other direct-acting antiviral agents including deleobuvir (an NS5B inhibitor).[63,64]

7.4.8   Asunaprevir (BMS-650032)

Asunaprevir (Bristol-Myers Squibb, Figure 7.1) is a linear tripeptidic inhibitor that contains acyl sulfonamide, isoquinoline and *t*-butyl carbamate moieties at the P1, P2*, and P4 sites of the natural substrate, respectively.[30] Asunaprevir exhibited subnanomolar binding affinity for HCV NS3 protease genotype 1 (GT1b, $IC_{50} = 0.3$ nM) and low nanomolar antiviral potency in a replication assay (GT1b replicon, $EC_{50} = 1.2$ nM).[30,65] The exposure profile of this compound across different animal species (mouse, rat, dog and monkey) revealed a high exposure in liver versus plasma concentrations. Asunaprevir is a twice-daily HCV protease inhibitor that is currently in Phase III trials. It is being developed in combination with PEG-IFN/RBV[66,67] and with other direct-acting antiviral agents including daclatasvir (an NS5A inhibitor)[47] and BMS-791325 (an NS5B polymerase inhibitor).[68]

7.4.9   GS-9451

GS-9451 (Gilead, Figure 7.1) is also a linear protease inhibitor that that contains a P4 *cis*-cyclopropylpentyl carbamate, a large P2-quinoline group and a P1 C-terminal 1-amino-2-vinylcyclopropylcarboxylic acid.[69] The fused cyclopropane-pentyl carbamate was introduced as a P4 group to pick up potential lipophilic interactions with the protease. The polar morpholine moiety was incorporated in the P2-quinoline group to improve aqueous solubility and PK. As a result, GS-9451 exhibited single digit nanomolar potency (GT1b, $IC_{50} = 1.4$ nM, GT1b replicon, $EC_{50} = 9.0$ nM) and a desirable PK profile (62% of oral bioavailability in rat, liver/plasma ratio of ∼40 in rat after IV dosing).[69,70] GS-9451 is a once-daily HCV protease inhibitor that is in Phase II trials. It is being developed in IFN-free regimens[71] with other direct-acting antiviral agents including tegobuvir (an NS5B inhibitor)[53] and sofosbuvir (a nucleotide analog inhibitor of HCV polymerase).[48]

7.4.10   ABT-450 and ACH-1625

ABT-450 (structure not disclosed, Abbott / Enanta) is a once-daily, ritonavir-boosted macrocyclic HCV PI.[72] This compound is being developed in Phase III trials in IFN-free all-oral regimens with several other direct-acting antiviral agents[73] including ABT-267 (an NS5A inhibitor)[74] and ABT-333 (a non-nucleoside polymerase inhibitor).[75] ACH-1625 (structure not reported, Achillion) is a once-daily, linear HCV PI currently in Phase II clinical trials.[76]

7.5 GSK and Anacor HCV Protease Inhibitor Discovery Efforts

Section 7.3 described a number of C-terminal covalent (ketoamide 'warheads') or non-covalent moieties that greatly enhance HCV protease inhibitory potency by interacting with the oxyanion hole and surrounding enzyme subsites. The discovery of ciluprevir prompted further efforts to improve potency and PK by replacing the carboxylic acid with bioisosteres such as tetrazole, acylcyanamide, acylsulfonamide, phosphonate and cyclopropyl acylsulfonamide, with some of these functionalities present in more recent clinical compounds.[27,29,38] Section 7.5 will summarize our attempts to optimize and utilize a covalent boron-based warhead in the context of key linear and cyclic HCV PI structures described earlier. Although these HCV PIs were not progressed into clinical development, the work nonetheless provided an *in vitro* proof of concept for this mechanism and is summarized here to aid in considering similar 'warheads' for other macromolecular targets medicinal chemists tackle and to illustrate the effect of macrocyclization on the properties of boron-containing inhibitors.

7.5.1 Design of HCV PIs Incorporating Cyclic Boronate (CB) and Benzoxaborole (BXB) Moieties

The design of novel boron-based warheads, used in the context of the linear and macrocyclic HCV PIs,[77–80] has been an active area of drug discovery. Boronic acid-based HCV NS3 protease inhibitors have been described.[81] Classical α-amino boronic acids have been studied extensively as inhibitors of various proteases and developed into Velcade™, used to treat relapsed multiple myeloma by intravenous or subcutaneous administration.[82] Diverse benzoxaboroles with broad applications to different disease indications have also been reported.[83–86] The benzoxaboroles combine the *P*-orbital reactivity of boron with chemical stability and selectivity, and the resulting compounds demonstrate good intrinsic drug-like properties. Several benzoxaborole-based compounds have entered human clinical trials for anti-fungal, anti-inflammatory, antibacterial and anti-trypanosomiasis indications, exemplified by Kerydin™ (AN2690),[83] AN2728,[84] AN3365 (GSK2251052),[85] and AN5568 (SCYX-7158)[86] (Figure 7.6).

Compounds described in this section incorporate cyclic boronates and benzoxaboroles as putative warheads at the P1 position, targeting the HCV protease active-site Ser 139, as well as positions P1' and P4 in search of other covalent and non-covalent opportunistic interactions with the enzyme.

7.5.1.1 Linear and Macrocyclic HCV PIs with CB Warheads in Position P1

As a proof of concept, linear and macrocyclic HCV PIs with cyclic α-amino oxaborole (CB) moieties in position P1 were constructed first. Telaprevir and

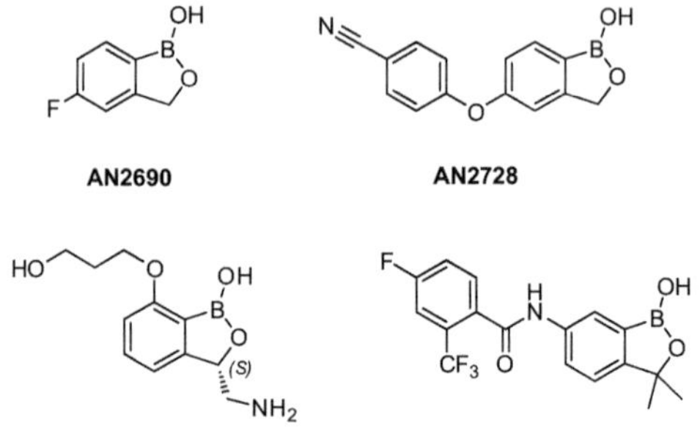

AN2690 AN2728

AN3365 (GSK2251052) AN5568 (SCYX-7158)

Figure 7.6 Benzoxaborole-based clinical compounds.

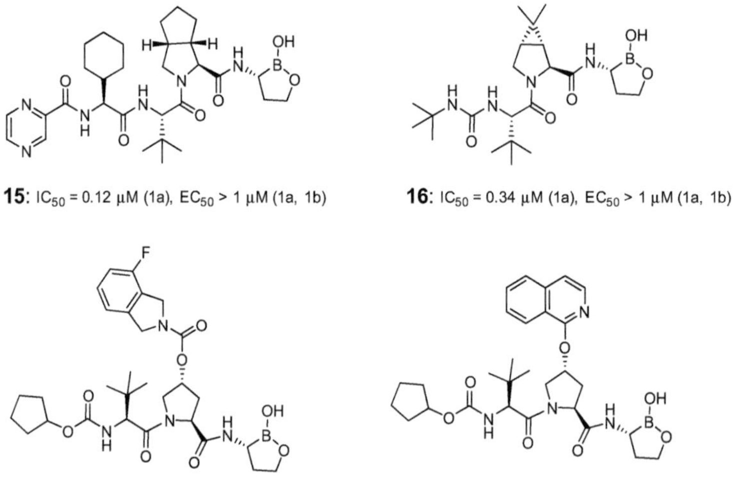

15: IC_{50} = 0.12 μM (1a), EC_{50} > 1 μM (1a, 1b)

16: IC_{50} = 0.34 μM (1a), EC_{50} > 1 μM (1a, 1b)

17: IC_{50} = 0.023 μM (1a), EC_{50} > 1 μM (1a, 1b)

18: IC_{50} = 0.12 μM (1a), EC_{50} > 1 μM (1a, 1b)

Figure 7.7a Cyclic boronate-based NS3 protease inhibitors.

boceprevir-based P1-CB HCV PIs shown in Figure 7.7a were evaluated using a FRET assay with the HCV GT1a NS3 protease domain.[87] When the α-amino oxaborole was placed onto a telaprevir template, the resulting compound, **15**, exhibited good enzyme potency ($IC_{50} = 0.12$ μM). The boceprevir-based inhibitor, **16**, was 3-fold less potent than **15** ($IC_{50} = 0.34$ μM). The best potency was observed when the CB moiety was incorporated into an analog bearing a P2 isoindoline moiety, **17** ($IC_{50} = 0.023$ μM), while lower potency was observed when the P2 isoindoline was replaced by the isoquinoline, as in analog **18** ($IC_{50} = 0.12$ μM). These CB-based linear inhibitors were much less active ($EC_{50} > 1$ μM) in the cell-based GT1a and 1b HCV replicon assays, leading to the hypothesis that this may reflect poor membrane-penetrating properties of compounds **15–18**.

To potentially improve cell permeability, a series of macrocycles **19–27**, exemplified in Figure 7.7b, featuring the P1–CB warhead attached to a

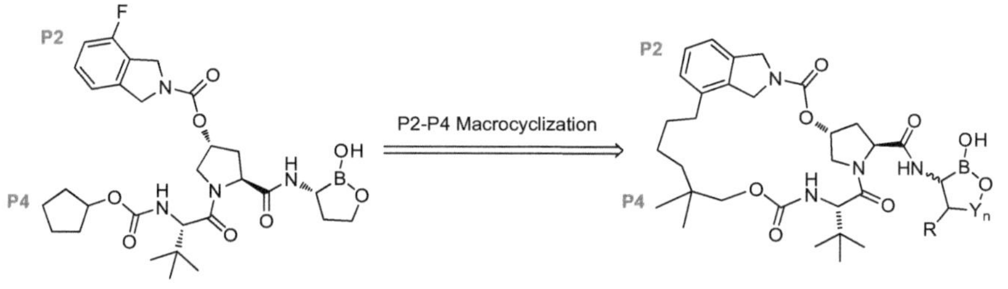

Figure 7.7b Evolution of P1-CB linear HCV PIs to P1–CB macrocyclic HCV PIs.

vaniprevir–derived P2–P4 macrocyclic motif was synthesized and evaluated (Table 7.1).[88]

As shown in Table 7.1, the prototypical compound **19** inhibited GT1a NS3 enzyme with an IC_{50} of 0.043 μM and EC_{50}s of 0.78 μM and 0.52 μM in cell-based GT1a and GT1b HCV replicon assays, respectively. The data for analogs **19–23** in Table 7.1 suggest a minimal influence of the ring size of the α-amino cyclic boronate on the enzymatic and replicon activities for this series of compounds. Thus, compound **23**, derived from a 7-membered cyclic boronate, showed comparable enzymatic potency ($IC_{50} = 0.047$ μM) to **19** and was somewhat more potent in the GT1a and 1b replicon assays, with EC_{50}s of 0.38 μM and 0.22 μM, respectively. Interestingly, inhibitors **19** and **23** exhibited comparable replicon potency compared to two acyclic serine-trap inhibitors, telaprevir (GT1b replicon, $EC_{50} = 0.35$ μM) and boceprevir (GT1b replicon, $EC_{50} = 0.2$ μM), and significantly improved potency in the replicon assays compared to the acyclic α-amino cyclic boronate inhibitor **17**. Similar trends were also observed for other macrocyclic inhibitors in this series, such as **22**. The HCV PIs bearing CB and BXB moieties were not cytotoxic in cellular assays (data not shown).

The influence of chirality at the α-position of the cyclic boronates on potency was also investigated. As shown in Table 7.1, the (R)-α-amino cyclic boronates were much more potent than the corresponding (S)-α-amino isomers. For example, (R)-α-amino oxaborole **19** was 30-fold more active against GT1a NS3, and over 14-fold more potent in the GT1a and 1b replicon assays, compared to its (S)-isomer **24**. Similarly, (R)-6- and 7-membered cyclic boronates **22** and **23** were significantly more active than their (S)-α-amino isomers, **26** and **27**, in both enzyme and replicon assays. Introducing a small methyl group at the β-position of the α-amino cyclic boronate in compounds **20** or **21** resulted in a several-fold decrease in both enzyme and cell-based replicon potency, suggesting that β-alkyl substituents are not well tolerated due to a steric clash with the S1 pocket of the protease.

The X-ray crystal structure of linear boronate inhibitor **18** bound to NS3 protease has been solved and is shown in Figure 7.8a.[87] The general binding mode of **18** is very similar to that of α-ketoamide inhibitors such as boceprevir. The peptide backbone from the inhibitor adopts an extended

Table 7.1 *In vitro* activity of P1-CB macrocyclic inhibitors against HCV GT1a NS3, and GT1a and 1b replicon.

Compound	Cyclic boronate R	NS3/4A 1a IC$_{50}$ (μM)	HCV replicon GT1a EC$_{50}$ (μM)	HCV replicon GT1b EC$_{50}$ (μM)
Linear analog 17	Not applicable	$\leq$0.023	8.7	>10
19		0.043	0.78	0.52
20		0.13	1.9	1.7
21		0.11	0.98	4.2
22		0.062	1.3	2.8
23		0.047	0.38	0.22
24		1.4	11	>50
25		25	33	30
26		1.3	12	>25
27		0.30	3.7	3.9

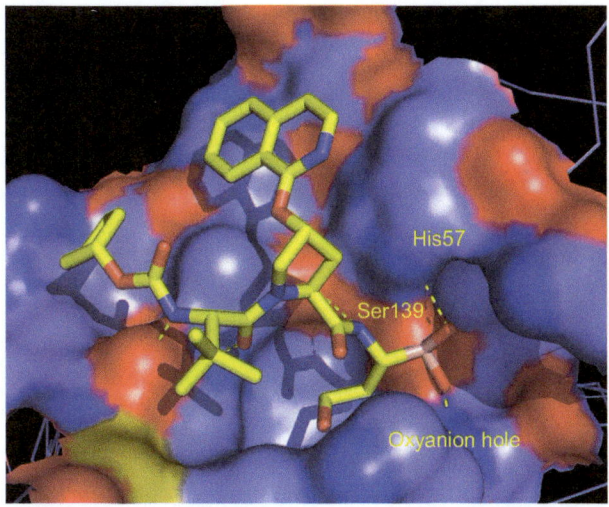

Figure 7.8a X-ray crystal structure of linear boronate inhibitor **18** complexed with HCV NS3 serine protease.

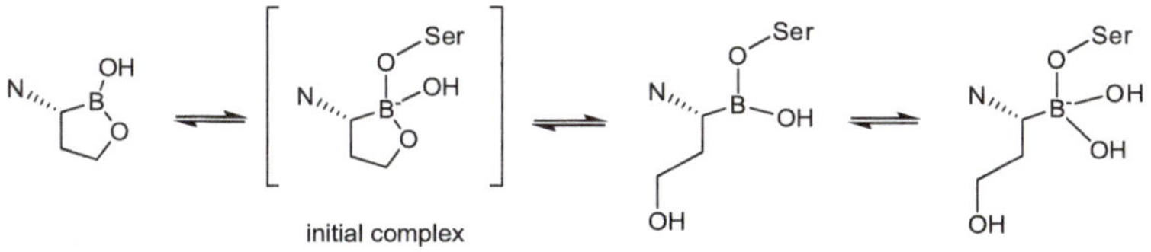

Figure 7.8b Putative HCV protease inhibition pathway for cyclic boronate warheads.

beta-strand conformation and forms three pairs of hydrogen bonds with the protein, while the P1–P4 side chains are properly oriented to fill in the S1–S4 subsites, respectively. As expected, the boron warhead is covalently linked to the hydroxyl group of Ser139 and is locked in the negatively charged tetrahedral form mimicking the transition state. However, the oxygen-boron bond inside the 5-membered oxaborole ring of inhibitor **18** is cleaved, resulting in the hydroxyethyl side chain in the S1 pocket.

In order to investigate if the catalytic Ser139 residue plays a role in the ring opening event, the X-ray crystal structure of linear inhibitor **18** bound to an NS3 protease S139A mutant was also solved (not shown). At the binding site of the mutant, inhibitor **18** maintained the expected extended conformation with P2–P4 in their respective subsites. However, with Ser139 absent in this mutant enzyme, electron density clearly shows that the 5-membered oxaborole ring at the S1 subsite was intact. This suggests that the nucleophilic attack of the catalytic Ser139 residue on the oxaborole in P1–CB compounds is the key mechanistic feature of this inhibitor class (Figure 7.8b).

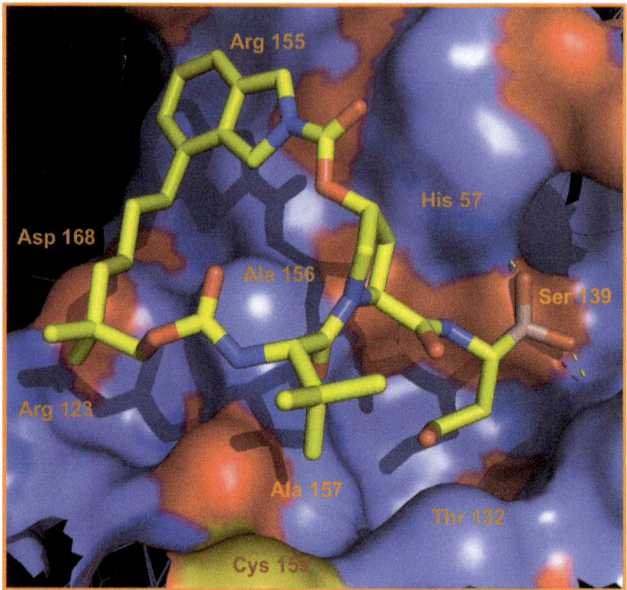

Figure 7.9 X-ray crystal structure of macrocyclic boronate inhibitor **19** complexed with HCV NS3 serine protease.

A very similar binding mode, as well as analogous cleavage of the oxaborole ring to the hydroxyethyl side chain, was observed in the X-ray crystal structure of the macrocyclic CB inhibitor **19** bound to NS3 protease (Figure 7.9).[88] Similarly, when the catalytic Ser139 was absent in the mutant enzyme, the cyclic boronate ring stayed intact at the S1 subsite. The cellular potency increase of cyclic inhibitor **19** *vs.* its linear comparator **17** could be associated with the P2-P4 cyclization, resulting in a more organized structure and/or added lipophilicity, although this hypothesis has not been experimentally verified.

7.5.1.2   P1′–BXB Macrocyclic HCV PIs

Results described in the previous section prompted exploration of a P1′ acylsulfamoyl benzoxaborole moiety.[89] Molecular modeling of a BXB-containing danoprevir-derived structure, **28**, docked into the HCV protease (Figure 7.10a) confirmed that while compounds in this class were not likely to develop specific BXB-Ser139 covalent interactions, the BXB group could form polar interactions with Thr42 and the positively charged Lys136 side chain, thereby potentially improving inhibitory potency. Thus, a scan for new potential BXB interactions with the protease was undertaken by exploring the impact of different regioisomers of acylsulfamoyl benzoxaboroles on the inhibitory activity of two distinct macrocyclic series represented by compounds **29–32** (Figure 7.10b).

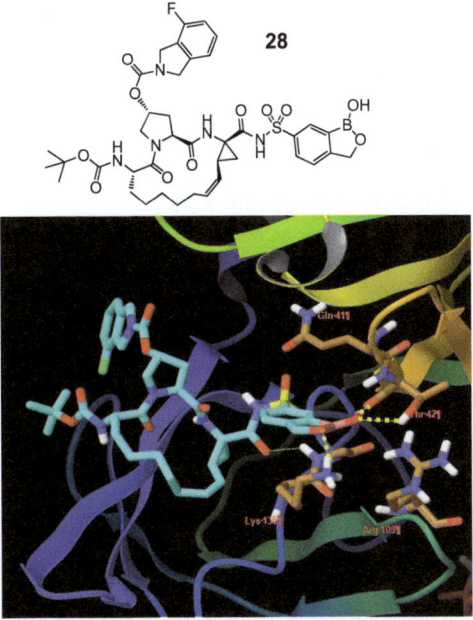

Figure 7.10a Modeling of a hypothetical benzoxaborole inhibitor derived from danoprevir with HCV NS3 protease. Potential polar interactions for P1′-benzoxaborole include main chain and side chain of Thr 42, and positively charged Lys 136.

Reprinted with permission from X. Li, Y.-K. Zhang, Y. Liu, S. Zhang, C. Z. Ding, Y. Zhou, J. J. Plattner, S. J. Baker, L. Liu, W. Bu, W. M. Kazmierski, L. L. Wright, G. K. Smith, R. L. Jarvest, M. Duan, J.-J. Ji, J. P. Cooper, M. D. Tallant, R. M. Crosby, K. Creech, Z.-J. Ni, W. Zou and J. Wright, *Bioorg. Med. Chem. Lett.*, 2010, **20**, 7493.

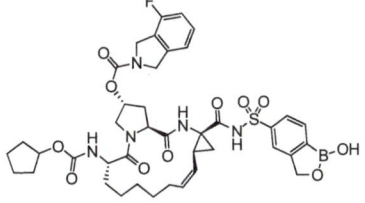

29: IC$_{50}$ = 0.4 nM (1a), EC$_{50}$ = 78 nM (1a) & 20 nM (1b)　　**30:** IC$_{50}$ = 0.6 nM (1a), EC$_{50}$ = 66 nM (1a) & 15 nM (1b)

31: IC$_{50}$ = 0.8 nM (1a), EC$_{50}$ = 66 nM (1a) & 8 nM (1b)　　**32:** IC$_{50}$ = 0.8 nM (1a), EC$_{50}$ = 70 nM (1a) & 12 nM (1b)

Figure 7.10b P1′-BXB P2-P4 and P1-P3 macrocyclic HCV PIs.

The P2–P4 macrocyclic compounds **29** and **30** and P1-P3 macrocyclic inhibitors **31** and **32** potently inhibited GT1a NS3 enzyme with an IC_{50} range of 0.4–0.8 nM (Figure 7.10b). This compares well with ciluprevir, simeprevir (TMC-435) and danoprevir (Table 7.3, $IC_{50} = 0.7$–10 nM). However, inhibitors **29–32** were considerably less potent in replicon assays (GT1b $EC_{50} = 8.0$–20 nM, GT1a $EC_{50} \sim 70$ nM) compared to these three reference compounds with their EC_{50} range of 0.2–1.5 nM (Table 7.3).

Geometric orientation of the acylsulfamoyl benzoxaborole group was not found to substantially influence inhibitory activity (**29** *vs.* **30**, **31** *vs.* **32**). This finding is consistent with the shallow enzyme binding pocket utilizing a number of relatively weak interactions. Along these lines, two distinct cyclization modes (P1–P3 and P2–P4) and many amino acid replacements could be accommodated. The P2–P4 (**29** and **30**) and P1–P3 (**31** and **32**) inhibitors were essentially equipotent, indicating that both macrocyclization modes are effective when individual residues were also optimized for each P1–P3 and P2–P4 motif.

7.5.1.3   *P4–BXB Linear and Macrocyclic HCV PIs*

Another design strategy was based on the molecular modeling suggestion that the BXB moiety in a P4–BXB–danoprevir derivative could interact with the Ser122, Arg123, Arg155 and Asp168 residues of HCV protease (not shown). Thus, P4-BXB derivatives **33–39** (Table 7.2) were synthesized in the context of a P1–P3 macrocycle.[90] Among the key findings resulting from this set of compounds, urea **33**, while essentially equipotent to danoprevir in the enzyme and GT1b replicon assays, was much less potent in the GT1a replicon assay ($EC_{50} = 159$ nM, Table 7.2). Optimization of the BXB linker with carbamates **34** and **35**, amide **39** and homologated urea **36** explored various BXB orientations and distances from the macrocycle with the hope of facilitating the serendipitous discovery of BXB interactions with HCV protease. While no major effect of these structural changes was observed on enzyme GT1a potency, there was a substantial potency range observed for these analogs in the HCV replicon assays (Table 7.2). Significantly, a 143- to 177-fold potency improvement was observed between inhibitors **38** and **35**. These two compounds differ by the nature of the linker (carbamate *vs.* urea), BXB substitution pattern and BXB positional isomery, and it is likely that all of these factors contributed to the improved cellular potency of **38**. For example, in the pair **34** and **35** the *meta-*, rather than the *para-* relationship of boron to the linker, was also preferred (by a factor of 5–10x). Since the compounds in Table 7.2 were about equipotent in the enzyme assay, but strongly differentiated in the cellular assay, it is likely that physical properties and related membrane permeability play a key role in their cell activity. Although it was felt that further potency improvement with additional substituted BXB analogs could be possible, it seemed unlikely that cellular potency could be sufficiently improved as compared to clinical compounds.

Table 7.2 *In vitro* activity of P4-BXB macrocyclic HCV PIs against HCV GT1a NS3, and GT1a and 1b replicon.

Compound	R	NS3/4 GT1a IC_{50} (nM)	HCV replicon EC_{50} (nM) GT1a	GT1b
33		0.4	159	3.7
34		1.6	661	15.0
35		2.4	3548	172
36		0.4	160	0.9
37		<0.2	35	1.5
38		0.4	20	1.2
39		1.0	201	3.2

The influence of P2 isoquinoline and quinoline substituents, present in asunaprevir and simeprevir (Figure 7.1), respectively, was also examined in the P4-BXB series (Figure 7.11). While isoquinolines **40** and **42** were somewhat less potent in the replicon assay than **38**, the quinoline-containing analogs **41** and **43** were substantially more potent (Figure 7.11) and compared well in potency to clinical reference compounds (Table 7.3).

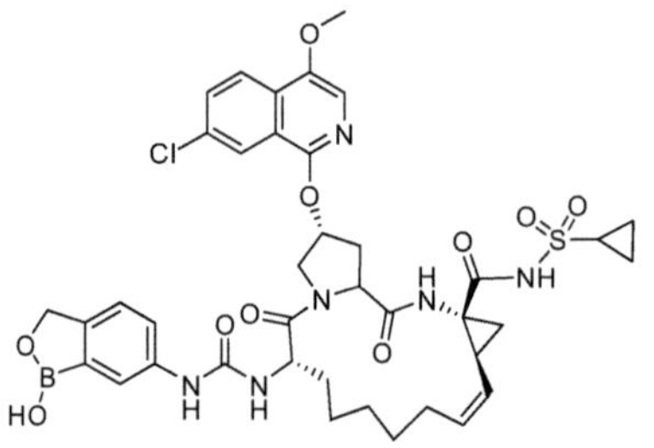

40: IC_{50} = 0.6 nM (1a), EC_{50} = 60.3 nM (1a) & 3.9 nM (1b)   **41:** IC_{50} = 5.6 nM (1a), EC_{50} = 12.5 nM (1a) & 1.2 nM (1b)

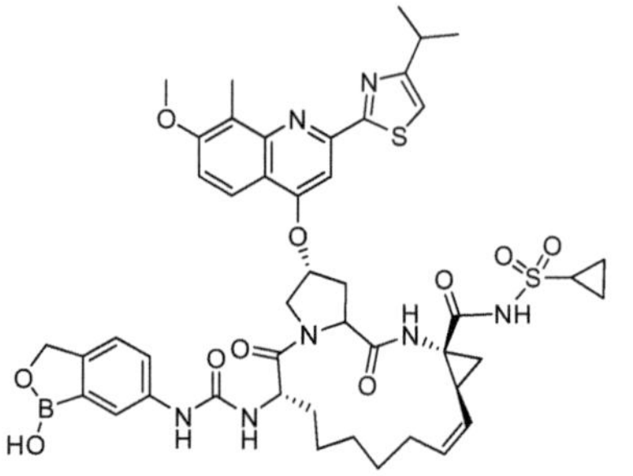

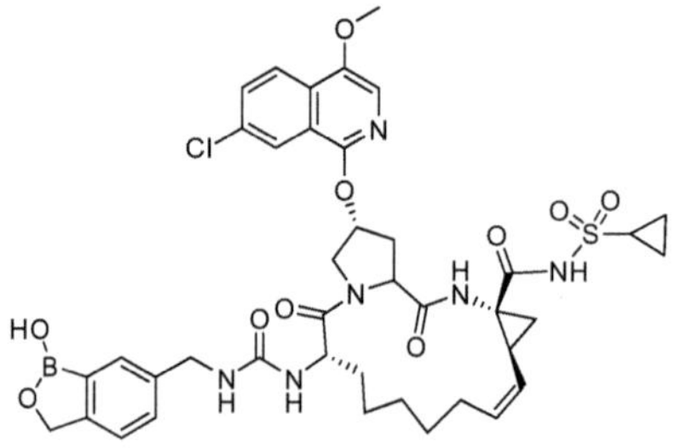

42: IC_{50} = 0.4 nM (1a), EC_{50} = 50.1 nM (1a) & 3.9 nM (1b)   **43:** IC_{50} = 4.1 nM (1a), EC_{50} = 4.2 nM (1a) & 0.5 nM (1b)

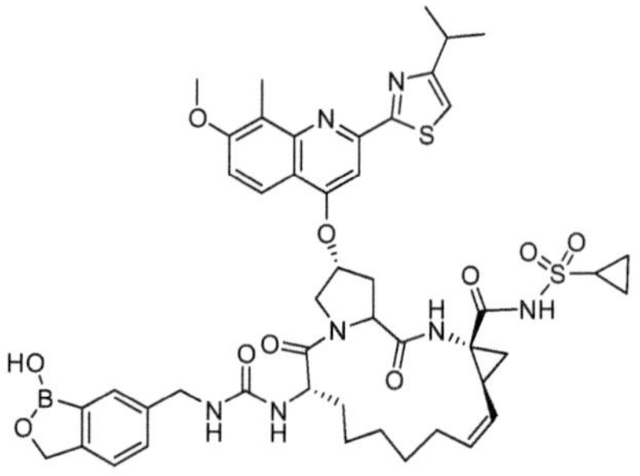

Figure 7.11   P4-BXB macrocyclic HCV PIs with diverse P2 substituents.

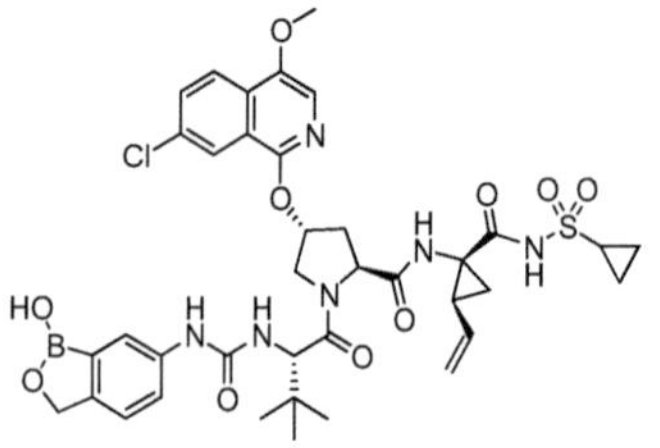

44: IC_{50} = 2.2 nM (1a), EC_{50} = 160 nM (1a) & 24 nM (1b)   **45:** IC_{50} = 2.0 nM (1a), EC_{50} = 130 nM (1a) & 25 nM (1b)

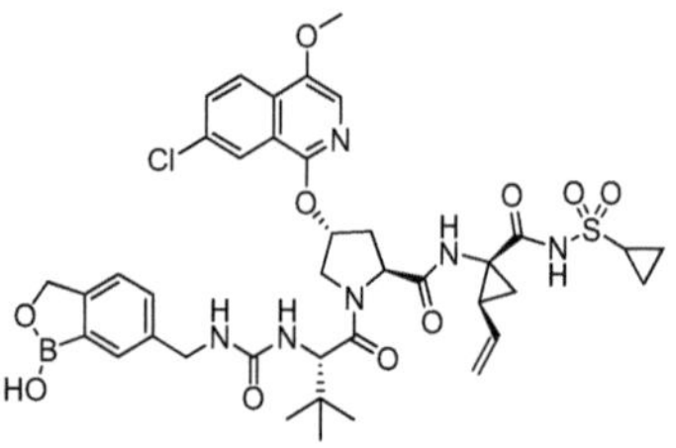

Figure 7.12   P4-BXB linear HCV PIs.

Finally, the macrocyclic, P2 isoquinoline inhibitors **40** and **42** were also substantially more potent than their respective linear urea P4-BXB analogs, **44** and **45** (Figure 7.12),[91] consistent with the generally beneficial effects of macrocyclization observed for HCV PIs.

The *in vivo* rat pharmacokinetic properties of P1'-BXB and P4-BXB inhibitors **31, 33, 36** and **43** were evaluated. While stable in rat plasma and rat liver microsomes, these compounds were generally characterized by low bioavailability, high clearance and high volume of distribution.

The exploration of boron-based HCV protease inhibitors described in Section 7.5.1 resulted in some very highly potent molecules, especially the

BXB-based **41** and **43**, even if these were apparently not able to develop additional boron-based interactions with the enzyme and thus did not offer immediate advantage over non-boron compounds. However, with the P1–CB based inhibitors **18** and **19** a proof of concept was reached with the CB moieties indeed interacting with Ser139. The unforeseen consequence of this interaction was the CB ring opening, which liberated a hydrophilic P1–hydroxy moiety. This was thought to reduce the inhibitory potency of analogs over the putative intact CB interacting with Ser139, since it is known that the HCV protease S1 subsite prefers hydrophobic moieties. It is believed that the experience and data gathered in the HCV PI explorations may lead to the successful use of CB and BXB moieties in other medicinal chemistry endeavors and it is thus hoped that this detailed account will help achieve this goal.

7.5.2 Macrocyclic Non-boron HCV PIs

7.5.2.1 P4–Urea Series

Careful investigation of the by-products obtained during the synthesis of boron derivative **43** revealed a small amount of the dihydroxy derivative **46** (Figure 7.13), likely formed *via* deboronation of **43**. Isolation and evaluation of **46** established it as a potent inhibitor (GT1a enzyme $IC_{50} = 0.5$ nM, GT1a/b replicon $EC_{50} = 15.5/1.1$ nM) compared with other advanced HCV PIs (Table 7.3). While the P4–urea motif has been described in the context of the linear[92] and macrocyclic[93] series, compounds in these references were either not very potent in the replicon assay or specific data were not reported. Considering the very high potency of **46** in the replicon assays, this serendipitous discovery prompted further evaluation of the macrocyclic P4-urea series.

Using a parallel chemistry approach, a number of urea analogs were synthesized, as exemplified by **47–50** (Table 7.3), to discover compounds with a superior potency profile against PI-resistant HCV mutants A156S, A156T, A156V, D168A, D168V and R155K.[94]

While N′,N′-cyclic urea compounds **47–50** were not strongly differentiated in the wild-type GT1a protease and GT1a/b stable replicon assays, their potencies against mutants D168A, D168V and R155K in the transient replicon assays were strongly differentiated and noticeably improved versus the BXB analog **43** (Table 7.3). Inhibitors **48–50** were also more potent than ciluprevir, telaprevir, simeprevir and danoprevir in the stable and/or transient mutant replicon assays (Table 7.3).

Inhibitors **48–50** were also evaluated in an *in vivo* rat PK model (Table 7.4). All compounds exhibited higher liver clearance compared to simeprevir (reported values 505 and 2300 $mL \cdot h^{-1} \cdot kg^{-1}$ at 2 and 4 mg kg^{-1} iv, respectively). The dose-normalized (DN) AUC values for **48–50** were also lower relative to simeprevir (0.194 $h \cdot \mu g \cdot kg \cdot mL^{-1} \cdot mg^{-1}$) and danoprevir ($0.317$ $h \cdot \mu g \cdot kg \cdot mL^{-1} \cdot mg^{-1}$).

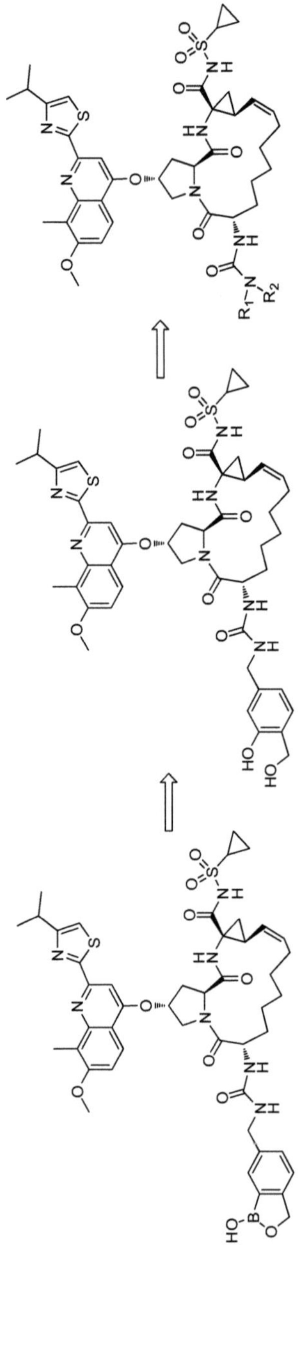

Figure 7.13 Evolution of potent P4-BXB **43** to the P4-urea derivatives.

Table 7.3 *In vitro* activity of P4-urea compounds and advanced HCV PIs in GT1a enzyme assay, stable and transient replicon assays.

Compound	N(R1,R2)	NS3/4A 1a IC$_{50}$ (nM)	Replicon EC$_{50}$ (nM) 1a	Replicon EC$_{50}$ (nM) 1b	GT1b transient replicon, EC$_{50}$ (nM) wt	A156 S	A156 T	A156 V	D168 A	D168 V	R155 K
43	(structure)	2	3.4	0.8	0.9	0.2	7	9	249	144	49
46	(structure)	0.5	15.5	1.1	n.d.[a]	n.d.[a]	n.d.[a]	n.d.[a]	n.d.[a]	n.d.[a]	n.d.[a]
47	(structure)	2	1.8	0.5	0.4	0.4	6	16	873	2261	66
48	(structure)	4	0.8	0.4	0.1	0.2	2	8	60	97	20
49	(structure)	2	0.8	0.5	0.1	0.1	1	6	15	58	14
50	(structure)	5	0.4	0.5	0.04	0.1	2	7	32	79	6
ciluprevir		2	2.2	0.5	1	3	604	627	205	438	241
telaprevir		500	540	372	34	883	1136	1965	638	207	1778
simeprevir		10	2	1	1	0.3	86	344	149	140	56
danoprevir		0.7	2	1.5	0.2	2	10	8	39	26	82

[a]No data.

Table 7.4 Pharmacokinetic parameters of compounds **48–50** in male Sprague-Dawley rats.

	Compound		
	48	**49**	**50**
CL (mL h^{-1} kg^{-1}), iv (1 mg kg^{-1})	9618	5462	5004
PO DNAUC (h μg kg mL^{-1} mg^{-1})	0.008	0.014	0.053
% F	4.2	4	9.4
Liver Concentration (Rat, PO solution, 5 mg kg^{-1})			
AUC (h*μg mL^{-1})	n.d.^{a}	n.d.^{a}	308
Terminal t$_{1/2}$ (h)	n.d.^{a}	n.d.^{a}	8.1

^{a}No data.

However, the piperidinyl urea **50** exhibited long half-life (t$_{1/2}$ = 8.1 h) in the rat liver when dosed po at 5 mg kg^{-1}, resulting in a liver AUC$_\infty$ of 308 h · μg mL^{-1} and a liver/plasma AUC ratio of 1158. This is markedly higher than the liver/plasma ratio reported for simeprevir and danoprevir (32–65 and ~10.5, respectively). Thus, although **50** was not as bioavailable as danoprevir or simeprevir in a classical sense, it targeted liver, the main HCV reservoir, to a much greater degree than either of these drugs. The calculated liver AUC$_\infty$/GT1a EC$_{50}$ ratio for **50** at 5 mg kg^{-1} oral dose was about 20-fold greater than the estimated ratio for danoprevir, even before higher oral dosing (30 mg kg^{-1})[39] is taken into consideration for the latter compound.

7.5.2.2 Non P4–Urea Series

Following the P4 urea discovery, other P4 linkers were also explored, as exemplified by inhibitors **51–58** (Table 7.5).[95] A cyclopropyl rather than isopropyl substituent on the P2* moiety was utilized in this series due to the accessibility of the synthetic intermediate (both were found equivalent in terms of potency and PK). The carbamate, urea, amide and oxalamide linkers in respective inhibitors **51**, **53**, **54** and **57** supported sub-nanomolar potencies in both GT1a and GT1b stable replicon assays. Compared to these compounds, amine **52**, cyclic carbamate **55**, lactam **56** and cyanoguanidine **58** exhibited a significant potency loss in stable GT1a and GT1b and/or transient GT1b replicon assays (Table 7.5). Compounds **51**, **53** and **54** were evaluated in an *in vivo* rat PK model (Table 7.6) and, similarly to urea **50**, were found to have high *in vivo* clearance and low oral exposure. As such, compounds in this series did not offer advantage over **50**.

7.5.2.3 P3–Oxo Series

The SAR in the P4–P3 linker region was further explored with a novel oxo-linker macrocyclic series represented by compounds **59–64** (Table 7.7).[96] Substituents incorporated into **59–64** were to a large degree based on the presumed preference for a hydrophobic motif in the P4–P3 position (with

Table 7.5 The *in vitro* activity of compounds **51–58** in GT1a enzyme, stable and transient replicon assays.

Compound	R^{1}R^{2}N-	NS3/4A 1a IC$_{50}$ (nM)	Replicon EC$_{50}$ (nM)		GT1b transient replicon, EC$_{50}$ (nM)						
			1a	1b	Wt	A156 S	A156 T	A156 V	D168 A	D168 V	R155 K
51		6.3	0.4	0.4	0.02	0.08	1.9	1.5	a	a	6.0
52		1.3	0.7	1.0	1.0	1.2	20	41	229	1660	155
53		0.6	0.3	0.2	0.03	0.1	1.0	5.5	19	51	4.0
54		2.0	0.2	0.1	0.04	0.3	20	85	91	263	44
55		2.5	17	14	27	3.5	107	151	1820	3020	977

Table 7.5 (*Continued*)

Compound	R^{1}R^{2}N-	NS3/4A 1a IC$_{50}$ (nM)	Replicon EC$_{50}$ (nM)		GT1b transient replicon, EC$_{50}$ (nM)						
			1a	1b	Wt	A156 S	A156 T	A156 V	D168 A	D168 V	R155 K
56		20	42	24	8.7	6.2	219	646	1349	3981	794
57		1.0	0.5	0.4	0.02	0.1	5.5	6.2	49	151	14
58		2.5	2.5	0.7	0.3	0.5	27	78	331	832	123

^{a}No data.

Table 7.6 PK parameters of inhibitors **51**, **53** and **54** in male Sprague-Dawley rats.

	Compound		
	51	**53**	**54**
CL $(mL\ h^{-1}\ kg^{-1})$, iv $(1\ mg\ kg^{-1})$	2736	9093	8635
PO DNAUC $(h\ \mu g\ kg\ mL^{-1}\ mg^{-1})$	0.04	0.01	0.01
%F	10.0	7.4	8.2

the exception of hydroxy analog **63** and imidazole derivative **64,** which were synthetic intermediates). The more hydrophobic P4–P3 compounds in this class were generally not as potent as the urea **50.** Conversely, the hydroxyl derivative **63** was the most potent inhibitor in this series (Table 7.7), similar to urea **50** in most potency assays.

In Section 7.5 some of the optimization efforts initially based on the potential of the CB and BXB moieties to develop interactions either with the active site or other parts of the HCV protease have been summarized. While these compounds were not progressed to the clinic, some valuable medicinal chemistry observations were made that can be useful for future efforts involving the inhibition of serine and perhaps cysteine proteases, and in all likelihood other enzymes and receptors. For example, the six-membered α-amino cyclic boronate core from some of the CB-containing HCV PIs has found application in the cyclic boronate-based β-lactamase inhibitor RPX7009 (Rempex Pharmaceuticals), which is currently in Phase I clinical trials.[97] Moreover, following up serendipitous observations from a deboronation product led to an attractive non-boron cyclic urea series. In this series, urea **50** was demonstrated to be more potent against the HCV protease mutants, in particular the key R155K mutant. In addition, **50** had a high liver AUC and AUC/EC$_{50}$ ratio compared to other clinical compounds, and thus fulfilled many of the key targeted optimization properties for a commercial HCV protease inhibitor. Although a plausible clinical candidate, compound **50** was not advanced to the clinic due to strategic considerations. It should also be noted that this exploration led to the discovery of the novel and truncated hydroxyl macrocycle **63,** also characterized by some attractive potency data.

7.6 Selected Examples of Inhibitor Macrocyclization for Related Targets

In the search for novel and effective therapeutics for the treatment of HCV, HCV protease inhibitors are not the only class of enzyme inhibitor to which macrocyclization strategy has been applied. Thus, macrocyclic inhibitors of the HCV NS5B polymerase have also been explored (Section 7.6.1). In addition, macrocyclic analogs of acyclic inhibitors of proteases including. Factor XIa, HIV protease, renin and beta-secretase have been investigated. Examples of each of these are briefly discussed in Section 7.6.2.

Table 7.7 The *in vitro* activity of **59–64** in GT1a enzyme, stable and transient replicon assays.

Compound	R	NS3/4A 1a IC$_{50}$ (nM)	Replicon EC$_{50}$ (nM)		GT1b transient replicon, EC$_{50}$ (nM)						
			1a	1b	wt	A156 S	A156 T	A156 V	D168 A	D168 V	R155 K
59		31.0	5.0	0.8	1.2	2.5	84.6	322.5	462.2	1071.5	323.6
60		107.2	251.2	79.4	63.1	29.4	397.2	434.4	514.0	693.5	3981.0
61		195.0	50.1	39.8	63.1	118.6	70.8	73.7	88.1	131.8	170.5
62		56.2	10.0	3.2	7.1	9.7	90.2	657.7	2152.8	3981.1	1484.5
63		6.8	1.0	0.8	1.3	0.1	2.6	3.2	62.8	45.7	60.3
64		3.2	0.8	0.5	0.5	0.1	2.8	3.9	70.0	151.0	47.9

7.6.1 HCV NS5B Polymerase Inhibitors

The HCV NS5B protein is an RNA polymerase that is an essential enzyme for viral replication. It is an attractive target for drug discovery and multiple inhibitor binding sites have been identified, including the active site and several allosteric sites.[98] Among the allosteric sites is one that has been characterized by several series of indole inhibitors, some of which have yielded crystal structures. One of these structures, containing the inhibitor **65** (Figure 7.14), formed the starting point for a macrocyclization campaign.[50,99–101]

Compound **65** had less than desirable physicochemical properties, some PK limitations, and a structural liability of acylglucuronide formation. The macrocyclization strategy was employed to address these issues by linking solvent exposed positions of the indole inhibitor, while maintaining and optimizing three key interaction features: a salt-bridge, the hydrophobic binding of the cyclohexyl group and the indole-aryl torsional angle of the inhibitor template.[100]

Initial macrocyclic analogs showed enhanced potency relative to non-cyclic precursors and subsequent lead optimization of the linker, salt-bridge binder (to an acylsulfonamide), and aryl substituents led to the identification of candidate TMC647055 (Figure 7.14).[50,100,101] This 17-membered macrocyclic compound had excellent potency against the HCV GT1b replicon ($EC_{50} = 82$ nM), acceptable rat and dog PK (F = 66–87%), including good liver exposure in the rat, and was shown not to result in the formation of an unstable acylglucuronide. While the compound is highly protein bound, the macrocyclization strategy achieved its goals, and TMC647055 is currently in Phase II clinical studies. It is being developed for the treatment of HCV infection in combination with other direct-acting antiviral agents such as simeprevir (an NS3 protease inhibitor, Figure 7.1)[38] and GSK2336805 (an HCV NS5A inhibitor).[49]

7.6.2 Non-HCV Protease Inhibitors

The macrocyclization of linear precursor molecules of medicinal interest has long been a favorite approach for the discovery of novel molecules with

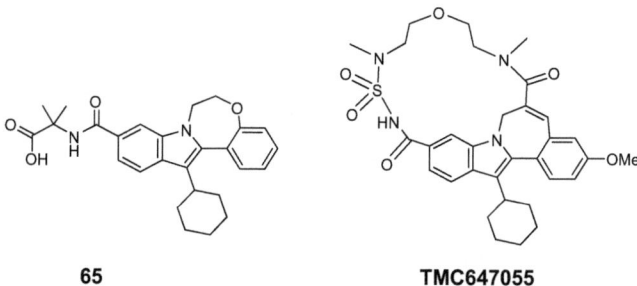

65   **TMC647055**

Figure 7.14 HCV NS5B inhibitor macrocyclization starting template and final clinical candidate.

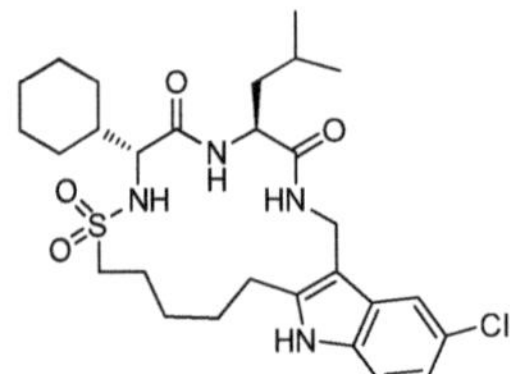

Figure 7.15   Examples of macrocyclic non-HCV protease inhibitors.

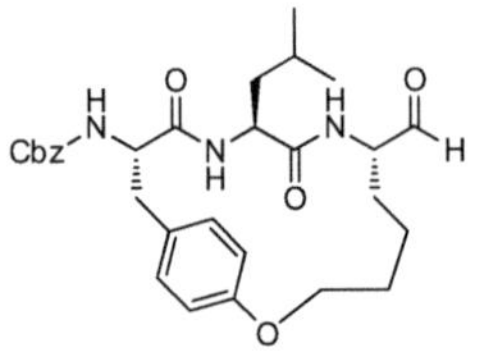

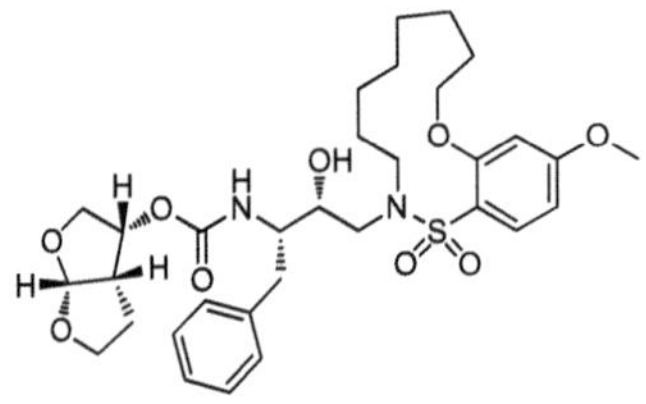

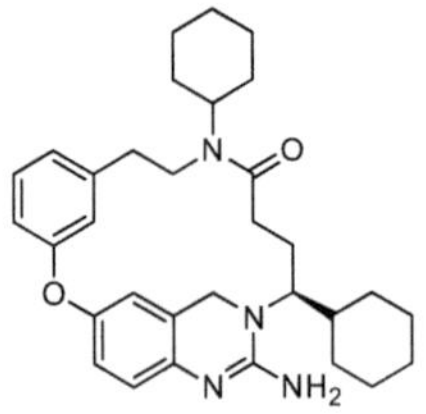

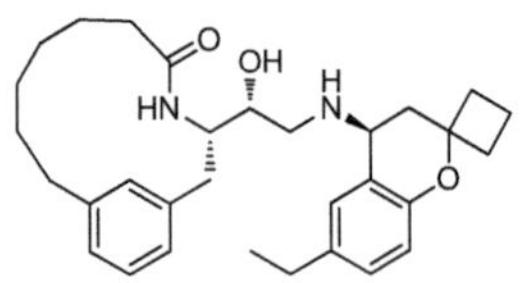

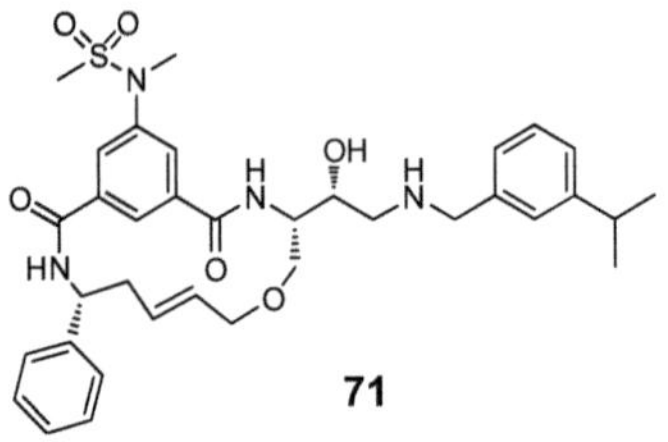

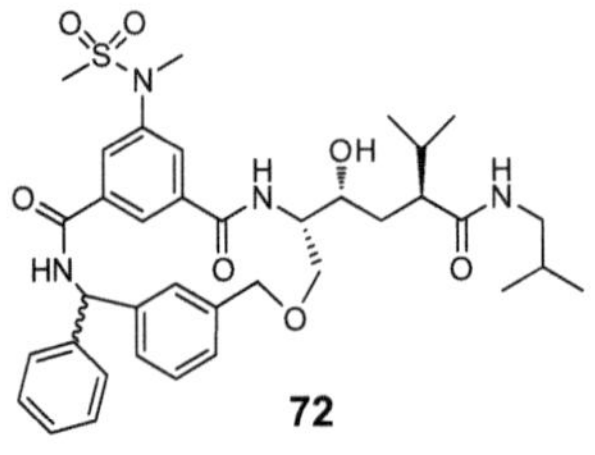

improved properties.[102–104] Selected recent examples of other proteolytic enzyme inhibitor optimization by macrocylization are shown in Figure 7.15.

The modeling of a peptidic linear inhibitor of Factor XIa, a trypsin-like serine protease involved in the blood coagulation cascade, bound to Factor XIa, suggested a macrocyclization mode that resulted in less peptidic, macrocyclic lead compounds such as indole **66**.[105] A similar approach applied to a linear inhibitor of calpain, a cysteine protease involved in a cortical cataractogenesis, resulted in potent macrocycles including **67**.[106] The macrocyclization strategy was also successfully applied to the discovery of novel inhibitors of various aspartic acid proteases. A darunavir-based series of macrocyclic HIV protease inhibitors, exemplified by **68**, designed to fill the hydrophobic pocket in the S1′–S2′ subsites has been demonstrated to lead to significant potency improvement compared to acyclic homologues.[107] Inhibition of beta-secretase (BACE) also proved to be a very fertile arena for the discovery of a number of potent macrocyclic inhibitors (**69–71**).[108–111] Finally, macrocycles such as **72** have demonstrated that a several-fold potency improvement could be realized by the cyclization of linear renin inhibitors.[112]

7.7 Conclusion

Among the respective linear and macrocyclic pairs of HCV protease inhibitors **17** and **19, 44** and **40, 45** and **42**, the macrocylic compounds demonstrated both greater enzymatic and cellular potency. The macrocyclic PIs are characterized by improved pharmacokinetic properties compared to the early, linear HCV PIs telaprevir and boceprevir (however, the new generation linear inhibitors faldaprevir and GS-9451 are being developed as qd agents). The macrocyclic HCV PIs also demonstrate an improved PI-resistant profile compared to the linear PIs. A major challenge in the development of the future generation of HCV PIs is the rapid emergence of resistant mutants which limit HCV treatment efficacy and durability. The structural characteristics of HCV NS3 protease have resulted in inhibitors that rely on multiple weak interactions for tight binding to the protease, and in some cases a single key mutation may lead to a significant loss of activity and thus drug resistance. Most primary drug-resistance mutations in HCV NS3 protease occur around the active site in those regions where drugs extend beyond the substrate binding site (R155, A156 and D168), as these residue changes have minimal impact on inhibitor binding and viral fitness. In our study, macrocyclic P4-urea inhibitors (such as **48–50**) have been shown to be much more potent in both stable and PI-resistant mutant transient replicon assays than telaprevir and the leading second generation inhibitors danoprevir and simeprevir. Recently, linear and macrocyclic versions of asunaprevir, danoprevir, vaniprevir, and MK-5172 were evaluated against wild-type and R155K, V36M/R155K, A156T and D168A HCV mutants in enzymatic and antiviral assays.[35] In each inhibitor series, macrocyclic PIs exhibited improved enzyme and replicon potency compared to the corresponding linear analogs against drug-resistant mutants. For example, the P1-P3 macrocyclic analog **5172-mcP1P3** (Figure 7.16) showed 18-fold improvement against wild-type protease and 4- to 24-fold improvement against resistant mutants in replicon assays, compared to its linear analog **5172-linear**. The P2–P4 macrocyclic inhibitor **MK-5172** exhibited a 16-fold potency improvement against wild-type protease and 0.5–37 fold against resistant mutants in replicon

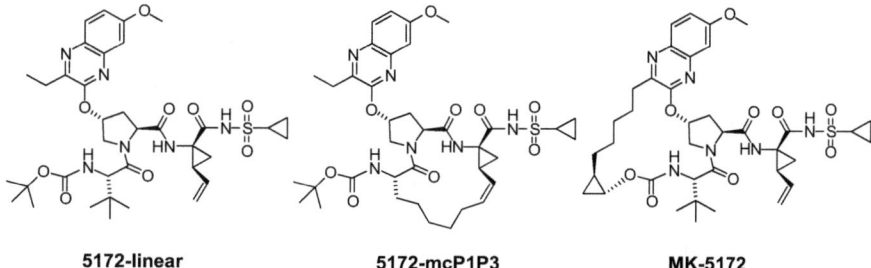

5172-linear   **5172-mcP1P3**   **MK-5172**

Figure 7.16 Linear and macrocyclic HCV PIs illustrating the roles of macrocyclization in addressing mutant potency.[35]

assays, compared to linear analog **5172-linear**. Furthermore, the cyclization mode of the macrocycle was critical for retaining activity against PI-resistant mutants. The P1-P3 macrocyclic PIs are less susceptible to resistance (A156T $EC_{50} = 3.96$ nM in replicon assays for **5172-mcP1P3** vs. $EC_{50} = 23.1$ nM for **5172-linear**). The P1–P3 macrocyclic core is distal from the sites of primary drug resistance mutation and this allows the P2 moiety to be flexible to adapt to structural or electronic changes in a binding pocket that harbors resistance mutations. On the other hand, the P2–P4 macrocyclic PIs are more susceptible to drug resistance (A156T $EC_{50} = 46.6$ nM in replicon assays for **MK-5172** vs. $EC_{50} = 23.1$ nM for **5172-linear**). This may be due to the P2 moiety constraint reducing the inhibitor's ability to adapt to changes resulting from HCV protease mutations. In addition, the recently published crystal structures of several inhibitors in complex with the major drug resistant mutants have revealed the molecular basis underlying the unique resistance profiles of these inhibitors,[34–36] and will provide useful information for further designing macrocyclic PIs against a wider spectrum of HCV PI-resistant mutants.

Tremendous progress has been made in the discovery and development of macrocyclic HCV PIs over the past decade. The macrocyclic HCV PI simeprevir was recently approved for the treatment of genotype 1 infected patients in combination with PEG-IFN/RBV. Other macrocyclic HCV PIs, danoprevir, vaniprevir and MK-5172, are expected to complete clinical trials soon. In the next few years, the fruit of macrocyclization strategies in generating highly active HCV PIs against a wider range of HCV genotypes and PI-resistant mutants will continue to be tested for effective clinical efficacy in human clinical trials. These macrocyclic PIs when combined with other direct-acting antivirals (DAAs) such as NS5B polymerase, NS5A, or cyclophilin inhibitors have the potential to create an all-oral, IFN-free regimens for the treatment of HCV infection. This would be a tremendous breakthrough in providing effective treatment cure to millions of patients.

Acknowledgments

We thank our many GSK, Anacor, BioDuro (China), and ACME Bioscience (Palo Alto, CA) colleagues who participated in all aspects of this program. Especially, we acknowledge Stephen Baker, Wei Bu, Joel Cooper, Renae Crosby, Katrina Creech, Luz Carballo, Maire Convery, Maosheng Duan, Charles Ding, Bill McDowell, Malcolm Ellis, Colin Edge, Dazhong Fan, Margaret Gartland, Richard Grimes, Julia Hubbard, Robert Hamatake, Jing-Jing Ji, Yang Liu, Qun Li, Liang Liu, Liang Liao, Linos Lazarides, Jackie Mordaunt, Zhi-Jie Ni, Pamela Nassau, Lewis Pennicott, Xuelei Qian, Paul Rowland, Martin Slater, Gary Smith, Don Somers, Tadeusz Skarzynski, Andrew Spaltenstein, Matthew Tallant, Pia Thommes, Gemma White, Lois Wright, Jon Wright, Amy Wang, Min Wu, Yong-Kang Zhang, Suoming Zhang, Wuxin Zou and Yasheen Zhou for their valuable contributions and discussions.

References

1. A. D. Kwong, *ACS Med. Chem. Lett.*, 2014, **5**, 214.
2. Q. L. Choo, G. Kuo, A. J. Weiner, L. R. Overby, D. W. Bradley and M. Houghton, *Science*, 1989, **244**, 359.
3. A. D. Kwong, R. S. Kauffman, P. Hurter and P. Mueller, *Nat. Biotechnol.*, 2011, **29**, 993.
4. R. B. Perni, S. J. Almquist, R. A. Byrn, G. Chandorkar, P. R. Chaturvedi, L. F. Courtney, C. J. Decker, K. Dinehart, C. A. Gates, S. L. Harbeson, A. Heiser, G. Kalkeri, E. Kolaczkowski, K. Lin, Y.-P. Luong, B. G. Rao, W. P. Taylor, J. A. Thomson, R. D. Tung, R. D, Y. Wei, A. D. Kwong and C. Lin, *Antimicrob. Agents Chemother.*, 2006, **50**, 899.
5. S. Venkatraman, S. L. Bogen, A. Arasappan, F. Bennett, K. Chen, E. Jao, Y. T. Liu, R. Lovey, S. Hendrata, Y. Huang, W. Pan, T. Parekh, P. Pinto, V. Popov, R. Pike, S. Ruan, B. Santhanam, B. Vibulbhan, W. Wu, W. Yang, J. Kong, X. Liang, J. Wong, R. Liu, N. Butkiewicz, R. Chase, A. Hart, S. Agrawal, P. Ingravallo, J. Pichardo, R. Kong, B. Baroudy, B. Malcolm, Z. Guo, A. Prongay, V. Madison, L. Broske, X. Cui, K. C. Cheng, Y. Hsieh, J. M. Brisson, D. Prelusky, W. Korfmacher, R. White, S. Bogdanowich-Knipp, A. Pavlovsky, P. Bradley, A. K. Saksena, A. Ganguly, J. Piwinski, V. Girijavallabhan and F. G. Njoroge, *J. Med. Chem.*, 2006, **49**, 6074.
6. B. A. Malcolm, R. Liu, F. Lahser, S. Agrawal, B. Belanger, N. Butkiewicz, R. Chase, F. Gheyas, A. Hart, D. Hesk, P. Ingravallo, C. Jiang, R. Kong, J. Lu, J. Pichardo, A. Prongay, A. Skelton, X. Tong, S. Venkatraman, E. Xia, V. Girijavallabhan and F. G. Njoroge, *Antimicrob. Agents Chemother.*, 2006, **50**, 1013.
7. J. Vermehren and C. Sarrazin, *Eur. J. Med. Res.*, 2011, **16**, 303.
8. R. Bartenschlager, V. Lohmann, T. Wilkinson and J. O. Koch, *J. Virol.*, 1995, **69**, 7519.
9. R. Bartenschlager, V. Lohmann and F. Penin, *Nat. Rev. Microbiol.*, 2013, **11**, 482.
10. E. Foy, K. Li, R. Sumpter, Jr, Y.-M. Loo, C. L. Johnson, C. Wang, P. M. Fish, M. Yoneyama, T. Fujita, S. M. Lemon and M. Gale, Jr, *Proc. Natl. Acad. Sci. USA*, 2005, **102**, 2986.
11. K. Li, E. Foy, J. C. Ferreon, M. Nakamura, A. C. M. Ferreon, M. Ikeda, S. C. Ray, M. Gale, Jr and S. M. Lemon, *Proc. Natl. Acad. Sci. USA*, 2005, **102**, 2992.
12. Y. Yan, Y. Li, S. Munshi, V. Sardana, J. L. Cole, M. Sardana, C. Steinkuehler, L. Tomei, R. De Francesco, L. C. Kuo and Z. Chen, *Protein Sci.*, 1998, **7**, 837.
13. R. A. Love, H. E. Parge, J. A. Wickersham, Z. Hostomsky, N. Habuka, E. W. Moomaw, T. Adachi and Z. Hostomska, *Cell*, 1996, **87**, 331.
14. I. Schechter and A. Berger, *Biochem. Biophys. Res. Commun.*, 1967, **27**, 157.
15. A. Grakoui, D. W. McCourt, C. Wychowski, S. M. Feinstone and C. M. Rice, *J. Virol.*, 1993, **67**, 2832.

16. M. Llinàs-Brunet, M. Bailey, G. Fazal, S. Goulet, T. Halmos, S. Laplante, R. Maurice, M. Poirier, M-A. Poupart, D. Thibeault, D. Wernic and D. Lamarre, *Bioorg. Med. Chem. Lett.*, 1998, **8**, 1713.

17. M. Llinàs-Brunet, M. Bailey, R. Déziel, G. Fazal, V. Gorys, S. Goulet, T. Halmos, R. Maurice, M. Poirier, M. A. Poupart, J. Rancourt, D. Thibeault, D. Wernic and D. Lamarre, *Bioorg. Med. Chem. Lett.*, 1998, **8**, 2719.

18. M. Llinàs-Brunet, M. Bailey, G. Fazal, E. Ghiro, V. Gorys, S. Goulet, T. Halmos, R. Maurice, M. Poirier, M.-A. Poupart, J. Rancourt, D. Thibeault, D. Wernic and D. Lamarre, *Bioorg. Med. Chem. Lett*, 2000, **10**, 2267.

19. S. R. LaPlante, D. R. Cameron, N. Aubry, S. Lefebvre, G. Kukolj, R. Maurice, D. Thibeault, D. Lamarre and M. Llinas-Brunet, *M. J. Biol. Chem.*, 1999, **274**, 18618.

20. J. Rancourt, D. R. Cameron, V. Gorys, D. Lamarre, M. Poirier, D. Thibeault and M. Llinas-Brunet, *J. Med. Chem.*, 2004, **47**, 2511.

21. N. Goudreau, C. Brochu, D. R. Cameron, J.-S. Duceppe, A.-M. Faucher, J.-M. Ferland, C. Grand-Maître, M. Poirier, B. Simoneau and Y. S. Tsantrizos, *J. Org. Chem.*, 2004, **69**, 6185.

22. S. R. LaPlante, H. Nar, C. T. Lemke, A. Jakalian, N. Aubry and S. H. Kawai, *J. Med. Chem.*, 2014, **57**, 1777.

23. Y. S. Tsantrizos, G. Bolger, P. Bonneau, D., Cameron, N. Goudreau, G. Kukolj, S. R. LaPlante, M. Llinas-Brunet, H. Nar and D. Lamarre, *Angew. Chem., Int. Ed.*, 2003, **42**, 1356.

24. N. J. Liverton, M. K. Holloway, J. A. McCauley, M. T. Rudd, J. W. Butcher, S. S. Carroll, J. DiMuzio, C. Fandozzi, K. F. Gilbert, S. S. Mao, C. J. McIntyre, K. T. Nguyen, J. J. Romano, M. Stahlhut, B. L. Wan, D. B. Olsen and J. P. Vacca, *J. Am. Chem. Soc.*, 2008, **130**, 4607.

25. J. A. McCauley, C. J. McIntyre, M. T. Rudd, K. T. Nguyen, J. J. Romano, J. W. Butcher, K. F. Gilbert, K. J. Bush, M. K. Holloway, J. Swestock, B. L. Wan, S. S. Carroll, J. M. DiMuzio, D. J. Graham, S. W. Ludmerer, S. S. Mao, M. W. Stahlhut, C. M. Fandozzi, N. Trainor, D. B. Olsen, J. P. Vacca and N. J. Liverton, *J. Med. Chem.*, 2010, **53**, 2443.

26. M. T. Rudd, J. A. McCauley, J. W. Butcher, J. J. Romano, C. J. McIntyre, K. T. Nguyen, K. F. Gilbert, K. J. Bush, M. K. Holloway, J. Swestock, B.-L. Wan, S. S. Carroll, J. M. DiMuzio, D. J. Graham, S. W. Ludmerer, M. W. Stahlhut, C. M. Fandozzi, N. Trainor, D. B. Olsen, J. P. Vacca and N. J. Liverton, *ACS Med. Chem. Lett.*, 2011, **2**, 207.

27. S. Harper, J. A. McCauley, M. T. Rudd, M. Ferrara, M. DiFilippo, B. Crescenzi, U. Koch, A. Petrocchi, M. K. Holloway, J. W. Butcher, J. J. Romano, K. J. Bush, K. F. Gilbert, C. J. McIntyre, K. T. Nguyen, E. Nizi, S. S. Carroll, S. W. Ludmerer, C. Burlein, J. M. DiMuzio, D. J. Graham, C. M. McHale, M W. Stahlhut, D. B. Olsen, E. Monteagudo, S. Cianetti, C. Giuliano, V. Pucci, N. Trainor, C. M. Fandozzi, M. Rowley, P. J. Coleman, J. P. Vacca, V. Summa and N. J. Liverton, *ACS Med. Chem. Lett.*, 2012, **3**, 332.

28. C. Lin, A. D. Kwong and R. B. Perni, *Infect. Disord. Drug Targets*, 2006, **6**, 3.

29. Y. Jiang, S. W. Andrews, K. R. Condroski, B. Buckman, V. Serebryany, S. Wenglowsky, A. L. Kennedy, M. R. Madduru, B. Wang, M. Lyon, G. A. Doherty, B. T. Woodard, C. Lemieux, M. G. Do, H. Zhang, J. Ballard, G. Vigers, B. J. Brandhuber, P. Stengel, J. A. Josey, L. Beigelman, L. Blatt and S. D. Seiwert, *J. Med. Chem.*, 2014, **57**, 1753.

30. P. M. Scola, L.-Q. Sun, A. X. Wang, J. Chen, N. Sin, B. L. Venables, S.-Y. Sit, Y. Chen, A. Cocuzza, D. M. Bilder, S. V. D'Andrea, B. Zheng, P. Hewawasam, Y. Tu, J. Friborg, P. Falk, D. Hernandez, S. Levine, C. Chen, F. Yu, A. K. Sheaffer, G. Zhai, D. Barry, J. O. Knipe, Y.-H. Han, R. Schartman, M. Donoso, K. Mosure, M. W. Sinz, T. Zvyaga, A. C. Good, R. Rajamani, K. Kish, J. Tredup, H. E. Klei, Q. Gao, L. Mueller, R. J. Colonno, D. M. Grasela, S. P. Adams, J. Loy, P. C. Levesque, H. Sun, H. Shi, L. Sun, W. Warner, D. Li, J. Zhu, N. A. Meanwell and F. McPhee, *J. Med. Chem.*, 2014, **57**, 1730.

31. P. M. Scola, Alan. X. Wang, A. C. Good, L.-Q. Sun, K. D. Combrink, J. A. Campbell, J. Chen, Y. Tu, N. Sin, B. L. Venables, S.-Y. Sit, Y. Chen, A. Cocuzza, D. M. Bilder, S. D'Andrea, B. Zheng, P. Hewawasam, M. Ding, J. Thuring, J. Li, D. Hernandez, F. Yu, P. Falk, G. Zhai, A. K. Sheaffer, Ch. Chen, M. S. Lee, D. Barry, J. O. Knipe, W. Li, Y.-H. Han, S. Jenkins, C. Gesenberg, Q. Gao, M. W. Sinz, K. S. Santone, T. Zvyaga, R. Rajamani, H. E. Klei, R. J. Colonno, D. M. Grasela, E. Hughes, C. Chien, S. Adams, P. C. Levesque, D. Li, J. Zhu, N. A. Meanwell and F. McPhee, *J. Med. Chem*, 2014, **57**, 1708.

32. D. Lamarre, P. C. Anderson, M. Bailey, P. Beaulieu, G. Bolger, P. Bonneau, M. Bös, D. R. Cameron, M. Cartier, M. G. Cordingley, A. M. Faucher, N. Goudreau, S. H. Kawai, G. Kukolj, L. Lagacé, S. R. LaPlante, H. Narjes, M. A. Poupart, J. Rancourt, R. E. Sentjens, R. St George, B. Simoneau, G. Steinmann, D. Thibeault, Y. S. Tsantrizos, S. M. Weldon, C. L. Yong and M. Llinàs-Brunet, *Nature*, 2003, **426**, 186.

33. M. Llinàs-Brunet, M. D. Bailey, G. Bolger, C. Brochu, A. M. Faucher, J. M. Ferland, M. Garneau, E. Ghiro, V. Gorys, C. Grand-Maître, T. Halmos, N. Lapeyre-Paquette, F. Liard, M. Poirier, M. Rhéaume, Y. S. Tsantrizos and D. Lamarre, *J. Med. Chem.*, 2004, **47**, 1605.

34. K. P. Romano, A. Ali, C. Aydin, D. Soumana, A. Ozen, L. M. Deveau, C. Silver, H. Cao, A. Newton, C. J. Petropoulos, W. Huang and C. A. Schiffer, *PLoS Pathog.*, 2012, **8**, e1002832.

35. A. Ali, C. Aydin, R. Gildemeister, K. P. Romano, H. Cao, A. Özen, D. Soumana, A. Newton, C. J. Petropoulos, W. Huang and C. A. Schiffer, *ACS Chem. Biol.*, 2013, **8**, 1469.

36. J. A. O'Meara, C. T. Lemke, C. Godbout, G. Kukolj, L. Lagacé, B. Moreau, D. Thibeault, P. W. White and M. Llinàs-Brunet, *J. Biol. Chem.*, 2013, **288**, 5673.

37. *Antiviral Drugs: From Basic Discovery Through Clinical Trials*, ed. W. M. Kazmierski, Hoboken, N.J., Wiley, 2011.

38. A. Rosenquist, B. Samuelsson, P. O. Johansson, M. D. Cummings, O, Lenz, P. Raboisson, K. Simmen, S. Vendeville, H. de Kock, M. Nilsson, A. Horvath, R. Kalmeijer, G. de la Rosa and M. Beumont-Mauviel, *J. Med. Chem.*, 2014, **57**, 1673.

39. S. D. Seiwert, S. W. Andrews, Y. Jiang, V. Serebryany, H. Tan, K. Kossen, P. T. Rajagopalan, S. Misialek, S. K. Stevens, A. Stoycheva, J. Hong, S. R. Lim, X. Qin, R. Rieger, K. R. Condroski, H. Zhang, M. G. Do, C. Lemieux, G. P. Hingorani, D. P. Hartley, J. A. Josey, L. Pan, L. Beigelman and L. M. Blatt, *Antimicrob. Agents Chemother.*, 2008, **52**, 4432.

40. M. B. Reddy, Y. Chen, J. O. Haznedar, J. Fretland, S. Blotner, P. Smith and J. Q. Tran, *Clin. Pharmacokinet.*, 2012, **51**, 457.

41. E. J. Gane, R. Rouzier, A. Wiercinska-Drapalo, D. G. Larrey, P. N. Morcos, B. J. Brennan, S. Le Pogam, I. Nájera, R. Petric, J. Q. Tran, R. Kulkarni, Y. Zhang, P. Smith, E. S. Yetzer and N. S. Shulman, *Antimicrob. Agents Chemother.*, 2014, **58**, 1136.

42. J. Guedj, H. Dahari, E. Shudo, P. Smith and A. S. Perelson, *Hepatology*, 2012, **55**, 1030.

43. P. Raboisson, H. de Kock, A. Rosenquist, M. Nilsson, L. Salvador-Oden, T. I. Lin, N. Roue, V. Ivanov, H. Wähling, K. Wickström, E. Hamelink, M. Edlund, L. Vrang, S. Vendeville, W. Van de Vreken, D. McGowan, A. Tahri, L. Hu, C. Boutton, O. Lenz, F. Delouvroy, G. Pille, D. Surleraux, P. Wigerinck, B. Samuelsson and K. Simmen, *Bioorg. Med. Chem. Lett.*, 2008, **18**, 4853.

44. T. I. Lin, O. Lenz, G. Fanning, T. Verbinnen, F. Delouvroy, A. Scholliers, K. Vermeiren, A. Rosenquist, M. Edlund, B. Samuelsson, L. Vrang, H. de Kock, P. Wigerinck, P. Raboisson and K. Simmen, *Antimicrob. Agents Chemother.*, 2009, **53**, 1377.

45. M. W. Fried, M. Buti, G. J. Dore, R. Flisiak, P. Ferenci, I. Jacobson, P. Marcellin, M. Manns, I. Nikitin, F. Poordad, M. Sherman, S. Zeuzem, J. Scott, L. Gilles, O. Lenz, M. Peeters, V. Sekar, G. De Smedt and M. Beumont-Mauviel, *Hepatology*, 2013, **58**, 1918.

46. S. Maekawa and N. Enomoto, *J. Gastroenterol.*, 2014, **49**, 163.

47. M. Belema, O. D. Lopez, J. A. Bender, J. L. Romine, D. R. St Laurent, D. R. Langley, J. A. Lemm, D. R. O'Boyle 2nd, J. H. Sun, C. Wang, R. A. Fridell and N. A. Meanwell, *J. Med. Chem.*, 2014, **57**, 1643.

48. M. J. Sofia, D. Bao, W. Chang, J. Du, D. Nagarathnam, S. Rachakonda, P. G. Reddy, B. S. Ross, P. Wang, H. R. Zhang, S. Bansal, C. Espiritu, M. Keilman, A. M. Lam, H. M. Steuer, C. Niu, M. J. Otto and P. A. Furman, *J. Med. Chem.*, 2010, **53**, 7202.

49. W. M. Kazmierski, A. Maynard, M. Duan, S. Baskaran, J. Botyanszki, R. Crosby, S. Dickerson, M. Tallant, R. Grimes, R. Hamatake, M. Leivers, C. D. Roberts and J. Walker, *J. Med. Chem.*, 2014, **57**, 2058.

50. M. D. Cummings, T. I. Lin, L. Hu, A. Tahri, D. McGowan, K. Amssoms, S. Last, B. Devogelaere, M. C. Rouan, L. Vijgen, J. M. Berke, P. Dehertogh, E. Fransen, E. Cleiren, L. van der Helm, G. Fanning,

O. Nyanguile, K. Simmen, P. Van Remoortere, P. Raboisson and S. Vendeville, *J. Med. Chem.*, 2014, **57**, 1880.

51. X. C. Sheng, A. Casarez, R. Cai, M. O. Clarke, X. Chen, A. Cho, W. E. Delaney 4th, E. Doerffler, M. Ji, M. Mertzman, R. Pakdaman, H. J. Pyun, T. Rowe, Q. Wu, J. Xu and C. U. Kim, *Bioorg. Med. Chem. Lett.*, 2012, **22**, 1394.

52. S. Zeuzem, P. Buggisch, K. Agarwal, P. Marcellin, D. Sereni, H. Klinker, C. Moreno, J. P. Zarski, Y. Horsmans, H. Mo, S. Arterburn, S. Knox, D. Oldach, J. G. McHutchison, M. P. Manns and G. R. Foster, *Hepatology*, 2012, **55**, 749.

53. I. H. Shih, I. Vliegen, B. Peng, H. Yang, C. Hebner, J. Paeshuyse, G. Pürstinger, M. Fenaux, Y. Tian, E. Mabery, X. Qi, G. Bahador, M. Paulson, L. S. Lehman, S. Bondy, W. Tse, H. Reiser, W. A. Lee, U. Schmitz, J. Neyts and W. Zhong, *Antimicrob. Agents Chemother.*, 2011, **55**, 4196.

54. N. J. Liverton, S. S. Carroll, J. Dimuzio, C. Fandozzi, D. J. Graham, D. Hazuda, M. K. Holloway, S. W. Ludmerer, J. A. McCauley, C. J. McIntyre, D. B. Olsen, M. T. Rudd, M. Stahlhut and J. P. Vacca, *Antimicrob. Agents Chemother.*, 2010, **54**, 305.

55. E. Lawitz, M. Rodriguez-Torres, A. Stoehr, E. J. Gane, L. Serfaty, S. Bhanja, R. J. Barnard, D. An, J. Gress, P. Hwang and N. Mobashery, *J. Hepatol.*, 2013, **59**, 11.

56. M. P. Manns, E. Gane, M. Rodriguez-Torres, A. Stoehr, C. T. Yeh, P. Marcellin, R. T. Wiedmann, P. M. Hwang, L. Caro, R. J. Barnard and A. W. Lee, *Hepatology*, 2012, **56**, 884.

57. V. Summa, S. W. Ludmerer, J. A. McCauley, C. Fandozzi, C. Burlein, G. Claudio, P. J. Coleman, J. M. Dimuzio, M. Ferrara, M. Di Filippo, A. T. Gates, D. J. Graham, S. Harper, D. J. Hazuda, C. McHale, E. Monteagudo, V. Pucci, M. Rowley, M. T. Rudd, A. Soriano, M. W. Stahlhut, J. P. Vacca, D. B. Olsen, N. J. Liverton and S. S. Carroll, *Antimicrob. Agents Chemother.*, 2012, **56**, 4161.

58. C. A. Coburn, P. T. Meinke, W. Chang, C. M. Fandozzi, D. J. Graham, B. Hu, Q. Huang, S. Kargman, J. Kozlowski, R. Liu, J. A. McCauley, A. A. Nomeir, R. M. Soll, J. P. Vacca, D. Wang, H. Wu, B. Zhong, D. B. Olsen and S. W. Ludmerer, *ChemMedChem*, 2013, **8**, 1930.

59. M. Llinàs-Brunet, M. D. Bailey, N. Goudreau, P. K. Bhardwaj, J. Bordeleau, M. Bös, Y. Bousquet, M. G. Cordingley, J. Duan, P. Forgione, M. Garneau, E. Ghiro, V. Gorys, S. Goulet, T. Halmos, S. H. Kawai, J. Naud, M. A. Poupart and P. W. White, *J. Med. Chem.*, 2010, **53**, 6466.

60. P. W. White, M. Llinàs-Brunet, M. Amad, R. C. Bethell, G. Bolger, M. G. Cordingley, J. Duan, M. Garneau, L. Lagacé, D. Thibeault and G. Kukolj, *Antimicrob. Agents Chemother.*, 2010, **54**, 4611.

61. K. Rutter, H. Hofer, S. Beinhardt, M. Dulic, M. Gschwantler, A. Maieron, H. Laferl, A. F. Stättermayer, T. M. Scherzer, R. Strassl, H. Holzmann, P. Steindl-Munda and P. Ferenci, *Aliment. Pharmacol. Ther.*, 2013, **38**, 118.

62. M. S. Sulkowski, T. Asselah, J. Lalezari, P. Ferenci, H. Fainboim, B. Leggett, F. Bessone, S. Mauss, J. Heo, Y. Datsenko, J. O. Stern, G. Kukolj, J. Scherer, G. Nehmiz, G. G. Steinmann and W. O. Böcher, *Hepatology*, 2013, **57**, 2143.

63. S. Zeuzem, T. Asselah, P. Angus, J. P. Zarski, D. Larrey, B. Müllhaupt, E. Gane, M. Schuchmann, A. W. Lohse, S. Pol, J. P. Bronowicki, S. Roberts, K. Arasteh, F. Zoulim, M. Heim, J. O. Stern, G. Nehmiz, G. Kukolj, W. O. Böcher and F. J. Mensa, *Antivir. Ther.*, 2013, **18**, 1015.

64. S. R. Laplante, M. Bös, C. Brochu, C. Chabot, R. Coulombe, J. R. Gillard, A. Jakalian, M. Poirier, J. Rancourt, T. Stammers, B. Thavonekham, P. L. Beaulieu, G. Kukolj and Y. S. Tsantrizos, *J. Med. Chem.*, 2014, **57**, 1845.

65. F. McPhee, A. K. Sheaffer, J. Friborg, D. Hernandez, P. Falk, G. Zhai, S. Levine, S. Chaniewski, F. Yu, D. Barry, C. Chen, M. S. Lee, K. Mosure, L. Q. Sun, M. Sinz, N. A. Meanwell, R. J. Colonno, J. Knipe and P. Scola, *Antimicrob. Agents Chemother.*, 2012, **56**, 5387.

66. A. S. Lok, D. F. Gardiner, C. Hézode, E. J. Lawitz, M. Bourlière, G. T. Everson, P. Marcellin, M. Rodriguez-Torres, S. Pol, L. Serfaty, T. Eley, S. P. Huang, J. Li, M. Wind-Rotolo, F. Yu, F. McPhee, D. M. Grasela and C. Pasquinelli, *J. Hepatol.*, 2014, **60**, 490.

67. J. P. Bronowicki, S. Pol, P. J. Thuluvath, D. Larrey, C. T. Martorell, V. K. Rustgi, D. W. Morris, Z. Younes, M. W. Fried, M. Bourlière, C. Hézode, K. R. Reddy, O. Massoud, G. A. Abrams, V. Ratziu, B. He, T. Eley, A. Ahmad, D. Cohen, R. Hindes, F. McPhee, B. Reilly, P. Mendez and E. Hughes, *Antivir. Ther.*, 2013, **18**, 885.

68. R. G. Gentles, M. Ding, J. A. Bender, C. P. Bergstrom, K. Grant-Young, P. Hewawasam, T. Hudyma, S. Martin, A. Nickel, A. Regueiro-Ren, Y. Tu, Z. Yang, K. S. Yeung, X. Zheng, S. Chao, J. H. Sun, B. R. Beno, D. M. Camac, C. H. Chang, M. Gao, P. E. Morin, S. Sheriff, J. Tredup, J. Wan, M. R. Witmer, D. Xie, U. Hanumegowda, J. Knipe, K. Mosure, K. S. Santone, D. D. Parker, X. Zhuo, J. Lemm, M. Liu, L. Pelosi, K. Rigat, S. Voss, Y. Wang, Y. K. Wang, R. J. Colonno, M. Gao, S. B. Roberts, Q. Gao, A. Ng, N. A. Meanwell and J. F. Kadow, *J. Med. Chem.*, 2014, **57**, 1855.

69. X. C. Sheng, T. Appleby, T. Butler, R. Cai, X. Chen, A. Cho, M. O. Clarke, J. Cottell, W. E. Delaney 4th, E. Doerffler, J. Link, M. Ji, R. Pakdaman, H. J. Pyun, Q. Wu, J. Xu and C. U. Kim, *Bioorg. Med. Chem. Lett.*, 2012, **22**, 2629.

70. H. Yang, M. Robinson, A. C. Corsa, B. Peng, G. Cheng, Y. Tian, Y. Wang, R. Pakdaman, M. Shen, X. Qi, H. Mo, C. Tay, S. Krawczyk, X. C. Sheng, C. U. Kim, C. Yang and W. E. Delaney 4th, *Antimicrob. Agents Chemother.*, 2014, **58**, 647.

71. E. J. Lawitz, J. M. Hill, T. Marbury, M. P. Demicco, W. Delaney, J. Yang, L. Moorehead, A. Mathias, H. Mo, J. G. McHutchison, M. Rodriguez-Torres and S. C. Gordon, *Antivir. Ther.*, 2013, **18**, 311.

72. A. F. Carrion, J. Gutierrez and P. Martin, *Expert Opin. Pharmacother.*, 2014, **15**, 711.
73. K. V. Kowdley, E. Lawitz, F. Poordad, D. E. Cohen, D. R. Nelson, S. Zeuzem, G. T. Everson, P. Kwo, G. R. Foster, M. S. Sulkowski, W. Xie, T. Pilot-Matias, G. Liossis, L. Larsen, A. Khatri, T. Podsadecki and B. Bernstein, *N. Engl. J. Med.*, 2014, **370**, 222.
74. D. A. Degoey, J. T. Randolph, D. Liu, J. Pratt, C. Hutchins, P. Donner, A. C. Krueger, M. Matulenko, S. Patel, C. E. Motter, L. Nelson, R. Keddy, M. Tufano, D. D. Caspi, P. Krishnan, N. Mistry, G. Koev, T. J. Reisch, R. Mondal, T. Pilot-Matias, Y. Gao, D. W. Beno, C. J. Maring, A. Molla, E. Dumas, A. Campbell, L. Williams, C. Collins, R. Wagner and W. M. Kati, *J. Med. Chem.*, 2014, **57**, 2047.
75. F. Poordad, E. Lawitz, K. V. Kowdley, D. E. Cohen, T. Podsadecki, S. Siggelkow, M. Heckaman, L. Larsen, R. Menon, G. Koev, R. Tripathi, T. Pilot-Matias and B. Bernstein, *N. Engl. J. Med.*, 2013, **368**, 45.
76. A. Agarwal, B. Zhang, E. Olek, H. Robison, L. Robarge and M. Deshpande, *Antivir. Ther.*, 2012, **17**, 1533.
77. S. Venkatraman and F. G. Njoroge, *Curr. Top. Med. Chem.*, 2007, **7**, 1290.
78. S. Avolio and V. Summa, *Curr. Top. Med. Chem.*, 2010, **10**, 1403.
79. Y. S. Tsantrizos, *Acc. Chem. Res.*, 2008, **41**, 1252.
80. P. W. White, M. Llinas-Brunet and M. Bos, *Prog. Med. Chem.*, 2006, **44**, 65.
81. Venkatraman, W. Wu, A. Prongay, V. Girijavallabhan and G. T. Njoroge, *Bioorg. Med. Chem. Lett.*, 2009, **19**, 180.
82. P. G. Richardson, C. Mitsiades, T. Hideshima and K. C. Anderson, *Annu. Rev. Med.*, 2006, **57**, 33.
83. S. J. Baker, Y.-K. Zhang, T. Akama, A. Lau, H. Zhou, V. Hernandez, W. Mao, M. R. K. Alley, V. Sanders and J. J. Plattner, *J. Med. Chem.*, 2006, **49**, 4447.
84. T. Akama, S. J. Baker, Y.-K. Zhang, V. Hernandez, H. Zhou, V. Sanders, Y. Freund, R. Kimura, K. R. Maples and J. J. Plattner, *Bioorg. Med. Chem. Lett.*, 2009, **19**, 2129.
85. V. Hernandez, T. Crépin, A. Palencia, S. Cusack, T. Akama, S. J. Baker, W. Bu, L. Feng, Y. R. Freund, L. Liu, M. Meewan, M. Mohan, W. Mao, F. L. Rock, H. Sexton, A. Sheoran, Y. Zhang, Y. K. Zhang, Y. Zhou, J. A. Nieman, M. R. Anugula, el. M. Keramane, K. Savariraj, D. S. Reddy, R. Sharma, R. Subedi, R. Singh, A. O'Leary, N. L. Simon, P. L. De Marsh, S. Mushtaq, M. Warner, D. M. Livermore, M. R. Alley and J. J. Plattner, *Antimicrob. Agents Chemother.*, 2013, **57**, 1394.
86. R. T. Jacobs, B. Nare, S. A. Wring, M. D. Orr, D. Chen, J. M. Sligar, M. X. Jenks, R. A. Noe, T. S. Bowling, L. T. Mercer, C. Rewerts, E. Gaukel, J. Owens, R. Parham, R. Randolph, B. Beaudet, C. J. Bacchi, N. Yarlett, J. J. Plattner, Y. Freund, C. Ding, T. Akama, Y.-K. Zhang, R. Brun, M. Kaiser, I. Scandale and R. Don, *PLoS Negl. Trop. Dis.*, 2011, **5**, e1151.

87. X. Li, Y.-K. Zhang, Y. Liu, C. Z. Ding, Q. Li, Y. Zhou, J. J. Plattner, S. J. Baker, X. Qian, D. Fan, L. Liao, Z.-J. Ni, G. V. White, J. E. Mordaunt, L. X. Lazarides, M. J. Slater, R. L. Jarvest, P. Thommes, M. Ellis, C. M. Edge, J. A. Hubbard, D. Somers, P. Rowland, P. Nassau, B. McDowell, T. J. Skarzynski, W. M. Kazmierski, R. M. Grimes, L. L. Wright, G. K. Smith, W. Zou, J. Wright and L. E. Pennicott, *Bioorg. Med. Chem. Lett.*, 2010, **20**, 3550.

88. X. Li, Y.-K. Zhang, Y. Liu, C. Z. Ding, Y. Zhou, Q. Li, J. J. Plattner, S. J. Baker, S. Zhang, W. M. Kazmierski, L. L. Wright, G. K. Smith, R. M. Grimes, R. M. Crosby, K. L. Creech, L. H. Carballo, M. J. Slater, R. L. Jarvest, P. Thommes, J. A. Hubbard, M. A. Convery, P. M. Nassau, W. McDowell, T. J. Skarzynski, X. Qian, D. Fan, L, Liao, Z.-J. Ni, L. E. Pennicott, W. Zou and J. Wright, *Bioorg. Med. Chem. Lett.*, 2010, **20**, 5695.

89. X. Li, Y. -K. Zhang, Y. Liu, S. Zhang, C. Z. Ding, Y. Zhou, J. J. Plattner, S. J. Baker, L. Liu, W. Bu, W. M. Kazmierski, L. L. Wright, G. K. Smith, R. L. Jarvest, M. Duan, J.-J. Ji, J. P. Cooper, M. D. Tallant, R. M. Crosby, K. Creech, Z. -J. Ni, W. Zou and J. Wright, *Bioorg. Med. Chem. Lett.*, 2010, **20**, 7493.

90. C. Z. Ding, Y.-K. Zhang, X. Li, Y. Liu, S. Zhang, Y. Zhou, J. J. Plattner, S. J. Baker, L. Liu, M. Duan, R. L. Jarvest, J. Ji, W. M. Kazmierski, M. D. Tallant, L. L. Wright, G. K. Smith, R. M. Crosby, A. A. Wang, Z.-J. Ni, W. Zou and J. Wright, *Bioorg. Med. Chem. Lett.*, 2010, **20**, 7317.

91. X. Li, S. Zhang, Y.-K. Zhang, Y. Liu, C. Z. Ding, Y. Zhou, J. J. Plattner, S. J. Baker, W. Bu, L. Liu, W. M. Kazmierski, M. Duan, R. M. Grimes, L. L. Wright, G. K. Smith, R. L. Jarvest, J. J. Ji, J. P. Cooper, M. D. Tallant, R. M. Crosby, K. Creech, Z. J. Ni, W. Zou and J. Wright, *Bioorg. Med. Chem. Lett.*, 2011, **21**, 2048.

92. M. Llinàs-Brunet, M. D. Bailey, E. Ghiro, V. Gorys, T. Halmos, M. Poirier, J. Rancourt and N. Goudreau, *J. Med. Chem.*, 2004, **47**, 6584.

93. Y. S. Tsantrizos, D. R. Cameron, A.-M. Faucher, E. Ghiro, N. Goudreau, T. Halmos and M. Llinas-Brunet, *Boehringer Ingelheim Ca Ltd, U.S. Pat. Appl.*, US 2004/0002448, 2010.

94. W. M. Kazmierski, R. Hamatake, M. Duan, L. L. Wright, G. K. Smith, R. L. Jarvest, J.-J. Ji, J. P. Cooper, M. D. Tallant, R. M. Crosby, K. Creech, X. Li, S. Zhang, Y.-K. Zhang, Y. Liu, C. Z. Ding, Y. Zhou, J. J. Plattner, S. J. Baker, W. Bu and L. Liu, *J. Med. Chem.*, 2012, **55**, 3021.

95. X. Li, Y. Liu, Y. K. Zhang, J. J. Plattner, S. J. Baker, W. Bu, L. Liu, Y. Zhou, C. Z. Ding, S. Zhang, W. M. Kazmierski, R. Hamatake, M. Duan, L. L. Wright, G. K. Smith, R. L. Jarvest, J. J. Ji, J. P. Cooper, M. D. Tallant, R. M. Crosby, K. Creech and A. Wang, *Bioorg. Med. Chem. Lett.*, 2012, **22**, 7351.

96. M. Duan, W. Kazmierski, R. Crosby, M. Gartland, J. Ji, M. Tallant, A. Wang, R. Hamatake, L. Wright, M. Wu, Y.-K. Zhang, C. Z. Ding, X. Li, Y. Liu, S. Zhang, Y. Zhou, J. J. Plattner and S. J. Baker, *Bioorg. Med. Chem. Lett.*, 2012, **22**, 2993.

97. M. S. Butler, M. A. Blaskovich and M. A. Cooper, *J. Antibiot.*, 2013, **66**, 571.
98. M. J. Sofia, W. Chang, P. A. Furman, R. T. Mosley and B. S. Ross, *J. Med. Chem.*, 2012, **55**, 2481.
99. M. D. Cummings, T.-I. Lin, L. Hu, A. Tahri, D. McGowan, K. Amssoms, S. Last, B. Devogelaere, M.-C. Rouan, L. Vijgen, J. M. Berke, P. Dehertogh, E. Fransen, E. Cleiren, L. van der Helm, G. Fanning, K. Van Emelen, O. Nyanguile, K. Simmen, P. Raboisson and S. Vendeville, *Angew. Chem. Int. Ed.*, 2012, **51**, 4637.
100. D. McGowan, S. Vendeville, T.-I Lin, A. Tahri, L. Hu, M. D. Cummings, K. Amssoms, J. M. Berke, M. Canard, E. Cleiren, P. Dehertogh, S. Last, E. Fransen, E. Van Der Helm, I. Van den Steen, L. Vijgen, M.-C. Rouan, G. Fanning, O. Nyanguile, K. Van Emelen, K. Simmen and P. Raboisson, *Bioorg. Med. Chem. Lett.*, 2012, **22**, 4431.
101. S. Vendeville, T.-I Lin, L. Hu, A. Tahri, D. McGowan, M. D. Cummings, K. Amssoms, M. Canard, S. Last, I. Van den Steen, B. Devogelaere, M.-C. Rouan, L. Vijgen, J. M. Berke, P. Dehertogh, E. Fransen, E. Cleiren, L. van der Helm, G. Fanning, K. Van Emelen, O. Nyanguile, K. Simmen and P. Raboisson, *Bioorg. Med. Chem. Lett.*, 2012, **22**, 4437.
102. J. Mallinson and I. Collins, *I. Future Med. Chem.*, 2012, **4**, 1409.
103. E. Marsault and M. L. Peterson, *J. Med. Chem.*, 2011, **54**, 1961.
104. E. M. Driggers, S. P. Hale, J. Lee and N. K. Terrett, *Nat. Rev. Drug Discov.*, 2008, 7, 608.
105. S. Hanessian, A. Larsson, T. Fex, W. Knecht and N. Blomberg, *Bioorg. Med. Chem. Lett.*, 2010, **20**, 6925.
106. B. G. Stuart, J. M. Coxon, J. D. Morton, A. D. Abell, D. Q. McDonald, S. G. Aitken, M. A. Jones and R. Bickerstaffe, *J. Med. Chem.*, 2011, **54**, 7503.
107. A. K. Ghosh, S. Kulkarni, D. D. Anderson, L. Hong, A. Baldridge, Y. F. Wang, A. A. Chumanevich, A. Y. Kovalevsky, Y. Tojo, M. Amano, Y. Koh, J. Tang, I. T. Weber and H. Mitsuya, *J. Med. Chem.*, 2009, **52**, 7689.
108. Y. Huang, E. D. Strobel, C. Y. Ho, C. H. Reynolds, K. A. Conway, J. A. Piesvaux, D. E. Brenneman, G. J. Yohrling, H. M. Arnold, D. Rosenthal, R. S. Alexander, B. A. Tounge, M. Mercken, M. Vandermeeren, M. H. Parker, A. B. Reitz and E. W. Baxter, *Bioorg. Med. Chem. Lett.*, 2010, **20**, 3158.
109. S. J. Stachel, C. A. Coburn, S. Sankaranarayanan, E. A. Price, B. L. Pietrak, Q. Huang, J. Lineberger, A. S. Espeseth, L. Jin, J. Ellis, M. K. Holloway, S. Munshi, T. Allison, D. Hazuda, A. J. Simon, S. L. Graham and J. P. Vacca, *J. Med. Chem.*, 2006, **49**, 6147.
110. L. D. Pennington, D. A. Whittington, M. D. Bartberger, S. R. Jordan, H. Monenschein, T. T. Nguyen, B. H. Yang, Q. M. Xue, F. Vounatsos, R. C. Wahl, K. Chen, S. Wood, M. Citron, V. F. Patel, S. A. Hitchcock and W. Zhong, *Bioorg. Med. Chem. Lett.*, 2013, **23**, 4459.

111. V. Sandgren, T. Agback, P. O. Johansson, J. Lindberg, I. Kvarnström, B. Samuelsson, O. Belda and A. Dahlgren, *Bioorg. Med. Chem.*, 2012, **20**, 4377.
112. C. Sund, O. Belda, D. Wiktelius, C. Sahlberg, L. Vrang, S. Sedig, E. Hamelink, I. Henderson, T. Agback, K. Jansson, N. Borkakoti, D. Derbyshire, A. Eneroth and B. Samuelsson, *Bioorg. Med. Chem. Lett.*, 2011, **21**, 358.

CHAPTER 8

Macrocyclic Inhibitors of GPCR's, Integrins and Protein–Protein Interactions[†]

PHILIPP ERMERT,[a] KERSTIN MOEHLE[b] AND
DANIEL OBRECHT*[a]

[a] Polyphor Ltd, Hegenheimermattweg 125, CH-4123, Allschwil, Switzerland;
[b] University of Zurich, Winterthurerstrasse 190, CH-8057, Zurich,
Switzerland
*Email: daniel.obrecht@polyphor.com

8.1 Macrocycles Are Privileged Structures in Drug Discovery

In recent years medium-sized natural and synthetic macrocycles in the molecular weight range of ~ 500–4000 Daltons have sparked renewed interest in the pharmaceutical industry particularly in their quest to address difficult therapeutic targets including extra- and intra-cellular protein–protein interactions. The expectations are that macrocycles, due to their size, semi-rigid nature and special ADME properties, may bridge an important gap in the diversity space between small molecules and large biopharmaceuticals. Several excellent reviews describing the privileged properties of medium-sized macrocycles for drug discovery have appeared.[1–4] Important attributes of such macrocycles are their increased propensity to bind

[†] Dedicated to Sir Jack Baldwin, FRS. In memory of Professor Dr Robert E. Ireland.

RSC Drug Discovery Series No. 40
Macrocycles in Drug Discovery
Edited by Jeremy Levin
© The Royal Society of Chemistry 2015
Published by the Royal Society of Chemistry, www.rsc.org

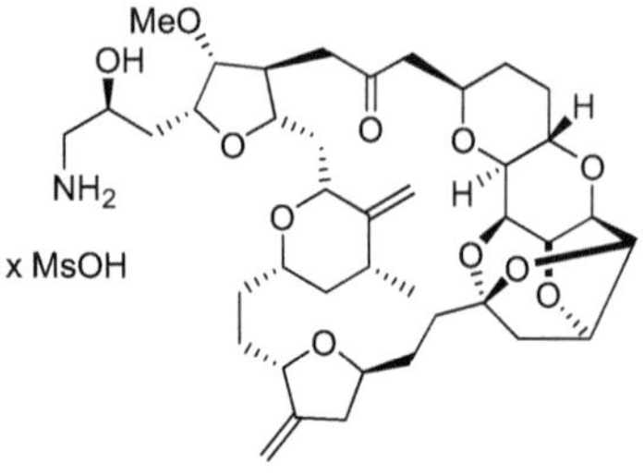

1 (Eribulin mesylate, Halaven)

Figure 8.1

specifically to larger and dynamic protein surfaces due to their size and semi-rigid nature compared to small molecules.[1] These attributes are well known to translate into drug-like properties well beyond the "Rule of 5" as exemplified in several cases.[2]

Macrocyclic natural products have been a rich source of inspiration for drug discovery for many decades and have provided a number of important drugs, especially in the anti-infective[4,5] and anticancer[6] therapeutic areas (see Chapter 1). However, from a medicinal chemistry point of view natural product drug discovery has also been extremely challenging, laborious and costly as exemplified by the discovery of eribulin (**1**) (Halaven™,[7] Figure 8.1). Renewed interest in macrocyclic natural product-inspired medicinal chemistry is nurtured by successful applications of powerful macrocycle-based hit finding technologies in combination with elaborated, modular high throughput macrocycle synthesis technologies yielding natural product-like complexity without compromising efficiency of compound optimization in medicinal chemistry or, at later stages, in scale-up for pre-clinical and clinical development.[1–4]

This chapter will focus on macrocyclic approaches targeting GPCRs, integrins and protein–protein interactions. Several of the successful approaches shown are based on cyclic peptides and cyclic peptide mimetics mimicking the bioactive conformations of the native peptide ligands. Approaches where non-peptide based macrocycles were developed will also be discussed. Several examples will highlight the semi-rigid nature of macrocycles where bound (bioactive) and unbound conformations differ significantly. It is most likely the conformational semi-rigidity, in addition to other attributes, that make macrocycles special for addressing complex biological targets.

8.2 Classes of Macrocycles

8.2.1 Cyclic Peptides and Depsipeptides; Cyclic Peptide Mimetics

Among the macrocyclic natural and synthetic drugs the cyclic peptides[8] and cyclic depsipeptides[9] play a central role in particular as anti-infective[4,5] and

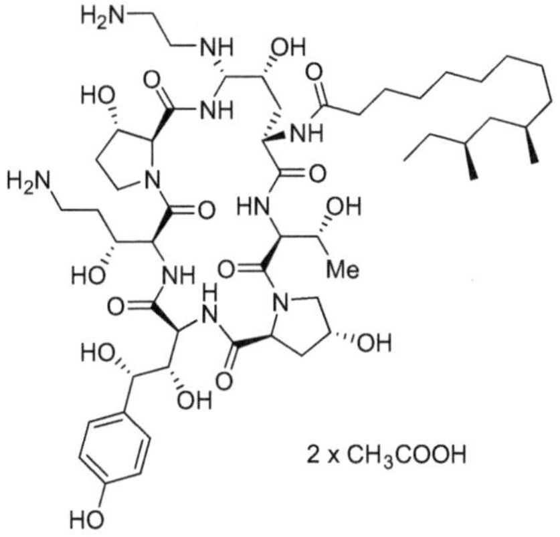

2 (Caspofungin; CANCIDAS)

Figure 8.2

anti-cancer drugs.[6] Compounds such as vancomycin, daptomycin, colistin, caspofungin (**2**, Figure 8.2), cyclosporine A, FK506, rapamycin, didemnin B are only a few well known examples.[1,4] Cyclic peptides and depsipeptides are generally synthesized by nature and by man as linear precursors through the modular assembly of simple key building blocks (amino acids, hydroxy-acids) using high yielding coupling reactions. However, it is only after cyclization of the generally unstructured linear precursors into the macro-cyclic analogs that the molecules adopt their bioactive conformations. Na-ture's fundamental principle to restrict conformations by cyclization is also found in polyketides (macrolides) and terpenoids (steroids). The synthesis of conformationally constrained peptides through backbone or side-chain cyclization became popular in the early 1980s.[10,11] Early work focused on constraining the unstructured natural linear peptidergic GPCR ligands (5–30 amino acids) into their bioactive, usually β-turn-like or α-helix-like, con-formations by means of cyclization.[10] Several successful examples of these approaches will be presented in Section 8.3. Also, several macrocyclic ap-proaches focusing on the design and synthesis of entire functional epitopes, such as mimetics of β-hairpins (see Section 8.2.2)[12,13] and α-helices will be highlighted.

8.2.2 Protein Epitope Mimetics (PEM)

An important class of peptide-derived macrocycles mimicking an entire functional epitope are Protein Epitope Mimetics (PEMs)[12,13] of the general formula **3** (Figure 8.3). PEM molecules are cyclopeptide-like molecules composed of a conformation-inducing template and a peptide chain of 4–20 amino acids, mimicking β-hairpin- and α-helical functional epitopes of proteins, the most important exposed protein epitopes involved in many

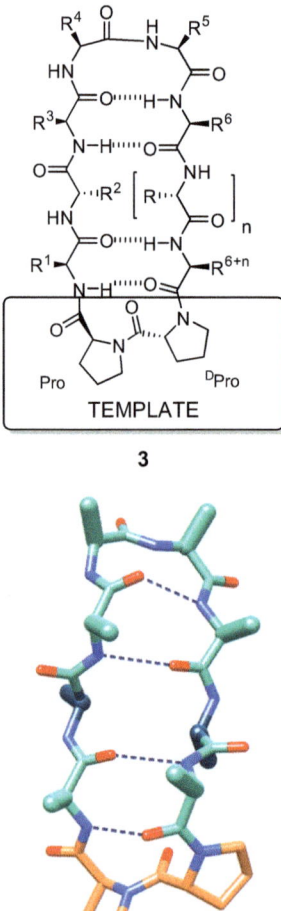

Figure 8.3 NMR structure of a template-bound β-hairpin mimetic. The side chains
are represented as Cα-Cβ cylinders pointing up and down (turquoise).
Hydrogen bonds are represented with dotted lines.

protein–protein interactions. The technology is very versatile and offers
many possibilities for varying the ring size, the amino acid building blocks
including amino acid isosteres, and finally the template in order to modulate activity, selectivity and ADME properties of the PEM molecules.[12]

The hairpin scaffold can also be exploited to mimic naturally occurring α-
helical epitopes. It has been shown that the distances between the Cα atoms
of two residues, i and i+2, along one strand is very close to that between the
two Cα atoms of two residues, i and i+4, on one face of the helix. This
approach was successfully used to design and synthesize potent PEM inhibitors of the HDM2-p53 interaction.[14,15] Residues Phe(1), 6-Cl-Trp(3), and
Leu(4) in the PEM molecule 4 ($IC_{50} = 140$ nM, Figure 8.4) mimic the key
helical pharmacophore Phe(19), Trp(23) and Leu(26)[16] in the tumor

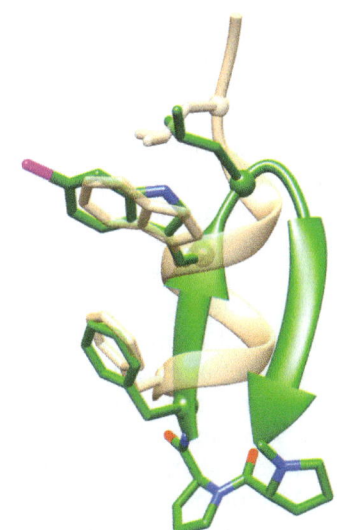

4; HDM2: IC$_{50}$ = 140 nM

Figure 8.4 Superposition of the X-ray crystal structures of HDM2 (not shown) in complex with a β-hairpin PEM molecule and p53 helical peptide.

suppressor p53 as determined by X-ray crystallography.[15] Inhibition of the p53-HDM2 interaction appears to be a promising strategy for increasing p53 associated tumor-suppressor activity in tumor cells.[17]

The PEM approach has been successfully applied to several drug discovery programs on different target classes such as GPCRs, proteases and transporters.[12] For example, transferring 7 or 11 residues of the Bowman-Birk reactive loop onto a ^{D}Pro-^{L}Pro template resulted in potent inhibitors of trypsin.[18] This PEM scaffold was recently used to generate a diverse library of serine protease inhibitors from which potent and highly selective inhibitors of human neutrophil elastase (hNE) were identified. Optimization of the initial hits led to POL6014 ($K_i = 1.4$ nM), which is a potent, selective and reversible inhibitor of hNE for use as an inhaled therapeutic for the treatment of lung diseases such as alpha-antitrypsin deficiency (AAT), cystic fibrosis (CF), acute lung injury (ALI), and chronic obstructive pulmonary disease (COPD).[19] POL6326 and POL7080, which successfully entered clinical development are discussed in Sections 8.3.4 and 8.5.7, respectively.

8.2.3   Non Peptide-based Macrocycles

Several approaches in the macrocyclic area have focused on the synthesis of macrocycles with backbones having a reduced number of peptide bonds in order to modulate physicochemical properties to obtain increased cell permeability and oral bioavailability. One of the first approaches was based on the general formula 5 (MATCH™, Figure 8.5), which integrates a tripeptide sequence and a tether into a macrocyclic structure.[20] The initial aim was to constrain key pharmacophores of peptidergic GPCR ligands (typically three amino acid residues) in order to find potent and selective GPCR modulators. Modulators of ghrelin (Section 8.3.8) and motilin (Section 8.3.11) will be discussed in more detail.

A further diversity-oriented approach to synthesize macrocyclic structures with natural product-like complexity using efficient, high-throughput synthesis was developed by researchers at the Broad Institute.[21,22] A 7936-membered library (individual compounds) consisting of all eight possible stereoisomers of the general formula 6 (Figure 8.6) was synthesized using solid-phase methodology on SynPhase lanterns. Simple chiral and achiral building blocks were systematically assembled using a build/couple/pair (B/C/P) strategy to obtain a maximally diverse set of macrocyclic compounds with natural product-like complexity.[22] This strategy was successfully applied for the synthesis of ML238 (7; Figure 8.6), a sub-nanomolar inhibitor of malaria parasite asexual blood-stage growth[23] (blood-stage malaria Dd2, $GI_{50} = 0.54$ nM).

Independently, the MacroFinder® technology platform was developed. This approach is based on non-peptidic macrocycles in the molecular weight range of 400–800 Da and was developed by Polyphor.[24] Macrocycles of ring

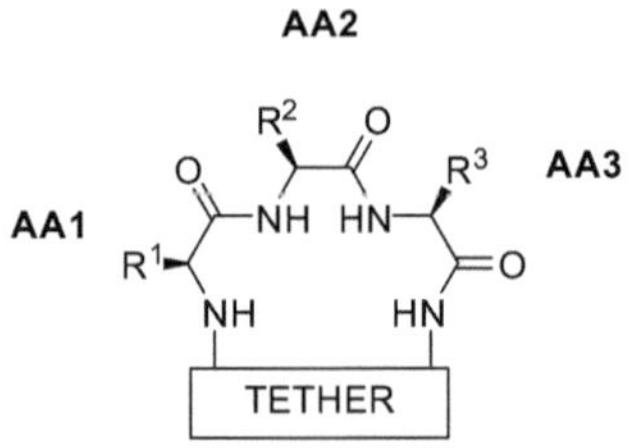

Figure 8.5

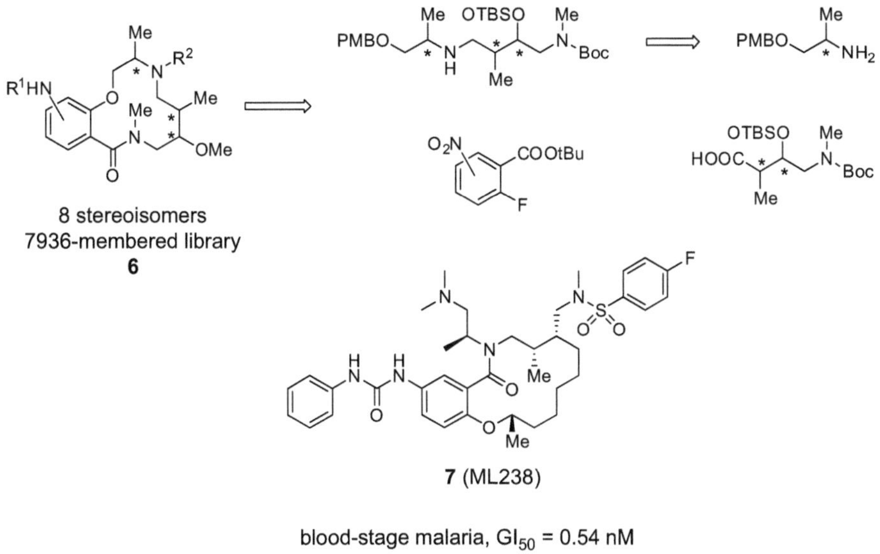

8 stereoisomers
7936-membered library
6

7 (ML238)

blood-stage malaria, GI_{50} = 0.54 nM

Figure 8.6

sizes of 12–30 are efficiently obtained by fully modular assembly of chiral and achiral building blocks using a high-throughput mixed solid phase/solution phase synthesis process. Special conformation-inducing building blocks (*e.g.* proline and o,m,p-substituted aromatic building blocks) are integrated into the macrocylic backbone in order to stabilize distinct backbone conformations, allowing a high degree of directed conformational fine tuning and positioning of appended substituents into β-turn-like and α-helix-like conformations. A highly diverse library of ~10 000 unique and individually purified macrocycles integrating several pharmacophores derived from ligands of GPCRs, ion channels and transporters, protease inhibitors, and modulators of protein–protein interactions, was successfully synthesized and tested against several therapeutically interesting targets. By screening a subset of the MacroFinder® library and follow-up of initial hits by parallel synthesis, the potent antagonist **8** (Figure 8.7) of the motilin receptor was identified after only two focused and fast rounds of optimization.

8.3 Macrocycles Targeting G-Protein Coupled Receptors (GPCRs)

8.3.1 Introduction

G-Protein-coupled receptors represent a large superfamily of signaling proteins composed of seven transmembrane helices, which can be grouped into three classes (class A: aminergic or rhodopsin-like; class B: secretin-like; C: neurotransmitter receptors).[25] The structural diversity of the natural ligands

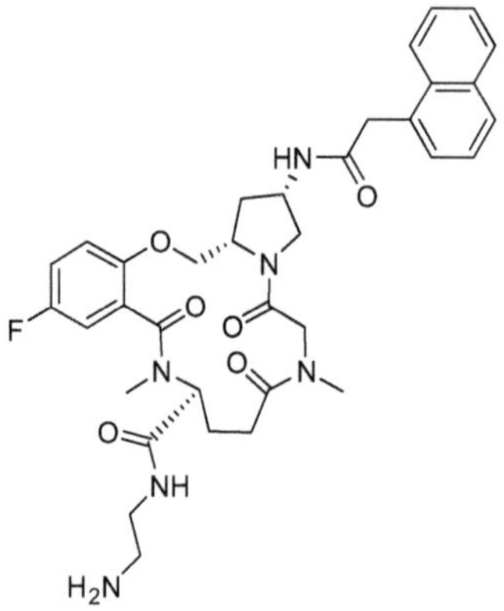

8 (Motilin receptor
antagonist, IC_{50} = 23 nM)

Figure 8.7

is high, comprising peptide and protein hormones (*e.g.* angiotensin, bradykinin, somatostatin), biogenic amines (*e.g.* adrenaline, serotonin, histamine), nucleosides and nucleotides (*e.g.* ATP, ADP), lipids and eicosanoids (*e.g.* leukotrienes, prostaglandins), and others.[26] There are several hundred GPCRs, excluding olfactory receptors, encoded in the human genome,[27] of which only about 30 represent targets for drugs that are currently on the market.[26] There are $\sim$160 orphan GPCRs for which the natural ligands are unknown. Whereas up to the 1980s GPCR drug discovery had been extremely successful ($\sim$25% of top-selling drugs target GPCRs), success stories in the era of high-throughput screening of large compound libraries were more scarce.[28] In the last five to six years remarkable progress in the structural biology of GPCRs has triggered a new era of structured-based GPCR drug design.[29] Crystal structures of the adenosineA2A receptor,[30] the D3 dopamine receptor,[31] the chemokine receptor CXCR4,[32] the histamine H1 receptor,[33] the sphingosine 1 phosphate receptor,[34] the muscarinic M2 and M3 receptors,[35,36] and most recently also the B-class receptors corticotropin-releasing factor receptor 1 (CRF_1R)[37] and the glucagon receptor ($GCGR$[38]) are key achievements in this respect.

As many peptidergic GPCR ligands are flexible linear peptides ($\sim$5–40 amino acid residues), cyclization strategies generating macrocyclic peptides[10,39] and peptidomimetics[40] in order to lock the ligands into the bioactive conformation have been extremely fruitful. In the following sections some of the most successful approaches and examples of macrocyclic GPCR modulators will be described.

8.3.2 Bradykinin Receptor Antagonists

Human bradykinin is a linear nonapeptide (Arg-Pro-Pro-Gly-Phe-Ser-Pro-Phe-Arg) that is released during inflammation and has several pharmacological effects.[25,41] In addition to algesic and pro-inflammatory effects bradykinin induces endothelium-dependent vasodilation and vascular and bronchial smooth muscle contraction.[42] Bradykinin mediates its actions *via* two GPCRs, designated B1 and B2. Most of the early inflammatory effects are related to the interaction with the B2 receptor. The four C-terminal residues of bradykinin (Ser-Pro-Phe-Arg) bound to the B2 receptor in the presence of dodecyl maltoside micelles (DDM; membrane-mimicking environment) adopt a β-turn conformation as determined by solid-state NMR spectroscopy.[43] Macrocyclic bradykinin antagonists mimicking the C-terminal β-turn have been designed, inspired by the structure of the linear peptide HOE140 ([D]Arg-Arg-Pro-Hyp-Gly-Thi-Ser-[D]Tic-Oic-Arg; $IC_{50} = 1.07$ nM; guinea pig ileum preparation),[44] synthesized and characterized.[42] For example, compound **14** (Figure 8.8) shows a pA_2 value of 7.4 (slope 1.11, rabbit jugular vein). NMR studies demonstrated that **14** adopts a type II' β-turn conformation in solution with the arginine NH forming a hydrogen bond with the carbonyl of the Thi residue thus demonstrating that macrocyclic peptides can be used to mimic β-turn conformations. Cyclo-peptide **14** shows selectivity for the B2 receptor with respect to the B1 receptor. Neither **14**, the cyclic analogs **12** and **13** (Table 8.1), nor the linear analogs **9**, **10** and **11** showed activity on B1 receptor preparations. Cycle size

Table 8.1 Bradykinin antagonist activity.[42]

Cpd	Structure	Rabbit jugular vein		Human umbilical vein
		pA_2 (pK_B)	slope	pK_B
9	Gly-Phe-[D]Tic-Oic-Arg	(6.07)		inactive at 10^{-5} M
10	Abu-Thi-[D]Tic-Oic-Arg	6.6	0.54	inactive at 10^{-5} M
11	Gly-Thi-[D]Tic-Oic-Arg	inactive at 10^{-5} M		4.79
12	c-[Gly-Phe-[D]Tic-Oic-Arg]	6.93	0.59	5.13
13	c-[Abu-Thi-[D]Tic-Oic-Arg]	6.49	0.89	inactive at 10^{-5} M
14	c-[Gly-Thi-[D]Tic-Oic-Arg]	7.39	1.11	4.93

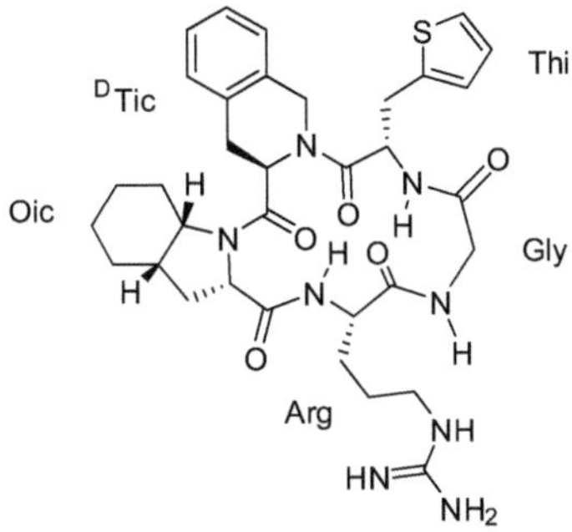

14 (Bradikinin receptor antagonist, pA_2 = 7.39; Sevier)

Figure 8.8

was important for activity. Replacement of the glycine in **14** by 4-aminobu-tyric acid (Abu) as in **13** resulted in an almost 10-fold loss of activity. A comparison of the pA$_2$ values of the cyclopeptides **12–14** determined on rabbit jugular vein with pK$_B$ values determined on human umbilical vein illustrates the large species differences for the potency of these compounds.

8.3.3 C5a Antagonists

The C5a anaphylatoxin and its receptor C5aR (CD88, a 350-residue GPCR) are important components of the complement system that plays a central role in the generation of innate and adaptive immune responses to in-fectious agents, foreign antigens, virus-infected cells, and tumor cells.[45] C5a induces expression of adhesion molecules and chemotaxis of C5aR-ex-pressing neutrophils, eosinophils, basophils, and monocytes and is associ-ated with several important immuno-inflammatory conditions. Disregulation of C5a is implicated in conditions such as rheumatoid arth-ritis and osteoarthritis, tissue graft rejection, psoriasis, ischemic heart dis-ease, gingivitis, atherosclerosis, fibrosis, cystic fibrosis, lung injury, systemic lupus erythematosus, reperfusion injury, septic and anaphylactic shock, burns, major trauma, adult respiratory distress syndrome, and Alzheimer's disease. Targeting the C5a/C5a receptor pair has been extremely chal-lenging,[46] leading to only one approved drug (eculizumab, an anti-C5a antibody)[45] during the last twenty years[47] despite significant efforts in pur-suing small molecules, peptides and antibodies.[45] Eculizumab (Soliris®) is a recombinant humanized monoclonal antibody and was approved in 2007 for the treatment of paroxysmal nocturnal hemoglobinuria (PMN).

C5a is a 74-amino acid glycoprotein. The structure in solution was found to be a 4-helix-bundle containing the receptor recognition domain with the C-terminus effector domain being responsible for receptor activation.[48–50] This latter domain was first described to be unstructured[48] and more re-cently to adopt an α-helical conformation spanning residues 69–74.[51] In-spired by these findings, macrocyclic peptides such as the derivative PMX-53 (**22**, Figure 8.9, Table 8.2) were developed.[52]

The linear hexapeptide **15** (Table 8.2) is a full antagonist that adopts a well defined structure in solution (DMSO) with an H-bond between ^{D}ChaNH and LysCO stabilizing an inverse γ-turn in a high population of conformers. The bulky side chain and the D-configuration of the cyclohexylalanine residue are important for antagonism.[49] Side-chain main-chain cyclization from Lys to the C-terminus resulted in the equipotent antagonist **16** (Table 8.2). Investigation of the structure activity relationship of a series of cyclic analogs of **15** demonstrated improved receptor affinity and antagonist potency for derivatives with ring sizes of 18 (cf. **18**) and 17 (cf. **19**), respectively. The most potent compounds, such as **22** (Table 8.2), contained Arg instead of ^{D}Arg as in compound **21**.[50] Further investigation of the structure activity relationship revealed a pharmacophore and demonstrated the importance of the pres-ence of an aromatic exocyclic residue (Phe or AcPhe) and that removal of the

Table 8.2 Structure–activity relationships of C5a antagonists.[50]

Cpd	Structure	Cycle size	Receptor affinity IC$_{50}$ [μM][a]	Antagonist potency IC$_{50}$ [μM][b]
15	MePhe-Lys-Pro-^{D}Cha-Trp-^{D}Arg	–	2.0	0.1
16	AcPhe-c[Lys-Pro-^{D}Cha-Trp-^{D}Arg]	19	3.2	0.1
17	Phe-c[Lys-Pro-^{D}Cha-Trp-Arg]	19	0.3	0.2
18	Phe-c[Orn-Pro-^{D}Cha-Trp-Arg]	18	0.06	0.03
19	Phe-c[Dab-Pro-^{D}Cha-Trp-Arg]	17	0.3	0.04
20	Phe-c[Dap-Pro-^{D}Cha-Trp-Arg]	16	10	2.4
21	AcPhe-c[Orn-Pro-^{D}Cha-Trp-^{D}Arg]	18	16	0.4
22	AcPhe-c[Orn-Pro-^{D}Cha-Trp-Arg]	18	0.3	0.02

[a]Concentration of peptide resulting in 50% inhibition of [^{125}I]C5a binding to intact polymorphonuclear leukocytes (PMNs).
[b]Concentration of peptide resulting in 50% inhibition of C5a (100 nM) induced release of myeloperoxidase from PMNs.

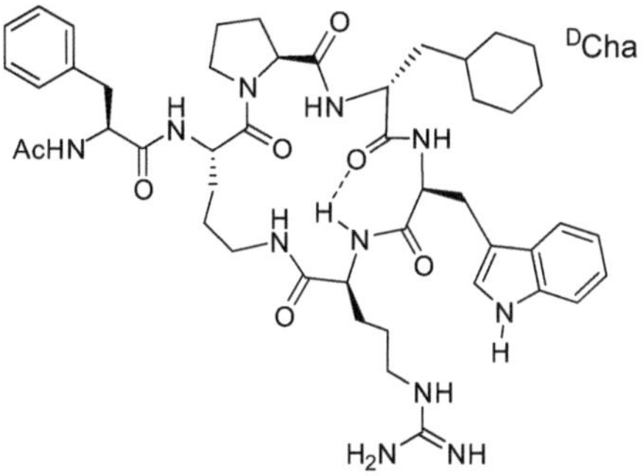

22 (PMX-53, 3D53), C5a antagonist,
receptor affinity: IC$_{50}$ = 0.3 μM,
antagonist potency: IC$_{50}$ = 0.02 μM

Figure 8.9

acetylated Phe resulted in complete loss of receptor affinity.[53] A comparison of NMR structures revealed that the turn conformations of the linear antagonist **15** as well as the terminal helical conformation of C5a are mimicked by the cyclic antagonist **22**.[53,49,50]

In a solution phase synthesis of cyclopeptide **22**, the macrolactam formation was achieved on a 100 g scale in 33% yield after RP-HPLC purification at a concentration of 10^{-1} M. The yield, however, was not improved by further dilution.[52]

The cyclopeptide **22** (PMX-53, 3D53) was described to be a receptor selective C5a antagonist,[50] stable to peptide degradation in blood or gastric fluid and orally active.[46,53,54] PMX-53 was assessed in several pre-clinical efficacy models of monoarticular arthritis, LPS-induced neutropenia, ulcerative colitis, dermal and peritoneal inflammation, and assorted ischemia/reperfusion injuries.[45] Furthermore, PMX-53 was well tolerated in Phase I clinical trials, both in healthy volunteers and in patients with psoriasis and arthritis.[55]

8.3.4   Chemokine Receptor Modulators: CXCR4

Chemokines (chemotactic cytokines) are small (5–20 kDa) proteins that regulate migration and adhesion of leukocytes[56,57] by binding to chemokine receptors. Currently more than 40 chemokines and 19 GPCRs are known and there is considerable redundancy in receptor–ligand interactions in the chemokine system. The importance of chemokines and chemokine receptors as pharmaceutical targets has grown considerably in recent years as they are key players in disease processes such as inflammation, autoimmune diseases, infectious diseases (HIV/AIDS), and cancer,[58,59] and a great number of chemokine antagonists have been described in the literature.[60] Although several chemokine receptor antagonists have progressed from discovery to the clinic, so far only maraviroc,[61] a CCR5 antagonist, and plerixafor (23, AMD3100, Figure 8.10),[62] a CXCR4 antagonist are registered as drugs.

The axis of CXCR4 and its unique ligand CXCL12 (SDF-1α) plays a critical role in embryogenesis of hematopoietic, nerve and endothelial tissues by regulation of tissue progenitor cell migration, homing and survival.[63] The CXCR4-CXCL12 axis is important in HIV, stem cell mobilization, autoimmune diseases, cancer[64] and tissue regeneration, and therefore modulators could have various important applications.[58] Several inhibitors of CXCR4 have been described in comprehensive reviews,[58,65] They fall into two main classes: the bicyclams and cyclams[66] (*e.g.* AMD3100 (23), Figure 8.10), and cyclopeptide-derived macrocycles (*e.g.* FC-131 (24)[67] and POL3026 (28,

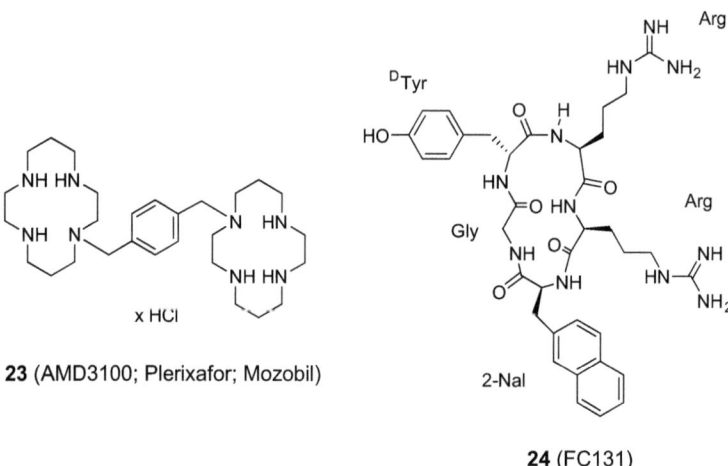

23 (AMD3100; Plerixafor; Mozobil)

24 (FC131)

Figure 8.10

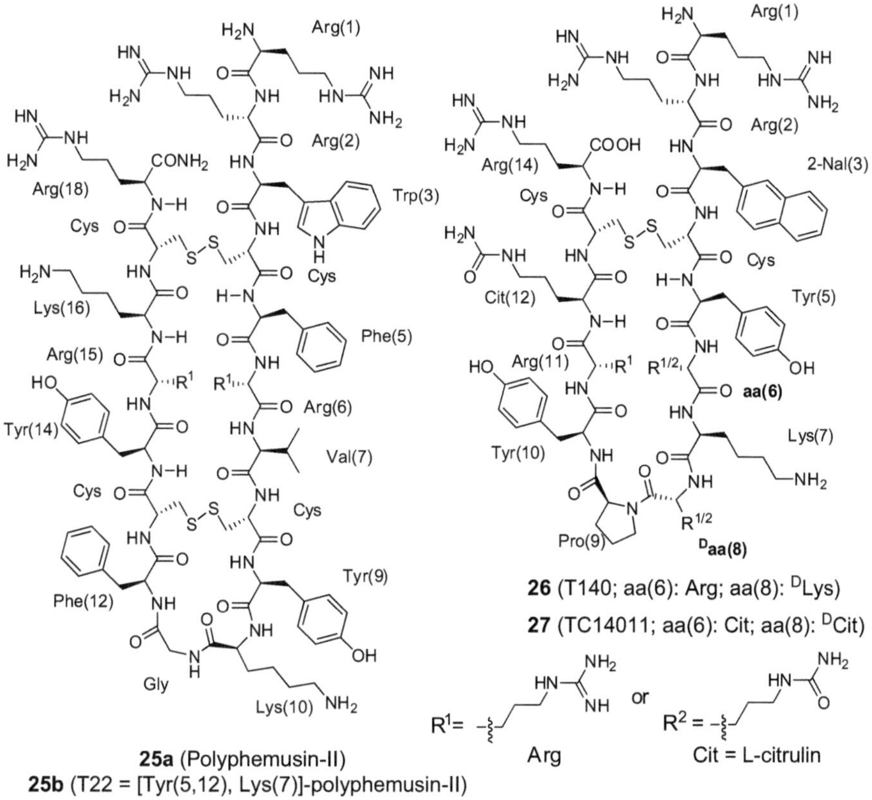

25a (Polyphemusin-II)
25b (T22 = [Tyr(5,12), Lys(7)]-polyphemusin-II)

26 (T140; aa(6): Arg; aa(8): ^{D}Lys)
27 (TC14011; aa(6): Cit; aa(8): ^{D}Cit)

Figure 8.11

Figure 8.12),[68] The discovery of polyphemusin II (**25a,** Figure 8.11), a naturally occurring 18-amino acid residue disulfide-bridged peptide isolated from the American horseshoe crab (*Limulus polyphemus*) and a closely related analog, T22 (**25b**),[69,70] triggered several investigations of macrocyclic peptide CXCR4 antagonists. These compounds adopt a β-hairpin conformation stabilized by two disulfide bonds as determined by NMR.[71] Subsequently, shortened analogs of T22 (**25b**) such as T140 (**26**) and TC14011(**27,** Figure 8.11)[72] were synthesized, which ultimately led to FC-131 and analogs.[73] The therapeutic potential of these early compounds was shown for the treatment of HIV,[74] cancer metastasis, and arthritis.[75]

The β-hairpin pharmacophore arrangement observed in polyphemusin II could be efficiently transplanted into a β-hairpin mimetic scaffold by applying PEM technology[12] (Section 8.2.2). After efficient optimization of activity and ADMET properties of the initial hits using high-throughput parallel synthesis, POL3026 (**28,** Figure 8.12) was obtained as a first highly potent ($IC_{50} = 1.2$ nM, Ca^{2+}-flux) and stable compound with favorable drug-like properties such as high stability in rat and human plasma ($t_{1/2} > 300$ Min.) and *in vivo* half life of 3.5 hours (sc administration of

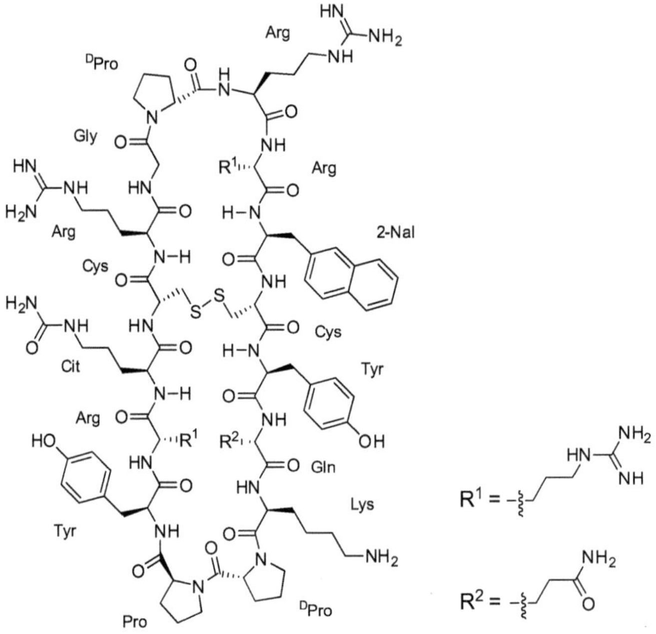

28 (POL3026)

Figure 8.12

1.5 mg kg^{-1} in beagle dogs).[68] The high potency was confirmed in a T-tropic HIV replication assay including a wide panel of T- and M- and T-dualtropic strains and subtypes in several culture models with EC$_{50}$ values in the sub-nanomolar range[68,76] making POL3026 (**28**) the most potent CXCR4 antagonist described to date. In an effort to progress compounds of the PEM CXCR4 series further, additional optimization rounds were performed and POL5551 and POL6326 were selected as the most promising candidates for testing in various animal models for efficacy, including stem cell mobilization and transplantation,[77,78] inhibition of neointimal hyperplasia in a murine model of stent implantation (wire injury),[79] and chemosensitization in hematological malignancies.[80] POL6326 (structure undisclosed) was finally selected as clinical candidate and progressed to the clinic for autologous hematopoetic stem cell (HSC) transplantation in multiple myeloma patients and interim results of the Phase II trial reveal that POL6326 is safe and well tolerated by all enrolled patients.[58,81]

8.3.5 Endothelin Antagonists

Endothelins (ET-1 to ET-3 and others) are a family of 21 amino acid residue peptides containing two conformationally constraining disulfide bonds.[25,41]

The endothelins interact with two endothelin receptors, ET_A and ET_B. Endothelins are highly potent vasoconstrictors and endothelin antagonists have the potential to be used clinically to treat pulmonary arterial hypertension (PAH), congestive heart failure, stroke, kidney failure, asthma, pain, and cancer.[82] The small molecule bosentan (Tracleer)[83] interacts with both ET_A and ET_B receptors and was the first endothelin antagonist to be used clinically for the treatment of PAH. Additional compounds are in clinical development or have reached the market.[82]

The residues 11–21 of ET adopt a helical structure placing the key pharmacophoric residues, Glu(10), Phe(14), Asp(18) and Trp(21), on one (α-helical) face as shown by X-ray structure.[41,84,85] NMR structures in various solvents also revealed a central helical region (residues 9–15) but, in contrast to the solid state structure, a flexible, structurally undefined C-terminal region (residues 16–21) was observed.[85]

The macrocyclic peptide BQ123 (**31**, Figure 8.13, Table 8.3), which mimics the key α-helical type I turn of the endothelins, was one of the first potent and specific ET_A antagonists described.[86,87] BQ123 exhibits an IC_{50} of 8.3 nM at the human ET_A receptor and an IC_{50} of 61 000 nM at the human ET_B receptor.[90] The pentapeptide analogs BE-18257A (**29**) and B (**30**) were isolated from the culture broth of *Streptomyces misakiensis*.[88,89] They inhibit the binding of [^{125}I]-ET-1 to the ET_A receptor with IC_{50} values (porcine smooth muscle membranes) of 3.0 and 1.4 μM, respectively.[86] Efforts to improve the potency and water solubility of these compounds resulted in the synthesis of potent, selective, and soluble ET_A receptor antagonists BQ-123 (**31**) and BQ-518 (**32**).[86,90]

In solution BQ-123 (**31**) adopts a single backbone conformation comprising a type II β-turn with Leu and ^{D}Trp as corner residues and an inverse γ-turn at proline.[91–94] Similar backbone conformations have been reported for the related peptides **29** and **30**.[87,90] The β,γ-backbone

Table 8.3 Selected activity and solubility data.[90]

Cpd	Structure	Receptor binding inhibition IC_{50} hET_A[b] [nM]	Receptor binding inhibition IC_{50} hET_B[c] [nM]	Antagonist Potency[g] pA$_2$	Solubility (Na salts in saline) [mg mL^{-1}]
29	c[^{D}Glu-Ala-^{D}Val-Leu-^{D}Trp]	(3000)[f]			
30	c[^{D}Glu-Ala-^{D}alloIle-Leu-^{D}Trp]	590	>100 000	5.9[d]	0.21
31	c[^{D}Asp-Pro-^{D}Val-Leu-^{D}Trp]	8.3	61 000	7.4[e]	>1000
32	c[^{D}Asp-Pro-^{D}Thg-Leu-^{D}Trp][a]	1.2	55 000	8.1[e]	4.0

[a]Thg = 2-(2-thienyl)glycine.
[b]Human neuroblastoma-derived cell-line SK-N-MC membranes.
[c]Human Girardi heart cell membranes.
[d]Rabbit iliac arteries.
[e]Porcine coronary arteries.
[f]Porcine aortic smooth muscle membranes.
[g]Antivasoconstriction.

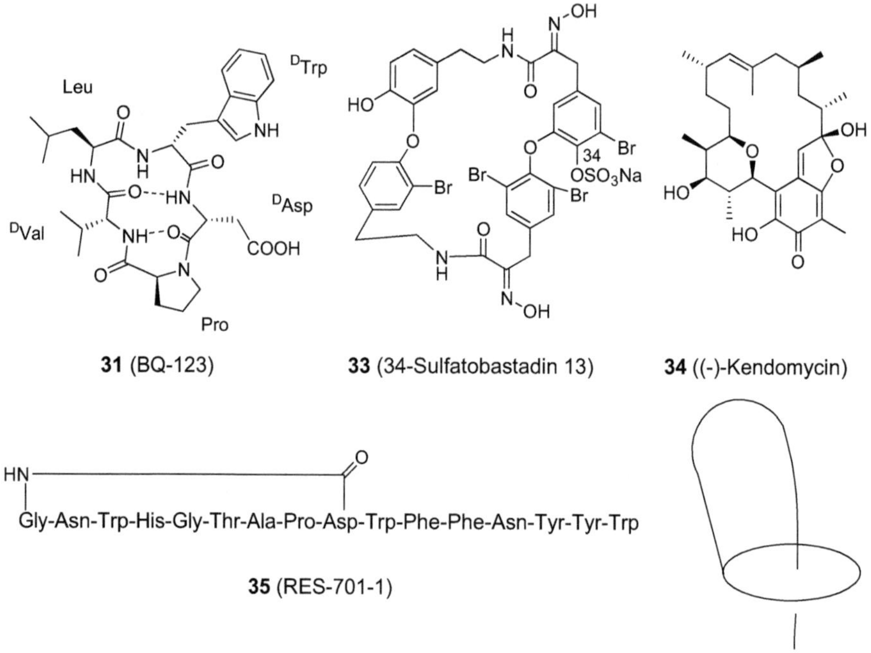

31 (BQ-123)   **33 (34-Sulfatobastadin 13)**   **34 ((-)-Kendomycin)**

35 (RES-701-1)

Figure 8.13

conformation has also been observed in other cyclic pentapetides, for example the C5a receptor antagonist **21**, as pointed out by Wong *et al.*,[49] and has been shown to be common for peptides with alternating L- and D-configured amino acids.

It was suggested that the cyclopeptides mimic the C-terminal part of the endothelins with the ^{D}Asp or ^{D}Glu side chain carboxylate assuming the role of the C-terminal carboxylate of endothelin which is important for binding.[87] Almost identical C-terminal sequences are seen for ET-1, ET-2 and ET-3.[84] The ET$_A$ receptor selectivity of the cyclopeptide antagonists was attributed to their ability to mimic a single conformation of the C-terminal region of endothelin.[87]

Two non-peptidic macrocyclic inhibitors of the ET$_A$ receptor have also been described. The bromotyrosine-derived macrolactam 34-sulfatobastadin 13 (**33**, Figure 8.13), isolated from the sponge *Ianthella* sp., weakly inhibits the binding of [^{125}I]-ET-1 to the ET$_A$ receptor with an IC$_{50}$ of 39 μM.[95] The polyketide (−)-kendomycin (**34**, TAN-2162, Figure 8.13) is a moderately potent inhibitor of both endothelin receptors (ET$_A$: IC$_{50}$ = 11.5 μM; ET$_B$: IC$_{50}$ = 2.9 μM), isolated from *Streptomyces* sp AL-71389.[96]

The class II lasso peptide RES-701-1 (**35**, Figure 8.13) is a potent ET$_B$ receptor selective antagonist which was isolated from the fermentation broth of *Streptomyces* sp. It inhibits the [^{125}I]-ET-1 binding to the ET$_B$ receptor expressed in CHO cells with IC$_{50}$ of 10 nM (ET$_A$: IC$_{50}$ > 5000 nM). It reduces intracellular Ca^{2+}-concentration induced by ET-1 in ET_B receptor expressing COS-7 cells.[97] RES-701-1 consists of 16 amino acids with a lactam bond between the N-terminal α-amino group of Gly(1) and the β-carboxylate of Asp(9) forming a 28-membered ring. With ^{1}H-NMR methods (DMSO) the remarkable folding of RES-701-1 was determined with the tail (Trp(10)–Trp(16)) passing through the ring region.[98]

8.3.6 Enkephalin Modulators

Enkephalins are natural penptapeptide (Tyr-Gly-Gly-Phe-Met = [Met]-enkephalin; Tyr-Gly-Gly-Phe-Leu = [Leu]-enkephalin) opioid receptor agonists with selectivity for the δ-opioid receptor (DOR) exhibiting morphine-like activity. δ-Selective agonists are expected to provide sufficient analgesic activity and reduced side effects as compared with morphine. Often, conformationally restricted peptides are more potent and selective than the more flexible linear parent peptides. Therefore, the search for δ-selective ligands included the synthesis of cyclic enkephalin analogs, which have been obtained through ring closure between a side-chain group and the C-terminal carboxyl group (*e.g.* 36 and 37, Figure 8.14) or between two side-chain groups (*e.g.* 38–44, Figure 8.14).

Lactam 36 was the first cyclic enkephalin analog prepared. It has a higher affinity for the μ-opioid receptor than for the δ-receptor.[99] The methylamine-bridged enkephalin (MABE) analog 37 exhibits nanomolar affinity for isolated μ- and δ-receptors and in an in vivo (rat) thermal escape assay an ED_{50} of 0.027 μg was determined, as compared with an ED_{50} of 2.4 μg for morphine.[100]

The cystine-bridged analog 38 shows good activity against both δ- and μ-receptors. Compound 39 (DPDPE), in contrast, is selective for the δ-receptor due to the presence of the *gem*-dimethyl groups of the β,β-dimethyl-Cys (penicillamine) residues.[101] The dicarba analogs of 38 were prepared by RCM of D-allylglycine residues and subsequent hydrogenation. The *cis*- (40a; hDOR binding $K_i = 0.43$ nM) and the *trans* isomer (40b; hDOR binding $K_i = 0.57$ nM)) show comparable, potent in vitro activities and binding affinities on both receptors with a slight, almost 10-fold, selectivity for the δ-receptor. The saturated product (40c) is 10-fold less potent.[102]

The mono-sulfide-bridged lanthionine enkephalin analogs 41–44 (Figure 8.14, Table 8.4) were described by Goodman and coworkers.[101,103] The functional *in vitro* activity of the compounds was found to parallel the binding affinities. The β,β-dimethyl group on the second residue is responsible for the δ-selectivity of 42 and 44. The D-configuration of the residue in position 5 increases the δ-selectivity in binding compared with the L-configuration. The δ-selective analogs 42 and 44 show weaker analgesic potency in a thermal escape assay than the non-selective analogs 41 and 43 that have picomolar potencies. This was interpreted[103] as an indication that the μ- and δ-receptors synergistically modulate the antinociceptive response.

Table 8.4 Selected activity data.[103]

Compound	K_i [nM][a] MOR	K_i [nM][a] DOR	K_i [nM][a] KOR	IC_{50} [nM] GPI[b]	IC_{50} [nM] MVD[b]	ED_{50} [nM][c]
41 H-Tyr-c[^{D}Ala$_L$- Gly-Phe-^{D}Ala$_L$]-OH	2.0	2.0	1600	0.56	1.58	0.0015
42 H-Tyr-c[^{D}Val$_L$- Gly-Phe-^{D}Ala$_L$]-OH	630	0.93	>10 000	730	2.33	0.26
43 H-Tyr-c[^{D}Ala$_L$- Gly-Phe-Ala$_L$]-OH	2.3	0.63	6400	1.06	0.35	0.0018
44 H-Tyr-c[^{D}Val$_L$- Gly-Phe-Ala$_L$]-OH	130	0.79	>1000	82	0.26	0.12
39 (DPDPE)	>10 000	2.2	>10 000	7300	4.1	130
morphine	17	150	260	59	644	15

[a]*In vitro* binding affinities at cloned receptors in CHO cell membranes; [^{3}H]-diprenorphine is reference ligand; MOR μ-opioid receptor; DOR δ-opioid receptor; KOR κ-opioid receptor.
[b]*In vitro* functional activity at guinea pig ileum (GPI) for μ-receptor and mouse vas deferens (MVD) for δ-receptors.
[c]*In vivo* activity; thermal escape latency assay.

8.3.7 *N*-Formyl Peptide Receptor 1 (FPR1) Antagonists

N-Formyl peptides are three to four amino acid-containing neutrophil and macrophage chemoattractant peptides (*e.g.* f-Met-Leu-Pro = fMLF) expressed by bacteria and humans which activate three GPCRs (FPR1, FPR2 and FPR3). FPR2 agonists have been widely described as potential agents with anti-inflammatory activity.[104] Recently, FPR1 has emerged as an important target in inflammation and human glioblastoma.[105] FPR1 was originally identified in phagocyctic leukocytes (neutrophils and monocytes) and mediates cell chemotaxis and activation in response to bacterial formylated chemotactic peptides. Hence, FPR1 plays an important role in the modulation of innate immune responses.[105] Furthermore, FPR1 has been described as one of the key receptors by which microbial pathogen-associated molecular patterns (PAMPs) activate innate immunocytes.[106] In contrast to agonists of FPR2, small molecule FPR1 antagonists are scarce.[107] Cyclosporin H (CsH; **45**, Figure 8.15), a close analog of the known immunosuppressive drug cyclosporine A (CsA; **46**) used in transplantation, is still the gold standard among the known FPR1 antagonists. CsH inhibits the binding of the agonist N-formyl-Met-Leu-Pro to FPR1 with an IC_{50} of 0.7 μM.[108] CsH was suggested to act as an inverse agonist.[109] Biological testing of 59 family members of the cyclosporin family in a standardized assay (with differentiated human leukemic cell line H-60 as FPR1-expressing cells and with *N*-acetyl-β-D-glucosaminidase release as readout) established a comprehensive structure activity relashionship, however, CsH remained the most potent compound in the series (IC_{50} = 0.15 μM).[110] Although CsH differs from CsA only at one position (^{D}MeVal(11) instead of MeVal(11); Figure 8.15), it is devoid of any of the immunosuppressive and antifungal activity of CsA. *N*10-desmethylated cyclosporins also showed good FPR1 activity, however, their conformations

side-chain C-terminus cyclized analogs

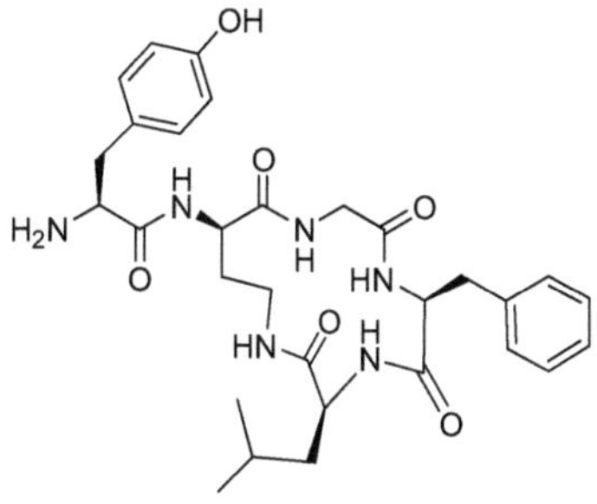

36 H-Tyr-c[^{D}Dab-Gly-Phe-Leu] 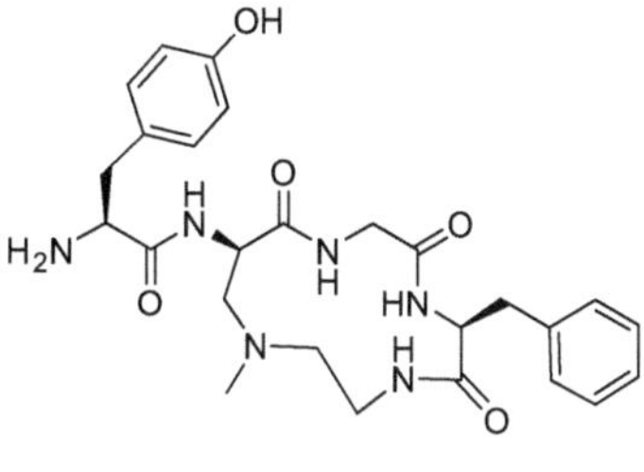   **37** (MABE)

disulfide-bridged analogs and their carba analogs

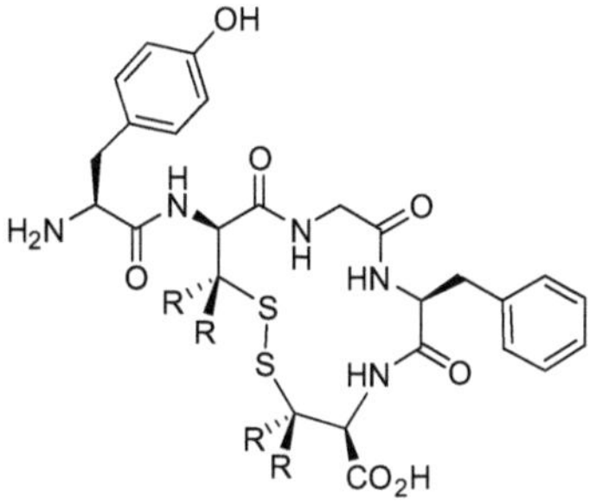

38 R = H; H-Tyr-c[^{D}Cys-Gly-Phe-^{D}Cys]-OH   **40**
39 (DPDPE) R = CH$_3$; H-Tyr-c[^{D}Pen-Gly-Phe-^{D}Pen]-OH

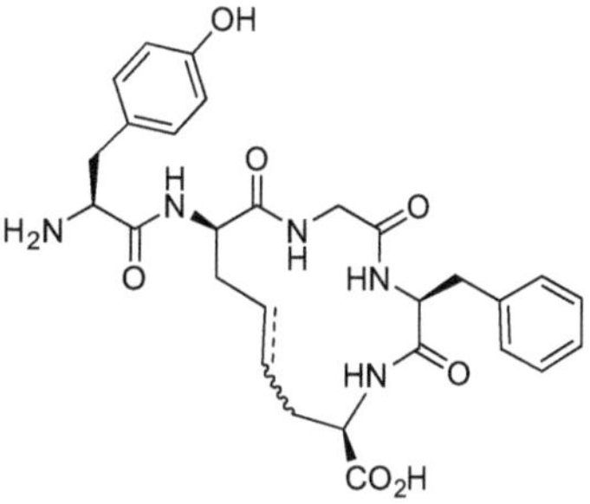

lanthionine analogs

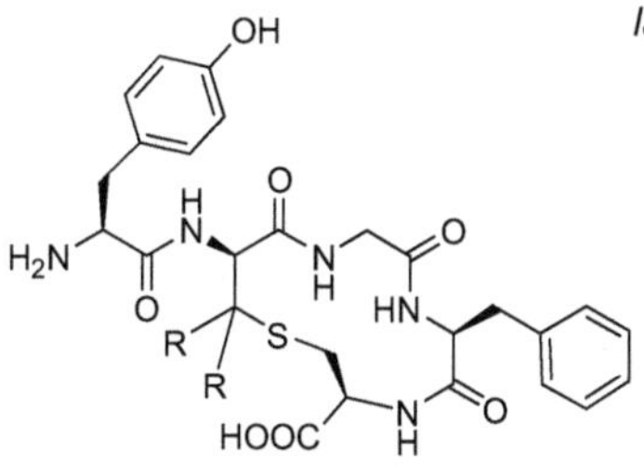

41 R = H; H-Tyr-c[^{D}Ala$_L$-Gly-Phe-^{D}Ala$_L$]-OH   **43** R = H;   H-Tyr-c[^{D}Ala$_L$-Gly-Phe-Ala$_L$]-OH
42 R = CH$_3$; H-Tyr-c[^{D}Val$_L$-Gly-Phe-^{D}Ala$_L$]-OH   **44** R = CH$_3$; H-Tyr-c[^{D}Val$_L$-Gly-Phe-Ala$_L$]-OH

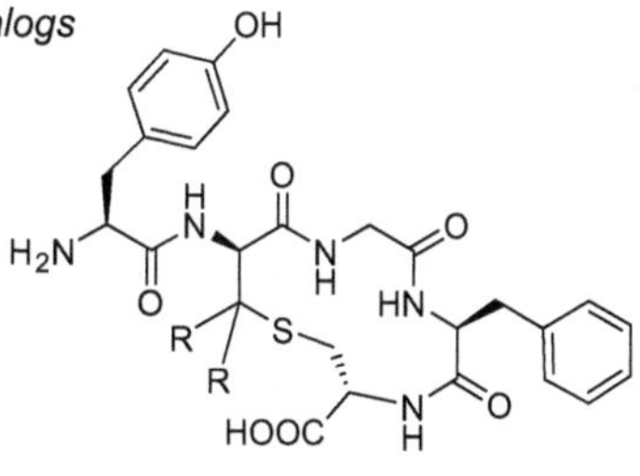

Figure 8.14

differed significantly from CsH, suggesting a different binding mode.[110] Synthetic analogs with FPR1 antagonist (or inverse agonist) activity have also been described in the patent literature, where mainly analogs of the MeBmt(1) (Figure 8.15) residue and small modifications at the Abu(2) and ^{D}Ala(8) positions (Figure 8.15)[111,112] or dihydroanalogs of CsH were prepared with comparable IC$_{50}$'s to CsH in the radionuclide binding assay (5–10 nM).[113]

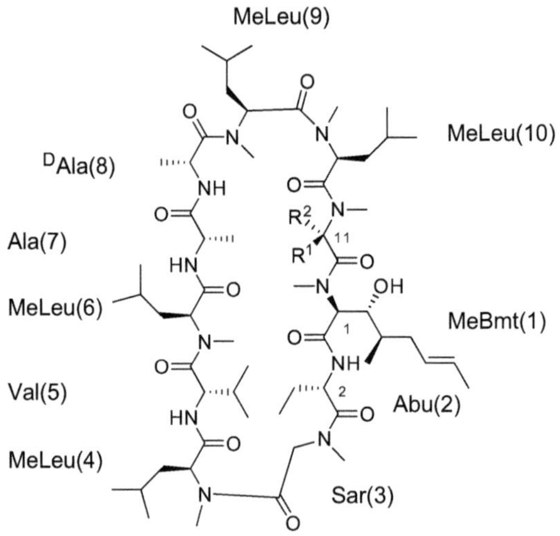

Cyclosporin H (**45**, R^1 = iPr; R^2 = H; ^{D}MeVal)
Cyclosporin A (**46**, R^1 = H; R^2 = iPr; MeVal)

Figure 8.15

8.3.8 Ghrelin Modulators

Ghrelin (GHRL; growth hormone secretagogue) is a 28-residue peptide that binds to the orphan growth hormone secretagogue receptor (GHS-R or GRLN)[114] and has an important role in the regulation of food intake.[25] Ghrelin is key to the proper function of the gut–brain–energy axis, is the only known natural orexigenic gastrointestinal peptide[2] and exhibits vasodilator activity in human vascular tissue. GHS-R also binds GHRP-6 and hexarelin.[115] Molecular modeling studies of GHRP-6 (His-^{D}Trp-Ala-Trp-^{D}Phe-Lys-NH$_2$) suggested a folded structure as a result of a β-turn conformation that was used to design compounds such as **47**, (L-692,429, mimetic of GHRP6; ED$_{50}$ = 60 nM; Figure 8.16) and a macrocyclic constrained analog **48** (ED$_{50}$ = 21 nM).[116–118]

An HTS screening campaign of a macrocyclic library (MATCH™)[20,2] identified the potent ghrelin agonist **49** (EC$_{50}$ = 68 nM,[2] EC$_{50}$ = 134 nM,[119] Figure 8.17). Hit to lead optimization focused on modifications in the tether region (hydrogenation of the double bond and introduction of R^1 = Me), AA1 (different alkyl and cycloalkyl substituents), AA2 (^{D}Ala preferred over Ala and Gly; R^2 = Me generally preferred over R^2 = H), and AA3 (different aromatic D-amino acids) (Figure 8.17).[119] These efforts led to the selection of **50** (TZP-101, ulimorelin, Figure 8.17) for further clinical development. Macrocycle **50** was evaluated in Phase III clinical trials for the treatment of post-operative ileus and acute gastroparesis. Development was discontinued after failing to meet efficacy endpoints in ULISES 007[120] and

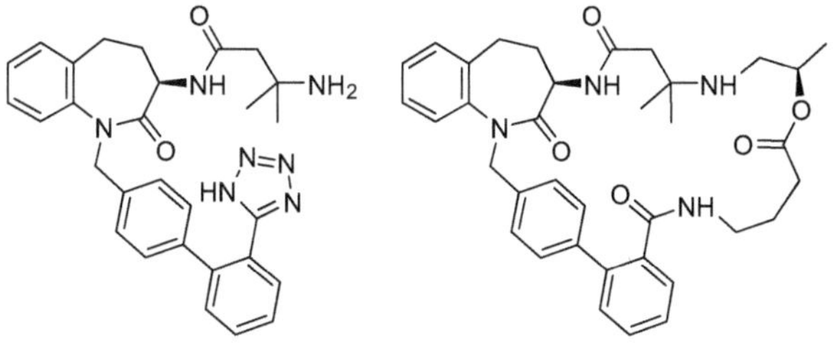

47 (L-692,429)

GRLN: ED_{50} = 60 nM

48

GRLN: ED_{50} = 21 nM

Figure 8.16

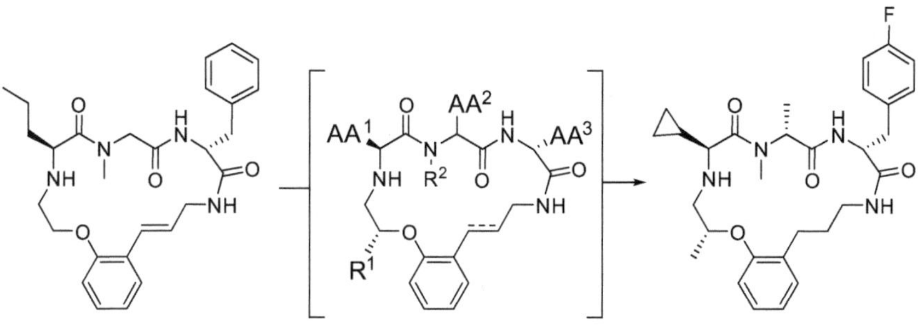

49

$(EC_{50} = 68 \text{ nM})^2$

$(EC_{50} = 134 \text{ nM})^{119}$

lead optimization
Ghrelin agonists

50 (TZP-101,Ulimorelin)

$(EC_{50} = 27 \text{ nM}; F = 16\% \text{ (rat)})^2$

$(EC_{50} = 29 \text{ nM})^{119}$

Figure 8.17

ULISES 008.[121] In these trials ulimorelin at doses of 160 and 480 μg kg^{-1} was not statistically different from placebo for the primary endpoint, the time to recovery of gastrointestinal (GI) function. A different analog (TZP-102, structure undisclosed) for oral use was being developed for diabetic gastroparesis and other chronic GI motility disorders but recently failed to meet efficacy endpoints in a Phase IIb clinical trial,[122] hence confirming the previous results obtained with **50**. Neither the 10 mg kg^{-1} nor the 20 mg kg^{-1} dose reached statistical significance versus placebo.

During the establishment of SAR it was found that replacement of the ^{D}(NMe)Ala of **50** with ^{L}(NMe)Ser changed the profile from an agonist to an antagonist (**51**; $K_i = 100$ nM; $IC_{50} = 500$ nM). More recently, a novel series, exemplified by compound **52** (Figure 8.18), with potent ghrelin antagonistic activity ($IC_{50} = 1$–10 nM) has been described.[123] The use of ghrelin antagonists such as TZP301 (exact structure undisclosed) for the treatment of type 2 diabetes and obesity has been validated in animal models.[2]

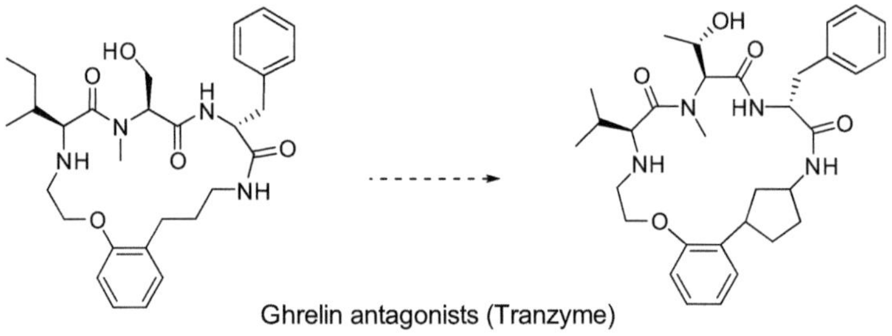

Ghrelin antagonists (Tranzyme)

51 $K_i = 100\,nM;$ $IC_{50} = 500\,nM$　　　　　　　　　**52** $IC_{50} = 1\text{-}10\,nM$

Figure 8.18

This example, on one hand, nicely shows how small changes in a macrocyclic scaffold can change an agonist into an antagonist and on the other hand underscores the validity of using diversity-oriented macrocyclic libraries to discover novel potent hit and lead compounds that are distinct from the natural ligands.

8.3.9 Melanocortin Receptor Modulators

The melanocyte stimulating hormones α-MSH, β-MSH and γ-MSH constitute, together with adrenocorticotropin hormone ACTH, the family of melanocortin peptides or melanotropins. The melanocortin peptides have a wide range of physiological functions including, among others, regulation of skin pigmentation and steroid formation as well as influencing energy balance, growth and body weight.[41,124] Their effects are mediated through five G-protein coupled receptors MC-1R to MC-5R. All of the MC receptors elevate c-AMP if activated and each has different ligand specificity and tissue distribution. Receptors 1,3,4, and 5 recognize α-MSH, β-MSH, and γ-MSH, while receptor 2 recognizes ACTH.[124] Important for biological activity is the conserved message or core sequence His(6)-Phe(7)-Arg(8)-Trp(9) that is present in all four hormones.[124,125]

MC-1R is expressed in the skin, and MC-2R in the adrenal gland. The MC-3 and MC-4 receptors are expressed in the brain and MC-5R in the brain and in peripheral tissues. The MC-4R receptor is involved in the regulation of food intake, energy balance, and body weight. Modulators of MC-4R were therefore considered to be potentially useful for the treatment of eating disorders (agonists to treat obesity, antagonists to treat anorexia).[124–126]

Selective modulators of receptor 4 were derived from cyclic peptide analogs **54** and **55** (Figure 8.19) of α-MSH (**53**). The cyclic peptide **54** (MT-II)[127] is a non-selective agonist at hMC-3R, hMC-4R and hMC-5R. The related peptide, **55** (SHU9119),[128] with ^{D}2-Nal instead of ^{D}Phe in position 7, is an antagonist at receptors 3 and 4 and an agonist at receptor 5.[124,125] The agonist **54** and the antagonist **55** were found by NMR to adopt

53 α-MSH Ac-Ser(1)-Tyr(2)-Ser(3)-Met(4)-Glu(5)-**His(6)-Phe(7)-Arg(8)-Trp(9)**-Gly(10)-Lys(11)-Pro(12)-Val(13)-NH$_2$

The numbering of amino acid residues of α-MSH is retained below.

54 MT-II   Ac-Nle(4)-c[Asp(5)-**His(6)-**^{D}**Phe(7)-Arg(8)-Trp(9)**-Lys(10)]-NH$_2$

55 SHU9119   Ac-Nle(4)-c[Asp(5)-**His(6)-**^{D}**2-Nal(7)-Arg(8)-Trp(9)**-Lys(10)]-NH$_2$

56 MBP10   c[COCH$_2$CH$_2$CO-^{D}**2-Nal(7)-Arg(8)-Trp(9)**-Lys(10)]-NH$_2$

57   c[COCH$_2$CH$_2$CO-**His(6)-**^{D}**Phe(7)-Arg(8)-Trp(9)**-Dab(10)]-NH$_2$

58   c[NH$_2$CH$_2$CH$_2$CO-**His(6)-**^{D}**Phe(7)-Arg(8)-Trp(9)**-Glu(10)]-NH$_2$

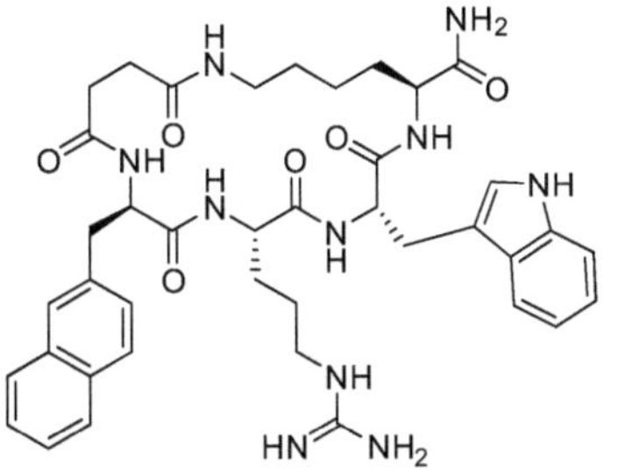

56 (MBP10)
Antagonist at MC-3R and MC-4R;
agonist at MC-5R
selectivity for MC-4R

Affinity: MC-3R: K$_i$ = 150 nM
              MC-4R: K$_i$ = 0.5 nM
              MC-5R: K$_i$ = 540 nM
selectivity ratio: 3R/4R = 300;
                        5R/4R = 1100

MC-5R: EC$_{50}$ = 530 nM

56 (MBP10)

Figure 8.19

similar, β-turn like conformations around the core sequence in aqueous solution. Stacking between the two aromatic groups in positions 6 and 7 was observed in **54** but not in **55**, indicating different spatial orientations of these side chains.[129]

Removal of the N-terminal Ac-Nle(4) segment of **55**, replacement of Asp(5) with succinate and omission of His(6) afforded the cyclic peptide **56** (20-membered ring, Figure 8.19), a hMC-4R antagonist with high affinity and selectivity.[124] ^{D}Phe analogs of **56**, for instance **57** and **58**, were found to be potent agonists at hMC-4R with selectivity over receptors 3 and 5.[130]

The related cyclopeptide **59** (BL3020-1, Figure 8.20) is an agonist at MC-4R (EC$_{50}$ = 4.0 nM). It exhibits increased metabolic stability and Caco-2 permeability as compared to its linear analog. Brain exposure of **59** was demonstrated after oral administration to rats.[131] A single dose of 0.5 mg kg^{-1} in male mice (n = 24) led to a decrease in food consumption of 46–48% as compared with an untreated control group. Repeated once daily oral dosing of 0.5 mg kg^{-1} day^{-1} for 12 days to mice (n = 9) reduced their weight gain after 10 days to 2.8% compared to their original weight, while the control group showed a weight gain of 7.5%.[131]

Cyclic MSH analogs with different receptor subtype selectivity were obtained by modification of the bridge of the macrocyclic peptides or by systematic *N*-methylation of amide groups. Replacement of the succinic acid

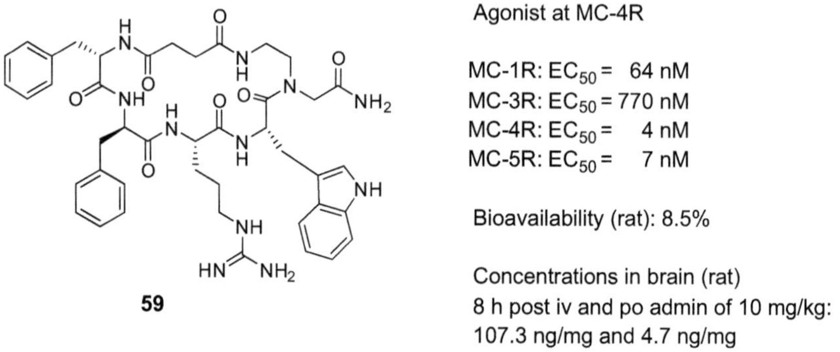

Agonist at MC-4R

MC-1R: $EC_{50} = $ 64 nM
MC-3R: $EC_{50} = $ 770 nM
MC-4R: $EC_{50} = $ 4 nM
MC-5R: $EC_{50} = $ 7 nM

Bioavailability (rat): 8.5%

Concentrations in brain (rat)
8 h post iv and po admin of 10 mg/kg:
107.3 ng/mg and 4.7 ng/mg

59

Figure 8.20

bridge of **56** by pyrazine-2,3-dicarboxylic acid resulted in the formation of a hMC-3R selective antagonist, **60** (Figure 8.21). Its analog with ^{D}Phe in position 7 is a selective agonist at the same receptor subtype.[132] The alkylthioaryl bridged cyclopeptide **61** (Figure 8.21) was derived from MT-II (**54**) and SHU9119 (**55**) and found to be a selective, competitive hMC-5R antagonist ($IC_{50} = 130$ nM; hMC-1,3,4R > 1 μM).[133] N-Methylation of MT-II (**54**) amide bonds afforded several derivatives that retained activity on hMC-1R and simultaneously lost binding affinity at the other MC-receptors. Peptide **62** (Figure 8.21), N-methylated on four amide bonds of the cyclic structure, is a potent and selective hMC-1R agonist and shows a preference in solution for one backbone conformation.[134]

Peptide **63** is an antagonist at mouse MC-R1 and MC-R4 and has no activity at MC-R3 and MC-R5. It was derived from agouti-related protein (AGRP). Agouti (ASP)[135] and agouti-related protein (AGRP)[136] are endogenous MC-R antagonists. The conserved Arg-Phe-Phe motif in both proteins is thought to mimic the MSH core Phe-Arg-Trp sequence. The hAGRP(109–118) sequence, derived from the full length hAGRP, is a disulfide bridged peptide with agonist activity at mouse MC-1R. Replacement of the disulfide with lactam bridges resulted in the cyclodecapeptide **63** with a 27-membered ring.[137]

8.3.10　μ-Opioid Receptor (MOR) Modulators

Macrocyclic modulators of the μ-opioid receptor include cyclic β-casomorphin- and enkephalin- analogs as well as so called atypical cyclic peptides derived from endomorphin-1.

β-Casomorphins are short peptides derived from the milk protein casein with the conserved N-terminal Tyr-Pro-Phe motif. They exhibit selectivity for the μ-receptor.[41] The cyclic β-casomorphin analog **64** (Figure 8.22) is a potent μ-agonist and weak δ-agonist.[138]

The presence of the N-terminal basic amino group of the tyrosine residue is seen as an important structural feature of opioid receptor agonists.

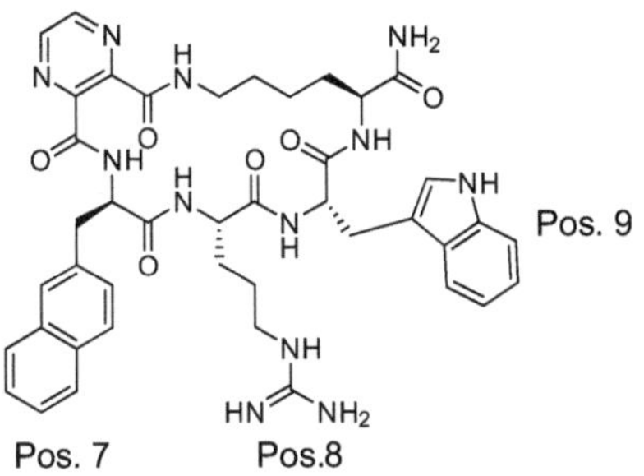

Pos. 9

Pos. 7   Pos.8

60
Antagonist at MC-3R
Selectivity for MC-3R
MC-1R: IC_{50} = 707 nM
MC-3R: IC_{50} = 23 nM
MC-4R: IC_{50} > 1000 nM
MC-5R: IC_{50} = 230 nM

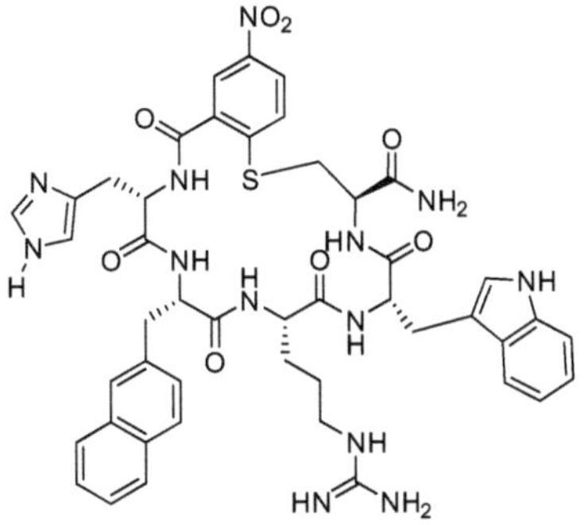

61
Antagonist at MC-5R
Selectivity for MC-5R
MC-1R: IC_{50} > 2000 nM
MC-3R: IC_{50} > 1000 nM
MC-4R: IC_{50} > 5000 nM
MC-5R: IC_{50} = 130 nM

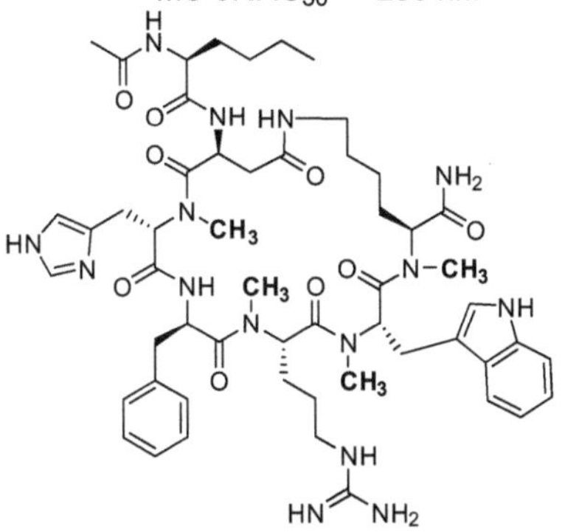

62
Agonist at MC-1R
Selectivity for MC-1R
Binding assay:
MC-1R: IC_{50} = 14 nM
MC-3R: IC_{50} = 2200 nM
MC-4R: no binding
MC-5R: no binding

c-AMP assay:
EC_{50} = 13 nM

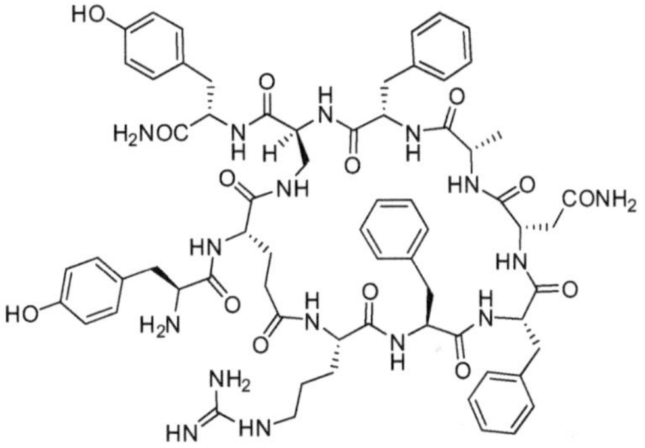

63
(Hairpin mimic of $R^{111}FF^{113}$
of AGRP (Agouti-related protein);
Antagonist of mMC1-R (pA_2 = 5.9)
and MC4-R (pA_2 = 6.9);
no activity on MC3-R and MC5-R;

Figure 8.21

The cysteine-containing enkephalin analog **65**[139] as well as the carbon tethered analogs **66** and **67** (Figure 8.23), with the dithio ether bridge replaced by methylene groups, exhibit agonist activity whereas dicarba analogs with replacement of the tyrosine residue by Dhp (**68**; Dhp = 3-(2,6-dimethyl-4-hydroxphenyl)propanoic acid) or [2S]-Mdp (**69**; [2S]-Mdp = [2S]-2-methyl-3-(2,6-dimethyl-4-hydroxphenyl)propanoic acid) manifest, as expected, antagonist activity at the µ-receptor. However, peptide **68** is a δ-agonist and compound **69** is a δ-antagonist.[140]

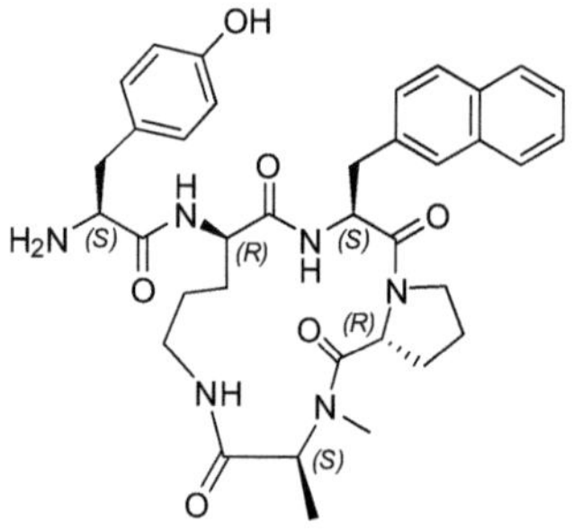

64 H-Tyr-c[^{D}Orn-2Nal-^{D}Pro-NMe-Ala]

Mimic of YPF in β-casomorphin;
MOR selective agonist (GPI: IC$_{50}$ = 35 nM)

Figure 8.22

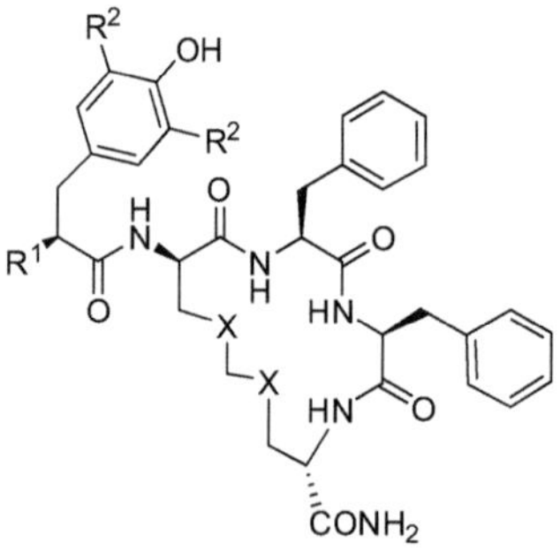

Opioid receptor binding data:

Compound	K$_i$[nM]		
	μ	δ	κ
65	0.016	1.8	2.5
66	1.04	2.24	11.3
67	1.54	1.20	15.8
68	8.95	39.2	> 500
69	18.3	18.7	302

65 X = S, R^1 = NH$_2$, R^2 = H;
66 X = CH$_2$, R^1 = NH$_2$, R^2 = H
67 X = CH$_2$, R^1 = NH$_2$, R^2 = CH$_3$
68 X = CH$_2$, R^1 = H, R^2 = CH$_3$
69 X = CH$_2$, R^1 = CH$_3$, R^2 = CH$_3$

Figure 8.23

Endomorphins 1 and 2 are μ-selective endogenous opioid receptor agonist peptides. In the more recent literature, endomorphin-1 derived cyclic peptides have been reported which activate the μ-opioid receptor although they lack an N-terminal free amino group. These atypical peptides, **70** and **71** (Figure 8.24), interact with the μ-opioid receptor through their hydrophobic groups.[141,142] Peptide **70** shows a K$_i$ value of 34 nM in a binding assay, μ-agonist properties in a functional assay (IC$_{50}$ = 29 nM)[141] and produces a dose-dependent preemptive anti-nociceptive effect (ED$_{50}$ = 1.24 mg kg^{-1}) if injected intraperitoneal (ip, dose 1.25–20 mg kg^{-1}) to mice 5 min before

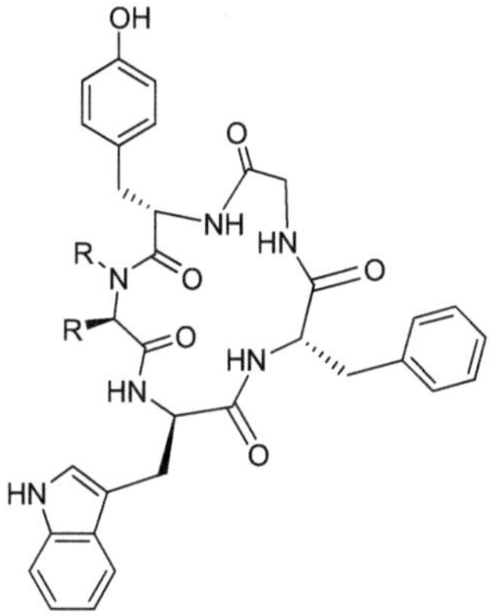

70 c[Tyr-^{D}Pro-^{D}Trp-Phe-Gly]

Affinity assay:
μ-opioid receptor: K_i = 34 nM

Functional assay:
μ-agonist; IC_{50} = 29 nM (E_{max} = 73%)

71 c[Tyr-Gly-^{D}Trp-Phe-Gly]

Affinity assay:
μ-opioid receptor: K_i = 3.6 nM

Functional assay:
μ-agonist; IC_{50} = 31 nM (E_{max} = 65%)

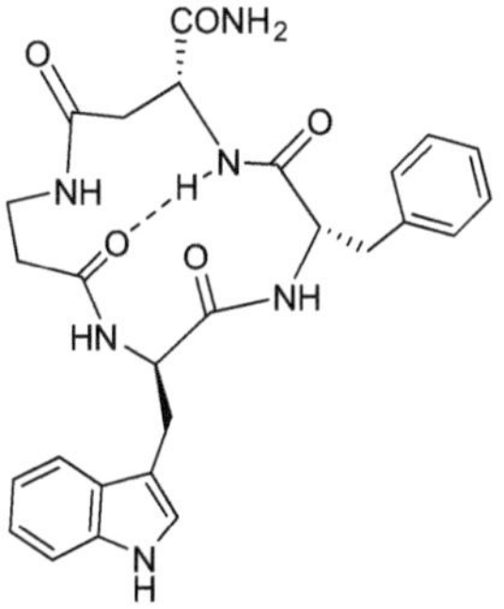

72 c[^{D}Asp-1-amide-β-Ala-^{D}Trp-Phe]

Affinity assay:
μ-opioid receptor: K_i = 5.9 nM

Functional assay:
μ-agonist; IC_{50} = 37 nM (E_{max} = 58%)

Figure 8.24

acetic acid is injected (20 mg kg^{-1}, ip).[143] NMR data indicate that **70** and **71** exist in solution as equilibrium mixtures of conformers. Molecular docking investigations suggest an inverse type II β-turn geometry centered on ^{D}Trp-Phe to be important for activity.[142] This model is corroborated by the synthesis of cyclopeptide **72**, which was not based on endomorphin-1 and which showed high affinity at the μ-receptor and partial agonist activity. Peptide **72** was found to adopt an inverse type II β-turn conformation around the ^{D}Trp-Phe residues in solution, stabilized by an H-bond between the β-Ala carbonyl and the ^{D}Asp NH group.[142]

8.3.11 Motilin Modulators

Motilin is a 22-amino acid residue peptide hormone that is expressed mainly in the gastrointestinal tract, in particular in the small intestine, and stimulates gastric motility. The motilin receptor (MTL-R or GP38)[144] is involved in the regulation of gastrointestinal motor activity.[2,25,41] Derivatives of the well-known antibiotic erythromycin A have been discovered as

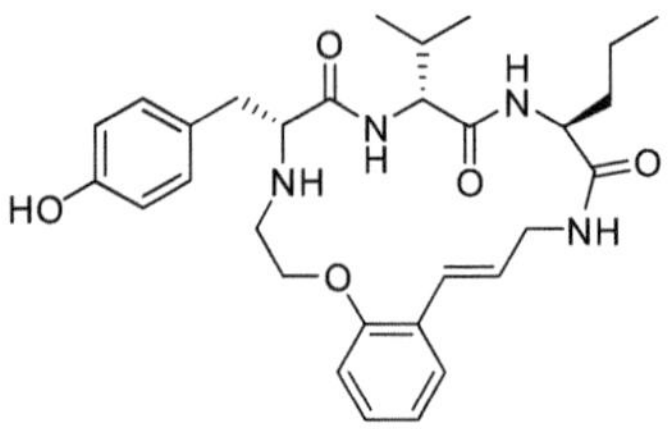

73 (MTL-R: IC$_{50}$ = 137 nM) 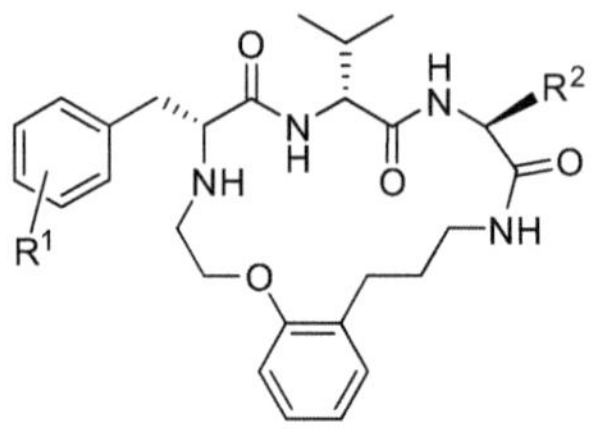   **74** (TZP-201, structure undisclosed)

Figure 8.25

agonists of MTL-R and were further developed clinically as agents to treat gastrointestinal distress.[145] Several NMR-based studies identified a β-turn type I conformation (Pro(3)-Thr(6)) at the N-terminus of motilin, followed by an α-helical stretch (Glu(9)-Lys(20)).[146] Biologically active cyclic peptides mimicking the N-terminal β-turn confirmed this structural hypothesis.[25,41]

From screening a library of 10 000 macrocyclic peptidomimetics (MATCH™)[147] a motilin antagonist, **73** (Figure 8.25), with good potency (IC$_{50}$ = 137 nM) was identified. Lead optimization resulted in a series of potent motilin antagonists with IC$_{50}$'s from 1 to 20 nM.[148] Of these, TZP-201 (structure undisclosed), an advanced compound from that series, was evaluated in an irinotecan-induced diarrhea in beagle dogs.[149,150] Diarrhea was induced in male beagle dogs by intravenous bolus injection of irinotecan (6 mg kg^{-1} day^{-1}) for two treatment cycles up to five consecutive days, separated by a 9-day wash-out period. Irinotecan induced severe diarrhea after four days of treatment. Dogs were treated with TZP-201 (2×2.5 mg kg^{-1} day^{-1} or 2×7.5 mg kg^{-1} day^{-1} infused over 45 min), loperamide (3×0.06 mg kg^{-1} day^{-1} po) or octreotide (3×0.007 mg kg^{-1} day^{-1}). Stool consistency was recorded for up to 28 days. TZP-201 treatment was more efficacious in reducing diarrhea than either loperamide or octreotide.[151]

8.3.12   Somatostatin Antagonists

Somatostatins or somatropin-release inhibitory factors (SRIFs) are 14 and 28 amino acid-derived peptides (SRIF14 and SRIF28) that are expressed in the CNS, GI tract and endocrine tissues and belong to a family of peptide hormones that are important in the regulation of endocrine and exocrine secretion in many tissues.[25,41,152] SRIF14 binds with high affinity to five GPCRs, sst1-5 (IC$_{50}$ = 0.2 nM for sst2). By binding to sst1-5 somatostatins inhibit the release of several hormones such as growth hormone, insulin, and adrenocorticotropic hormone (ACTH).

Early studies on cyclic hexapeptide analogs identified ^{D}Trp-Lys-Thr as the key pharmacophore in a type II or II' conformation which further resulted in a potent bicyclic analog **75** (IC$_{50}$ = 3.7 nM, sst2, Figure 8.26).[154] This example

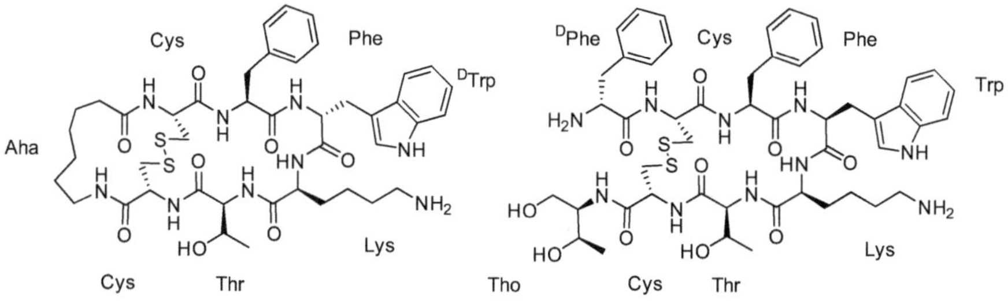

75 (Merck)   **76** (Octreotide; Novartis)

Figure 8.26

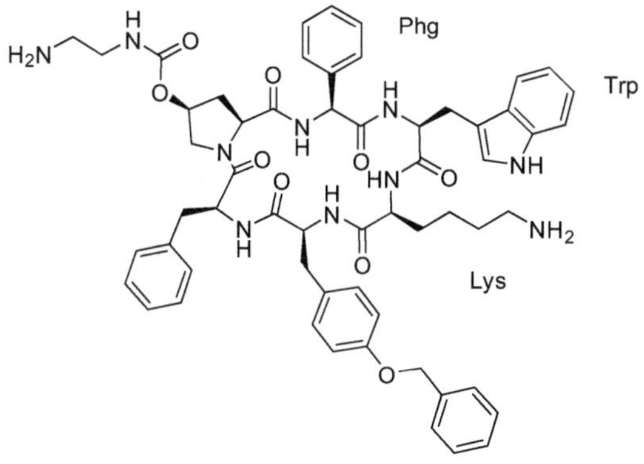

77 (Pasireotide, approved in 2012; Novartis)

Figure 8.27

was one of the first studies of a transfer of a β-turn motif into a macrocyclic structure. Similar studies finally led to the marketed products octreotide (Sandostatin, Novartis; **76**) and lanreotide (Somatuline, Ipsen) which were approved to treat disorders, including acromegaly, that are characterized by the excessive production of hormones, such as growth hormone. However, these first generation products showed high activity only against sst2.[152] Compound **76** (Octreotide) shows the following pK_i values: sst1 (6.6); sst2 (9.5); sst3 (8.3); sst4 (<6.0); sst5 (8.3).[153]

In an attempt to generate a SRIF14 analog mimicking more precisely the sst1–5 inhibitory spectrum of the natural hormone, pasireotide (**77**, Figure 8.27) was developed and was granted marketing approval by the European Commission and the FDA in 2012 for the treatment of Cushing's disease.[152] Pasireotide binds and activates four of the five SSTRs, in particular sst5 (pK_i values: sst1 (8.2); sst2 (9.0); sst3 (9.1); sst4 (<7.0); sst5 (9.9))[153] in corticotropic cells of ACTH-producing adenomas, leading to the inhibition of ACTH secretion.[152,155]

8.3.13 Tachykinins: Inhibitors of NK1

Tachykinins belong to a family of peptide hormones targeting three GPCRs, neurokinin receptors NK1-3. Among the more than 40 tachykinins known to date, substance P, substance K, neurokinins A and B, and neuromedin L are well known.[25,41] Structural studies on substance P and neurokinins A and B, suggested α-helical turns (β-turn type I) to be important for receptor binding.[25] Cyclic peptides mimicking the tachykinin pharmacophores resulted in potent and selective NK1 antagonists (*e.g.* **78**, $IC_{50} = 2$ nM, Figure 8.28).[156]

8.3.14 Vasopressin Receptor (V_{1a}) Agonists: FE202158

Arginine vasopressin (AVP, **79**, Figure 8.29) binds to three receptors $V_{1a}R$, $V_{1b}R$ and V_2R and also to the oxytocin receptor (OTR). $V_{1a}R$ is expressed in the liver (regulation of glycogenolysis), vascular smooth muscle cells (vasoconstriction), and in the brain. The $V_{1b}R$ receptor is expressed in the limbic system and the pituitary gland while V_2R is mainly expressed in the kidney where it regulates water and sodium excretion.[157]

AVP (**79**) is a nonapeptide forming a disulfide-bridged (Cys(1), Cys(6)) 20-membered ring. The presence of the ring is required for the agonist activity of AVP (**79**) analogs at $V_{1a}R$, but not for binding. AVP (**79**) is not receptor subtype selective. It acts on $V_{1a}R$ and V_2R with comparable potency.[158] The treatment of vasodilatory hypotension as observed in septic shock would however require a $V_{1a}R$-selective agonist with a short half-life.[159]

The synthesis of analogs of AVP modified in positions 2, 3, 4, and 8 afforded a series of compounds with a suitable profile, among them **80** (FE202158, Figure 8.29),[158] which was found to be a potent and selective full agonist at the human V_{1a} receptor (Table 8.5) and also a potent vasoconstrictor *in vivo* in rats, as shown by dose-dependent reduction of ear skin blood flow (ED_{50} of 4.0 pmol kg^{-1} min^{-1}; given by constant intravenous

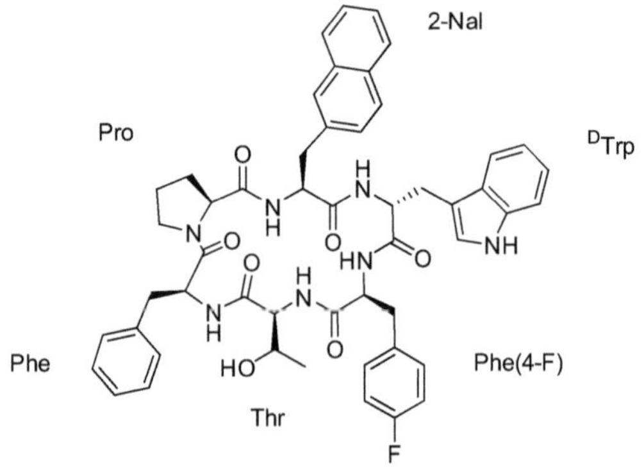

78 (NK1 antagonist, IC_{50} = 2 nM)

Figure 8.28

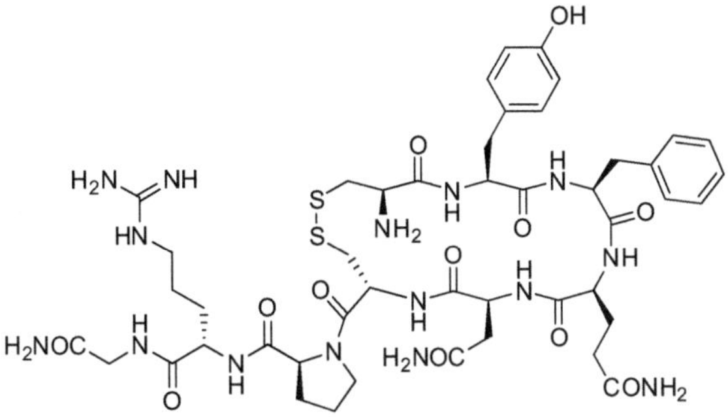

79 (Arginine vasopressin, AVP)

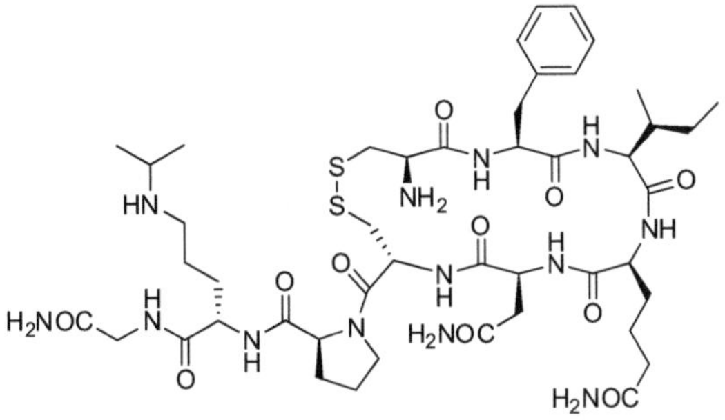

80 (FE 202158, Ferring), V_{1a} agonist

Figure 8.29

Table 8.5   Agonist activity of **79** (AVP) and **80** (FE202158).[158,159]

	79 (AVP)	**80** (FE202158)
EC_{50} $hV_{1a}R$	0.24 nM ($E_{max} = 100\%$)	2.4 nM ($E_{max} = 84\%$)
EC_{50} $hV_{1b}R$	4.3 nM	340 nM
EC_{50} hV_2R	0.05 nM	2656 nM
EC_{50} hOTR	22 nM	1057 nM

infusion), with no V_2R mediated antidiuretic activity.[159] Macrocycle **80** (FE202158) was chosen for clinical trials for the treatment of septic shock.[158]

8.4   Macrocycles Targeting Integrins

8.4.1   Introduction

Integrins are a large family of heterodimeric cell adhesion proteins involved in cell growth, proliferation and migration.[160] They each consist of one α- and β-subunit and to date 18 α-subunits and 8 β-subunits are known.[160,161] The list of ligands that bind to integrins includes bone matrix proteins, collagens, fibronectins, fibrinogen, laminins, thrombospondins, vitronectin, and von Willebrand factor,[162] frequently containing the RGD motif.

Approved drugs are available targeting the three integrins αIIbβ3 (abcix-imab, epifibatide, and tirofiban), α4-subunit (tysabri), and αLβ2 or LFA1 (efalizumab).[160,161] In recent years several successful examples of macro-cyclic inhibitors of integrins have appeared (*vide infra*).[163,164]

8.4.2 Cilengitide (81): Inhibitor of αvβ3, αvβ5, α5β1

Cilengitide (**81**, Figure 8.30) is a cyclic RGD pentapeptide, c(RGDf(*N*Me)V), which was discovered in the early 1990s by Kessler *et al.*[165] by successfully applying three chemical strategies to RGD: (1) reduction of conformational freedom by cyclization; (2) spatial screening of cyclic peptides; and(3) *N*-methyl scan. The compound shows sub-nanomolar antagonistic activity for the αvβ3 receptor and nanomolar affinities for αvβ5 and α5β1 receptors, with high selectivity over the platelet receptor αIIbβ3. It is 100–1000 times more active than the parent linear peptide. The conformation of the RGD-motif in cilengitide proved critical for the observed high selectivity for αvβ3 over αIIbβ3.[166,167] The X-ray structures of cilengitide (**81**) in complex with αvβ3 have been solved.[168,169] Remarkably, the conformation determined in solution turned out to be identical to the one described for Cilengitide bound to the αvβ3 integrin, shown in Figure 8.31.[165] Cilengitide (**81**) is being

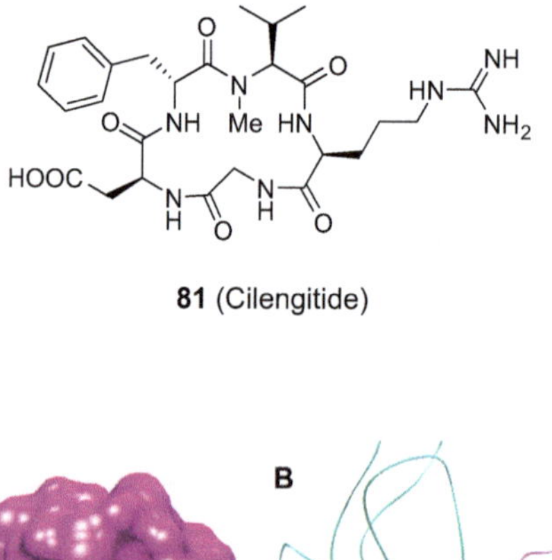

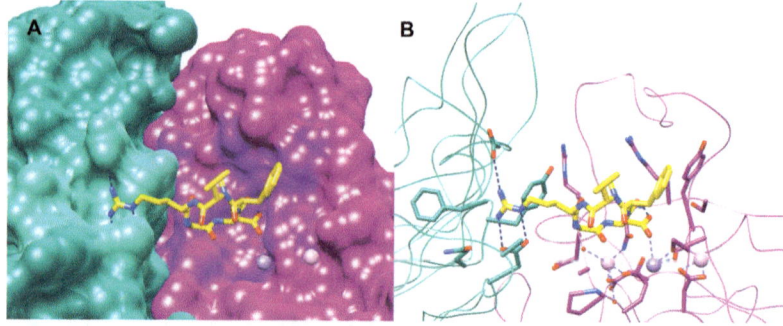

81 (Cilengitide)

Figure 8.30

Figure 8.31 A: Surface representation of Integrin αvβ3 in complex with Cilengitide shown as stick model (yellow).[168] The Mn^{2+} ions are shown as spheres. B: Residues interacting with Cilengitide are shown in stick represen-tation. Hydrogen bonds and salt bridges are represented with dotted lines.

developed by Merck-Serono (Darmstadt, Germany) and is currently in Phase III clinical trials for the treatment of glioblastomas[170] and in Phase II trials for several other tumors. Unfortunately it was recently disclosed that the primary endpoint of the Phase III CENTRIC trial to treat glioblastoma multiforme (GBM) was not met.[171]

8.4.3   Inhibitors of αIIbβ3 (Platelet Receptor)

The integrin receptor αIIbβ3 and its ligand fibrinogen play a key role in platelet aggregation and blood coagulation. The interaction between fibrinogen and its receptor is mediated by an RGD motif and therefore, RGD containing cyclic peptides and small molecule RGD mimetics have been the focus for discovering novel drugs to prevent platelet aggregation. These efforts have resulted in three approved drugs (abciximab, epifibatide, and tirofiban).[161]

Several approaches to cyclic RGD-containing peptides have been described in the literature.[167,172–174] Conformational analysis of disulfide- and RGD-containing cyclic pentapeptide **82** (Figure 8.32)[175] by NMR led to the design of the template-bridged macrocyclic RGD-containing peptide **83** (Figure 8.32), which was a highly potent inhibitor of αIIbβ3.[174] Whereas **82** binds with an affinity of 0.1 µM to αIIbβ3, the template-bridged analog **83** binds with an IC_{50} of approximately 0.1 nM and shows also good activity in a platelet aggregation assay at oral doses as low as 0.1 mg kg^{-1}.[174] The oral activity of **83** was assessed by testing and analysing blood samples from unanesthetized canines taken at different time points in a platelet aggregation inhibitory assay, after oral administration of 0.1 mg kg^{-1}. At 6 h the compound elicited a 45% inhibition of platelet aggregation (at 1 mg kg^{-1} a 100% inhibition was observed at the 6 h time point).[174]

Both cilengitide (**81**) and **83** demonstrate that by appropriately modulating the RGD conformation, highly potent and selective macrocyclic RGD-containing peptides with good drug-like properties can be obtained.

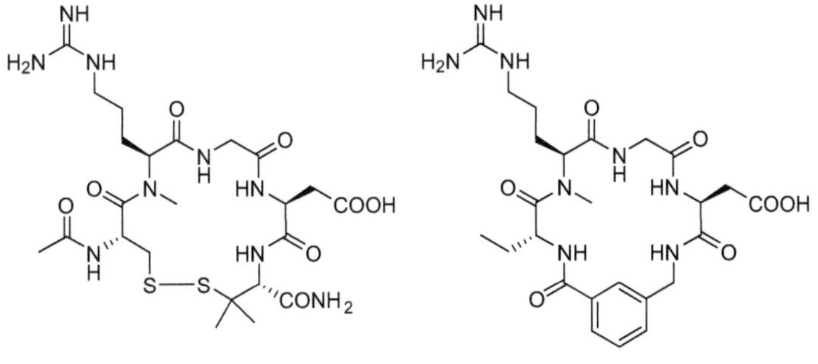

82   **83**

Inhibitors of αIIbβ3

Figure 8.32

8.4.4 HUN-7293: Inhibitor of VCAM

Cell adhesion molecules such as ICAM-1, VCAM-1 and E-selectin play key roles in the immune response. With the aim of identifying inhibitors of VCAM-1 expression, two independent screens were run[176] which identified two structurally related fungal cyclic depsipeptide natural products, HUN-7293 (**84**: R = CH$_2$CH$_2$CN) and **85** (R = H, Figure 8.33). A total synthesis of HUN-7293 was achieved[177] as well as a general synthesis approach which allowed the synthesis of analogs of the natural product[178] and the establishment of a structure activity relationship. HUN-7293 (**84**) has potent inhibitory activity for VCAM-1 (IC$_{50}$ = 1 nM) and modest selectivity over ICAM-1 (IC$_{50}$ = 24 nM; ratio ICAM-1/VCAM-1 = 24).[178] Alanine-scanning identified the relative importance of each individual residue of **84** for biological activity and provided **86** (R = Me, Figure 8.33), which showed potent activity for VCAM-1 activation (IC$_{50}$ = 2.3 nM) with higher selectivity over ICAM-1 (IC$_{50}$ = 178 nM; ratio ICAM-1/VCAM-1 = 77).[178] The same compound proved to be a natural product in its own right and was named HUN-7293B. Other interesting compounds were **87** (IC$_{50}$ = 2.3 nM) and **88**, the latter of which is an *N*-methyl-leucine epimer (C$_2^3$) of HUN-7293. The 3D-structures of HUN-7293 were determined by X-ray as well as in solution by NMR[179] and were very similar.

8.5 Macrocycles Targeting Protein–Protein Interactions (PPIs)

8.5.1 The Nature of PPIs

Extra- and intracellular protein–protein interactions largely dictate the processes by which extra-cellular signals are relayed from the plasma to specific intra-cellular sites. The activation of protein kinases and phosphatases as key signaling mediators are regulated by scaffold, anchoring, and adaptor proteins that contribute to the specificity of these signal transduction events.[180] Modular domains recognize relatively short peptide consensus sequences, such as WW domains recognizing proline-rich peptides, EH

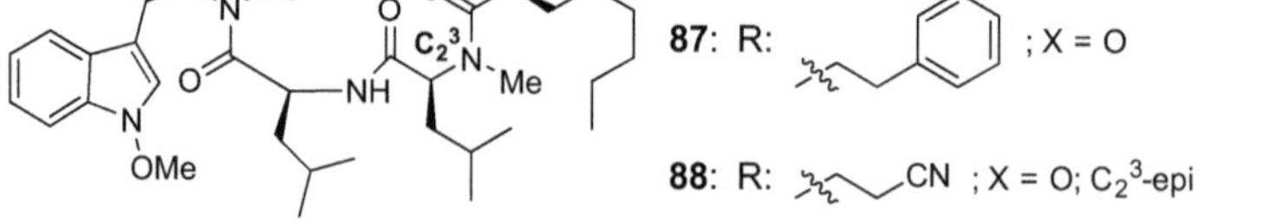

Figure 8.33

domains binding to peptides containing the NPF motif, SH2 and PTB domains binding to peptides containing a phosphorylated tyrosine, and PDZ domains recognizing certain C-terminal peptides sequences.[180,181] In addition, several conserved embryonic signaling pathways such as Hedgehog (Hh),[182] Wingless (Wnt)[183,184] and Notch,[185] which play an important role in the development of cancers[186,187] are also mediated by extra- and intra-cellular protein–protein interactions.

Targeting therapeutically relevant intra-cellular protein–protein interactions with small molecules has become an important topic in drug discovery as many cell signaling pathways are mediated by the specific formation of protein complexes and whole clusters. However, finding small molecule inhibitors of such protein–protein interactions has traditionally proven to be difficult.[188]

The tremendous challenges and opportunities associated with the discovery of small molecule PPI inhibitors have been described in several reviews.[188–191] One significant challenge of targeting PPIs with small molecules is that the interfaces of interacting proteins are typically large, $\sim$1500–3000 Å^2.[188] However, Wells and colleagues have shown that within these large surfaces there are areas of high energy interactions ("hot spots")[192] that are significantly smaller (700–1300 Å^2) and potentially amenable to small to medium-sized molecules. By studying the anatomy of "hot spots"[193] it was concluded that these high energy interactions are mainly mediated by the amino acid residues trypthophan, arginine, and tyrosine, surrounded by hydrophobic residues such as leucine and isoleucine. Analysis of a number of X-ray structures of natural and synthetic macrocyclic products (*e.g.* rapamycin[194]) in the 1–2 kDa range bound to their protein targets show that these molecules are able to bind to surfaces as large as 1000 Å^2.

The dynamic nature of protein surfaces[195] poses a second major challenge for inhibitor design. However, the semi-rigid nature of macrocycles should favor interactions with a flexible protein target interface by induced fit. A particularly striking example in this respect is cyclosporin A (**46**, Figure 8.36), where the conformations observed in the unbound form in organic solvents or in the crystal[196] differ significantly from the bound conformations with cyclophilin[197] and in the ternary complex with cyclophilin and calcineurin (Figure 8.34).[198,199]

Taken together all of these arguments underscore the potential of macrocycles as privileged structures to modulate PPIs.

8.5.2 SH2 Domains: Macrocyclic Modulators of Grb2

Src homology 2 (SH2) domains are protein modules which recognize phosphotyrosine sites and are parts of proteins that couple protein-tyrosine kinases (PTKs) to intracellular signaling pathways.[200,201] The growth factor-bound protein 2 (Grb2) is a SH2 domain-receptor signaling domain that participates in the signaling of many oncogenic growth factor PTKs, including erb-B-dependent breast cancers and Met-dependent kidney

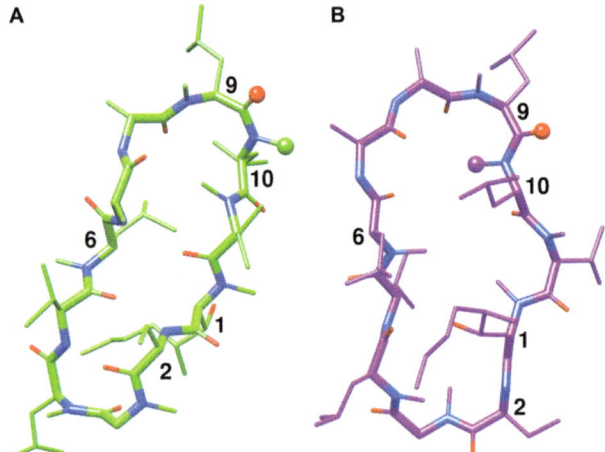

Figure 8.34 A: X-ray structure of Cyclosporin A in the free (unbound) state.[196] B: X-ray structure of Cyclosporin A bound to calcineurin and cyclo-philin.[199] The most striking feature of the unbound state is a *cis* 9,10 peptide bond found in the crystal and in solution conformation of CsA. However, the cyclophilin-bound form exhibits all *trans* peptide bonds.

cancers.[202] The discovery of potent small molecule inhibitors of Grb2 SH2 domain-signaling antagonists has proven very challenging for various reasons. Grb2 SH2 is a typical intra-cellular PPI target and recognizes the highly polar, anionic and poorly cell-permeable consensus sequence phospho-Tyr-X-Asn-X. An X-ray structure of a phospho-tyrosine-containing peptide derived from BCR-Abl (sequence174-180: KPF-pY-VNV) bound to Grb2 SH2[203] revealed a β-turn conformation in the peptide and was instrumental for the design of smaller macrocyclic molecules. Burke *et al.* designed and synthesized a series of open-chain and macrocyclic Grb SH2 mimetics such as **89** (IC$_{50}$ = 9 nM, ELISA assay; IC$_{50}$ = 20 nM SPR assay, Figure 8.35).[204,205] Compound **89** also showed activity (IC$_{50}$ = 5 μM) in a whole cell assay with MDA-MB-453 breast cancer cell line where the erb-2 gene is amplified.[204] The cyclohexylglycine residue at the i+2 position of the β-turn of **89** greatly stabilizes the bioactive conformation. Through macrocyclization using a ring-closing metathesis reaction, this conformation was subsequently further stabilized in compound **90** (IC$_{50}$ = 2 nM, ELISA assay, Figure 8.35). Different phospho-tyrosine replacements (**90**: X = –CH$_2$PO(OH)$_2$; **91**: X = –CH$_2$(COONa)$_2$) were investigated in order to improve cell permeability and whole cell activity. Interestingly, the whole cell activity for **90**, which was sub-micromolar in MDA-MB-453 cells, was significantly improved over the open-chained analog **89**.[206] Compound **91** was the most potent non-phosphorous containing phospho-tyrosine mimetic with good whole cell activity. Finally, further exploration of the SAR gave macrocycle **92** (Figure 8.35) with exquisite binding properties (K$_d$ ~ 60–90 pM) and excellent whole cell activity (inhibition of MDA-MB cell growth; IC$_{50}$ = 0.6 μM).[207,208]

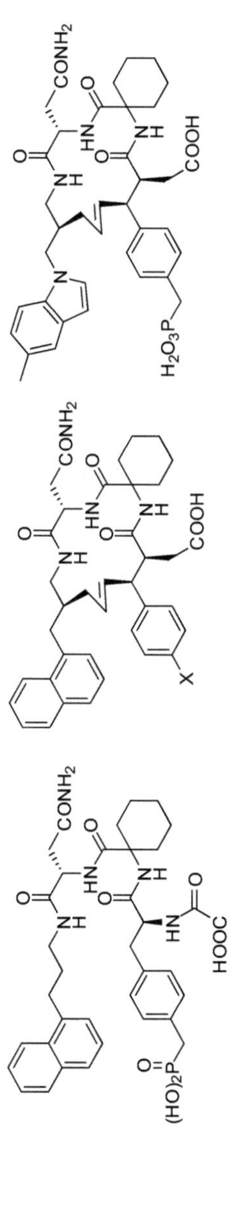

89 (IC$_{50}$ = 20 nM, SPR)
(IC$_{50}$ = 9 nM, ELISA)

90 X= -CH$_2$PO(OH)$_2$ (IC$_{50}$ = 2 nM, ELISA)

91 X= -CH(COONa)$_2$ (IC$_{50}$ = 4.3 nM, ELISA)

92 (K$_d$ = 60–90 pM; SPR)

Figure 8.35

In summary, this example nicely underscores the fact that macrocyclization is a powerful approach to stabilize a bioactive conformation as well as to favorably modulate cell permeability.

8.5.3 Peptidyl Prolyl Isomerases (PPIases)

Peptidyl prolyl isomerases (PPIases) commonly catalyse the *cis-trans* interconversion of proline-containing protein strands and play an important role in the proper folding of proteins.[209] PPIases consist of three families: cyclophilins, FK-506 binding proteins and parvulins. The macrocyclic natural products cyclosporin A (**46**), FK506 (**93**) and rapamycin (**94**, Figure 8.36) bind to the cyclophilin family (CypA, Cyp18)[210] and FKBP-12, respectively, thereby inhibiting rotamase activity.[211] These natural products were key for identifying the exact mechanism by which they exert their potent immunosuppressive activity. The cyclosporin A-cyclophilin complex binds to the human phosphatase calcineurin B (protein phosphatase 2B),[199] which inhibits dephosphorylation of nuclear factor of activated T-cells (NFAT) and ultimately blocks T-cell activation. Similarly, the FK506-FKBP12 (FK506-binding protein) complex binds to calcineurin[212] and blocks T-cell activation. In contrast, the rapamycin-FKBP12 complex binds to human FRAP (FKBP-rapamycin-associated protein)[194] or the mammalian target of rapamycin (mTOR).[213] The crystal structures of the three ternary complexes of cyclosporin A[199], FK506,[212] and rapamycin[194] with their targets provided significant insight on how macrocycles can modulate complex protein–protein interactions.

Besides its impressive immunosuppressive activity, rapamycin also exhibits potent antiproliferative activity. The rapamycin–FKBP complex

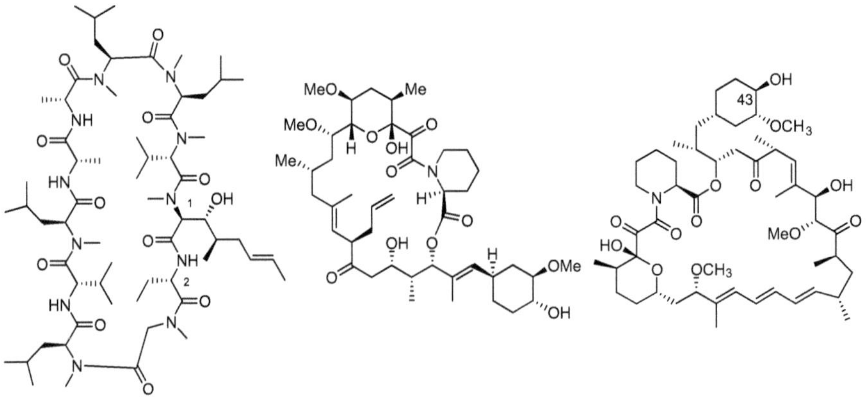

46 (Cyclosporin A)

binds to cyclophilin
and calcineurin

93 FK506 (Tacrolimus)

binds to FKBP12
and calcineurin

94 Rapamycin (Sirolimus)

binds to FKBP12
and mTOR (hFRAP)

Figure 8.36

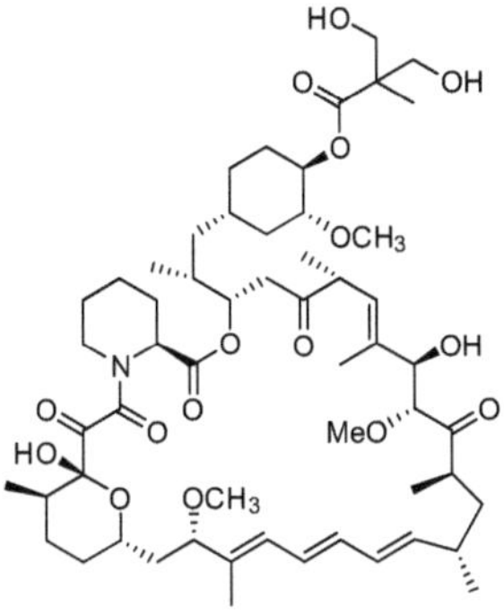

95 CCI-779 (Torisel)
(FKBP12; mTOR)

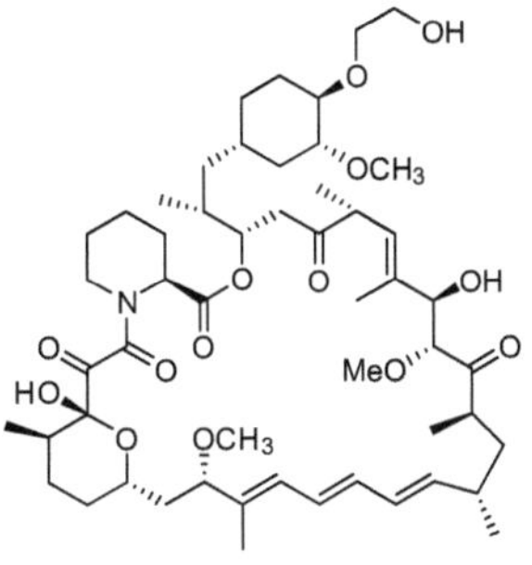

96 Everolimus (Affinitor)
(FKBP12; m-TOR)

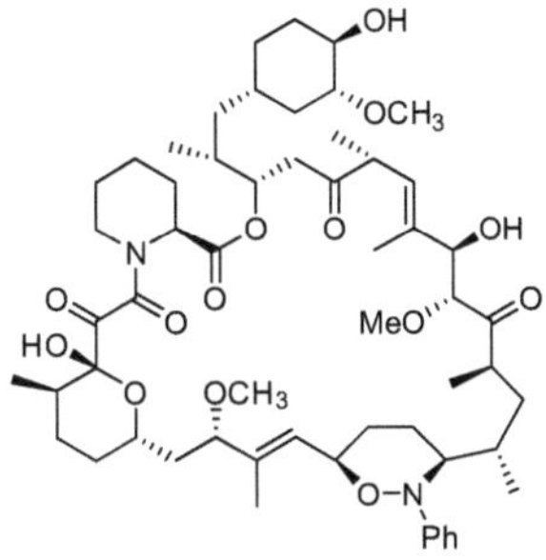

97 ILS-920
(FKBP52; CACNB1)

Figure 8.37

binds close to the kinase domain of mTOR and blocks mTOR-mediated signal transduction pathways resulting in cell cycle arrest (G1 phase).[213] Using a semi-synthetic strategy to modify the secondary alcohol at C-43 led to the discovery of CCI-779 (**95**) which exhibited potent antitumor activity and was approved in 2007 as Torisel® for the treatment of renal cell carcinoma,[214] and to Everolimus (Affinitor®; **96**, Figure 8.37) for use in treating several cancers.[215,216] In addition to their immunosuppressant activity, ligands of FKBP12 such as FK506 and rapamycin show neuroprotective activity in animal models of ischemia, and therefore there was significant interest in finding analogs showing neuroprotection but devoid of immunosuppressive effects. In an attempt to generate analogs with modified properties, rapamycin was transformed in a two-step procedure (hetero Diels-Alder reaction with PhN=O and subsequent hydrogenation) into ILS-920 (**97**).[214] In contrast to FK506 and rapamycin, ILS-920 showed no immunosuppressive activity in an IL-2 stimulated human CD4+ T-cell proliferation assay. In addition, ILS-920 showed significantly higher affinity for FKBP52 than FKBP12 and potently inhibits L-type Ca^{2+}-channels (CACNB1; β1-subunit). ILS-920 promoted survival of E16 primary rat cortical neurons in culture and stimulated neurite outgrowth in that system.[217] In addition, **97** demonstrated neuroprotection in a rat mCAO focal ischemia model in a dose dependent manner (at 10 mg kg^{-1} the reduction of the infarct volume was 23%, at 30 mg kg^{-1} 36%).[217]

8.5.4 Macrocyclic Modulators of PDZ Domains

The PDZ domain-containing protein family consists of over 250 members which are involved in many important biological functions such as the control of cell migration and invasion, cell proliferation, cell polarity, cell attachment and cell-cell contact, apoptosis and immune cell recognition and

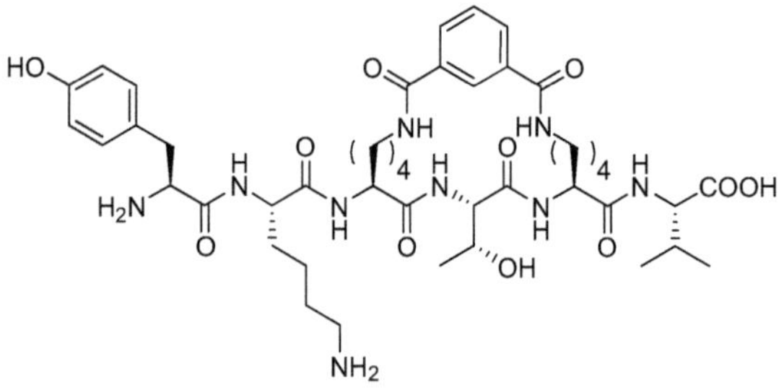

98 (mimic of Y-K-K-T-K-V)

Figure 8.38

signaling.[218] PDZ domains themselves are regions of usually 80–90 amino acid residues that share common stretches of amino acids (GLGF-motif) forming a hydrophobic binding pocket and are privileged sites for protein-protein recognition and association. They are generally considered to act as scaffolding molecules, around which multi-protein signaling complexes are assembled.

The post-synaptic density protein 95 (PSD-95) was the first PDZ-containing protein described and regulates signaling in glutaminergic neurons by acting as a molecular scaffold for protein complex formation at the post-synaptic density of dendritic spines.[219] PDZ domains of PSD-95 are involved in the regulation of kainate receptors. Inhibitors of this interaction may lead to novel medicines for the treatment of drug addiction and epilepsy.[220] A series of macrocyclic peptides designed to target PDZ domains of PSD-95 were synthesized and tested for their binding to the third PDZ domain (PDZ3) of PSD-95. Compound **98** (Figure 8.38) showed the highest affinity for PDZ3 ($K_d = 3.8$ μM; by calorimetric titration). Compound **98** was also tested in a cell-based assay (PSD-95 promotes clustering of GluR6 kainate receptors when coexpressed in HEK293 cells).[221] The cyclic compound **98** was significantly more active in inhibiting clustering of kainite receptors after 14 h than the parent linear compound reflecting its higher potency and enzymatic stability.[220]

8.5.5 Inhibitors of Menin-MLL1 Interaction

Targeting the menin-mixed lineage leukemia gene1 protein (MLL1) interaction with a macrocyclic peptide derivative constitutes a recent impressive example of inhibiting a typical protein protein interaction.[222] Chromosomal translocations in the *MLL1* gene are observed in >70% of leukemia in infants, and in 5–10% of acute myeloid leukemia (AML) in adults.[223] These rearrangements lead to the fusion of the N-terminal part of MLL1 to roughly 60 diverse interacting proteins.[224] The target was biologically validated by a small molecule inhibitor of the menin-MLL1 interaction which was found by high throughput screening.[225,226] This molecule reverses MLL fusion-protein

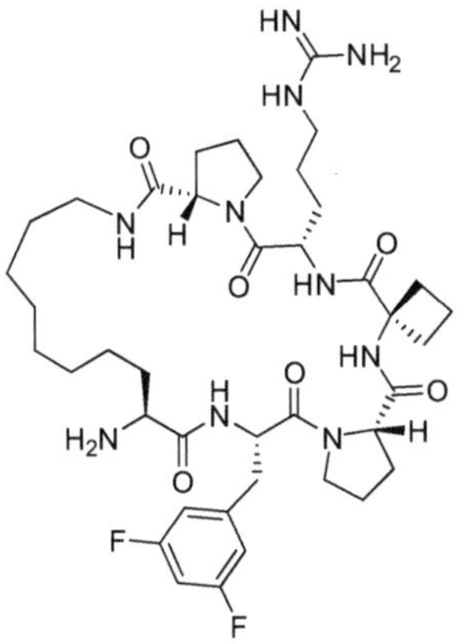

99 (MLL1, K_i = 4.7 nM)

Figure 8.39

mediated leukemic transformation by down regulating the expression of target genes required for MLL oncogenic activity, and blocks proliferation and induces apoptosis in cell carrying the MML translocations.[225]

A highly conserved octapeptide (Arg-Trp-Arg-Phe-Pro-Ala-Arg-Pro) in MLL1 mediates the interaction with menin as determined by an X-ray structure of the MLL1-menin complex.[222] Based on the observed conformation of the key octapeptide sequence, macrocyclic compounds such as **99** (Figure 8.39) mimicking the key pharmacophore were designed and synthesized. Macrocycle **99** (K_i = 4.7 nM) was >600 times more potent than the corresponding acyclic peptide.[222]

8.5.6 Sonic Hedgehog (Shh) Modulators

The hedgehog signaling pathway is essential in embryonic development and its dysfunction at the adult state is associated with cancer development.[182] Full length sonic hedgehog (Shh), the most widely characterized homologue, is auto-cleaved to an active 20 kDa N-terminal fragment (ShhN) which binds to its 12-transmembrane receptor Patched (Ptc1). Binding of Shh to Ptc1 reverses its inhibitory effect on Smo (Smoothened), which activates transcription of target genes such as *Gli1* and *Pct1*. By small-molecule microarray screening of a macrocyclic library generated by diversity-oriented synthesis (DOS),[227] an initial hit (**100**, Figure 8.40) inhibiting the interaction of ShhN and Pct1 was found (K_D = 9 µM, determined by SPR).[228] As part of a medicinal chemistry program to explore macrocycles with improved activity, compound **101** (robotnikinin, Figure 8.40) was identified. This macrocycle displayed a K_D of 3.1 µM as determined by SPR, a significantly longer off rate than observed for **100**.[227] This is the first example of a small molecule that binds to purified ShhN protein and interferes with the ShhN-Ptc1 interaction

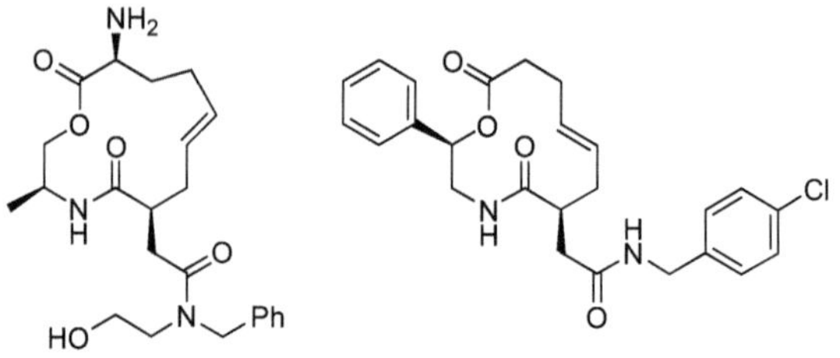

100   **101** (Robotnikinin)

Figure 8.40

and does not compete with the cyclopamine-Smo interaction. Potent antagonists of Smo such as GDC-0449 (Vismodegib, Erivedge)[229] have shown promising efficacy in clinical trials for the treatment of basal cell carcinoma (BCC) and pancreatic cancer.[230] Vismodegib was approved in December 2012 by the FDA for the treatment of BCC.[231]

8.5.7 Transporters: Novel Macrocycles Targeting LptD

There is an urgent need for new antibiotics with novel mechanisms of action due to the rapid emergence of multidrug-resistant (MDR) pathogens, especially against MDR *Enterococcus faecium, Staphylococcus aureus, Klebsiella pneumonia, Acinetobacter baumannii, Pseudomonas aeruginosa*, and *Enterobacter species*, also referred to as the so called ESKAPE pathogens.[232] The discovery of novel antibiotics, especially against MDR Gram-negative species has been scarce.[233,234] Antimicrobial peptides (AMPs) are important constituents of innate immunity and have attracted a lot of attention due to their low propensity to generate bacterial resistance.[235] However, the clinical development of AMPs as systemic drugs has been extremely challenging due to unfavorable ADMET properties.[236] By transplanting the key pharmacophore of protegrin I (**102**) [237] onto a suitable PEM scaffold (Section 8.2.2) a library of PEM molecules was designed and synthesized and tested for antimicrobial activity.[238,239] Some initial hits showed antimicrobial activity comparable to protegrin I, however, in contrast to protegrin I they were not hemolytic. Other compounds of the library were completely selective for *Pseudomonas aeruginosa (Pa)*. Applying PEM Technology (Section 8.2.2) to these initial *Pa*-selective hits generated, after several rounds of optimization, a novel class of antibiotics with potent activity against *Pa*. POL7001 (**103**, Figure 8.41) was highly active against a broad panel of *Pseudomonas* strains including many MDR clinical isolates (MIC$_{90}$ = 0.25 µg/ml).[240] Excellent efficacy of POL7001 (**103**) was also shown in a mouse septicemia infection model after dosing subcutaneously at 1 and 5 hours after inoculation with either *Pa* ATCC9027 or ATCC27853 with an ED$_{50}$ in the range of 0.25–0.28 mg/kg (gentamycin as control in the same model gave ED$_{50}$s of 3.1 mg kg^{-1} and 2.9 mg kg^{-1}, respectively).[240] In parallel to further optimization, mechanism of action studies were initiated. These antibiotics did

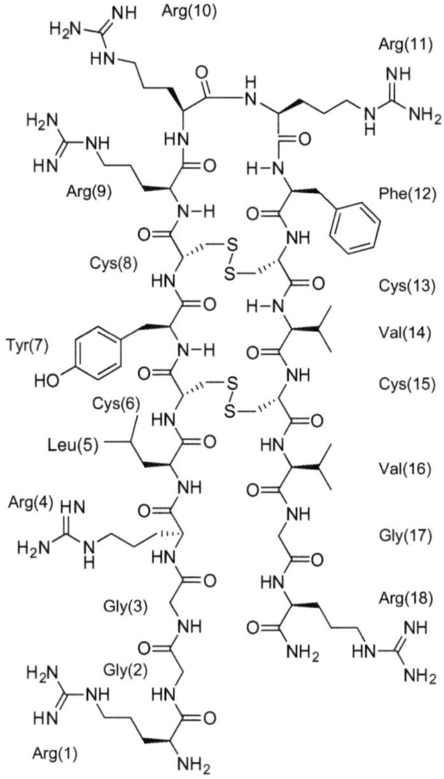

102 (Protegrin-I)

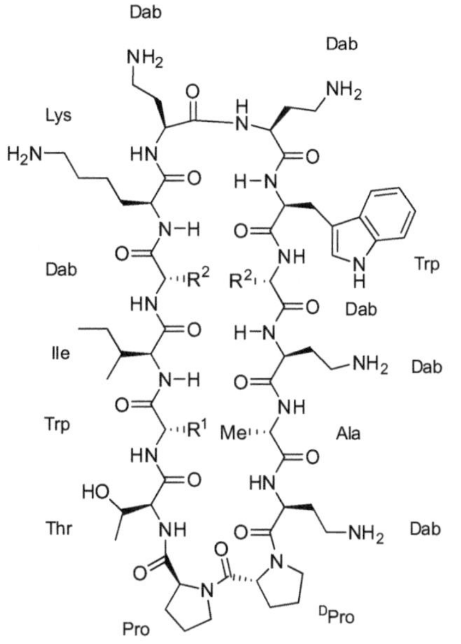

103 (POL 7001)

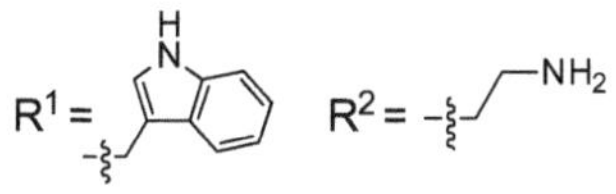

(Dab, L-2, 4-diamino-butyric acid)

Figure 8.41

not interfere with protein or DNA biosynthesis. In addition, the compounds were bactericidal, but not hemolytic or membranolytic on bacterial membranes, and not cytotoxic. Forward genetic and biochemical studies pointed towards the outer membrane protein transporter LptD (OstA, Imp), a novel antibacterial target. Photo-affinity labeling studies confirmed LptD as the likely target of POL7001 and its analogs.[240] LptD is a β-barrel protein critically involved in transporting lipopolysaccharide (LPS) from the periplasm to the outer leaflet of the outer membrane, and is highly conserved in Gram-negative bacteria. After final optimization, POL7080 (structure undisclosed) was selected as clinical candidate and has successfully completed Phase I clinical studies, started Phase II and was recently outlicensed to Roche.

8.6   Summary and Outlook

This review has summarized some highlights of macrocyclic drug discovery in the area of GPCRs, integrins, and protein–protein interactions spanning roughly the last 30 years. One of the most fruitful approaches is to conformationally lock pharmacophores derived from natural peptide ligands into the context of a constrained macrocycle ("lock of the bioactive conformation"). It is interesting to note that in the case of integrins the same pharmacophore (*e.g.* RGD) displayed in different macrocycles and conformations shows different biological and selectivity profiles. The same can be observed in the GPCR area.

Due to their semi-rigid nature, macrocycles display unique properties. They can adapt their conformation during binding to a flexible protein target surface ("induced fit"), and due to their size they can interact with larger protein interfaces ("hot spots"). In addition, macrocycles can display favorable ADME properties well beyond the "Rule of 5" in particular exhibiting favorable cell penetrating properties and oral bioavailability. New macrocyclic discovery technologies and modular high throughput medicinal chemistry methodologies will further contribute to the growing interest of the drug discovery community in this attractive class of molecules. Taken together, there is a strong belief that natural and synthetic macrocycles will have a bright future in the drug discovery of complex biological targets.

The authors would like to thank Drs E. Chevalier, F. Jung, B. Romagnoli, O. Sellier-Kessler, M. Thommen, and S. Weinbrenner for their contributions and proofreading of the manuscript.

References

1. E. M. Driggers, S. P. Hale, J. Lee and N. K. Terrett, *Nat. Rev. Drug Discovery*, 2008, **7**, 608.
2. E. Marsault and M. L. Peterson, *J. Med. Chem.*, 2011, **54**, 1961.
3. J. Mallinson and I. Collins, *Future Med. Chem.*, 2012, **4**, 1409.
4. D. Obrecht, J. A. Robinson, F. Bernardini, C. Bisang, S. J. DeMarco, K. Moehle and F. O. Gombert, *Curr. Med. Chem.*, 2009, **16**, 42.
5. F. von Nussbaum, M. Brands, B. Hinzen, S. Weigand and D. Habich, *Angew. Chem. Int. Ed.*, 2006, **45**, 5072.
6. G. M. Suarez-Jimenez, A. Burgos-Hernandez and J. M. Ezquerra-Brauer, *Mar. Drugs*, 2012, **10**, 963.
7. M. J. Yu, W. Zheng, B. M. Seletsky, B. A. Littlefield and Y. Kishi, *Annu. Rep. Med. Chem.*, 2011, **46**, 227.
8. C. J. White and A. K. Yudin, *Nat. Chem.*, 2011, **3**, 509.
9. C. E. Ballard, H. Yu and B. Wang, *Curr. Med. Chem.*, 2002, **9**, 471.
10. V. J. Hruby, *Life Sci.*, 1982, **31**, 189.
11. H. Kessler, *Angew. Chem. Int. Ed. Engl.*, 1982, **21**, 512.
12. D. Obrecht, E. Chevalier, K. Moehle and J. A. Robinson, *Drug Discovery Today: Technologies*, 2012, **9**, e63.
13. J. A. Robinson, S. DeMarco, F. Gombert, K. Moehle and D. Obrecht, *Drug Discovery Today*, 2008, **13**, 944.
14. R. Fasan, R. L. Dias, K. Moehle, O. Zerbe, J. W. Vrijbloed, D. Obrecht and J. A. Robinson, *Angew. Chem. Int. Ed.*, 2004, **43**, 2109.

15. R. Fasan, R. L. Dias, K. Moehle, O. Zerbe, D. Obrecht, P. R. Mittl, M. G. Grutter and J. A. Robinson, *ChemBioChem*, 2006, 7, 515.

16. P. H. Kussie, S. Gorina, V. Marechal, B. Elenbaas, J. Moreau, A. J. Levine and N. P. Pavletich, *Science*, 1996, **274**, 948.

17. P. Chene, *Nat. Rev. Cancer*, 2003, 3, 102.

18. A. Descours, K. Moehle, A. Renard and J. A. Robinson, *ChemBioChem*, 2002, 3, 318.

19. E. Chevalier, O. Sellier-Kessler, F. Jung, S. DeMarco, G. Lemercier, J. Zumbrunn, C. Ludin, C. Bisang, K. Moehle, H. Henze, F. O. Gombert and D. Obrecht, *Amer. J. Respir. Crit. Care Med.*, 2009, **179**, [1_MeetingAbstracts], A5652.

20. E. Marsault, H. R. Hoveyda, R. Gagnon, M. L. Peterson, M. Vezina, C. Saint-Louis, A. Landry, J. F. Pinault, L. Ouellet, S. Beauchemin, S. Beaubien, A. Mathieu, K. Benakli, Z. Wang, M. Brassard, D. Lonergan, F. Bilodeau, M. Ramaseshan, N. Fortin, R. Lan, S. Li, F. Galaud, V. Plourde, M. Champagne, A. Doucet, P. Bherer, M. Gauthier, G. Olsen, G. Villeneuve, S. Bhat, L. Foucher, D. Fortin, X. Peng, S. Bernard, A. Drouin, R. Deziel, G. Berthiaume, Y. L. Dory, G. L. Fraser and P. Deslongchamps, *Bioorg. Med. Chem. Lett.*, 2008, **18**, 4731.

21. E. Comer, H. Liu, A. Joliton, A. Clabaut, C. Johnson, L. B. Akella and L. A. Marcaurelle, *Proc. Natl. Acad. Sci., U. S. A.*, 2011, **108**, 6751.

22. M. E. Fitzgerald, C. A. Mulrooney, J. R. Duvall, J. Wei, B. C. Suh, L. B. Akella, A. Vrcic and L. A. Marcaurelle, *ACS Comb. Sci.*, 2012, **14**, 89.

23. R. W. Heidebrecht, C. Mulrooney, C. P. Austin, R. H. Barker, J. A. Beaudoin, K. C.-C. Cheng, E. Comer, S. Dandapani, J. Dick, J. R. Duvall, E. H. Ekland, D. A. Fidock, M. E. Fitzgerald, M. Foley, R. Guha, P. Hinkson, M. Kramer, A. K. Lukens, D. Masi, L. A. Marcaurelle, X. Z. Su, C. J. Thomas, M. Weiwer, R. C. Wiegand, D. Wirth, M. Xia, J. Yuan, J. Zhao, M. Palmer, B. Munoz and S. Schreiber, *ACS Med. Chem. Lett.*, 2012, 3, 112.

24. C. Cain, *BioCentury*, 2012, **38**, A7.

25. J. D. Tyndall, B. Pfeiffer, G. Abbenante and D. P. Fairlie, *Chem. Rev.*, 2005, **105**, 793.

26. T. Klabunde and G. Hessler, *ChemBioChem*, 2002, 3, 928.

27. J. C. Venter, M. D. Adams, E. W. Myers, P. W. Li, R. J. Mural, G. G. Sutton, H. O. Smith, M. Yandell, C. A. Evans, R. A. Holt, J. D. Gocayne, P. Amanatides, R. M. Ballew, D. H. Huson, J. R. Wortman, Q. Zhang, C. D. Kodira, X. H. Zheng, L. Chen, M. Skupski, G. Subramanian, P. D. Thomas, J. Zhang, G. L. Gabor Miklos, C. Nelson, S. Broder, A. G. Clark, J. Nadeau, V. A. McKusick, N. Zinder, A. J. Levine, R. J. Roberts, M. Simon, C. Slayman, M. Hunkapiller, R. Bolanos, A. Delcher, I. Dew, D. Fasulo, M. Flanigan, L. Florea, A. Halpern, S. Hannenhalli, S. Kravitz, S. Levy, C. Mobarry, K. Reinert, K. Remington, J. Bu-Threideh, E. Beasley, K. Biddick, V. Bonazzi, R. Brandon, M. Cargill, I. Chandramouliswaran, R. Charlab,

K. Chaturvedi, Z. Deng, F. Di, V, P. Dunn, K. Eilbeck, C. Evangelista,
A. E. Gabrielian, W. Gan, W. Ge, F. Gong, Z. Gu, P. Guan, T. J. Heiman,
M. E. Higgins, R. R. Ji, Z. Ke, K. A. Ketchum, Z. Lai, Y. Lei, Z. Li, J. Li,
Y. Liang, X. Lin, F. Lu, G. V. Merkulov, N. Milshina, H. M. Moore,
A. K. Naik, V. A. Narayan, B. Neelam, D. Nusskern, D. B. Rusch,
S. Salzberg, W. Shao, B. Shue, J. Sun, Z. Wang, A. Wang, X. Wang,
J. Wang, M. Wei, R. Wides, C. Xiao, C. Yan, A. Yao, J. Ye, M. Zhan,
W. Zhang, H. Zhang, Q. Zhao, L. Zheng, F. Zhong, W. Zhong, S. Zhu,
S. Zhao, D. Gilbert, S. Baumhueter, G. Spier, C. Carter, A. Cravchik,
T. Woodage, F. Ali, H. An, A. Awe, D. Baldwin, H. Baden, M. Barnstead,
I. Barrow, K. Beeson, D. Busam, A. Carver, A. Center, M. L. Cheng,
L. Curry, S. Danaher, L. Davenport, R. Desilets, S. Dietz, K. Dodson,
L. Doup, S. Ferriera, N. Garg, A. Gluecksmann, B. Hart, J. Haynes,
C. Haynes, C. Heiner, S. Hladun, D. Hostin, J. Houck, T. Howland,
C. Ibegwam, J. Johnson, F. Kalush, L. Kline, S. Koduru, A. Love,
F. Mann, D. May, S. McCawley, T. McIntosh, I. McMullen, M. Moy,
L. Moy, B. Murphy, K. Nelson, C. Pfannkoch, E. Pratts, V. Puri,
H. Qureshi, M. Reardon, R. Rodriguez, Y. H. Rogers, D. Romblad,
B. Ruhfel, R. Scott, C. Sitter, M. Smallwood, E. Stewart, R. Strong,
E. Suh, R. Thomas, N. N. Tint, S. Tse, C. Vech, G. Wang, J. Wetter,
S. Williams, M. Williams, S. Windsor, E. Winn-Deen, K. Wolfe, J. Zaveri,
K. Zaveri, J. F. Abril, R. Guigo, M. J. Campbell, K. V. Sjolander,
B. Karlak, A. Kejariwal, H. Mi, B. Lazareva, T. Hatton, A. Narechania,
K. Diemer, A. Muruganujan, N. Guo, S. Sato, V. Bafna, S. Istrail,
R. Lippert, R. Schwartz, B. Walenz, S. Yooseph, D. Allen, A. Basu,
J. Baxendale, L. Blick, M. Caminha, J. Carnes-Stine, P. Caulk,
Y. H. Chiang, M. Coyne, C. Dahlke, A. Mays, M. Dombroski,
M. Donnelly, D. Ely, S. Esparham, C. Fosler, H. Gire, S. Glanowski,
K. Glasser, A. Glodek, M. Gorokhov, K. Graham, B. Gropman, M. Harris,
J. Heil, S. Henderson, J. Hoover, D. Jennings, C. Jordan, J. Jordan,
J. Kasha, L. Kagan, C. Kraft, A. Levitsky, M. Lewis, X. Liu, J. Lopez,
D. Ma, W. Majoros, J. McDaniel, S. Murphy, M. Newman, T. Nguyen,
N. Nguyen and M. Nodell, *Science*, 2001, **291**, 1304.

28. P. Gribbon and A. Sewing, *Drug Discovery Today*, 2005, **10**, 17.
29. B. K. Shoichet and B. K. Kobilka, *Trends Pharmacol. Sci.*, 2012, **33**, 268.
30. V. P. Jaakola, M. T. Griffith, M. A. Hanson, V. Cherezov, E. Y. T. Chien,
    J. R. Lane, A. P. IJzerman and R. C. Stevens, *Science*, 2008, **322**, 1211.
31. E. Y. T. Chien, W. Liu, Q. Zhao, V. Katritch, G. Won Han, M. A. Hanson,
    L. Shi, A. H. Newman, J. A. Javitch, V. Cherezov and R. C. Stevens,
    Science, 2010, **330**, 1091.
32. B. Wu, E. Y. Chien, C. D. Mol, G. Fenalti, W. Liu, V. Katritch,
    R. Abagyan, A. Brooun, P. Wells, F. C. Bi, D. J. Hamel, P. Kuhn,
    T. M. Handel, V. Cherezov and R. C. Stevens, *Science*, 2010, **330**, 1066.
33. T. Shimamura, M. Shiroishi, S. Weyand, H. Tsujimoto, G. Winter,
    V. Katritch, R. Abagyan, V. Cherezov, W. Liu, G. W. Han, T. Kobayashi,
    R. C. Stevens and S. Iwata, *Nature*, 2011, **475**, 65.

34. M. A. Hanson, C. B. Roth, E. Jo, M. T. Griffith, F. L. Scott, G. Reinhart, H. Desale, B. Clemons, S. M. Cahalan, S. C. Schuerer, M. G. Sanna, G. W. Han, P. Kuhn, H. Rosen and R. C. Stevens, *Science*, 2012, **335**, 851.

35. K. Haga, A. C. Kruse, H. Asada, T. Yurugi-Kobayashi, M. Shiroishi, C. Zhang, W. I. Weis, T. Okada, B. K. Kobilka, T. Haga and T. Kobayashi, *Nature*, 2012, **482**, 547.

36. Y. Aachoui, I. A. Leaf, J. A. Hagar, M. F. Fontana, C. G. Campos, D. E. Zak, M. H. Tan, P. A. Cotter, R. E. Vance, A. Aderem and E. A. Miao, *Science*, 2013, **339**, 975.

37. K. Hollenstein, J. Kean, A. Bortolato, R. K. Y. Cheng, A. S. Doré, A. Jazayeri, R. M. Cooke, M. Weir and F. H. Marshall, *Nature*, 2013, **499**, 438.

38. F. Y. Siu, M. He, C. de Graaf, G. W. Han, D. Yang, Z. Zhang, C. Zhou, Q. Xu, D. Wacker, J. S. Joseph, W. Liu, J. Lau, V. Cherezov, V. Katritch, M-W. Yang and R. C. Stevens, *Nature*, 2013, **499**, 444.

39. H. Kessler, R. Gratias, G. Hessler, M. Gurrath and G. Müller, *Pure Appl. Chem.*, 1996, **68**, 1201.

40. S. Hanessian, G. Naughton-Smith, H. G. Lombart and W. D. Lubell, *Tetrahedron*, 1997, **53**, 12789.

41. G. Ruiz-Gomez, J. D. Tyndall, B. Pfeiffer, G. Abbenante and D. P. Fairlie, *Chem. Rev.*, 2010, **110**, PR1.

42. C. Thurieau, M. Feletou, P. Hennig, E. Raimbaud, E. Canet and J. L. Fauchere, *J. Med. Chem.*, 1996, **39**, 2095.

43. J. J. Lopez, A. K. Shukla, C. Reinhart, H. Schwalbe, H. Michel and C. Glaubitz, *Angew. Chem. Int. Ed.*, 2008, **47**, 1668.

44. F. J. Hock, K. Wirth, U. Albus, W. Linz, H. J. Gerhards, G. Wiemer, S. Henke, G. Breipohl, W. Konig, J. Knolle and B. A. Schölkens, *Br. J. Pharmacol.*, 1991, **102**, 769.

45. J. P. Powers, D. J. Dairaghi and J. C. Jaen, *Annu. Rep. Med. Chem.*, 2011, **46**, 171.

46. T. M. Woodruff, K. S. Nandakumar and F. Tedesco, *Mol. Immunol.*, 2011, **48**, 1631.

47. A. J. Hutchison and J. E. Krause, *Annu. Rep. Med. Chem.*, 2004, **39**, 139.

48. E. R. Zuiderweg, D. G. Nettesheim, K. W. Mollison and G. W. Carter, *Biochemistry*, 1989, **28**, 172.

49. A. K. Wong, A. M. Finch, G. K. Pierens, D. J. Craik, S. M. Taylor and D. P. Fairlie, *J. Med. Chem.*, 1998, **41**, 3417.

50. A. M. Finch, A. K. Wong, N. J. Paczkowski, S. K. Wadi, D. J. Craik, D. P. Fairlie and S. M. Taylor, *J. Med. Chem.*, 1999, **42**, 1965.

51. X. Zhang, W. Boyar, M. J. Toth, L. Wennogle and N. C. Gonnella, *Proteins*, 1997, **28**, 261.

52. R. C. Reid, G. Abbenante, S. M. Taylor and D. P. Fairlie, *J. Org. Chem.*, 2003, **68**, 4464.

53. D. R. March, L. M. Proctor, M. J. Stoermer, R. Sbaglia, G. Abbenante, R. C. Reid, T. M. Woodruff, K. Wadi, N. Paczkowski, J. D. Tyndall, S. M. Taylor and D. P. Fairlie, *Mol. Pharmacol.*, 2004, **65**, 868.

54. T. M. Woodruff, A. J. Strachan, N. Dryburgh, I. A. Shiels, R. C. Reid, D. P. Fairlie and S. M. Taylor, *Arthritis Rheum.*, 2002, **46**, 2476.

55. J. Kohl, *Curr. Opin. Mol. Ther.*, 2006, **8**, 529.

56. B. Moser, M. Wolf, A. Walz and P. Loetscher, *Trends in Immunol.*, 2004, **25**, 75.

57. B. Moser and K. Willimann, *Ann. Rheum. Dis.*, 2004, **63**, Suppl 2, ii84.

58. K. Dembowsky, B. Romagnoli, J. Zimmermann, E. Chevalier, C. Ludin and D. Obrecht, *CXCR4 Antagonists in, Novel Developments in Stem Cell Mobilization: Focus on CXCR4*, ed. S. Fruehauf, W. J. Zeller and G. Calandra, *Springer*, New York, Dordrecht, Heidelberg, London, 2012, ch. 16, p. 303.

59. A. Zlotnik, O. Yoshie and H. Nomiyama, *Genome Biol.*, 2006, **7**, 243.

60. J. E. Pease and R. Horuk, *J. Med. Chem.*, 2012, **55**, 9363.

61. R. D. Macarthur and R. M. Novak, *Clin. Infect. Dis.*, 2008, **47**, 236.

62. S. P. Fricker, *Expert. Opin. Investig. Drugs*, 2008, **17**, 1749.

63. A. Peled, O. Wald and J. Burger, *Expert. Opin. Investig. Drugs*, 2012, **21**, 341.

64. J. A. Burger and A. Peled, *Leukemia*, 2009, **23**, 43.

65. Y. Lavrovsky, Y. A. Ivanenkov, K. V. Balakin, D. A. Medvedeva and A. V. Ivachtchenko, *Mini Rev. Med. Chem.*, 2008, **8**, 1075.

66. G. J. Bridger, R. T. Skerlj, P. E. Hernandez-Abad, D. E. Bogucki, Z. Wang, Y. Zhou, S. Nan, E. M. Boehringer, T. Wilson and J. Crawford, *J. Med. Chem.*, 2010, **53**, 1250.

67. T. Narumi, R. Hayashi, K. Tomita, K. Kobayashi, N. Tanahara, H. Ohno, T. Naito, E. Kodama, M. Matsuoka, S. Oishi and N. Fujii, *Org. Biomol. Chem.*, 2010, **8**, 616.

68. S. J. DeMarco, H. Henze, A. Lederer, K. Moehle, R. Mukherjee, B. Romagnoli, J. A. Robinson, F. Brianza, F. O. Gombert, S. Lociuro, C. Ludin, J. W. Vrijbloed, J. Zumbrunn, J. P. Obrecht, D. Obrecht, V. Brondani, F. Hamy and T. Klimkait, *Bioorg. Med. Chem.*, 2006, **14**, 8396.

69. M. Masuda, H. Nakashima, T. Ueda, H. Naba, R. Ikoma, A. Otaka, Y. Terakawa, H. Tamamura, T. Ibuka and T. Murakami, *Biochem. Biophys. Res. Commun.*, 1992, **189**, 845.

70. H. Nakashima, M. Masuda, T. Murakami, Y. Koyanagi, A. Matsumoto, N. Fujii and N. Yamamoto, *Antimicrob. Agents Chemother.*, 1992, **36**, 1249.

71. H. Tamamura, M. Kuroda, M. Masuda, A. Otaka, S. Funakoshi, H. Nakashima, N. Yamamoto, M. Waki, A. Matsumoto and J. M. Lancelin, *Biochim. Biophys. Acta*, 1993, **1163**, 209.

72. H. Tamamura, A. Omagari, S. Oishi, T. Kanamoto, N. Yamamoto, S. C. Peiper, H. Nakashima, A. Otaka and N. Fujii, *Bioorg. Med. Chem. Lett.*, 2000, **10**, 2633.

73. K. Kobayashi, S. Oishi, R. Hayashi, K. Tomita, T. Kubo, N. Tanahara, H. Ohno, Y. Yoshikawa, T. Furuya, M. Hoshino and N. Fujii, *J. Med. Chem.*, 2012, **55**, 2746.

74. N. Fujii, H. Nakashima and H. Tamamura, *Expert Opin. Investig. Drugs*, 2003, **12**, 185.

75. H. Tamamura and N. Fujii, *Expert Opin. Ther. Targets*, 2005, **9**, 1267.

76. G. Moncunill, M. Armand-Ugon, I. Clotet-Codina, E. Pauls, E. Ballana, A. Llano, B. Romagnoli, J. W. Vrijbloed, F. O. Gombert, B. Clotet, S. De Marco and J. A. Este, *Mol. Pharmacol.*, 2008, **73**, 1264.

77. D. Karpova, K. Dauber, G. Spohn, D. Chudziak, B. Romagnoli, K. Patel, E. Chevalier and H. Bonig. *Exp. Hematol.*, 2011, 39 (Suppl 1), S15. (ISEH Annual Meeting Abstracts) 2011. 01108534 (Oral Presentation).

78. D. Karpova, K. Dauber, G. Spohn, D. Chudziak, E. Wiercinska, M. Schulz, B. Romagnoli, E. Chevalier, K. Patel and H. Bonig, *ASH Annual Meeting Abstracts, Blood*, 2012, **701**, 4100(Poster presentation).

79. K. Hamesch, P. Subramanian, X. Li, A. Thiemann, K. Heyll, K. Dembowsky, E. Chevalier, C. Weber and A. Schober, *Cardiovasc. Res.*, 2012, **93**, S62.

80. Y. C. Chen, Z. Zeng, Y. Shi, R. Jacamo, C. Ludin, K. Dembowsky, P. S. Frenette, M. Konopleva and M. Andreeff, *Blood*, 2010, **116**, 2179.

81. S. Schmitt, N. Weinhold, K. Dembowsky, K. Neben, M. Witzens-Harig, M. Braun, J. Klemmer, P. Wuchter, C. Ludin and A. D. Ho, *Blood*, 2010, **116**, Abstract 824: Oral session.

82. M. H. Bolli, J. Marfurt, C. Grisostomi, C. Boss, C. Binkert, P. Hess, A. Treiber, E. Thorin, K. Morrison, S. Buchmann, D. Bur, H. Ramuz, M. Clozel, W. Fischli and T. Weller, *J. Med. Chem.*, 2004, **47**, 2776.

83. L. J. Rubin and S. Roux, *Expert Opin. Investig. Drugs*, 2002, **11**, 991.

84. R. W. Janes, D. H. Peapus and B. A. Wallace, *Nat. Struct. Biol.*, 1994, **1**, 311.

85. B. A. Wallace, R. W. Janes, D. A. Bassolino and S. R. Krystek, *Jr, Protein Sci.*, 1995, **4**, 75.

86. K. Ishikawa, T. Fukami, T. Nagase, K. Fujita, T. Hayama, K. Niiyama, T. Mase, M. Ihara and M. Yano, *J. Med. Chem.*, 1992, **35**, 2139.

87. M. Coles, V. Sowemimo, D. Scanlon, S. L. A. Munro and D. J. Craik, *J. Med. Chem.*, 1993, **36**, 2658.

88. S. Nakajima, K. Niiyama, M. Ihara, K. Kojiri and H. Suda, *J. Antibiot.*, 1991, **44**, 1348.

89. S. Miyata, N. Fukami, M. Neya, S. Takase and S. Kiyoto, *J. Antibiot.*, 1992, **45**, 788.

90. T. Fukami, T. Nagase, K. Fujita, T. Hayama, K. Niiyama, T. Mase, S. Nakajima, T. Fukuroda, T. Saeki, M. Nishikibe, M. Ihara, M. Yano and K. Ishikawa, *J. Med. Chem.*, 1995, **38**, 4309.

91. J. W. Bean, C. E. Peishoff and K. D. Kopple, *Int. J. Pept. Protein Res.*, 1994, **44**, 223.

92. R. A. Atkinson and J. T. Pelton, *FEBS Lett.*, 1992, **296**, 1.

93. M. D. Reily, V. Thanabal, D. O. Omecinsky, J. B. Dunbar Jr, A. M. Doherty and P. L. DePue, *FEBS Lett.*, 1992, **300**, 136.

94. S. R. Krystek Jr, D. A. Bassolino, R. E. Bruccoleri, J. T. Hunt, M. A. Porubcan, C. F. Wandler and N. H. Andersen, *FEBS Lett.*, 1992, **299**, 255.

95. N. K. Gulavita, A. E. Wright, P. J. McCarthy, S. A. Pomponi, M. Kelly-Borges, M. Chin and M. A. Sills, *J. Nat. Prod.*, 1993, **56**, 1613.

96. Y. Funahashi, T. Ishimaru, N. Kawamura, *Takeda Chem Ind Ltd, Japan. JP Pat. Appl.*, 08231552.

97. Y. Morishita, S. Chiba, E. Tsukuda, T. Tanaka, T. Ogawa, M. Yamasaki, M. Yoshida, I. Kawamoto and Y. Matsuda, *J. Antibiot.*, 1994, **47**, 269.

98. R. Katahira, K. Shibata, M. Yamasaki, Y. Matsuda and M. Yoshida, *Bioorg. Med. Chem.*, 1995, **3**, 1273.

99. P. W. Schiller and J. DiMaio, *Nature*, 1982, **297**, 74.

100. K. Shreder, L. Zhang, T. Dang, T. L. Yaksh, H. Umeno, R. DeHaven, J. Daubert and M. Goodman, *J. Med. Chem.*, 1998, **41**, 2631.

101. M. Goodman, C. Zapf and Y. Rew, *Biopolymers*, 2001, **60**, 229.

102. A. Mollica, G. Guardiani, P. Davis, S. W. Ma, F. Porreca, J. Lai, L. Mannina, A. P. Sobolev and V. J. Hruby, *J. Med. Chem.*, 2007, **50**, 3138.

103. Y. Rew, S. Malkmus, C. Svensson, T. L. Yaksh, N. N. Chung, P. W. Schiller, J. A. Cassel, R. N. DeHaven and M. Goodman, *J. Med. Chem.*, 2002, **45**, 3746.

104. F. N. Gavins, *Trends Pharmacol. Sci.*, 2010, **31**, 266.

105. M. Liu, J. Zhao, K. Chen, X. Bian, C. Wang, Y. Shi and J. M. Wang, *Int. Immunopharmacol.*, 2012, **14**, 283.

106. Q. Zhang, M. Raoof, Y. Chen, Y. Sumi, T. Sursal, W. Junger, K. Brohi, K. Itagaki and C. J. Hauser, *Nature*, 2010, **464**, 104.

107. J. Unitt, M. Fagura, T. Phillips, S. King, M. Perry, A. Morley, C. MacDonald, R. Weaver, J. Christie, S. Barber, R. Mohammed, M. Paul, A. Cook and A. Baxter, *Bioorg. Med. Chem. Lett.*, 2011, **21**, 2991.

108. K. Wenzel-Seifert and R. Seifert, *J. Immunol.*, 1993, **150**, 4591.

109. R. Seifert and K. Wenzel-Seifert, *Life Sci.*, 2003, **73**, 2263.

110. F. Loor, F. Tiberghien, T. Wenandy, A. Didier and R. Traber, *J. Med. Chem.*, 2002, **45**, 4613.

111. Y. S. Or, T. Lazarova and B. C. Hamann, *Enanta Pharmaceuticals, Inc., USA. PCT Int. Appl.*, WO02069902.

112. Y. S. Or and T. Lazarova, *Enanta Pharmaceuticals, Inc., USA, PCT Int. Appl.*, WO03030834.

113. J. D. Benson, *Nikan Pharmaceuticals, LLC., USA. PCT Int. Appl.*, WO2010141584.

114. M. Rosicka, M. Krsek, Z. Jarkovska, J. Marek and V. Schreiber, *Physiol. Res.*, 2002, **51**, 435.

115. O. Gualillo, F. Lago, J. Gomez-Reino, F. F. Casanueva and C. Dieguez, *FEBS Lett.*, 2003, **552**, 105.

116. R. J. DeVita, R. Bochis, A. J. Frontier, A. Kotliar, M. H. Fisher, W. R. Schoen, M. J. Wyvratt, K. Cheng, W. W. Chan, B. Butler, T. M. Jacks, G. J. Hickey, K. D. Schleim, K. Leung, Z. Chen, S. L. Chiu, W. P. Feeney, P. K. Cunningham and R. G. Smith, *J. Med. Chem.*, 1998, **41**, 1716.

117. W. R. Schoen, J. M. Pisano, K. Prendergast, M. J. Wyvratt Jr, M. H. Fisher, K. Cheng, W. W. Chan, B. Butler, R. G. Smith and R. G. Ball, *J. Med. Chem.*, 1994, **37**, 897.

118. R. J. DeVita, A. J. Frontier, W. R. Schoen, M. J. Wyvratt, M. H. Fisher, K. Chen, W. S. Chan, B. S. Butler and R. G. Smith, *Helv. Chim. Acta*, 1997, **80**, 1244.

119. H. R. Hoveyda, E. Marsault, R. Gagnon, A. P. Mathieu, M. Vézina, A. Landry, Z. Wang, K. Benakli, S. Beaubien, C. Saint-Louis, M. Brassard, J. F. Pinault, L. Ouellet, S. Bhat, M. Ramaseshan, X. Peng, L. Foucher, S. Beauchemin, P. Bhérer, D. F. Veber, M. L. Peterson and G. L. Fraser, *J. Med. Chem.*, 2011, **54**, 8305.

120. Tranzyme Press Release, 12 March 2012.

121. Tranzyme Press Release, 25 May 2012.

122. Tranzyme Press Release, 15 November 2012.

123. H. Hoveyda, E. Marsault, H. Thomas, G. Fraser, S. Beaubien, A. Mathieu, J. Beignet, M. A. Bonin, S. Phoenix, D. Drutz, M. Petersen, S. Beauchemin, M. Brassard and M. Venzina, *Tranzyme Pharma, Inc., USA, PCT Int. Appl.*, WO2011053821.

124. M. A. Bednarek, T. MacNeil, R. N. Kalyani, R. Tang, L. H. Van der Ploeg and D. H. Weinberg, *J. Med. Chem.*, 2001, **44**, 3665.

125. P. Grieco, A. Lavecchia, M. Cai, D. Trivedi, D. Weinberg, T. MacNeil, L. H. Van der Ploeg and V. J. Hruby, *J. Med. Chem.*, 2002, **45**, 5287.

126. R. P. Nargund, A. M. Strack and T. M. Fong, *J. Med. Chem.*, 2006, **49**, 4035.

127. F. A. Al-Obeidi, A. M. Castrucci, M. E. Hadley and V. J. Hruby, *J. Med. Chem.*, 1989, **32**, 2555.

128. V. J. Hruby, D. Lu, S. D. Sharma, A. L. Castrucci, R. A. Kesterson, F. A. Al-Obeidi, M. E. Hadley and R. D. Cone, *J. Med. Chem.*, 1995, **38**, 3454.

129. J. Ying, K. E. Kover, X. Gu, G. Han, D. B. Trivedi, M. J. Kavarana and V. J. Hruby, *Biopolymers*, 2003, **71**, 696.

130. M. A. Bednarek, T. MacNeil, R. Tang, R. N. Kalyani, L. H. Van der Ploeg and D. H. Weinberg, *Biochem. Biophys. Res. Commun.*, 2001, **286**, 641.

131. S. Hess, Y. Linde, O. Ovadia, E. Safrai, D. E. Shalev, A. Swed, E. Halbfinger, T. Lapidot, I. Winkler, Y. Gabinet, A. Faier, D. Yarden, Z. Xiang, F. P. Portillo, C. Haskell-Luevano, C. Gilon and A. Hoffman, *J. Med. Chem.*, 2008, **51**, 1026.

132. A. V. Mayorov, M. Cai, E. S. Palmer, M. M. Dedek, J. P. Cain, A. R. Van Scoy, B. Tan, J. Vagner, D. Trivedi and V. J. Hruby, *J. Med. Chem.*, 2008, **51**, 187.

133. P. Grieco, M. Cai, L. Liu, A. Mayorov, K. Chandler, D. Trivedi, G. Lin, P. Campiglia, E. Novellino and V. J. Hruby, *J. Med. Chem.*, 2008, **51**, 2701.

134. L. Doedens, F. Opperer, M. Cai, J. G. Beck, M. Dedek, E. Palmer, V. J. Hruby and H. Kessler, *J. Am. Chem. Soc.*, 2010, **132**, 8115.

135. D. Lu, D. Willard, I. R. Patel, S. Kadwell, L. Overton, T. Kost, M. Luther, W. Chen, R. P. Woychik, W. O. Wilkison and R. D. Cone, *Nature*, 1994, **371**, 799.

136. M. M. Ollmann, B. D. Wilson, Y. K. Yang, J. A. Kerns, Y. Chen, I. Gantz and G. S. Barsh, *Science*, 1997, **278**, 135.

137. R. Thirumoorthy, J. R. Holder, R. M. Bauzo, N. G. Richards, A. S. Edison and C. Haskell-Luevano, *J. Med. Chem.*, 2001, **44**, 4114.

138. K. A. Carpenter, P. W. Schiller, R. Schmidt and B. C. Wilkes, *Int. J. Pept. Protein Res.*, 1996, **48**, 102.

139. M. J. Przydzial, I. D. Pogozheva, J. C. Ho, K. E. Bosse, E. Sawyer, J. R. Traynor and H. I. Mosberg, *J. Pept. Res.*, 2005, **66**, 255.

140. I. Berezowska, C. Lemieux, N. N. Chung, B. C. Wilkes and P. W. Schiller, *Chem. Biol. Drug Des.*, 2009, **74**, 329.

141. G. Cardillo, L. Gentilucci, A. Tolomelli, R. Spinosa, M. Calienni, A. R. Qasem and S. Spampinato, *J. Med. Chem.*, 2004, 47, 5198.

142. L. Gentilucci, A. Tolomelli, R. DeMarco, S. Spampinato, A. Bedini and R. Artali, *ChemMedChem*, 2011, **6**, 1640.

143. A. Bedini, M. Baiula, L. Gentilucci, A. Tolomelli, R. DeMarco and S. Spampinato, *Peptides*, 2010, **31**, 2135.

144. S. D. Feighner, C. P. Tan, K. K. McKee, O. C. Palyha, D. L. Hreniuk, S. S. Pong, C. P. Austin, D. Figueroa, D. MacNeil, M. A. Cascieri, R. Nargund, R. Bakshi, M. Abramovitz, R. Stocco, S. Kargman, G. O'Neill, L. H. Van der Ploeg, J. Evans, A. A. Patchett, R. G. Smith and A. D. Howard, *Science*, 1999, **284**, 2184.

145. Z. Itoh, *Peptides*, 1997, **18**, 593.

146. A. Andersson and L. Maler, *J. Biomol. NMR*, 2002, **24**, 103.

147. E. Marsault, H. R. Hoveyda, M. L. Peterson, C. Saint-Louis, A. Landry, M. Vezina, L. Ouellet, Z. Wang, M. Ramaseshan, S. Beaubien, K. Benakli, S. Beauchemin, R. Deziel, T. Peeters and G. L. Fraser, *J. Med. Chem.*, 2006, **49**, 7190.

148. E. Marsault, K. Benakli, S. Beaubien, C. Saint-Louis, R. Déziel and G. Fraser, *Bioorg. Med. Chem. Lett*, 2007, **17**, 4187.

149. Tranzyme, Press Release, 24 October 2007. www.tranzyme.com.

150. H. Thomas, C. Chen and E. Marsault, *Mol. Cancer Ther.*, 2007, **6**, 3606S.

151. H. Thomas, C. Chen and E. Marsault, *Neurogastroenterol. Motil.*, 2007, **19**, supplement 3, p. 35, CS19.

152. R. A. Feelders, U. Yasothan and P. Kirkpatrick, *Nat. Rev. Drug Discovery*, 2012, **11**, 597-598.

153. I. Lewis, W. Bauer, R. Albert, N. Chandramopuli, J. Pless, G. Weckbecker and C. Bruns, *J. Med. Chem.*, 2003, **46**, 2334.

154. D. F. Veber, R. M. Freidinger, D. S. Perlow, W. J. Paleveda Jr, F. W. Holly, R. G. Strachan, R. F. Nutt, B. H. Arison, C. Homnick, W. C. Randall, M. S. Glitzer, R. Saperstein and R. Hirschmann, *Nature*, 1981, **292**, 55.

155. C. Bruns, I. Lewis, U. Briner, G. Meno-Tetang and G. Weckbecker, *Eur. J. Endocrinol.*, 2002, **146**, 707.

156. R. Hirschmann, W. Yao, M. A. Cascieri, C. D. Strader, L. Maechler, M. A. Cichy-Knight, J. Hynes Jr, R. D. Van Rijn, P. A. Sprengeler and A. B. Smith III, *J. Med. Chem.*, 1996, **39**, 2441.

157. T. Ryckmans, *Annu. Rep. Med. Chem.*, 2009, **44**, 129.

158. K. Wisniewski, R. Galyean, H. Tariga, S. Alagarsamy, G. Croston, J. Heitzmann, A. Kohan, H. Wisniewska, R. Laporte, P. J. Riviere and C. D. Schteingart, *J. Med. Chem.*, 2011, **54**, 4388.

159. R. Laporte, A. Kohan, J. Heitzmann, H. Wisniewska, J. Toy, E. La, H. Tariga, S. Alagarsamy, B. Ly, J. Dykert, S. Qi, K. Wisniewski, R. Galyean, G. Croston, C. D. Schteingart and P. J. Riviere, *J. Pharmacol. Exp. Ther.*, 2011, **337**, 786.

160. N. Hogg, I. Patzak and F. Willenbrock, *Nat. Rev. Immunol.*, 2011, **11**, 416.

161. D. Cox, M. Brennan and N. Moran, *Nat. Rev. Drug Discovery*, 2010, **9**, 804.

162. E. F. Plow, T. A. Haas, L. Zhang, J. Loftus and J. W. Smith, *J. Biol. Chem.*, 2000, **275**, 21785.

163. R. O. Hynes, *Cell*, 2002, **110**, 673.

164. J. D. Humphries, A. Byron and M. J. Humphries, *J. Cell Sci.*, 2006, **119**, 3901.

165. C. Mas-Moruno, F. Rechenmacher and H. Kessler, *Anticancer Agents Med. Chem.*, 2010, **10**, 753.

166. M. Gurrath, G. Muller, H. Kessler, M. Aumailley and R. Timpl, *Eur. J. Biochem.*, 1992, **210**, 911.

167. M. Pfaff, K. Tangemann, B. Muller, M. Gurrath, G. Muller, H. Kessler, R. Timpl and J. Engel, *J. Biol. Chem.*, 1994, **269**, 20233.

168. J. P. Xiong, T. Stehle, R. Zhang, A. Joachimiak, M. Frech, S. L. Goodman and M. A. Arnaout, *Science*, 2002, **296**, 151.

169. T. Xiao, J. Takagi, B. S. Coller, J. H. Wang and T. A. Springer, *Nature*, 2004, **432**, 59.

170. K. Kurozumi, T. Ichikawa, M. Onishi, K. Fujii and I. Date, *Neurol. Med. Chir. (Tokyo)*, 2012, **52**, 539.

171. Merck KDaA, Press Release, February 25, 2013.

172. R. S. McDowell and T. R. Gadek, *J. Am. Chem. Soc.*, 1992, **114**, 9245.

173. A. C. Bach, C. J. Eyermann, J. D. Gross, M. J. Bower, R. L. Harlow, P. C. Weber and W. F. DeGrado, *J. Am. Chem. Soc.*, 1994, **116**, 3207.

174. S. Jackson, W. DeGrado, A. Dwivedi, A. Parthasarathy, A. Higley, J. Krywko, A. Rockwell, J. Markwalder, G. Wells, R. Wexler, S. Mousa and R. Harlow, *J. Am. Chem. Soc.*, 1994, **116**, 3220.

175. T. Ammosova, R. Berro, M. Jerebtsova, A. Jackson, S. Charles, Z. Klase, W. Southerland, V. R. Gordeuk, F. Kashanchi and S. Nekhai, *Retrovirology*, 2006, **3**, 78.

176. E. P. Schreiner, M. Kern, A. Steck and C. A. Foster, *Bioorg. Med. Chem. Lett.*, 2004, **14**, 5003.

177. D. L. Boger, H. Keim, B. Oberhauser, E. P. Schreiner and C. A. Foster, *J. Am. Chem. Soc.*, 1999, **121**, 6197.

178. Y. Chen, M. Bilban, C. A. Foster and D. L. Boger, *J. Am. Chem. Soc.*, 2002, **124**, 5431.

179. U. Hommel, H. P. Weber, L. Oberer, H. U. Naegeli, B. Oberhauser and C. A. Foster, *FEBS Lett.*, 1996, **379**, 69.

180. T. Pawson and J. D. Scott, *Science*, 1997, **278**, 2075.
181. J. Teyra, S. S. Sidhu and P. M. Kim, *FEBS Lett.*, 2012, **586**, 2631.
182. T. L. Lin and W. Matsui, *Onco. Targets Ther.*, 2012, **5**, 47.
183. K. Watanabe and X. Dai, *Proc. Natl. Acad. Sci. U. S. A.*, 2011, **108**, 5929.
184. D. Holsworth and S. Krauss, *Annu. Rep. Med. Chem.*, 2012, **47**, 393.
185. K. Brennan and R. B. Clarke, *Ther. Adv. Med. Oncol.*, 2013, **5**, 17.
186. F. C. Kelleher, *Carcinogenesis*, 2011, **32**, 445.
187. S. Gupta, N. Takebe and P. Lorusso, *Ther. Adv. Med. Oncol.*, 2010, 2, 237.
188. J. A. Wells and C. L. McClendon, *Nature*, 2007, **450**, 1001.
189. D. A. Erlanson, A. C. Braisted, D. R. Raphael, M. Randal, R. M. Stroud, E. M. Gordon and J. A. Wells, *Proc. Natl. Acad. Sci., U. S. A.*, 2000, **97**, 9367.
190. M. R. Arkin, M. Randal, W. L. DeLano, J. Hyde, T. N. Luong, J. D. Oslob, D. R. Raphael, L. Taylor, J. Wang, R. S. McDowell, J. A. Wells and A. C. Braisted, *Proc. Natl. Acad. Sci., U. S. A.*, 2003, **100**, 1603.
191. W. L. DeLano, *Curr. Opin. Struc. Biol.*, 2002, **12**, 14.
192. T. Clackson and J. A. Wells, *Science*, 1995, **267**, 383.
193. A. A. Bogan and K. S. Thorn, *J. Mol. Biol.*, 1998, **280**, 1.
194. J. Choi, J. Chen, S. L. Schreiber and J. Clardy, *Science*, 1996, **273**, 239.
195. S. Sogabe, F. Stuart, C. Henke, A. Bridges, G. Williams, A. Birch, F. K. Winkler and J. A. Robinson, *J. Mol. Biol.*, 1997, **273**, 882.
196. H. R. Loosli, H. Kessler, H. Oschkinat, H. P. Weber, T. J. Petcher and A. Widmer, *Helv. Chim. Act.*, 1985, **68**, 682.
197. M. F. O'Donohue, A. W. Burgess, M. D. Walkinshaw and H. R. Treutlein, *Protein Sci.*, 1995, **4**, 2191.
198. Q. Huai, H. Y. Kim, Y. Liu, Y. Zhao, A. Mondragon, J. O. Liu and H. Ke, *Proc. Natl. Acad. Sci., U. S. A.*, 2002, **99**, 12037.
199. L. Jin and S. C. Harrison, *Proc. Natl. Acad. Sci., U. S. A.*, 2002, **99**, 13522.
200. B. A. Liu, K. Jablonowski, M. Raina, M. Arce, T. Pawson and P. D. Nash, *Mol. Cell*, 2006, **22**, 851.
201. P. Filippakopoulos, S. Muller and S. Knapp, *Curr. Opin. Struct. Biol.*, 2009, **19**, 643.
202. A. M. Tari and G. Lopez-Berestein, *Semin. Oncol.*, 2001, **28**, 142.
203. J. Rahuel, B. Gay, D. Erdmann, A. Strauss, C. Garcia-Echeverria, P. Furet, G. Caravatti, H. Fretz, J. Schoepfer and M. G. Grutter, *Nat. Struct. Biol.*, 1996, **3**, 586.
204. C. Q. Wei, B. Li, R. Guo, D. Yang and T. R. Burke Jr, *Bioorg. Med. Chem. Lett.*, 2002, **12**, 2781.
205. Z. J. Yao, C. R. King, T. Cao, J. Kelley, G. W. Milne, J. H. Voigt and T. R. Burke Jr, *J. Med. Chem.*, 1999, **42**, 25.
206. C. Q. Wei, Y. Gao, K. Lee, R. Guo, B. Li, M. Zhang, D. Yang and T. R. Burke Jr, *J. Med. Chem.*, 2003, **46**, 244.
207. Z. D. Shi, K. Lee, H. Liu, M. Zhang, L. R. Roberts, K. M. Worthy, M. J. Fivash, R. J. Fisher, D. Yang and T. R. Burke Jr, *Biochem. Biophys. Res. Commun.*, 2003, **310**, 378.
208. Z. D. Shi, K. Lee, C. Q. Wei, L. R. Roberts, K. M. Worthy, R. J. Fisher and T. R. Burke Jr, *J. Med. Chem.*, 2004, **47**, 788.

209. P. T. Flaherty and P. Jain, *Annu. Rep. Med. Chem.*, 2011, **46**, 337.
210. G. Fischer, *Angew. Chem. Int. Ed. Engl.*, 1994, **33**, 1415.
211. S. L. Schreiber, *Science*, 1991, **251**, 283.
212. J. P. Griffith, J. L. Kim, E. E. Kim, M. D. Sintchak, J. A. Thomson, M. J. Fitzgibbon, M. A. Fleming, P. R. Caron, K. Hsiao and M. A. Navia, *Cell*, 1995, **82**, 507.
213. S. N. Sehgal, *Transplant. Proc.*, 2003, **35**, S7.
214. M. Abou-Gharbia, *J. Med. Chem.*, 2009, **52**, 2.
215. B. M. Slomovitz, K. H. Lu, T. Johnston, R. L. Coleman, M. Munsell, R. R. Broaddus, C. Walker, L. M. Ramondetta, T. W. Burke, D. M. Gershenson and J. Wolf, *Cancer*, 2010, **116**, 5415.
216. P. M. LoRusso, *Oncology*, 2013, **84**, 43.
217. B. Ruan, K. Pong, F. Jow, M. Bowlby, R. A. Crozier, D. Liu, S. Liang, Y. Chen, M. L. Mercado, X. Feng, F. Bennett, D. von Schack, L. McDonald, M. M. Zaleska, A. Wood, P. H. Reinhart, R. L. Magolda, J. Skotnicki, M. N. Pangalos, F. E. Koehn, G. T. Carter, M. Abou-Gharbia and E. I. Graziani, *Proc Natl. Acad. Sci., U. S. A.*, 2008, **105**, 33.
218. V. K. Subbaiah, C. Kranjec, M. Thomas and L. Banks, *J. Biochem.*, 2011, **439**, 195.
219. G. Udugamasooriya, D. Saro and M. R. Spaller, *Org. Lett.*, 2005, **7**, 1203.
220. A. Piserchio, G. D. Salinas, T. Li, J. Marshall, M. R. Spaller and D. F. Mierke, *Chem. Biol.*, 2004, **11**, 469.
221. E. P. Garcia, S. Mehta, L. A. Blair, D. G. Wells, J. Shang, T. Fukushima, J. R. Fallon, C. C. Garner and J. Marshall, *Neuron*, 1998, **21**, 727.
222. H. Zhou, L. Liu, J. Huang, D. Bernard, H. Karatas, A. Navarro, M. Lei and S. Wang, *J. Med. Chem.*, 2013, **56**, 1113.
223. A. V. Krivtsov and S. A. Armstrong, *Nat. Rev. Cancer*, 2007, **7**, 823.
224. C. Meyer, E. Kowarz, J. Hofmann, A. Renneville, J. Zuna, J. Trka, A. R. Ben, E. Macintyre, B. E. De, B. M. De, E. Delabesse, M. P. de Oliveira, H. Cave, E. Clappier, J. J. van Dongen, B. V. Balgobind, M. M. van den Heuvel-Eibrink, H. B. Beverloo, R. Panzer-Grumayer, A. Teigler-Schlegel, J. Harbott, E. Kjeldsen, S. Schnittger, U. Koehl, B. Gruhn, O. Heidenreich, L. C. Chan, S. F. Yip, M. Krzywinski, C. Eckert, A. Moricke, M. Schrappe, C. N. Alonso, B. W. Schafer, J. Krauter, D. A. Lee, S. U. Zur, K. G. Te, R. Sutton, S. Izraeli, L. Trakhtenbrot, N. L. Lo, G. Tsaur, L. Fechina, T. Szczepanski, S. Strehl, D. Ilencikova, M. Molkentin, T. Burmeister, T. Dingermann, T. Klingebiel and R. Marschalek, *Leukemia*, 2009, **23**, 1490.
225. J. Grembecka, S. He, A. Shi, T. Purohit, A. G. Muntean, R. J. Sorenson, H. D. Showalter, M. J. Murai, A. M. Belcher, T. Hartley, J. L. Hess and T. Cierpicki, *Nat. Chem. Biol.*, 2012, **8**, 277.
226. A. Shi, M. J. Murai, S. He, G. Lund, T. Hartley, T. Purohit, G. Reddy, M. Chruszcz, J. Grembecka and T. Cierpicki, *Blood*, 2012, **120**, 4461.
227. L. F. Peng, B. Z. Stanton, N. Maloof, X. Wang and S. L. Schreiber, *Bioorg. Med. Chem. Lett.*, 2009, **19**, 6319.

228. B. Z. Stanton, L. F. Peng, N. Maloof, K. Nakai, X. Wang, J. L. Duffner, K. M. Taveras, J. M. Hyman, S. W. Lee and A. N. Koehler, *Nat. Chem. Biol.*, 2009, **5**, 154.

229. K. D. Robarge, S. A. Brunton, G. M. Castanedo, Y. Cui, M. S. Dina, R. Goldsmith, S. E. Gould, O. Guichert, J. L. Guzner, J. Halladay, W. Jia, C. Khojasteh, M. F. T. Koehler, K. Kotkow, H. La, R. L. Lalonde, K. Lau, L. Lee, D. Marshall, J. C. Marsters, L. J. Murray, C. Qian, L. L. Rubin, L. Salphati, M. S. Stanley, J. H. A. Hubbard, D. P. Sutherlin, S. Ubhayaker, S. Wang, S. Wong and M. Xie, *Bioorg. Med. Chem. Lett.*, 2009, **19**, 5576.

230. E. De Smaele, E. Ferretti and A. Gulino, *Curr. Opin. Investig. Drugs*, 2010, **11**, 707.

231. S. Sandhiya, G. Melvin, S. S. Kumar and S. A. Dkhar, *J. Pharmacol. Pharmacother.*, 2013, **4**, 4.

232. L. B. Rice, *J. Infect. Dis.*, 2008, **197**, 1079.

233. D. Obrecht, F. Bernardini, G. Dale and K. Dembowsky, *Annu. Rep. Med. Chem.*, 2011, **46**, 245.

234. D. T. Moir, T. J. Opperman, M. M. Butler and T. L. Bowlin, *Curr. Opin. Pharmacol.*, 2012, **12**, 535-544.

235. E. B. Hadley and R. E. Hancock, *Current Topics in Medicinal Chemistry*, 2010, **10**, 1872.

236. M. Vaara, *Curr. Opin. Pharmacol.*, 2009, **9**, 1.

237. D. A. Steinberg, M. A. Hurst, C. A. Fujii, A. H. Kung, J. F. Ho, F. C. Cheng, D. J. Loury and J. C. Fiddes, *Antimicrob. Agents Chemother.*, 1997, **41**, 1738.

238. S. C. Shankaramma, Z. Athanassiou, O. Zerbe, K. Moehle, C. Mouton, F. Bernardini, J. W. Vrijbloed, D. Obrecht and J. A. Robinson, *ChemBioChem*, 2002, **3**, 1126.

239. J. A. Robinson, S. C. Shankaramma, P. Jetter, U. Kienzl, R. A. Schwendener, J. W. Vrijbloed and D. Obrecht, *Bioorg. Med. Chem.*, 2005, **13**, 2055.

240. N. Srinivas, P. Jetter, B. J. Ueberbacher, M. Werneburg, K. Zerbe, J. Steinmann, B. Van der Meijden, F. Bernardini, A. Lederer, R. L. A. Dias, P. E. Misson, H. Henze, J. Zumbrunn, F. O. Gombert, D. Obrecht, P. Hunziker, S. Schauer, U. Ziegler, A. Käch, L. Eberl, K. Riedel, S. J. DeMarco and J. A. Robinson, *Science*, 2010, **327**, 1010.

CHAPTER 9

Macrocyclic α-Helical Peptide Drug Discovery

TOMI K. SAWYER,*,† VINCENT GUERLAVAIS, KRZYSZTOF DARLAK AND ERIC FEYFANT‡

Aileron Therapeutics, Cambridge, MA 02139
*Email: sawyerkrt@aol.com

9.1 Introduction

Macrocyclization of peptides has inspired both basic research and drug discovery focused on Nature's three dimensional (3D) molecular recognition underlying intracellular protein–protein interactions as well as extracellular peptide/protein–protein interactions. Secondary structural features of such intermolecular interactions have been intensively studied[1–15] and shown to involve α-helical, β-strand and reverse-turn motifs of the protein 'ligand' binding with its cognate protein 'target'. Hence, the design of proteomimetics has captivated the imagination of drug hunters to challenge so-called 'undruggable' target space that otherwise exists because of the paucity of successful options based upon classical small-molecule or protein approaches. Although the wide scope of such work is beyond the limits of this chapter, it is timely to capture the extraordinary progress that has been achieved with respect to macrocyclic α-helical peptides and, in particular, hydrocarbon-stapled peptides.[3,12,16–29] As detailed in subsequent subsections of this chapter, an extraordinary multidisciplinary knowledge base

†Present address: Merck & Company, Boston, MA 02115, USA.
‡Present address: Schrodinger, Cambridge, MA 02141, USA.

RSC Drug Discovery Series No. 40
Macrocycles in Drug Discovery
Edited by Jeremy Levin
© The Royal Society of Chemistry 2015
Published by the Royal Society of Chemistry, www.rsc.org

of macrocyclic α-helical peptides (again, for hydrocarbon-stapled peptides especially) is emerging that embraces new insights in biology, biophysical and computational chemistry, structural diversity and synthesis, and drug design. Ultimately, macrocyclic α-helical peptides represent a new drug class that embodies a unique amalgamation of biological/pharmacological attributes, including proteolytic stability, cellular permeability, and sustained pharmacokinetic properties, which have enabled the advancement of such molecules through iterative lead optimization into the clinic. The recent milestone announcement by Aileron Therapeutics for a stapled peptide drug ALRN-6924, a novel dual specific MDM2/MDMX antagonist for p53-dependent cancer therapy, underscores such extraordinary progress. Furthermore, such macrocyclic α-helical peptides, especially hydrocarbon-stapled peptides, exemplify a promising new synthetic biologic 'privileged scaffold' for innovative drug discovery to exploit the high fidelity of Nature's molecular recognition within the expansive scope of α-helical interfacing protein-protein target space.

9.2 α-Helical Interfaces in Protein–Protein Drug Target Space

Significant advances in structural biology and computational chemistry technologies have enabled the visualization of innumerable drug–target interactions at high resolution. Noteworthy in this regard has been the unveiling and increasing understanding of α-helical interfaces that exist for a majority of intermolecular protein–protein interactions, and such is well exemplified from comprehensive analyses of the Protein Data Bank (www.rcsb.org).[1–3,14,21] Representative of intracellular α-helical protein–protein interactions of more than 1600 non-redundant, unique, high resolution 3-dimensional structures found in the Protein Data Bank are those having therapeutic relevance for cancer, inflammatory, and immune diseases such as BIM BH3:Mcl-1,[30] BAD:Bcl-Xl,[31] p53:MDM2,[32] MAML:Notch,[33] HIF-1α:p300,[34] Myc-Max,[35] eIF4G:eIF4E,[36] TIF2:GCCR,[37] Scr-2:RORγ,[38] and IKKβ:NEMO[39] (Figure 9.1). Most importantly, it is this abundance of compelling therapeutic opportunities corresponding to such α-helical interfaces in protein–protein drug space that has propelled the concept of a new drug modality based upon macrocyclic α-helical peptide design.[3,12,16–29] In particular, stapled peptides have been developed as novel molecular probes within academia and, notably, Aileron Therapeutics is advancing the stapled peptides into drug development and future clinical testing.

9.2.1 Stapled Peptide Modulation of Drug Target Space

For the past decade, stapled peptides have emerged as a novel class of drugs (see ref. 19–24,27–29 and 62 for reviews) for the modulation a plethora of intracellular targets (i.e. Bcl2-family,[19,22–24,43,47,48,58,67–71,76,77,83,92,93,98

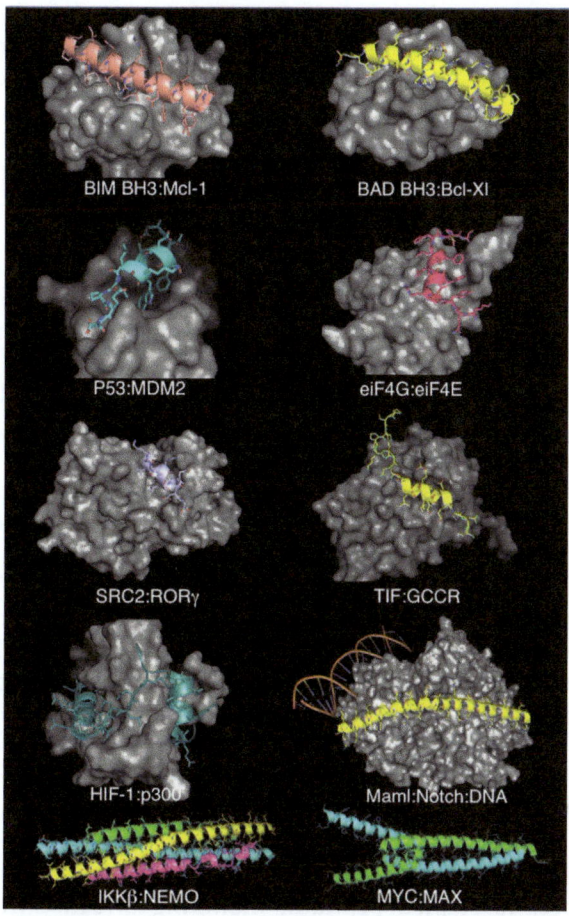

Figure 9.1 Some representative 3D structures of intracellular α-helical protein–protein interactions determined by X-ray crystallography and deposited in the Protein Data Bank.

p53:MDM2/X,[42,57,65,66,72,79,81,82,87,89,94,95] MAML:Notch,[49] eIF4E,[158] ERα/ERβ,[50] IRS1,[84] HIF-1:p300,[56,90] RAS:SOS,[59] Rab-GTPase,[96] β-catenin,[64,78,80] protein kinase-A,[91] RPA,[97] HIV-1 integrase,[85,86] and HIV-1 capsid,[44,45,88]) and extracellular targets (*i.e.* HIV-1 gp41/gp120,[46,88] HCV E2,[102] galanin,[101] neuropeptide-Y,[101] ABCA1 transporter,[51] N-methyl-D-aspartic acid receptor,[99] and vitamin D receptor[103]) of therapeutic significance for many disease areas (*e.g.* cancer, metabolic disorders, and infectious diseases). Such work exemplifies the intensity of basic and translational research within academia as well as drug discovery within pharmaceutical/biotechnology industry. Specific examples from the above studies will be highlighted in terms of stapled peptide chemistry, structure–activity relationships, and biological properties in the sections below related to intracellular and extracellular drug targets. In particular, the recent breakthrough studies on the dual

MDM2/MDMX antagonist stapled peptide ATSP-7041[81,82] (*vide infra*) provides an in-depth and rigorous *in vitro* and *in vivo* proof-of-concept for drug development of this promising class of macrocyclic α-helical peptide therapeutics.

9.2.2 Understanding the Cell Penetration Properties of Macrocyclic α-Helical Peptides

Unquestionably, there is significant interest in understanding the cell penetration properties of macrocyclic α-helical peptides. Such work is now the focus of ongoing basic research that will leverage sophisticated biochemical, cellular and biophysical methods to address the complexity of molecular mechanisms involved in cell penetration by stapled peptides. For example, highly potent macrocyclic α-helical peptides such as the stapled peptide ATSP-7041[81,82] provide opportunistic tool molecules to interrogate cell penetration relative to cellular uptake mechanisms and peptide biophysical properties, including the establishment of benchmarks and standardized procedures.

In sharp contrast to cell-penetrating peptides (CPPs),[105–117] which have been predominantly shown to serve as carriers for various cargo molecules conjugated to them, macrocyclic α-helical peptides possess overlapping target-specific pharmacophoric and intrinsic cell-penetrating properties within the same peptide sequence. The current understanding of differences in cell penetration between CPPs and macrocyclic α-helical peptides (*e.g.* stapled peptides) is that there are likely very different biological mechanisms involved and a comparative experimental analysis will be necessary to fully investigate each modality. In fact, such studies will be very important to accelerate the expansion of peptide drug discovery into intracellular druggable space.

With respect to stapled peptides, mounting evidence from numerous studies[19–24,43,44,47–49,56,57,64,66–98] has implicated active transport processes to underlie cellular uptake as demonstrated by intracellular on-target engagement and/or fluorescence microscopy (*i.e.* visualization of fluorescently labeled stapled peptide analogs). Furthermore, the design and iterative optimization of macrocyclic α-helical peptides has provided a knowledge base to systematically correlate biophysical properties (*e.g.* lipophilicity, charge, length, α-helicity, amphipathicity, and solubility) with cell penetration and, ultimately, *in vitro* biological potency and *in vivo* pharmacological efficacy. In this regard, the stapled peptide ATSP-7041[81,82] provides an intriguing benchmark molecule for such structure–property analysis.

9.3 Structural Diversity and Chemistry of Macrocyclic α-Helical Peptides

As previously noted, the α-helix is a major secondary structure found in Nature and exists at the interface of a plethora of protein–protein interactions.[1–3,21,26] Such α-helices may be further categorized as linear, kinked, and curved, of which the latter is the predominant type. Historically, numerous strategies have emerged to create novel synthetic α-helical secondary structure proteomimetics.[19–24,43,44,47,48,56,57,64,66–104,118–122] Albeit not detailed in this focused review, such strategies have included N-terminal helical-inducing capping moieties,[123–125] non-peptide foldamers/oligomers[126,127] and small-molecule mimetics.[128–136] Unquestionably, the most rewarding strategy has been proven to be the synthesis of macrocyclic α-helical peptides utilizing a variety of linkers, including disulfide,[118] thioether,[60,66,75] diester,[120] lactam,[119,121,122] hydrocarbon,[19,20,23,28,29,40–43,52,53,56,61–63,81,139–143,159] triazole[54,55,64,95] and pyrazole[65] as exemplified by compounds **1–26** (*vide infra*).

Pioneering studies on macrocyclic α-helical peptides first demonstrated[118,119] the effective use of disulfide-bridged and bis-lactam-bridged macrocyclic peptides **1** and **2** (Figure 9.2), respectively, and focused on model systems wherein α-helicity properties were confirmed by circular dichroism and/or NMR spectroscopy. The diester- and lactam-bridged macrocyclic peptides **3** and **4** further exemplified achievements in harnessing the helical sequences of G-protein coupled receptor agonists corresponding to glucagon-like peptide-1 and parathyroid hormone.[120,121] Likewise, a

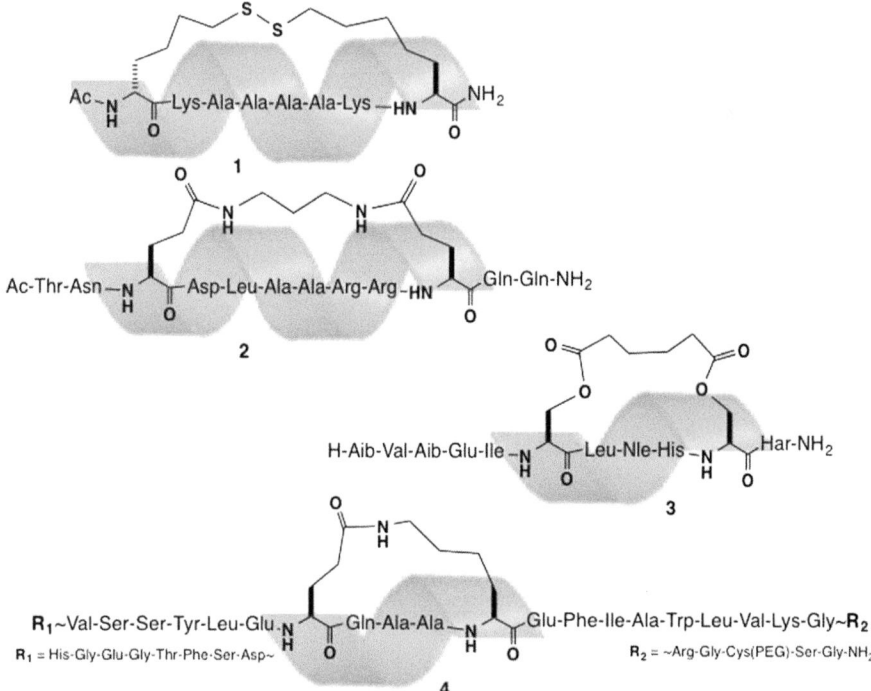

Figure 9.2 Examples of macrocyclic α-helical peptides using disulfide, lactam, and diester linkages for biophysical studies and drug discovery.

lactam-bridged peptide (not shown) was found to demonstrate a propensity for adopting an α-helical structure within a BH3 sequence.[122]

The most robust methodologies used to generate macrocyclic α-helical peptide strategies[19–24,40–104] include ring-closing metathesis and azide–alkyne cycloaddition, and such have established a growing armamentarium of stapled peptides 5–26 (Figures 9.3–9.8). Specifically, the stapled peptide 5 (Figure 9.3) illustrates a prototype using O-allylation of two serine residues to subsequently perform ring-closing metathesis.[40] The p53 stapled peptide 6[42] and stapled BID BH3 peptide 7[43] (Figure 9.3) provide two early examples of hydrocarbon-stapled peptides having double-turn (i,i+7) and single-turn (i,i+4) macrocylization approaches, respectively. Stapled peptides 6 and 7 also reveal both stereochemical and side-chain length requirements of their particular novel Cα,α-dialkylated amino acid building blocks that confer α-helicity and enable ring-closing metathesis as well-investigated by Verdine and colleagues.[28,41–43,52,62,140–142] Furthermore, both of these stapled peptides exhibit cell-penetrating properties.[42,43]

The stapled HIV-1 Gag capsid domain peptide 8[44,45] and double-stapled HIV-1 gp41 peptide 9[46] (Figure 9.4) exemplify hydrocarbon-stapled peptides acting at intracellular and extracellular targets, respectively. Furthermore, the double-stapled peptide 9 exhibits significant stability against proteolytic degradation and is a prototype for larger helical peptides in overcoming metabolic and pharmacokinetic boundaries. Unsurprisingly, such stability is

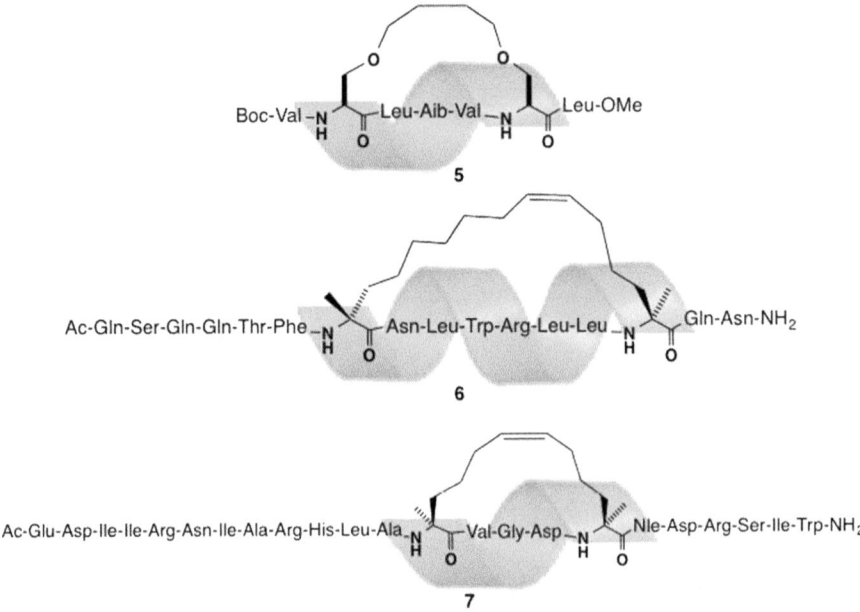

Figure 9.3 Examples of stapled peptides using ring-closing metathesis chemistry. α,α-lkylated hydrocarbon-stapled peptides are highlighted as key progenitor molecules designed for p53 and Bcl-2 family therapeutic targets.

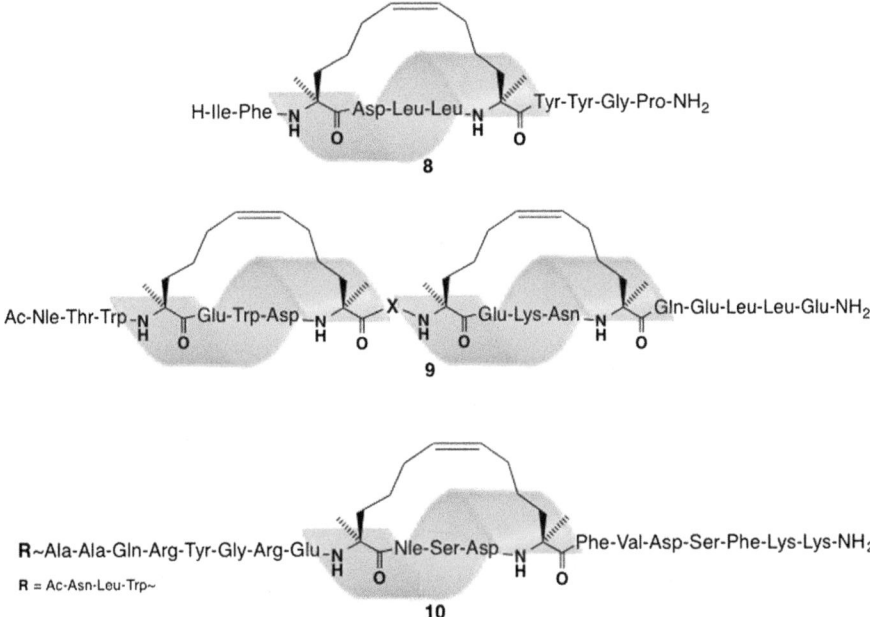

Figure 9.4 Design of α,α-alkylated hydrocarbon-stapled peptides for HIV and glucokinase therapeutic targets.

a consequence of minimizing the propensity of extended-like conformations that would otherwise be requisite for substrate binding to proteases. The stapled BAD BH3 peptide **10**[47] exhibits unique cell-penetrating properties for a phosphorylated peptide relative to what might be predicted from modifying molecules of any type with phosphate moieties, and such work provides compelling motivation to further investigate the potential for other phosphorylated peptides of therapeutic significance.

In addition, the stapled Notch peptide **11**[49] (Figure 9.5) is an example of a strongly hydrophilic helical peptide with cell-penetrating properties, which incorporates a single-turn, hydrocarbon-bridged macrocycle. Moreover, the stapled co-activator peptide **12**, which binds the estrogen receptor,[50] and stapled apolipoprotein A-1 fragment peptide **13**, which binds and increases cholesterol efflux by the ABCA1 transporter,[51] have recently been described (Figure 9.5). Novel single-turn i,i+3 α-helical and i,i+3 3_{10}-helical (defined as having three amino acid residues/turn and ten atoms comprising the intramolecular H-bonding substructure) peptide stabilization using ring-closing metathesis methodology has also been achieved, as exemplified by stapled peptide models **14**[52] and **15**,[53] respectively (Figure 9.5). In the case of compound **14**, the *R*-configuration of the i-residue and *S*-configuration of the i+3 residue was key to stabilization of α-helicity, whereas for compound **15**, extended sequence of Aib residues and macrocyclization correlated with stabilization of 3_{10}-helicity.

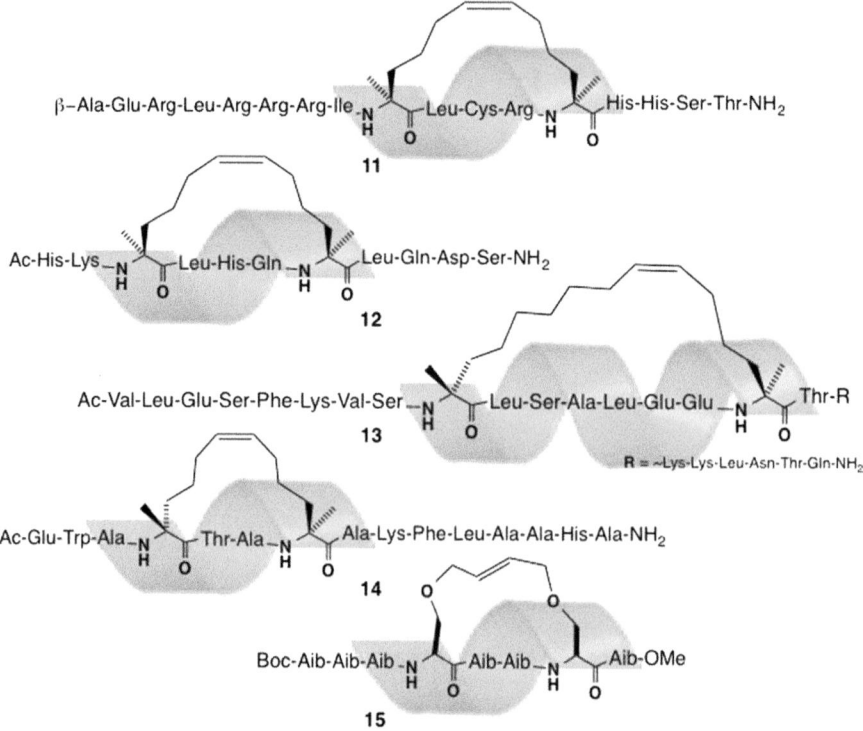

Figure 9.5　Design of α,α-alkylated hydrocarbon-stapled peptides for Notch and ABCA1 transporter. Both i,i + 3 α-helical and 3_{10} helical model peptides are highlighted.

Azide-alkyne cycloaddition (generally referred to as "click" chemistry), which has also been applied to macrocyclization of both α-helical and 3_{10}-helical peptides, exemplified by **16**[54] and **17**[55] respectively (Figure 9.6), provides facile synthetic methodology and is expected to contribute to future design and structure–activity studies of such click-stapled peptides. α-helical-inducing, hydrogen-bond surrogate (HBS) strategies leveraging N-terminal macrocyclization to create an internal H-bond replacement by covalent linkage, including ring-closing metathesis as well as thio-ether chemistries, have been described by Arora and colleagues to successfully advance cell-penetrating stapled HIF-1, p53 and SOS peptides **18**,[56,90] **19**,[57] **20**[59] and **21**[60] (Figure 9.6).

Especially compelling for the synthesis of highly conformationally rigid peptides are the tandem stapled (also referred to as "stitched") peptides such as **22**[63] (Figure 9.7). Recently, alkyne–azide cycloaddition (triazole-stapling) has been successfully applied to BCL9 α-helical peptides such as **23**.[64] Furthermore, a double-click strategy to create novel functionalized bis-triazolo-aryl staples has been recently exemplified by the stapled p53 peptide **24**.[95]

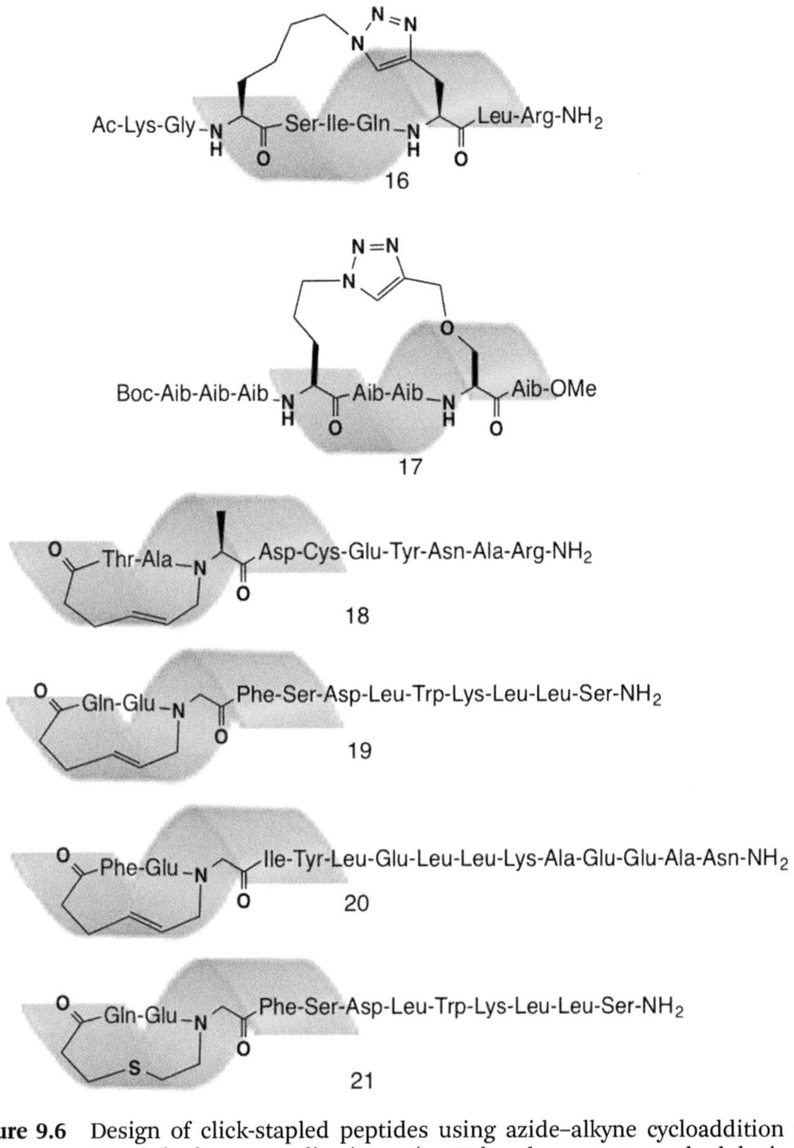

Figure 9.6 Design of click-stapled peptides using azide–alkyne cycloaddition and N-terminal macrocyclization using H-bond surrogate methodologies for various intracellular therapeutic targets.

The structural diversity of macrocyclic α-helical peptides continues to expand with novel chemistry methodologies. For example, a photoinduced 1,3-dipolar cycloaddition approach for macrocyclization has been introduced as illustrated by the pyrazoline-stapled p53 peptide **25**[65] (Figure 9.8). Interestingly, a bis-thioether macrocyclized α-helical p53 peptide, **26,** was determined to exhibit good cellular uptake when conjugated with a

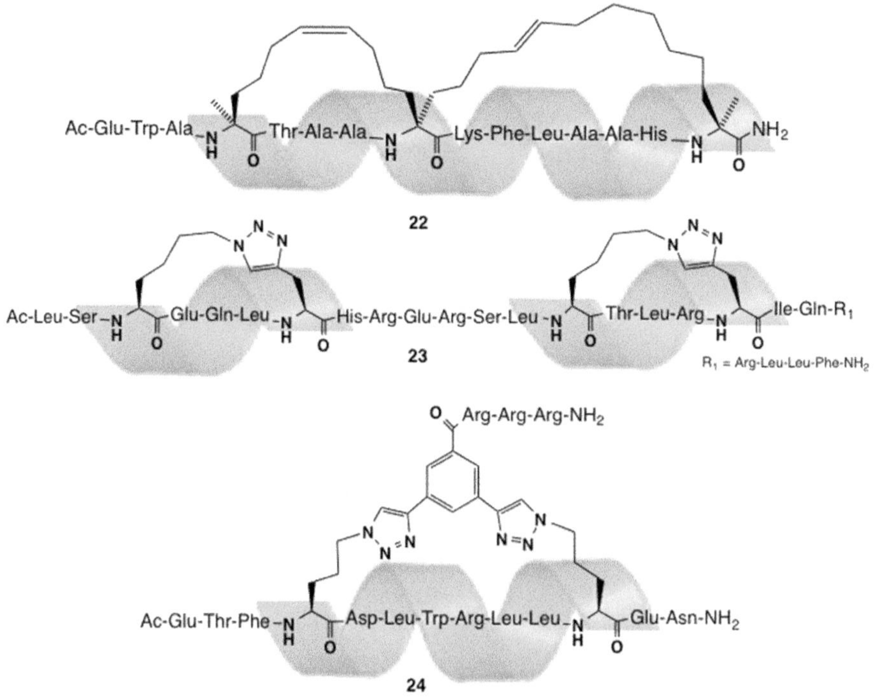

22

23

R₁ = Arg-Leu-Leu-Phe-NH₂

24

Figure 9.7 Design of tandem hydrocarbon-stapled ("stitched") peptides and expansion of click-stapling chemistry, including bis-triazolo-aryl-stapling, to various intracellular targets.

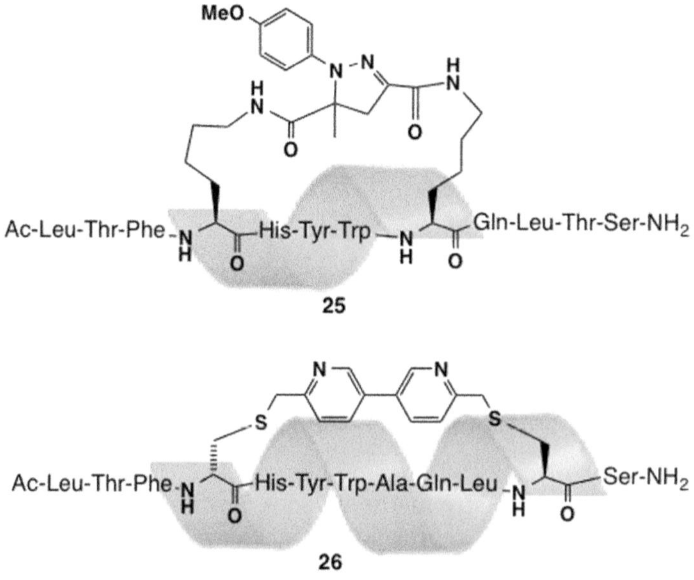

25

26

Figure 9.8 Design of pyrazoline-stapled and bis-thioether macrocyclized peptides for p53.

polyamine moiety.[66] In this case the polyamine moiety was selected to enhance intracellular delivery based on past work on lipophilic small-molecules and negatively charged siRNA as well as for increasing α-helicity through favorable charge–dipole interactions by introducing a positive-charge at the C-terminus. Furthermore, and related to bis-thioether macro-cyclization, a perfluoro-cysteine S_NAr chemistry approach to unprotected peptide stapling has been recently reported.[75]

Beyond the above first examples of varying types of macrocyclic α-helical peptides, especially stapled peptides, to illustrate the structural diversity of this emerging new class, it is ultimately the 3D-structural and biophysical properties (*vide infra*) of such molecules that will be key to a greater understanding of their biochemical, cellular, and *in vivo* pharmacological activities. Exemplifying the 3D-structural diversity of varying subclasses of hydrocarbon-stapled peptides are 6 (double-turn), 7 (single-turn), **14** (stitch), **20** (i,i+3 single-turn) and **22** (H-bond surrogate), and their 3D-structures are shown in Figure 9.9. Unquestionably, there are many unique ways to stabilize helical peptides through stereospecific side chain-to-side chain macrocyclization as well as achiral N-terminal H-bond surrogate chemistries.

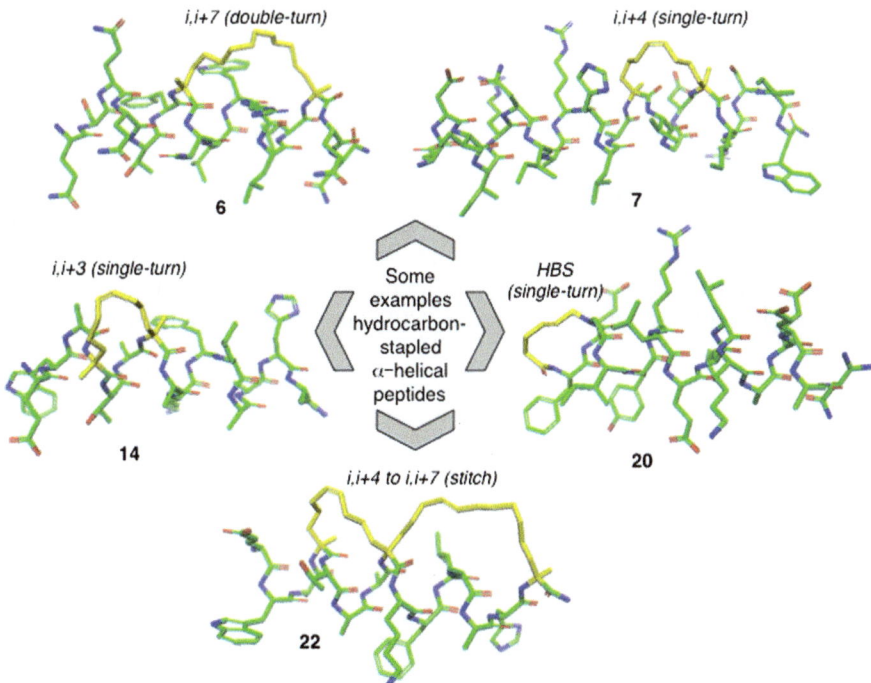

Figure 9.9 3D-structural diversity of varying subclasses of hydrocarbon-stapled peptides, including double-turn, single-turn, stitch, i,i + 3 single-turn and H-bond surrogate macrocyclizations.

9.3.1 Hydrocarbon Stapled Peptide Chemistry

As first described by Verdine and colleagues,[28,41,52,62] the term "hydrocarbon-stapling" generally refers to an all-hydrocarbon crosslink created from ring-closing metathesis of two terminal olefin side-chain modified amino acids also having α-methyl substitution. This macrocyclization approach includes single-turn, double-turn, stitch tandem, and multiple staple chemistries (*vide supra*). It is important to point out that hydrocarbon-stapled peptides have exemplified the first macrocylization strategy to confer both helical stability and cell penetration properties relative to previously described approaches. Specifically, such hydrocarbon-stapling chemistry combined two distinct strategies for α-helix stabilization, namely the helical-inducing effect of α-methylation[137,138] and intramolecular conformational constraint by side chain-to-side chain cyclization through ring-closing metathesis.[40,139] Furthermore, Verdine and colleagues systematically investigated both linker length and stereochemistry for the optimal design of the hydrocarbon-stapled peptides with respect to i,i+7, i,i+4 and i,i+3 helical stapling chemistries.[41,52,62,140–142] These groundbreaking studies reflected iterative analysis of varying the configuration and regiospecific insertion of the chiral α,α-dialkylated amino acids as well as varying hydrocarbon lengths of the terminal alkenyl side chains to identify by circular dichroism and related biophysical and target-based biochemical studies the optimal macrocyclic α-helical structures from ring-closing metathesis. As illustrated in the case of the i,i+7 (double-turn) hydrocarbon-stapled p53 peptide 6 (SAH-p53-8), the configurations of the first and second α,α-dialkyl amino acids are *R* and *S*, respectively, and a 33-membered macrocycle that incorporates eight amino acids and eleven carbon atoms derived from the optimized linker moiety. Further investigations of hydrocarbon-stapling chemistry have addressed the specific positioning of the olefin moiety of the cross-linker itself in terms of investigating ring closing metathesis efficiency and helical stabilization.[143]

The design of hydrocarbon-stapled peptides requires the synthesis of the α-methyl, α-alkenyl glycines (Figure 9.10) and various chemistry methods

(*R*)-2-((((9*H*-fluoren-9-yl)methoxy)carbonyl)amino)-   (*S*)-2-((((9*H*-fluoren-9-yl)methoxy)carbonyl)amino)-
2-methyldec-9-enoic acid   2-methylhept-6-enoic acid

R8   **S5**

Figure 9.10   Chemical structures of α,α-dialkyl-amino acids *S*5 and *R*8.

have been developed to prepare α,α-dialkyl-amino acids with high enantio-meric purity.[144] Exemplifying one asymmetric synthesis approach as first describing such hydrocarbon-stapling chemistry was that by Verdine and colleagues using a Williams chiral auxiliary to prepare the requisite α,α-dialkylated-amino acids.[145] Importantly, chiral cyclic enolates derived from alanine are well-known (*e.g.* Williams, Schölkopf, and Seebach reagents) to provide direct and reliable synthetic routes to α,α-disubstituted amino acids through diastereoselective α-alkylation reactions.[62,137,145]

Nevertheless, the aforementioned chemistries typically use anhydrous conditions at very low temperature and quite strong and sensitive bases are necessary. Also, the hydrolysis of the resulting α-alkylated heterocycles to release the amino acids can be problematic, since harsh reaction con-ditions are typically required. Furthermore, Verdine and colleagues re-ported that over-reduction of the olefin moiety during the dissolving metal reduction step of the Williams method may be problematic.[145] Hence, such challenges would complicate chemical development with respect to achieving economically feasible, large-scale manufacturing. An alternative and robust synthetic chemistry method is that of Belokon and colleagues,[146,147] as it can be optimized for multi-kilogram scale synthesis. As exemplified for the *R8* stapling amino acid (Scheme 9.1), the chiral auxiliary (*R*)-2-[*N*-(*N*′-benzylprolyl)amino]benzophenone (BPB) enables straightforward C-alkylation of the Nickel(II) Schiff base complex of alanine to prepare α,α-dialkylated-amino acids with good yields and high optical purity.

Subsequent to having the desired α,α-dialkylated amino acids available, the synthesis of hydrocarbon-stapled peptides is relatively straightforward and employs solid-phase peptide chemistry, as illustrated for ATSP-7041 (Scheme 9.2),[81,82] to provide a feasible route for chemical development. As further detailed below, the hydrocarbon-stapled peptide ATSP-7041 is a dual MDM2/MDMX antagonist that exhibits high potency *in vitro* and efficacy *in vivo* in p53-dependent cancer models.

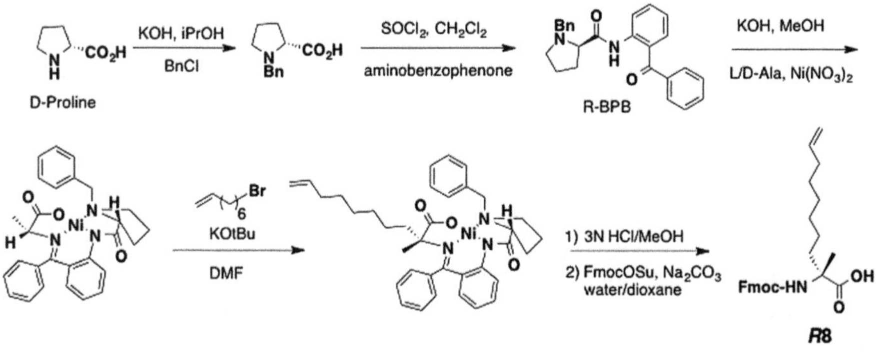

Scheme 9.1 Synthesis of the stapling amino acid *R8*.

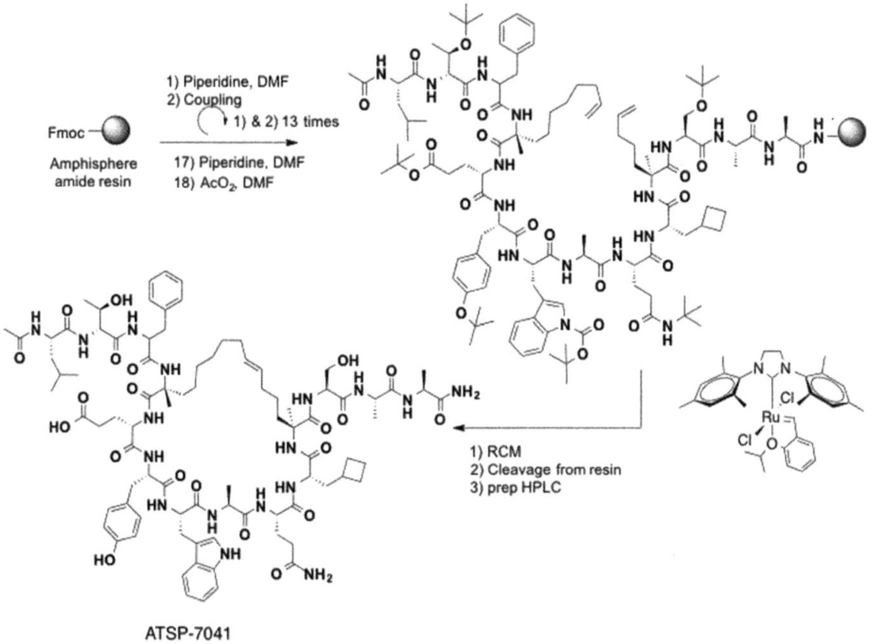

ATSP-7041

Scheme 9.2   Synthesis of dual MDM2/MDMX antagonist stapled peptide ATSP-7041.

9.4   Biophysical and Computational Analysis of Macrocyclic α-Helical Peptides

Biophysical and computational analysis of macrocyclic α-helical peptides (*e.g.* stapled peptides) have provided significant insights to their molecular recognition at α-helical protein–protein interfaces and their inherent conformational dynamics properties.[23,24,40–44,46,50,52–61,67–72,81,82,148–159] High-resolution molecular mapping of the binding sites of cognate targets for helical peptides provide the opportunity for iterative structure-based drug design, precise chemical modification of sidechains and the regiospecific placement of the stapling amino acids to create high affinity macrocyclic analogs. For instance, the macrocyclizing linker (staple) moiety itself may directly participate in molecular recognition with the target as revealed by X-ray crystallography for stapled peptide ligand complexes with Mcl-1,[70] the estrogen receptor,[50] MDM2[153] and MDMX.[81] Specifically, a high resolution structure of stapled peptide ATSP-7041 (Figure 9.11) shows the hydrocarbon linker moiety nestled to the binding surface of the target protein that is proximate to the hydrophobic pockets occupied by its Phe, Trp, and Leu side chains. In fact, a comparative structure–activity analysis of ATSP-7041 has shown that the collective effect of both macrocyclization and other specific modifications accounts for its high affinity to both MDM2 and MDMX relative to both its related linear parent phage display peptide and the small molecule Nutlin-3 (Figure 9.11).[81] Recently, biophysical and chemical

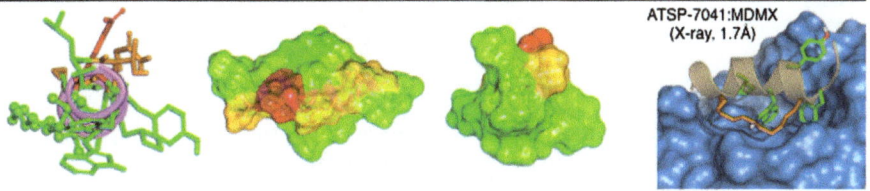

ATSP-7041

Peptides		14	15	16	17	18	19	20	21	22	23	24	25	26	27	28	29	30		MDM2 binding Ki (nM)	MDMX binding Ki (nM)
SAH-p53-8	Ac-	Gln	Ser	Gln	Gln	Thr	Phe	R8	Asn	Leu	Trp	Arg	Leu	Leu	S5	Gln	Asn		-NH2	25.9	105.7
ATSP-3848	Ac-				Leu	Thr	Phe	Glu	His	Tyr	Trp	Ala	Gln	Leu	Thr	Ser			-NH2	14.6	47.4
ATSP-3900	Ac-				Leu	Thr	Phe	R8	His	Tyr	Trp	Ala	Gln	Leu	S5	Ser			-NH2	1	18.3
ATSP-4641	Ac-				Leu	Thr	Phe	R8	Ala	Tyr	Trp	Ala	Gln	Leu	S5	Ser			-NH2	4.9	34.3
ATSP-6935	Ac-				Leu	Thr	Phe	R8	Glu	Tyr	Trp	Ala	Gln	Leu	S5	Ser			-NH2	1.2	8
ATSP-7041	Ac-				Leu	Thr	Phe	R8	Glu	Tyr	Trp	Ala	Gln	Cba	S5	Ser	Ala	Ala	-NH2	0.9	6.8
ATSP-7342	Ac-				Leu	Thr	Ala	R8	Glu	Tyr	Trp	Ala	Gln	Cba	S5	Ser	Ala	Ala	-NH2	536	>1000
Nutlin-3a																				52.3	>1000

ATSP-7041:MDMX (X-ray, 1.7Å)

Figure 9.11 Chemical structure, structure-activity and 3D biophysical properties of stapled peptide ATSP-7041, including a high resolution X-ray structure of it complexed with MDMX.
Adapted, in part, with permission from *Proc. Natl. Acad. Sci. U. S. A.* (ref. 81).

biology studies of stapled phospho-BAD BH3 peptide interactions with glucokinase have revealed its unique allosteric mechanism of activation.[48]

The individual contribution of side chain interactions to target binding may also be experimentally determined by stepwise alanine substitution (*i.e.* Ala-scanning) or other amino acid replacements to evaluate hydrophobicity, charge or other molecular properties. Such drug design strategies have also enabled the construction of mutant stapled peptide analogs that may serve as negative controls (*i.e.* molecules exhibiting very similar overall chemical and biophysical properties, but having significantly weaker affinity to bind the cognate target) to support cellular testing with respect to on-target mechanism of action.[23,24,67–71,81,82] An elegant study to correlate the contributions of individual side chains of a hydrocarbon-stapled peptide to target binding is that described for the dual MDM2/MDMX antagonist stapled peptide ATSP-3900[81,82] using the Ala-scanning method (Figure 9.12). Specifically, alanine substitution effected a 10- to 100-fold decrease in target binding affinity essentially only for the key hydrophobic side chains of Phe, Trp, and Leu of the stapled peptide, and such results correlated well with an X-ray structure of it complexed with MDMX.[82]

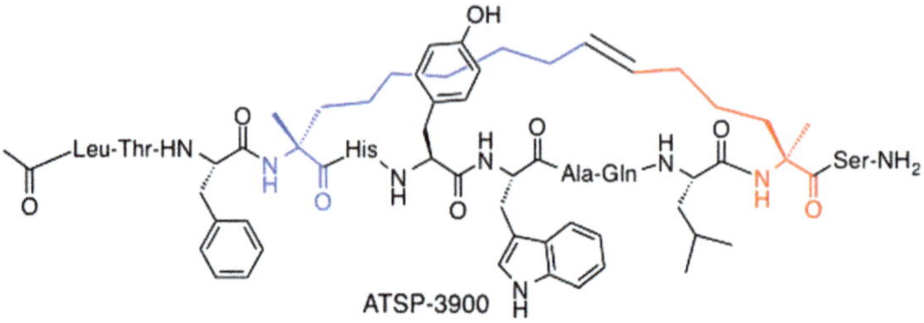

ATSP-3900

Peptides	14	15	16	17	18	19	20	21	22	23	24	25	26	27	28	29	30	MDM2 binding Ki (nM)	MDMX binding Ki (nM)	SJSA-1, 10% FBS Cellular Viability IC50 (µM)
SAH-p53-8 Ac-	Gln	Ser	Gln	Gln	Thr	Phe	R8	Asn	Leu	Trp	Arg	Leu	Leu	S5	Gln	Asn	-NH2	25.9	105.7	>30
ATSP-3900 Ac-				Leu	Thr	Phe	R8	His	Tyr	Trp	Ala	Gln	Leu	S5	Ser	-NH2		8	12.7	15
Analog A17				Ala	Thr	Phe	R8	His	Tyr	Trp	Ala	Gln	Leu	S5	Ser			3	7.3	12
Analog A18				Leu	Ala	Phe	R8	His	Tyr	Trp	Ala	Gln	Leu	S5	Ser			24.1	105.2	23
Analog A19				Leu	Thr	Ala	R8	His	Tyr	Trp	Ala	Gln	Leu	S5	Ser			228	13224	>30
Analog A21				Leu	Thr	Phe	R8	Ala	Tyr	Trp	Ala	Gln	Leu	S5	Ser			5	34	5.9
Analog A22				Leu	Thr	Phe	R8	His	Ala	Trp	Ala	Gln	Leu	S5	Ser			20.8	76.9	>30
Analog A23				Leu	Thr	Phe	R8	His	Tyr	Ala	Ala	Gln	Leu	S5	Ser			196	8600	>30
Analog A25				Leu	Thr	Phe	R8	His	Tyr	Trp	Ala	Ala	Leu	S5	Ser			17.5	12.5	17.2
Analog A26				Leu	Thr	Phe	R8	His	Tyr	Trp	Ala	Gln	Ala	S5	Ser			550	862	>30
Analog A28				Leu	Thr	Phe	R8	His	Tyr	Trp	Ala	Gln	Leu	S5	Ala			5	11.2	8
ATSP-7041 Ac-				Leu	Thr	Phe	R8	Glu	Tyr	Trp	Ala	Gln	Cba	S5	Ser	Ala	Ala -NH2	0.9	6.8	0.6

Figure 9.12 Alanine scanning and structure–activity properties of stapled peptide ATSP-3900 relative to MDM2 and MDMX binding.
Adapted, in part, with permission from *Proc. American Peptide Symp.* (ref. 82).

Molecular dynamics and modeling studies have also provided an understanding of both the intrinsic secondary structural stability of stapled helical peptides, as well as their intermolecular interactions with cognate targets. Exemplifying such work was an investigation of stapled peptide conformational stability at the atomistic level using computational chemistry methods to systematically measure α-helicity of BID-BH3 and RNAse peptides in terms of linear versus stapled analogs and mutants in which alanine was substituted at the two macrocyclizing amino acid sites.[150] In this study alanine substitutions were chosen based upon the known intrinsic α-helical propensity of this amino acid. The experimental results confirmed that hydrocarbon-stapling conferred higher α-helicity content and that both position and size of the linker (staple) moiety affected stability of the α-helical motif. Furthermore, this study determined that the principal energetic component of such stapled peptides for α-helicity propensity correlated with enthalpy from intramolecular H-bonding and backbone conformational terms.

Other noteworthy work focused on the biophysical and computational chemistry of stapled p53 peptide analogs of the SAH-p53-8 series (see compound **6**) have shown a predictive correlation of α-helicity with experimental circular dichroism,[151] and stapled p53 peptide binding to MDM2(X) further predicting direct contact between the hydrocarbon linker moiety of SAH-p53-8 (**6**) and the target protein.[152] Importantly, such predictions were subsequently verified by the determination of an X-ray crystal structure of the stapled p53 peptide SAH-p53-8 bound to MDM2.[153] Very recently, computational methodologies have been focused on probing the 3D-structural stability of both single- and double-stapled analogs of hydrocarbon-stapled p53 peptides in complex with MDM2,[157] and such studies provide insight to the future development of more powerful *in silico* approaches to predict macrocyclic peptide binding to target proteins to support lead generation and/or optimization. Furthermore, the implementation of conformational analysis by methods such as circular dischroism, NMR and hydrogen exchange-mass spectrometry[151,154,156] may provide increased understanding of the α-helical stability of stapled peptides and, ultimately, to enable correlation with their manifest biological properties (*i.e.* cell penetration, resistance to proteolysis, and *in vivo* pharmacokinetics).

9.5 Macrocyclic α-Helical Peptide Chemical Biology and Drug Design

The promise of macrocyclic α-helical peptide drug discovery fundamentally leverages innovative technologies and predictive knowledge gained from iterative, systematic drug design and chemical biology. Realistically, this has resulted from significant empirical basic and translational research. Both academic and industrial drug discovery campaigns have engaged to advance a new class of breakthrough medicines. As reflected in the literature and as comprehensively listed in the reference section of this chapter, about one hundred scientific articles and reviews on macrocyclic α-helical peptides have been published to date, and a vast majority of such work has been focused on hydrocarbon-stapled peptides. Therefore, and within the limits of this chapter, representative studies on macrocyclic α-helical peptides (*e.g.* stapled peptides) from both academic and industrial scientists are described hereinafter to address achievements, challenges, and opportunities to tackle both intracellular and extracellular drug space.

9.5.1 Intracellular Therapeutic Target Drug Discovery

An increasing number of studies have described the identification of stapled peptides for intracellular targets that exhibit potent target binding, *in vitro* efficacy and, in some cases, *in vivo* proof-of-concept (see ref. 19–24, 28, and 29 for reviews). The spectrum of such intracellular α-helical protein–protein interaction target space includes the BH3:Bcl-2 family,[19,22–24,43,47,48,58,67–71,76,77,83,92,93,98] p53:MDM2/X,[42,57,65,66,72,79,81,82,87,89,94,95] MAML:Notch,[49] eIF4E,[158] TIF2:ERβ,[50] IRS1,[84] Hif-1:p300,[56,90] SOS:Ras,[59] R6IP1:Rab GTPase,[96] Bcl9:β-catenin,[64] TCF4:β-catenin,[78] Axin:β-catenin,[80] AKAP:protein kinase-A,[91] RPA,[97] HIV-1 integrase:LEDGE/p75,[85,86] and HIV-1 Gag capsid:HIV-1 Gag CTD/gp120 V3.[44,45,88] Importantly, in comparison to small-molecule drug discovery, stapled peptides have shown the potential to achieve unique target family selectivity profiles that are of significant value for exploring intracellular mechanisms and/or to overcome known disease resistance mechanisms. One example of this includes the design of BID BH3, BIM BH3, BAD BH3 and Mcl-1 BH3 stapled helical peptides for Bcl-2 family targets[19,22–24,43,47,58,67–71,77,83,92,93,122] in which multi-specificity inclusive of Mcl-1 binding or exclusive to Mcl-1 binding has been successfully achieved, as well as direct BAX/BAK activation by a previously unknown allosteric mechanism. Another example includes the design of p53 and structurally related phage display-derived stapled helical peptides having high binding affinity to both MDM2 and MDMX that has been successfully achieved.[42,57,58,65,66,72,79,81,82,87,94,95]

In the case of BID BH3 stapled peptides, proof-of-concept studies demonstrating *in vivo* efficacy in a human leukemia xenograft model (10 mg kg^{-1} dosing intravenously qd for seven days) were achieved, subsequent to an iterative process to identify a molecule having enhanced proteolytic and serum stability, high binding affinity to anti-apoptotic protein Bcl-2, cell penetration and mitochondrial co-localization, and cytochrome C-driven cellular apoptosis.[43] Recent studies have further shown the successful development of BIM BH3 and BID BH3 stapled peptides which are capable of directly activating the pro-apoptotic protein BAX to affect apoptosis.[67–69] The mechanism for this activation involves an allosteric binding site on BAX for the BH3 stapled helical peptide and propagation of BAX to ultimately form homo-oligomeric pores inducing mitochondrial apoptosis.

Mcl-1 is a recognized major resistance factor in human cancer and Mcl-1 over-expression has been linked to the pathogenesis of several cancers. Its anti-apoptotic properties are mechanistically related to its neutralizing interaction with BIM, BAK, NOXA and PUMA.[160,161] Recently, a compelling Mcl-1 BH3 stapled peptide has been reported to exhibit highly specificity and affinity to bind Mcl-1 as well as effectively sensitizing cancer cells to caspase-dependent apoptosis *in vitro*.[71] An X-ray structure of Mcl-1 complexed with this Mcl-1 BH3 stapled peptide was also determined and showed intermolecular contact of its hydrocarbon staple moiety with Mcl-1, accounting for the specificity versus other Bcl-2 family proteins.

The transcription factor p53 further illustrates the promise of stapled helical peptides to address challenging oncology targets for small-molecule drug discovery, including those in which resistance has been implicated. In the case of hydrocarbon-stapled p53 peptides, proof-of-concept studies of SAH-p53-8 (**6**) have shown its target binding to each MDM2 and MDMX, *in vitro* p53-dependent cytotoxicity in MDMX-overexpressing osteosarcoma SJSA-X and choriocarcinoma JEG-3 cells, and *in vivo* tumor growth inhibition in a JEG-3 tumor model (10 mg kg^{-1} dosed intravenously daily for four days).[72] Mechanistically, such dual MDM2 and MDMX antagonist properties would block p53 sequestration by both E3 ubiquitin ligases and potentially overcome a known cause of cancer resistance to existing MDM2-specific small-molecule drugs to effect reactivation of p53 tumor suppressor pathways.[162–164]

Recently, the dual MDM2/MDMX antagonist ATSP-7041 (see Scheme 9.2 for its chemical structure and Figure 9.11 for biophysical and biological data), has been reported[81,82] and shown by rigorous *in vitro* and *in vivo* testing to be a promising progenitor lead compound for further drug development. Relative to SAH-p53-8, ATSP-7041 exhibited >50-fold increased cellular potency and this correlated with its high binding affinities (low nM) to both MDM2 and MDMX. ATSP-7041 demonstrated selective p53-dependent sub-micromolar cellular activities and a capacity to exhibit more durable, on-target effects on p53 signaling than the small molecule clinical candidate MDM2-selective inhibitor RG7112.[81] A fluorescently-labeled analog of ATSP-7041 showed robust cell-penetrating properties. Importantly, ATSP-7041 demonstrated potent *in vivo* efficacy in a MCF-7 tumor xenograft model (20 or 30 mg/kg dosing intravenously qod for 23 days). Most profoundly, ATSP-7041 is a negatively charged, hydrocarbon-stapled peptide and it possesses high solubility and amphipathic α-helicity that exposes an extended hydrophobic surface. It is hypothesized that these biophysical attributes of ATSP-7041 correlate with its cell penetration and pharmacokinetic properties. Such a working hypothesis is being further investigated as ATSP-7041 is a significant benchmark stapled peptide to understand both cell penetration and pharmacokinetic properties of this modality of macrocyclic α-helical peptides for intracellular targets of therapeutic interest.

Beyond Bcl2-family BH3 and MDM2/MDMX, numerous other intracellular targets (*e.g.* Notch, eIF4E, ERβ, IRS1, Hif-1, Ras, Rab, β-catenin, PKA, RPA, HIV-1 integrase, and HIV-1 Gag capsid) have been shown to be effectively modulated by hydrocarbon-stapled peptides. Although a more detailed description is beyond the scope of this chapter, these studies greatly demonstrate the promise of macrocyclic α-helical peptides for both interrogating so-called 'undruggable' target space to investigate disease mechanisms across many therapeutic areas and drug development to advance breakthrough medicines.

9.5.2 Extracellular Therapeutic Target Drug Discovery

Advances in both basic and translational research have been achieved for macrocyclic α-helical peptides (*e.g.* hydrocarbon-stapled peptides) directed at extracellular targets. Examples of these include HIV-1 gp41 fusion antagonists,[46] a galanin agonist,[101] a neuropeptide-Y agonist,[101] an ABCA1 transporter modulator,[51] *N*-methyl-D-aspartic acid receptor antagonists,[99] and vitamin D receptor-coactivator inhibitors.[103] Such studies illustrate the diversity of extracellular target space as well as compelling new therapies for the treatment of infectious diseases, neuroendocrine, and metabolic disease. In designing such macrocyclic α-helical peptides for extracellular targets, there is no challenge of cell penetration as is otherwise critically important for success in lead optimization involving intracellular targets. However, proteolysis may become a greater challenge for such peptides to the extent that they are lengthy (*e.g.* HIV-1 gp41 fusion antagonists[46]), and in such cases there is a rationale for multiple and tandem stapling (collectively referred to as "stitching") that might enhance helicity to overcome degradation by plasma and/or membrane-bound proteases.

9.6 Macrocyclic α-Helical Peptide Drug Development

As evidenced by numerous scientific publications over the past decade, there is high expectation that macrocyclic α-helical peptides (*e.g.* stapled peptides) will further contribute to the expansion of druggable intracellular and extracellular target space. In particular, the structural diversity and tunable biophysical properties of stapled peptides underscore the fact that they exemplify a promising new synthetic biologic "privileged scaffold" for innovative drug discovery to exploit the high fidelity of Nature's molecular recognition within the expansive scope of α-helical interfacing protein-protein target space.

Aileron Therapeutics has pioneered hydrocarbon-stapled peptides since its founding with a goal to advance drug development and achieve clinical proof-of-concept for this highly investigated class of macrocyclic α-helical peptides. Towards this goal, the hydrocarbon-stapled peptide ALRN-6924 is poised for clinical testing and, hopefully, to become a breakthrough medicine. This has also provided incentive to the field of peptide drug discovery as well as a milestone achievement more specifically for stapled peptides.[165] Unquestionably, continued progress in basic and translational research of macrocyclic α-helical peptides will further contribute to the impact that the collective work described in this chapter to the momentum of future peptide drug discovery in terms of multidisciplinary science, innovative technology and transformational medicine.[166–168]

Acknowledgments

The authors wish to thank their colleagues at Aileron Therapeutics, and many academic collaborators as well as the members of the scientific advisory board for their support to the advancing Aileron's Stapled Peptide drug pipeline and technology platform.

References

1. A. L. Jochim and P. S. Arora, *Mol. Biosyst.*, 2009, **5**, 924.
2. A. L. Jochim and P. S. Arora, *ACS Chem. Biol.*, 2010, **5**, 919.
3. B. N. Bullock, A. L. Joachim and P. S. Arora, *J. Am. Chem. Soc.*, 2011, **133**, 14220.
4. W. L. DeLano, *Curr. Opin. Struct. Biol.*, 2002, **12**, 14.
5. B. Ma, M. Elkayam, H. Wolfson and R. Nussinov, *Proc. Natl. Acad. Sci. U. S. A.*, 2003, **100**, 5772.
6. I. M. A. Nooren and J. M. Thornton, *EMBO J.*, 2003, **22**, 3486.
7. J. C. Obenauer and M. B. Yaffe, *Methods Mol. Biol.*, 2004, **261**, 445.
8. Y. Pommier and J. Cherfils, *Trends Pharm. Sci.*, 2005, **26**, 138.
9. D. P. Ryan and J. M. Matthews, *Curr. Opin. Struct. Biol.*, 2005, **15**, 441.
10. D. C. Fry and L. T. Vassilev, *J. Mol. Med.*, 2005, **83**, 955.

11. H. Remaut and G. Waksman, *Trends Biochem. Sci.*, 2006, **31**, 436.
12. M. J. de Vega, M. Martín-Martínez and R. González-Muñiz, *Curr. Top. Med. Chem.*, 2007, 7, 33.
13. B. Ma and R. Nussinov, *Curr. Top. Med. Chem.*, 2007, 7, 999.
14. Z. Keskin, A. Gursoy, B. Ma and R. Nussinov, *Chem. Rev.*, 2008, **108**, 1225.
15. H. Jubb, A. P. Higueruelo, A. Winter and T. L. Blundell, *Trends Pharmacol. Sci.*, 2012, **33**, 241.
16. R. P. McGeary and D. P. Fairlie, *Curr. Opin. Drug Disc. Dev.*, 1998, **1**, 208.
17. S. J. Hershberger, S. G. Lee and J. Chmielewski, *Curr. Top. Med. Chem.*, 2007, 7, 928.
18. Y. Che and G. R. Marshall, *Expert Opin. Ther. Targets*, 2008, **12**, 101.
19. G. H. Bird, F. Bernal, K. Pitter and L. D. Walensky, *Methods Enzymol.*, 2008, **446**, 369.
20. L. K. Henchey, A. L. Jochim and P. S. Arora, *Curr. Opin. Chem. Biol.*, 2008, **12**, 692.
21. D. A. Guarracino, B. N. Bullock and P. S. Arora, *Biopolymers*, 2011, **95**, 1.
22. G. L. Verdine and L. D. Walensky, *Clin. Cancer Res.*, 2007, **13**, 7264.
23. G. H. Bird, F. Bernal, K. Pitter and L. D. Walensky, *Methods Enzymol.*, 2008, **446**, 369.
24. K. Pitter, F. Bernal, J. Labelle and L. D. Walensky, *Methods Enzymol.*, 2008, **446**, 387.
25. A. Moretto, M. Crisma, F. Formaggio and C. Toniolo, *Biopolymers*, 2010, **94**, 721.
26. J. Garner and M. M. Harding, *Org. Biomol. Chem.*, 2007, **5**, 3577.
27. R. Dharanipragada, *Future Med. Chem.*, 2013, **5**, 831.
28. G. L. Verdine and G. J. Hilinski, *Methods Enzymol.*, 2012, **503**, 3.
29. G. L. Verdine and G. J. Hilinski, *Drug Discovery Today: Technol.*, 2012, **9**, e1.
30. E. Fire, S. V. Gullá, R. A. Grant and A. E. Keating, *Protein Sci.*, 2010, **19**, 507.
31. B. Ku, J. S. Woo, C. Liang, K. H. Lee, H. S. Hong, E. X, K. S. Kim, J. U. Jung and B. H. Oh, *PLoS Pathog.*, 2008, **4**, e25.
32. P. H. Kussie, S. Gorina, V. Marechal, B. Elenbaas, J. Moreau, A. J. Levine and N. P. Pavletich, *Science*, 1996, **274**, 948.
33. Y. Nam, P. Sliz, L. Song, J. C. Aster and S. C. Blacklow, *Cell*, 2006, **124**, 973.
34. S. A. Dames, M. Martinez-Yamout, R. N. De Guzman, H. J. Dyson and P. E. Wright, *Proc. Natl. Acad. Sci., U. S. A.*, 2002, **99**, 5271.
35. S. K. Nair and S. K. Burley, *Cell*, 2003, **112** 193.
36. J. Marcotrigiano, A. C. Gingras, N. Sonenberg and S. K. Burley, *Mol. Cell*, 1999, **3**, 707.
37. R. B. Bledsoe, V. G. Montana, T. B. Stanley, C. J. Delves, C. J. Apolito, D. D. McKee, T. G. Consler, D. J. Parks, E. L. Stewart, T. M. Wilson, M. H. Lambert, J. T. Moore, K. H. Pearce and H. E. Xu, *Cell*, 2002, **110**, 93.
38. L. Jin, D. Martynowski, S. Zheng, T. Wada, W. Xie and Y. Li, *Mol. Endocrinol.*, 2010, **24**, 923.

39. M. Rushe, L. Silvian, S. Bixler, L. L. Chen, A. Cheung, S. Bowes, H. Cuervo, S. Berkowitz, T. Zheng, K. Guckian, M. Pellegrini and A. Lugovskoy, *Structure*, 2008, **16**, 798.

40. H. E. Blackwell, J. D. Sadowsky, R. J. Howard, J. N. Sampson, J. A. Chao, W. E. Steinmetz, D. J. O'Leary and R. H. Grubbs, *J. Org. Chem.*, 2001, **66**, 5291.

41. C. E. Schafmeister, J. Po and G. L. Verdine, *J. Am. Chem. Soc.*, 2000, **122**, 5891.

42. F. Bernal, A. F. Tyler, S. J. Korsmeyer, L. D. Walensky and G. L. Verdine, *J. Am. Chem. Soc.*, 2007, **129**, 2456.

43. L. D. Walensky, A. L. Kung, I. Escher, T. J. Malia, S. Barbuto, R. D. Wright, G. Wagner, G. L. Verdine and S. J. Korsmeyer, *Science*, 2004, **305**, 1466.

44. H. Zhang, Q. Zhao, S. Bhattacharya, A. A. Waheed, X. Tong, A. Hong, S. Heck, F. Curreli, M. Goger, D. Cowburn, E. O. Freed and A. K. Debnath, *J. Mol. Biol.*, 2008, **378**, 565.

45. H. Zhang, F. Curreli, X. Zhang, S. Bhattacharya, A. A. Waheed, A. Cooper, D. Cowburn, E. O. Freed and A. K. Debnath, *Retrovirology*, 2011, **8**, 28.

46. G. H. Bird, N. Madani, A. F. Perry, A. M. Princiotto, J. G. Supko, X. He, E. Gavathiotis, J. G. Sodroski and L. D. Walensky, *Proc. Natl. Acad. Sci., U. S. A.*, 2010, **107**, 14093.

47. N. N. Danial, L. D. Walensky, C.-Y. Zhang, C. S. Choi, J. K. Fisher, A. J. A. Molina, S. R. Datta, K. I. Pitter, G. H. Bird, J. D Wikstrom, J. T. Deeney, K. Robertson, J. Morash, A. Kulkarni, S. Neschen, S. Kim, M. E. Greenberg, B. E. Corkey, O. S. Shirihai, G. I. Shulman, B. B. Lowell and S. J. Korsemeyer, *Nat. Med.*, 2008, **14**, 144.

48. B. Szlyk, C. R. Braun, S. Ljubicic, E. Patton, G. H. Bird, M. A. Osundiji, F. M. Matschinsky, L. D. Walensky and N. N. Danial, *Nat. Struct. Mol. Biol.*, 2014, **21**, 36.

49. R. E. Moellering, M. Cornejo, T. N. Davis, C. Del Biaco, J. C. Aster, S. C. Blacklow, A. L. Kung, D. G. Gilliland, G. L. Verdine and J. E. Bradner, *Nature*, 2009, **462**, 182.

50. C. Phillips, R. Bazin, A. Bent, N. L. Davies, R. Moore, A. D. Pannifer, A. R. Pickford, S. H. Prior, C. M. Read, L. R. Roberts, M. Schade, A. Scott, D. G. Brown, B. Xu and S. L. Irving, *J. Am. Chem. Soc.*, 2011, **133**, 9696.

51. D. O. Sviridov, I. Z. Ikpot, J. Stonik, S. K. Drake, M. Amar, D. O. Osei-Hwedieh, G. Piszczek, S. Turner and A. T. Remaley, *Biochem. Biophys. Res. Commun.*, 2011, **410**, 446.

52. Y. W. Kim, P. S. Kutchukian and G. L. Verdine, *Org. Lett.*, 2010, **12**, 3046.

53. A. K. Boal, I. Guryanov, A. Moretto, M. Crisma, E. L. Lanni, C. Toniolo, R. H. Grubbs and D. J. O'Leary, *J. Am. Chem. Soc.*, 2007, **129**, 6986.

54. S. Cantel, A. Le Chevalier Isaad, M. Scrima, J. J. Levy, R. D. DiMarchi, P. Rovero, J. A. Halperin, A. M. D'Ursi, A. M. Panini and M. Chorev, *J. Org. Chem.*, 2008, **73**, 5663.

55. O. Jacobsen, H. Maekawa, N.-H. Ge, C. H. Gorbitz, P. Rongved, O. P. Ottersen, M. Amiry-Moghaddam and J. Klaveness, *J. Org. Chem.*, 2011, **76**, 1228.

56. L. K. Henchey, S. Kushal, R. Dubey, R. N. Chapman, B. Z. Olenyuk and P. S. Arora, *J. Am. Chem. Soc.*, 2010, **132**, 941.

57. L. K. Henchey, J. R. Porter, I. Ghosh and P. S. Arora, *ChemBioChem.*, 2010, **11**, 2104.

58. J. R. Porter, M. R. Helmers, P. Wang, J. L. Furman, S. T. Joy, P. S. Arora and I. Ghosh, *Chem. Commun.*, 2010, **46**, 8020.

59. A. Patgiri, K. K. Yadav, P. S. Arora and D. Bar-Sagi, *Nat. Chem. Biol.*, 2011, **7**, 585.

60. A. B. Mahon and P. S. Arora, *Chem. Commun.*, 2011, **48**, 1416.

61. A. Patgiri, M. Z. Menzenski, A. B. Mahon and P. S. Arora, *Nat. Protoc.*, 2010, **5**, 1857.

62. Y. W. Kim, T. N. Grossmann and G. L. Verdine, *Nat. Protoc.*, 2011, **6**, 761.

63. G. L. Verdine and Y.-W. Kim, *Harvard University*, USA. *U.S. Pat. Appl.* 20100184645, 2010.

64. S. A. Kawamoto, A. Coleska, X. Ran, H. Yi, C. Y. Yang and S. Wang, *J. Med. Chem.*, 2012, **55**, 1137.

65. M. M. Madden, A. Muppidi, Z. Li, X. Li, J. Chen and Q. Lin, *Bioorg. Med. Chem. Lett.*, 2011, **21**, 1472.

66. A. Muppidi, Z. Li, J. Chen and Q. Lin, *Bioorg. Med. Chem. Lett.*, 2011, **21**, 7412.

67. L. D. Walensky, K. Pitter, J. Morash, K. J. Oh, S. Barbuto, J. Fisher, E. Smith, G. L. Verdine and S. J. Korsmeyer, *Mol. Cell*, 2006, **24**, 199.

68. E. Gavathiotis, M. Suzuki, M. L. Davis, K. Pitter, G. H. Bird, S. G. Katz, H. C. Tu, H. Kim, E. H. Cheng, N. Tjandra and L. D. Walensky, *Nature*, 2008, **455**, 1076.

69. E. Gavathiotis, D. E. Reyna, M. L. Davis, G. H. Bird and L. D. Walensky, *Mol. Cell*, 2010, **40**, 481.

70. C. R. Braun, J. Mintseris, E. Gavathiotis, G. H. Bird, S. P. Gygi and L. D. Walensky, *Chem. Biol.*, 2010, **17**, 1325.

71. M. L. Stewart, E. Fire, A. E. Keating and L. D. Walensky, *Nat. Chem. Biol.*, 2010, **6**, 595.

72. F. Bernal, M. Wade, M. Godes, T. N. Davis, D. G. Whitehead, A. L. Kung, G. M. Wahl and L. D. Walensky, *Cancer Cell*, 2010, **18**, 411.

73. T. L. Sun, Y. Sun, C. C. Lee and H. W. Huang, *Biophys. J.*, 2013, **104**, 1923.

74. L. Nevola, A. Martin-Quiros, K. Eckelt, N. Camarero, S. Tosi, A. Llobet, E. Giralt and P. Gorostiza, *Angew. Chem., Int. Ed.*, 2013, **52**, 7704.

75. A. M. Spokoyny, Y. Zou, J. J. Ling, H. Yu, Y-S. Lin and B. L. Pentelute, *J. Am. Chem. Soc.*, 2013, **135**, 5946.
76. J. L. LaBelle, S. G. Katz, G. H. Bird, E. Gavathiotis, M. L. Stewart, C. Lawrence, J. K. Fisher, M. Godes, K. Pitter, A. L. Kung and L. D. Walensky, *J. Clin. Invest.*, 2012, **122**, 2018.
77. N. A. Cohen, M. L. Stewart, E. Gavathiotis, J. L. Tepper, S. R. Bruekner, B. Koss, J. T. Opferman and L. D. Walensky, *Chem. Biol.*, 2012, **19**, 1175.
78. T. N. Grossmann, J. T. Yeh, B. R. Bowman, Q. Chu, R. E. Moellering and G. L. Verdine, *Proc. Natl. Acad. Sci., U. S. A.*, 2012, **109**, 17942.
79. C. J. Brown, S. T. Quah, J. Jong, A. M. Goh, P. C. Chiam, K. H. Khoo, M. L. Choong, M. A. Lee, L. Yurlova, K. Zolghadr, T. L. Joseph, C. S. Verma and D. P. Lane, *ACS Chem. Biol.*, 2013, **8**, 506.
80. H. K. Cui, B. Zhao, Y. Li, Y. Guo, H. Hu, L. Liu and Y. G. Chen, *Cell Res.*, 2013, **23**, 581.
81. Y. S. Chang, B. Graves, V. Guerlavais, C. Tovar, K. Packman, T. To, K. Olson, K. Kesavan, P. Gangurde, A. Mukherjee, T. Baker, K. Darlak, C. Elkin, Z. Filipovic, F. Z Qureshi, H. Cai, P. Berry, E. Feyfant, X. E. Shi, J. Horstick, A. Annis, N. Fotouhi, T. Manning, H. Nash, L. T. Vassilev and T. K. Sawyer, *Proc. Natl. Acad. Sci., U. S. A.*, 2013, **110**, E3445.
82. V. Guerlavais, K. Darlak, B. Graves, C. Tovar, K. Packman, K. Olson, K. Kesavan, P. Gangurde, J. Horstick, A. Mukherjee, T. Baker, X. E. Shi, S. Lentini, K. Sun, S. Irwin, E. Feyfant, T. To, Z. Filipovic, C. Elkin, J. Pero, S. Santiago, T. Bruton, T. Sawyer, A. Annis, N. Fotouhi, T. Manning, H. Nash, L. T. Vassilev, Y. S. Chang and T. K. Sawyer, *Proceedings of the 23rd American Peptide Symposium*, ed. M. Lebl, Prompt Scientific Publishing, San Diego, 2013, pp. 184–185.
83. T. Okamoto, K. Zobel, A. Fedorova, C. Quan, H. Yang, W. J. Fairbrother, D. C. Huang, B. J. Smith, K. Deshayes and P. E. Czabotar, *ACS Chem. Biol.*, 2013, **8**, 297.
84. Y. Hao, C. Wang, B. Cao, B. M. Hirsch, J. Song, S. D. Markowitz, R. M. Ewing, D. Sedwick, L. Liu, W. Zheng and Z. Wang, *Cancer Cell*, 2013, **23**, 583.
85. Y. Q. Long, S. X. Huang, Z. Zawahir, Z. L. Xu, H. Li, T. W. Sanchez, Y. Zhi, S. De Houwer, F. Christ, Z. Debyser and N. Neamati, *J. Med. Chem.*, 2013, **56**, 5601.
86. W. Nomura, H. Aikawa, N. Ohashi, E. Urano, M. Metifiot, M. Fujino, K. Maddali, T. Ozaki, A. Nozue, T. Narumi, C. Hashimoto, T. Tanaka, Y. Pommier, N. Yamamoto, J. A. Komano, T. Murakami and H. Tamamura, *ACS Chem. Biol.*, 2013, **8**, 2235.
87. B. Rao, S. Lain and A. M. Thompson, *Br. J. Cancer*, 2013, **109**, 2954.
88. H. Zhang, F. Curreli, A. A. Waheed, P. Y. Mercredi, M. Mehta, P. Bhargava, D. Scacalossi, X. Tong, S. Lee, A. Cooper, M. F. Summers, E. O. Freed and A. K. Debnath, *Retrovirology*, 2013, **10**, 136.
89. S. J. Wei, T. Joseph, S. Chee, L. Li, L. Yurlova, K. Zolghadr, C. Brown, D. Lane, C. Verma and F. Ghadessy, *PLoS One*, 2013, **8**, e81068.

90. S. Kushal, B. Bullock Lao, L. K. Henchey, R. Dubey, H. Mesallati, N. J. Traaseth, B. Z. Olenyuk and P. S. Arora, *Proc. Natl. Acad. Sci., U. S. A.*, 2013, **110**, 15602.

91. Y. Wang, T. G. Ho, D. Bertinetti, M. Neddermann, E. Franz, G. C. Mo, L. P. Schendowich, A. Sukhu, R. C. Spelts, J. Zhang, F. W. Herberg and E. J. Kennedy, *ACS Chem. Biol.*, 2014, **9**, 635.

92. G. H. Bird, E. Gavathiotis, J. L. Labelle, S. G. Katz and L. D. Walensky, *ACS Chem. Biol.*, 2014, **9**, 831.

93. T. Okamoto, D. Segal, K. Zobel, A. Fedorova, H. Yang, W. J. Fairbrother, D. C. S. Huang, B. J. Smith, K. Deshayes and P. E. Czabotar, *ACS Chem. Biol.*, 2014, **9**, 838.

94. L. Yurlova, M. Derks, A. Buchfellner, I. Hickson, M. Janssen, D. Morrison, I. Stansfield, C. J. Brown, F. J. Ghadessy, D. P. Lane, U. Rothbauer, K. Zolghadr and E. Krausz, *J. Biomol. Screen.*, 2014, **19**, 516.

95. Y. H. Lau, P. de Andrade, S.-T. Quah, M. Rossman, L. Laraia, N. Skold, T. J. Sum, P. J. E. Rowling, T. L. Joseph, C. Verma, M. Hyvonen, L. S. Itzhaki, A. R. Venkitaraman, C. J. Brown, D. P. Lane and D. R. Spring, *Chem. Sci.*, 2014, **5**, 1804.

96. J. Spiegel, P. M. Cromm, A. Itzen, R. S. Goody, T. N. Grossmann and H. Waldmann, *Angew. Chem., Int. Ed.*, 2014, **53**, 2498.

97. A. O. Frank, B. Vangamudi, M. D. Feldkamp, E. M. Souza-Fagundes, J. W. Luzwick, D. Cortez, E. T. Olejniczak, A. G. Waterson, O. W. Rossanese, W. J. Chazin and S. W. Fesik, *J. Med. Chem.*, 2014, **57**, 2455.

98. C. Reynolds, J. E. Roderick, J. L. Labelle, G. Bird, R. Mathieu, K. Bodaar, D. Colon, U. Pyati, K. E. Stevenson, J. Qi, M. Harris, L. B. Silverman, S. E. Sallan, J. E. Bradner, D. S. Neuberg, A. T. Look, L. D. Walensky, M. A. Kelliher and A. Gutierrez, *Leukemia*, 2014, DOI: 10.1038/leu.2014.78.

99. R. J. Platt, T. S. Han, B. R. Green, M. D. Smith, J. Skalicky, P. Gruszczynski, H. S. White, B. Olivera, G. Bulaj and J. Gajewiak, *J. Biol. Chem.*, 2012, **287**, 20727.

100. H. Chapuis, J. Slaninová, L. Bednárová, L. Monincová, M. Buděšínský and V. Čeřovský, *Amino Acids*, 2012, **43**, 2047.

101. B. R. Green, B. D. Klein, H. K. Lee, M. D. Smith, H. S. White and G. Bulaj, *Bioorg. Med. Chem.*, 2013, **21**, 303.

102. H. K. Cui, J. Qing, Y. Guo, Y. J. Wang, L. J. Cui, T. H. He, L. Zhang and L. Liu, *Bioorg, Med. Chem.*, 2013, **21**, 3547.

103. Y. Demizu, S. Nagoya, M. Shirakawa, M. Kawamura, N. Yamagata, Y. Sato, M. Doi and M. Kurihara, *Bioorg. Med. Chem. Lett.*, 2013, **23**, 4292.

104. T. K. Pham, D. H. Kim, B. J. Lee and Y. W. Kim, *Bioorg. Med. Chem. Lett.*, 2013, **23**, 6717.

105. H. J. Johansson, S. E. Andaloussi and Ü. Langel, *Methods Mol. Biol.*, 2011, **683**, 233.

106. R. M. Johnson, S. D. Harrison and D. Maclean, *Methods Mol. Biol.*, 2011, **683**, 535.
107. S. El-Andaloussi, T. Holm and Ü. Langel, *Curr. Pharm. Des.*, 2005, **11**, 3597.
108. E. Vivès, J. Schmidt and A. Pèlegrin, *Biochim. Biophys. Acta*, 2008, **1786**, 126.
109. C. Foerg and H. P. Merkle, *J. Pharm. Sci.*, 2008, **97**, 144.
110. R. L. Juliano, R. Alam, V. Dixit and H. M. Kang, *Wiley Interdiscip. Rev. Nanomed. Nanobiotechnol.*, 2009, **1**, 324.
111. M. Fotin-Mleczek, R. Fischer and R. Brock, *Curr. Pharm. Design*, 2005, **11**, 3613.
112. R. Fischer, M. Fotin-Mleczek, H. Hufnagel and R. Brock, *ChemBio-Chem.*, 2005, **6**, 2126.
113. M. Grdisa, *Curr. Med. Chem.*, 2011, **18**, 1373.
114. F. Duchardt, M. Fotin-Mlecezek, H. Schwarz, R. Fischer and R. Brock, *Traffic*, 2007, **8**, 848.
115. J. M. Gump and S. F. Dowdy, *Trends Mol. Med.*, 2007, **13**, 443.
116. W. P. Verdurmen and R. Brock, *Trends Pharmacol. Sci.*, 2011, **32**, 116.
117. G. P. H. Dietz and M. Bohr, *Mol. Cell. Neurosci.*, 2004, **27**, 85.
118. D. Y. Jackson, D. S. King, J. Chmielewski, S. Singh and P. G. Schultz, *J. Am. Chem. Soc.*, 1991, **113**, 9391.
119. J. C. Phelan, N. J. Skelton, A. C. Braisted and R. S. McDowell, *J. Am. Chem. Soc.*, 1997, **119**, 455.
120. A. Caporale, M. Sturlese, L. Gesiot, F. Zanta, A. Wittelsberger and C. Cabrele, *J. Med. Chem.*, 2010, **53**, 8072.
121. L. P. Miranda, K. A. Winters, C. V. Gegg, A. Patel, J. Aral, J. Long, J. Zhang, S. Diamond, M. Guido, S. Stanislaus, M. Ma, H. Li, M. J. Rose, L. Poppe and M. M. Veniant, *J. Med. Chem.*, 2008, **9**, 2758.
122. B. Yang, D. Liu and Z. Huang, *Bioorg. Med. Chem. Lett.*, 2004, **14**, 1403.
123. R. E. Austin, R. A. Maplestone, A. M. Sefler, K. Liu, W. N. Hruzewicz, C. W. Liu, H. S. Cho, D. E. Wemmer and P. A. Bartlett, *J. Am. Chem. Soc.*, 1997, **119**, 6461.
124. K. Muller, D. Obrecht, A. Knierzinger, C. Stankovic, C. Spiegler, W. Bannwarth, A. Trzeciak, G. Englert, A. M. Labhardt and P. Schonholzer, *Perspectives in Medicinal Chemistry*, ed. B. Testa and E. Kyburz, *Verlag Helv. Chim. Acta, Basel*, 1993, pp. 513–532.
125. D. S. Kemp, T. P. Curran, J. G. Boyd and T. J. Allen, *J. Org. Chem.*, 1991, **56**, 6672.
126. W. S. Horne, J. L. Price and S. H. Gellman, *Proc. Natl. Acad. Sci., U. S. A.*, 2008, **105**, 9151.
127. P. Tosovská and P. S. Arora, *Org. Lett.*, 2010, **12**, 1588.
128. B. P. Orner, J. T. Ernst and A. D. Hamilton, *J. Am. Chem. Soc.*, 2001, **123**, 5382.
129. H. Yin, G. Lee, K. A. Sedey, O. Kutzki, H. S. Park, B. P. Orner, J. T. Ernst, H. G. Wang, S. M. Sebti and A. D. Hamilton, *J. Am. Chem. Soc.*, 2006, **127**, 10191.

130. H. Oguri, A. Oomura, S. Tanabe and M. Hirama, *Tetrahedron Lett.*, 2005, **46**, 2179.
131. M. Sasaki and K. Tachibana, *Tetrahedron Lett.*, 2007, **48**, 3181.
132. S. Ujihara, T. Oishi, K. Torikai, K. Konoki, N. Matsumori, M. Murata, Y. Oshima and S. Aimoto, *Bioorg. Med. Chem. Lett.*, 2008, **18**, 6115.
133. P. Raboisson, J. J. Marugan, C. Schubert, H. K. Koblish, T. Lu, S. Zhao, M. R. Player, A. C. Maroney, R. L. Reed, N. D. Huebert, J. Lattanze, D. J. Parks and M. D. Cummings, *Bioorg. Med. Chem. Lett.*, 2005, **15**, 1857.
134. B. L. Grasberger, T. Lu, C. Schubert, D. J. Parks, T. E. Carver, H. K. Koblish, M. D. Cummings, L. V. LaFrance, K. L. Milkiewicz, R. R. Calvo, D. Maguire, J. Lattanze, C. F. Franks, S. Zhao, K. Ramachandren, G. R. Bylebyl, M. Zhang, C. L. Manthey, E. C. Petrella, M. W. Pantoliano, I. C. Deckman, J. C. Spurlino, A. C. Maroney, B. E. Tomczuk, C. J. Molloy and R. F. Bone, *J. Med. Chem.*, 2005, **48**, 909.
135. K. Leonard, J. J. Marugan, P. Raboisson, R. Calvo, J. M. Gushue, H. K. Koblish, J. Lattanze, S. Zhao, M. D. Cummings, M. R. Player, A. C. Maroney and T. Lu, *Bioorg. Med. Chem. Lett.*, 2006, **16**, 3463.
136. I. Saraogi, C. D. Incarvito and A. D. Hamilton, *Angew. Chem., Int. Ed.*, 2008, **47**, 9691.
137. C. Toniolo, M. Crisma, F. Formaggio, G. Valle, G. Cavicchioni, G. Precigoux, A. Aubry and J. Kampuis, *Biopolymers*, 1993, **33**, 1061.
138. I. L. Karle and P. Balaram, *J. Am. Chem. Soc.*, 1990, **29**, 6747.
139. A. K. Boal, I. Guryanov, A. Moretto, M. Crisma, E. L. Lanni, C. Toniolo, R. H. Grubbs and D. J. O'Leary, *J. Am. Chem. Soc.*, 2007, **129**, 6986.
140. Y.-W. Kim and G. L. Verdine, *Bioorg. Med. Chem. Lett.*, 2009, **19**, 2533.
141. Y.-W. Kim, P. S. Kutchukian and G. L. Verdine, *Org. Lett.*, 2010, **12**, 3046.
142. S. Y. Shim, Y.-W. Kim and G. L. Verdine, *Chem. Biol. Drug Des.*, 2013, **82**, 635.
143. T. K. Pham, J. Yoo and Y.-W. Kim, *Bull. Korean Chem. Soc.*, 2013, **34**, 2640.
144. C. Cativiela and M. D. Diaz-de-Villegas, *Tetrahedron: Asymmetry*, 2007, **18**, 569.
145. R. M. Williams and M.-N. Im, *J. Am. Chem. Soc.*, 1991, **113**, 9276.
146. Y. N. Belokon, V. I. Bakhmutov, N. I. Chernoglazova, K. A. Kochetkov, S. V. Vitt, N. S. Garbalinskaya and V. M. Belikov, *J. Chem. Soc., Perkin Trans. 1*, 1988, 305.
147. Y. N. Belokon, V. I. Tararov, V. I. Maleev, T. F. Savel'eva and M. G. Ryzhov, *Tetrahedron: Asymmetry*, 1998, **9**, 4249.
148. S. Bhattacharya, H. Zhang, A. K. Debnath and D. Cowburn, *J. Biol. Chem.*, 2008, **283**, 16274.
149. K. Hamacher, A. Hübsch and J. A. McCammon, *J. Chem. Phys.*, 2006, **124**, 164907.
150. P. S. Kutchukian, J. S. Yang, G. L. Verdine and E. I. Shakhnovich, *J. Am. Chem. Soc.*, 2009, **131**, 4622.

151. Z. Guo, U. Mohanty, J. Noehre, T. K. Sawyer, W. Sherman and G. Krilov, *Chem. Biol. Drug Des.*, 2010, **75**, 348.

152. T. L. Joseph, D. Lane and C. S. Verma, *Cell Cycle*, 2010, **9**, 4560.

153. S. Baek, P. S. Kutchukian, G. L. Verdine, R. Huber, T. A. Holak, K. W. Lee and G. M. Popowicz, *J. Am. Chem. Soc.*, 2012, **134**, 103.

154. S. Bhattacharya, H. Zhang, D. Cowburn and A. K. Debnath, *Biopolymers*, 2012, **97**, 253.

155. T. L. Joseph, D. P. Lane and C. S. Verma, *PLoS One*, 2012, 7, e43985.

156. X. E. Shi, T. E. Wales, C. Elkin, N. Kawahata, J. R. Engen and D. A. Annis, *Anal. Chem.*, 2013, **85**, 11185.

157. Z. Guo, K. Streu, G. Krilov and U. Mohanty, *Chem. Biol. Drug Des.*, 2014, **13**, 631.

158. D. Lama, S. T. Quah, C. S. Verma, R. Lakshminarayanan, R. W. Beuerman, D. P. Lane and C. J. Brown, *Sci. Rep.*, 2013, **3**, 3451.

159. G. L. Verdine and K. Hayashi, *Harvard University*, USA, *PCT Int. Appl.* WO2014/052647, 2014.

160. R. Beroukhim, C. H. Mermel, D. Porter, G. Wei, S. Raychaudhuri, J. Donovan, J. Barretina, J. S. Boehm, J. Dobson, M. Urashima, K. T. McHenry, R. M. Pinchback, A. H. Ligon, Y.-J. Cho, L. Haery, H. Greulich, M. Reich, W. Winckler, M. S. Lawrence, B. A. Weir, K. E. Tanaka, D. Y. Chiang, A. J. Bass, A. Loo, C. Hoffman, J. Prenser, T. Liefeld, Q. Gao, D. Yecies, S. Signoretti, E. Maher, F. J. Kaye, H. Sasaki, J. E. Tepper, J. A. Fletcher, J. Tabernero, J. Baselga, M.-S. Tsao, F. DeMichelis, M. A. Rubin, P. A. Janne, M. J. Daly, C. Nucera, R. L. Levine, B. L. Ebert, S. Gabriel, A. K. Rustgi, C. R. Antonescu, M. Ladanyi, A. Letai, S. A. Garraway, M. Loda, D. G. Beer, L. D. True, A. Okamoto, S. L. Pomeroy, S. Singer, T. R. Golub, E. S. Lander, G. Getz, W. R. Sellers and M. Meyerson, *Nature*, 2010, **463**, 899.

161. B. A. Quinn, R. Dash, B. Azab, S. Sarkar, S. K. Das, S. Kumar, R. A. Oyesanya, S. Dasgupta, P. Dent, S. Grant, M. Rahmani, D. T. Curiel, I. Dmitriev, M. Hedvat, J. Wei, B. Wu, J. L. Stebbins, J. C. Reid, M. Pellecchia, D. Sarkar and P. B. Fisher, *Expert Opin. Invest. Drugs*, 2011, **20**, 1397.

162. G. M. Popowicz, A. Domling and T. A. Holak, *Angew. Chem., Int. Ed.*, 2011, **50**, 2680.

163. M. Wade, Y. V. Wang and G. M. Wahl, *Trends Cell Biol.*, 2010, **20**, 299.

164. A. Gembarska, F. Luciani, C. Fedele, E. A. Russell, M. Dewaele, S. Villar, A. Zwolinska, S. Haupt, J. de Lange, D. Yip, J. Goydos, J. J. Haigh, Y. Haupt, L. Larue, A. Jochemsen, H. Shi, G. Moriceau, R. S. Lo, G. Ghanem, M. Shackleton, F. Bernal and J.-C. Marine, *Nat. Med.*, 2012, **18**, 1239.

165. S. Crunkhorn, *Nat. Rev. Drug Discov.*, 2013, **12**, 741.

166. P. Vlieghe, V. Lisowski, J. Martinez and M. Khrestchatisky, *Drug Discovery Today*, 2010, **15**, 40.

167. K. Bellmann-Sickert and A. G. Beck-Sickinger, *Trends Pharmacol. Sci.*, 2010, **31**, 434.

168. J. Audie and C. Boyd, *Curr. Pharm. Des.*, 2010, **16**, 567.

CHAPTER 10

Optimizing the Permeability and Oral Bioavailability of Macrocycles

ALAN M. MATHIOWETZ,*[a] SIEGFRIED S. F. LEUNG[b] AND
MATTHEW P. JACOBSON[c]

[a] Worldwide Medicinal Chemistry, Pfizer Inc., Cambridge, MA 02139, USA;
[b] Circle Pharma, Inc., San Francisco, CA 94107; [c] Department of
Pharmaceutical Chemistry, University of California
San Francisco, San Francisco, CA 94158, USA
*Email: alan.m.mathiowetz@pfizer.com

10.1 Introduction

Oral dosing is a highly preferred route of administration of drugs because, from the point of view of the patient, it is a relatively simple and familiar process. This simplicity belies the great complexity of processes required for an orally dosed medication to reach systemic circulation and, eventually, the targeted organs. Many of the physical, transport, and metabolic processes involved are influenced by the physicochemical properties of the drug molecule, so it has been possible to develop property guidelines to help medicinal chemists design drugs with an improved chance of being orally bioavailable. The guidelines define what is often called "Rule-of-5 space", named after one of the pioneering analyses performed in this field.[1] In the chemical universe outside of this Rule-of-5 space, the probability of achieving significant oral bioavailability decreases significantly, yet there are

RSC Drug Discovery Series No. 40
Macrocycles in Drug Discovery
Edited by Jeremy Levin
© The Royal Society of Chemistry 2015
Published by the Royal Society of Chemistry, www.rsc.org

therapeutic drivers for the discovery of drugs of this type. In the quest for Beyond Rule-of-5 oral drugs, macrocyclization has the potential to mitigate several detrimental properties. The sophisticated design rules and related synthetic challenges for identifying orally bioavailable macrocycles are beginning to emerge.

The classic "Rule of 5" paper by Lipinski and co-workers[1] describes simple physical property guidelines for organic molecules being pursued in drug discovery. Compounds adhering to these guidelines were shown to have increased odds of attaining oral bioavailability. While the physical property relationships for oral bioavailability have been refined and expanded,[1–7] Rule-of-5 compliant molecules remain a primary focus of medicinal chemistry, since the likelihood of achieving oral absorption drops off rapidly with molecular weight (MW) over 500 Daltons, and clearance increases with increasing logD.[2] Unfortunately, not all therapeutically interesting biological targets have binding pockets that are amenable to the high affinity binding of Rule-of-5 molecules.[8] Larger biologically derived drugs, especially antibodies, now make up a majority of the top-selling drugs.[9] These biologicals usually have properties far outside the Rule-of-5 property guidelines and rarely have significant oral bioavailability, depending instead upon injectable, intranasal, or other routes of administration. There is, however, a growing body of evidence that oral drugs, often macrocyclic, can be discovered in a "Middle Space" between Rule-of-5 compliant synthetic compounds and biologicals.[10] These select compounds are large enough to interact efficaciously with some larger surfaces that previously required biologicals, yet have the right balance of properties to achieve significant oral bioavailability.

Since chemistry space expands exponentially in proportion to heavy atom count,[11] the Middle Space of molecules between 500 and 1500 Daltons is enormously larger and more diverse than Rule-of-5 space. However, as the chemistry space grows larger, the proportion of molecules that are orally bioavailable becomes minute, and it becomes imperative to develop a greater understanding of which properties and synthetic strategies can lead to the efficient discovery of orally bioavailable molecules.

10.2 Pharmacokinetic Benefits of Macrocyclization

Macrocyclization can provide pharmacological benefits such as improved potency and selectivity and a larger protein binding surface for difficult targets such as protein–protein interactions,[12–14] and it also provides several benefits in the quest to attain oral bioavailability, a complex phenomenon governed by physical processes as well as a variety of biological transport and metabolic functions. Naturally, physical processes such as dissolution or diffusion are highly dependent on a molecule's physical properties, but even biological functions can be influenced significantly by the physical properties of drug molecules.

It is helpful to view oral bioavailability as combining intestinal absorption, passage through the intestinal or gut wall, and hepatic extraction as in Equation 10.1.[2]

$$F = F_a \times F_g \times F_h \tag{10.1}$$

F_a is the fraction of the compound absorbed, F_g is the fraction evading intestinal wall metabolism, and F_h is the fraction evading hepatic extraction.[2] Of these, F_g has not been widely studied until recently,[2,15] and more information is available to help understand the processes of hepatic extraction and intestinal absorption. Intestinal absorption itself involves many distinct processes: dissolution of a drug's physical formulation, avoidance of degradation by digestive enzymes (proteolytic degradation for the case of peptide drugs), passage along the gastrointestinal tract, and permeation through the intestinal lumen. Since macrocyclization dramatically affects the structure and physical properties of a molecule, it potentially can influence a wide variety of the factors that impact bioavailability.

Macrocyclization can potentially affect the metabolism, and therefore the hepatic extraction rate, of compounds in a number of ways. For example, the chemical structure of the cyclic backbone or pendant side chains can raise or lower logD, shown to be a major determinant of F_h.[2] Likewise, cyclization could introduce or eliminate metabolic soft spots. A more direct, consistently beneficial effect of macrocyclization is reduction in molecular flexibility,[12] believed to reduce the ability of molecules to enter CYP P450 active sites[2,7] and to be metabolized. For example, macrocycles developed for the inhibition of HCV NS3 protease (see Chapter 7) have demonstrated the value of macrocyclization in the reduction of systemic clearance.[12,16] Macrocyclic linkers can be varied in length, physical properties, and conformational shape and flexibility, all of which have the potential to modulate CYP P450 metabolism and systemic clearance. Table 10.1 demonstrates the impact of the linker on the CYP P450 metabolism, as measured in rat liver microsomes, for a series of Hsp90 inhibitors.[17] In addition, for the case of peptides, cyclization can eliminate systemic proteolytic degradation, thereby decreasing F_h for cyclic peptides.[18] A study of the acyclic decapeptide H-LLEDPVGTVA-NH2 compared to cyclic peptide, disulfide, and thioether variations[18] showed that the acyclic peptide had completely disappeared in 10% human serum after 24 hours, while the cyclic variants were still at least 90% intact. The most stable version, the thioether, was still 100% intact after 96 hours in 50% human serum.

Macrocyclization can potentially have an even greater impact on oral bioavailability by increasing the fraction absorbed (F_a). For peptides, cyclization can reduce or eliminate susceptibility to proteolytic degradation by gastric, intestinal, or brush border proteases,[19,20] thereby significantly increasing the fraction of peptides available for permeation. Table 10.2 shows the stability of two cyclic peptides in brush border membrane vesicles. Cyclic peptide **6** is only 25% degraded after 90 minutes. N-methylation

Table 10.1   A series of Hsp90 inhibitors from ref. 17.[a]

Structure	Ring size	RLM T/12 (min)	Solubility (μg mL^{-1})	MW	ClogP
1	11	15	>100	380	3.3
2	12	30	35	395	3.6
3	12	15	52	423	4.4
4	13	3	6	437	4.7
5	14	28	73	425	2.9

[a]Experimental microsomal stability half-life in Rat Liver Microsomes (RLM) and Solubility are shown, along with molecular weight (MW) and calculated logP (ClogP).

Table 10.2 Stability of peptides in brush border membrane vesicles.[19]

Structure	% Degraded (30 min)	% Degraded (90 min)
6	15	25
7	<5%	<5%

further stabilizes the cyclic peptide and 7 is almost completely stable.[20] The ability of macrocyclization to modulate solubility has also been demonstrated,[13] and may be due to a combination of properties such as reduced lipophilicity and incorporation of ionizable groups, which are not universal but may be incorporated into specific macrocycles, and disruption of molecular planarity,[21] which may be a more general benefit of macrocyclization. The Hsp 90 Inhibitors in Table 10.1 display a range of solubility depending upon lipophilicity (ClogP) and conformational flexibility. Nevertheless, it is likely that the biggest potential impact of macrocyclization on oral bioavailability is through its control of three-dimensional (3D) molecular shape and polarity, and the impact this has on permeability and intestinal absorption.

Nearly all macrocycles, whether derived from peptidic or nonpeptidic natural products, or synthesized as constrained analogs of smaller organics, have a more compact 3D fold and less conformational flexibility than their acyclic counterparts, potentially improving diffusion rates[22] and therefore permeability and ultimately absorption. Conformational constraints, if designed correctly,[23] can also enforce intramolecular hydrogen-bonding (IMHB), thereby reducing unfavorable desolvation as a drug progresses from the gastrointestinal fluid through the intestinal epithelium and into systemic circulation. Diffusion rates for eight pairs of macrocycles and acyclic controls are shown in Figure 10.1. The structures of three of these pairs are

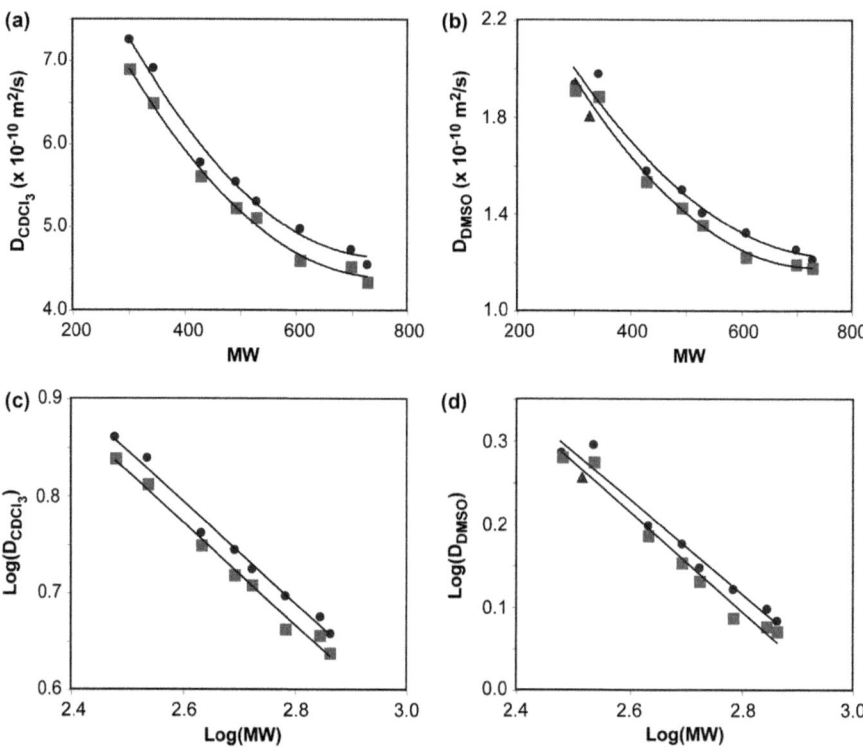

Figure 10.1 Diffusion rates for cyclic and acyclic compound pairs in CDCl$_3$ and DMSO.[22] (The macrocycles are plotted as circles while their acyclic controls are plotted as squares.)

shown in Table 10.3, exemplifying low, medium, and high MW molecules in the study.[22]

It is important to note that macrocyclization does not automatically confer these various benefits, summarized in Table 10.4; rather, only very specific macrocyclic constraints allow a molecule to adopt the precise fold required for improved solubility, stability and/or permeability, and these constraints must be synthetically cost-effective and, of course, consistent with the three-dimensional requirements for functional potency. It is a complex multi-dimensional challenge but, fortunately, one with a growing number of successful examples. Consistent success will eventually come from understanding a spectrum of knowledge: information about natural product macrocycles including cyclic peptides and macrolides, a great breadth of creative synthetic approaches, understanding of key physical properties and analytical methods to measure these, and computational methods that can predict essential properties. Permeability may be simultaneously the greatest challenge for Beyond Rule-of-5 molecules and the property where the most effective theoretical understanding is being built, and this is the focus here.

Table 10.3 Example small, medium, and large cyclic/acylic pairs[22] with diffusion data in CDCl$_3$ and DMSO plotted in Figure 10.1.

	Structure	MW
8		300
9		302
10		491
11		493
12		727

Table 10.3   (*Continued*)

Structure	MW
13	729

Table 10.4   Summary of potential impact of macrocyclization on oral bioavailability.

Property impacted	How to improve property	Ref.
Hepatic Extraction (F_h)	Reduce logD. Eliminate metabolic softspots. Reduce flexibility.	2, 7, 43
GI stability	(For peptides): provide resistance to gastric, intestinal, and brush border proteases	46
Solubility	Reduce lipophilicity. Incorporate ionizable groups. Disrupt planarity.	47, 49
Permeability	Reduce molecular volume. Reduce polarity (desolvation penalty). Form intramolecular H-bonds.	8, 9

10.3   Properties Related to Permeability and Oral Bioavailability

Numerous publications have appeared in recent years describing structural and physical properties that are related directly or indirectly to permeability, oral absorption, or oral bioavailability. These have recently been reviewed[24] and here we summarize several contributions (see Table 10.5).

The highly influential Rule-of-5 paper by Lipinski *et al.* was developed in order to provide medicinal chemists with "calculable parameters...that were likely related to absorption or permeability," presented in a way that would "focus on the chemists very strong pattern recognition and chemical structure recognition skills".[1] The authors analyzed a set of 2245 compounds from Phase II and later, using parameters previously indicated to be related to these properties: MW, related to intestinal and blood brain barrier

Table 10.5 Physicochemical properties associated with permeability, absorption, and/or oral bioavailability.

Property	Cutoffs	Ref.
Rule of 5	Alerts when two or more cutoffs exceeded: MW > 500, ClogP > 5.0 (or MLogP > 4.15), NH + OH > 5, or N + O > 10.	1
Polar Surface Area	Low absorption when van der Waals Polar Surface Area > 120 Å^2	3, 4
Rotatable Bonds	Rat oral bioavailability is improved when TPSA $\leq$ 140 Å^2 and rotatable bonds $\leq$ 10 or HBD + HBA $\leq$ 12 and rotatable bonds $\leq$ 10	7
Various related to absorption	Human F_a improves with: MW $\leq$ 500, TPSA $\leq$ 125 Å, HBD + HBA $\leq$ 9, Rotatable bonds $\leq$ 12, or ClogD$_{7.4}$ $\geq$ − 2.	2
Various related to clearance	Human F_h improves with cLogD$_{7.4}$ $\leq$ 3 and % rel RB $\leq$ 2.	2
3D Properties	Improved RRCK P_{app} with van der Waals 3D-PSA $\leq$ 100 Å and Radius of Gyration $\leq$ 7 when 0 < ClogP < 5.	6

permeability; ClogP (MLogP), related to absorption; and counts of NH + OH bonds, an approximation of hydrogen-bond donor ability related to permeability. The authors also identified counts of N and O atoms as a good approximation to hydrogen-bond acceptor count. For each of these properties, they determined values within which 90% of the database compounds fell. A system was created to alert chemists any time a registered compound exceeded two or more of these specific cutoffs, summarized in Table 10.5. Although the authors were aware that some orally bioavailable compounds fell outside the Rule-of-5, they suggested that nearly all of these contained structural features that made them substrates for active transporters,[1] and therefore were not passively absorbed.

At the same time, an alternative measure of polarity, the polar surface area (PSA), was shown to have a sigmoidal relationship with oral absorption.[3] Although the initial dataset was relatively small, containing F_a values for twenty drugs, the trend that was identified[3] and refined[4] has held up well in subsequent studies.[2,6] It was soon shown that topological polar surface area (TPSA), not requiring 3D structural information, was an excellent surrogate for PSA and correlated well with absorption and permeability.[5] This rapid calculation has become a very popular tool for quickly estimating the likelihood of a compound's permeability, but recent studies[6] have shown the importance of returning to the 3D formulation of PSA when studying large molecules, including macrocycles, in order to account for possible hiding of polarity within the molecule, *via* cyclization, intramolecular hydrogen-bonding, or both.

Rotatable bonds (RB) were introduced as a key predictor of oral bioavailability by Veber *et al.*[7] Upon analyzing over 1100 rat oral bioavailability data points, the authors concluded that oral bioavailability was improved for less flexible molecules, even when controlling for MW. The principal hypothesis given for this trend was that decreased molecular flexibility allowed for greater selectivity for the drug's intended target than for off-target proteins involved in clearance of the drug. This hypothesis was later supported in an analysis of human absorption and clearance data,[2] which showed that % relative rotatable bond count (normalized for MW) increased human hepatic clearance rates, but did not impact fraction absorbed.

The analysis of human oral bioavailability data by Varma *et al.*,[2] was an enlightening analysis of previously noted physicochemical properties. Their dataset was a carefully refined set of 309 drugs with human data from oral studies, delineated into the three stages as in Equation 10.1: the fraction of the compound absorbed (F_a), the fraction evading intestinal wall metabolism (F_g), and the fraction evading hepatic extraction (F_h). This work was able to distinguish the impact of molecular size properties (MW, rotatable bonds) from lipophilicity ($CLogD_{7.4}$). Thus, it was found that large size (*e.g.* MW > 500, RB > 12) impacts absorption but not clearance, whereas high lipophilicity (*e.g.* $CLogD_{7.4} > 3$), on the other hand, primarily impacts gut wall and hepatic extraction. It likewise confirmed that high polar surface area (> 125 Å^2) and greater numbers of hydrogen-bonding groups (> 9) were detrimental to permeability but did not affect metabolism.

These analyses and others have provided guidance for medicinal chemists seeking orally bioavailable drugs, but by definition they limit chemists to the small-molecule Rule-of-5 space. Recent attention has been given to understanding how larger molecules might escape the detrimental effects of excessive size, polarity and flexibility by adopting compact 3D folds that hide significant amounts of polarity from the solvent environment. Macrocycles such as Cyclosporine A (CsA) (see Table 10.6) have provided the impetus for this work; CsA has properties far outside the Rule-of-5 and TPSA guidelines, yet has human oral bioavailability approaching 30%. It is believed that intramolecular hydrogen bonds[25] are able to stabilize conformations that shield multiple polar atoms. This can be especially powerful for macrocycles that are able to form IMHBs in their lowest-energy conformations.[23] An analysis of over 35,000 molecules with passive permeability data[6] indicated that the 3D radius of gyration is a better descriptor of size for large molecules (MW > 550) than is MW itself. It is likely that a more sophisticated treatment of the 3D properties of molecules and the physics of permeability, solubility, and metabolism, will be necessary to understand more completely how to obtain oral bioavailability for molecules that lie beyond the Rule-of-5.

Table 10.6 Representatives beyond Rule-of-5 macrocycles with human oral bioavailability >10%.[a]

Structure	Name *Indication, Source*	Human % F	Ref.	MW *R-Gyr*	# Ro5 Viols	ClogP	TPSA *3D-PSA*
14	Rifampicin *Antibiotic, Semi-synthetic*	93	2	823 *5.4 Å*	3	3.7	220 Å² *153 Å²*
15	Roxithromycin *Antibiotic, Semi-synthetic*	78.5	66	837 *5.3 Å*	2	2.3	217 Å² *116 Å²*

Table 10.6 (*Continued*)

Structure	Name Indication, Source	Human % F	Ref.	MW R-Gyr	# Ro5 Viols	ClogP	TPSA 3D-PSA
16	Cyclosporine A *Immuno-suppressant, Natural product*	28	2	1203 6.4 Å	3	14.4	279 Å² 105 Å²
17	Rifabutin *Antibiotic, Semi-synthetic*	20	2	847	2	4.7	206 Å²

Tacrolimus
Immuno-suppressant,
Natural product

15 2 804 3 5.8 178 Å^2

18

Rapamycin
Immuno-suppressant,
Natural product

14 67 914 3 7.0 195 Å^2
        6.4 Å   144 Å^2

19

[a]2D properties were calculated from the structures shown, while 3D properties were computed from available X-ray crystal structures of rifampicin (CSD60-RIFAMP),[55] roxithromycin (CSD-FUXYOM),[56] cyclosporine A (CSD-DEKSAN),[57] and rapamycin (CSD-RAPMCN11).[58]

10.4 Computational Modeling of Absorption and Permeation

Permeation across the intestinal wall involves both passive and facilitated processes. Passive transport includes passive transcellular permeation and paracellular diffusion across cell junctions, while facilitated transport includes active influx and efflux processes that pump molecules in and out of the cells. In order to improve absorption of a molecule, engineering passive permeability is a preferred strategy over engineering affinity to an influx transporter. The expression levels of active transporters vary significantly between different tissues and individuals,[26] and the specificities and expression levels vary among mammals, which decreases the ability to predict human PK based on animal studies. In contrast, passive membrane permeability basically works the same with any eukaryotic membrane, although there may be minor quantitative differences due to different membrane compositions. As paracellular permeation is mainly pertinent to small and polar molecules, passive membrane permeability, which is crucial to transcellular diffusion, is therefore one of the key properties that needs to be optimized for developing bioavailable macrocycles.

The primary method for modeling permeability in drug discovery is by using quantitative-structure-property-relationships (QSPR). Such models represent empirical statistical relationships between physicochemical descriptors and existing experimental data,[6,27,28] such as *in vitro* permeability measurements,[29] intestinal absorption data,[30] bioavailability,[31] and blood–brain barrier penetration.[32] Common statistical analysis methods include multiple linear regression, partial least squares, neural networks, genetic algorithms, and support vector machines.[33] Physicochemical descriptors relevant to permeability include quantitative measures of hydrophobicity, polarity, ionization state, and size. The most common descriptors include MW, polar surface area (PSA), and counts of functional groups, such as hydrogen bond donors and acceptors, many of the same descriptors used in the Rule-of-5 and other simple guidelines discussed above.

This type of QSPR approach is widely adopted, especially for the development of small molecule therapeutics. However, the key limitation, as in the field of quantitative-structure-activity-relationships (QSAR) modeling of protein–ligand interactions, is transferability.[34] The accuracy of such statistical modeling depends strongly on the similarity between the query and the training set. This is a particularly relevant issue for predicting the permeability of macrocycles because many existing QSPR models were not trained with this chemical class, in part due to the limited amount of available data. However, macrocycles also present additional challenges due to their 3D complexity and conformational flexibility. For large and flexible molecules like macrocycles, their molecular properties, including hydrophobicity and shape, depend sensitively on the conformation(s) they adopt. Conformational flexibility in response to the environment is of great importance in studying ADME properties of macrocycles. For example, in the case of membrane permeation, a solute is expected to expose polar or hydrogen bonding features in water to maximize interactions with surrounding water molecules, but these polar features can be "shielded" in membranes by means of intramolecular hydrogen bonding.[23]

An alternate strategy is to predict membrane permeability by modeling the physics of membrane permeation. In principle, such models do not require training on existing experimental data and should have a broad domain of applicability. One approach is to model the process based on solubility–diffusion theory, in which the membrane permeability of the permeant is formulated as the reciprocal of the resistance experienced in the permeation process.[35] With the assumption that diffusional resistance is only contributed by the membrane and there is negligible resistance in the unstirred aqueous layer and the membrane interface, the permeation rate can be estimated from (1) the partition between the aqueous phase and the membrane, (2) the diffusion across the membrane, and (3) the distance of permeation. Common descriptors such as PSA and MW are reasonable surrogates for these properties, but it is possible to obtain more accurate estimates, as described below.

Given a planar membrane that propagates in the xy-plane and varies only in the z-axis along which permeation occurs, the membrane/water partition and the membrane diffusivity are dependent on the permeant's position in the membrane. The diffusional resistance in the membrane, R_m, can be written as:

$$R_m = \frac{1}{P_m} = \int_{water}^{d} \frac{dz}{K_{m/w}(z)D_m(z)} \tag{10.2}$$

where P_m is the permeability coefficient, $K_{m/w}$ is the membrane/water partition coefficient, D_m is diffusivity in the membrane, and d is the width of the membrane.

The most rigorous and computationally costly approach is to simulate the permeation process *via* all-atom simulations with all molecular components (permeant, lipids, water) represented in atomic detail explicitly.[36–39] The general approach is to calculate the potential of mean force (PMF) for the permeant traversing the membrane by performing molecular dynamics (MD) umbrella sampling simulations. The PMF along the membrane normal, thus the z axis, allows computation of the free energy moving along the permeation path, $\Delta G(z)$, from which the position-dependent partition coefficient can be calculated.

$$K_{m/w}(z) = \exp\left(\frac{-\Delta G(z)}{RT}\right) \tag{10.3}$$

The local diffusion coefficient can be computed from the corresponding friction coefficient, $\xi(z)$, along the z axis.

$$D_m(z) = \frac{RT}{\xi(z)} \tag{10.4}$$

By substituting the position-dependent terms in Equation 10.3 and Equation 10.4 into Equation 10.2, the permeability coefficient can be obtained by integrating along the permeation path:

$$\frac{1}{P_m} = \int_{water}^{d} \frac{\exp(\Delta G(z)/RT)dz}{D_m(z),} \tag{10.5}$$

Most simulation studies have focused on the permeation of small molecules.[36-39] These results have shown that such a demanding approach can produce a reasonable correlation with *in vitro* permeability data. While predicting the absolute permeability rate is still a challenge, these simulations have provided valuable insights into the fundamental physics of permeation. Based on the free energy profiles from MD simulations, unless the permeant is completely non-polar in nature or contains no polar atoms, such as benzene or ethane, the free energy maximum along the permeation path is usually located near the hydrophobic core (central region) of the lipid bilayer where the permeant is desolvated. The calculated diffusion profiles for small molecules show little variation through the course of permeation.

These findings support a simplified model in which the rate of permeation is limited by a homogenous "barrier region".[35] In this approximation, both the partition coefficient and the diffusivity term in Equation 10.2 are no longer position-dependent, allowing the model to be expressed in position-independent terms:

$$R_m = \frac{1}{P_m} = \frac{\delta_{barrier}}{K_{barrier}D_{barrier}}, \tag{10.6}$$

where $K_{barrier}$ is the barrier domain/water partition coefficient, $D_{barrier}$ is the diffusivity in the barrier domain, and $\delta_{barrier}$ is the effective barrier width. This simple model provides a way to estimate the permeability coefficient in a more straightforward and less computationally expensive manner.

The simpler version of the solubility–diffusion model described in Equation 10.6 has been combined with a conformational sampling algorithm by Jacobson *et al.*[40] Instead of explicitly simulating the permeation process, extensive conformational analyses are performed in (implicit) water and chloroform, which is used as a surrogate for the low dielectric of the membrane. This approximation significantly speeds the calculation, making it practical for comparisons of multiple compounds. Permeants are represented using molecular mechanics force fields, and both water and chloroform are represented by implicit solvent models. The conformational search allows the identification of favorable conformations in a high dielectric medium and a low dielectric medium, producing an "ensemble" of low energy conformations for subsequent evaluation to find the relevant "membranephilic" conformation with optimal predicted permeability.

Following the Barrier Domain Model developed by Xiang and Anderson,[41] the barrier/water partition coefficient, $K_{barrier}$, is estimated from the chloroform/water partition coefficient, $K_{c/w}$, and a volume-based size-selective factor, ξ_V, which accounts for anistropic characteristics of the membrane that are absent from the reference isotropic bulk solvent.

$$K_{\text{barrier}} = K_{c/w}\xi_V \tag{10.7}$$

The computed chloroform/water partition coefficient, which is the most significant term in the model for predicting relative permeabilities, accounts for (1) the free energy of desolvation, (2) the free energy of deionization (the permeant is assumed to be neutral in the membrane),[42] and (3) the entropic cost of adopting the "membranephilic" conformation. The free energy of transfer of the membranephilic conformation from water to the membrane appears to be the dominant term in permeation.[43] It is assumed[40,43] that there is only one such conformation in the membrane, whereas there are many in water, based in part on published observations[44] on cyclosporine A. While such approximation helps simplify the computational modeling and produces good correlation with experimental data,[40] exceptions would not be unconceivable. It is a current challenge how to properly account for multiple conformations. A study by Swift and Amaro[45] showed that this single-state approximation produces a better correlation to PAMPA permeability of small molecules than the "predominant-states" method, which includes additional conformations beyond the global minima. For the molecules they studied, the global minima accounted for more than 97% of the total free energy.[45]

The size-selectivity factor, which depends on the permeant's volume and the lateral pressure exerted by the membrane, is formulated as the reverse work done required to accommodate the permeant in the membrane. In this sense, it is analogous to the "cavitation" term in models of water solvation. Based on molecular dynamic simulations of membrane diffusion of small molecules, the calculated diffusion coefficients display small deviations across the membrane barrier.[46,47] Assuming that the rates of diffusion in the membrane barrier are similar to those of bulk solvent with similar viscosity, or at least that they correlate strongly, the barrier diffusion coefficient is estimated using the size-dependent Stokes–Einstein relation,[48] where k_B is the Boltzmann constant, T is temperature, η_m is membrane viscosity and r_p is the radius of the permeant.

$$D_{\text{barrier}} = \frac{k_B T}{6\pi\eta_m r_p} \tag{10.8}$$

If the effective membrane barrier width (d_{barrier}) is further assumed to be constant for all permeants, the permeability coefficient can be estimated based on three variables: one free energy term ($K_{c/w}$) and two size-dependent terms (ξ_V, D_{barrier}).

$$P_m = \frac{K_{c/w}\xi_V D_{\text{barrier}}}{d_{\text{barrier}}} \tag{10.9}$$

The resulting model (Equation 10.9), coupled with conformational sampling algorithms, allows efficient physics-based permeability predictions for small molecules and macrocycles.[23,40,49] The conformational sampling of macrocycles is significantly more challenging than for Rule-of-5 compliant small molecules. The larger size and greater number of rotatable bonds typically observed for macrocycles is one obvious reason. The macrocycle ring itself presents another challenge. While in principle the ring-closure condition decreases the effective number of rotatable bonds in the macrocyclic ring (by six: equal to the reduction in the number of degrees of freedom), the problem of effectively sampling all ring conformations consistent with a closed ring, with no steric clashes or excessive strain, is nontrivial. Luckily, an analogous challenge problem exists for sampling loop conformations in proteins, and a number of solutions have been presented. We have adopted an algorithm based on the loop prediction method of Jacobson *et al.*[50] In brief, the algorithm splits the macrocycle in half and samples conformations on both sides by a systematic search in torsion space, rapidly eliminating conformations with steric clashes. Then, all pairs of conformations from each side that lead to a closed ring are identified and filtered to eliminate those with excessive strain. Remaining closed ring conformations are clustered, and representative conformations from each cluster are subjected to further optimization of the side chains (non-ring degrees of freedom) and energy minimization.

Such a computational approach combining physics-based evaluation and conformational sampling has successfully been applied in screening large virtual libraries of cyclic hexapeptides (N > 1000) and identified permeable cyclic hexapeptides (MW ~ 750) that show *in vitro* membrane permeability (RRCK P_{app} ≥ 4.7 × 10^{-6} cm s^{-1}) and oral bioavailability in rat greater than 20%.[23,49]

10.5   Orally Bioavailable Macrocycles

10.5.1   Examples of Orally Bioavailable Macrocycles

In order to identify macrocycles (ring size ≥ 12) with human and/or rat oral bioavailability data, the ChEMBL[51] and GVKBIO GOSTAR[52] databases were utilized and this was supplemented by data from recent publications.[19,49,53] The combined dataset included 184 macrocycles. Twenty-two macrocycles had human oral bioavailability (*F*) and seven of these had an average *F* greater than 30%. Likewise, 168 macrocycles had rat oral bioavailability and only 47 of these (28%) had an average *F* greater than 30%. Rule-of-5 compliance had little effect on the rat oral bioavailability of these macrocycles: 10 of the 31 (32%) Rule-of-5 compliant macrocycles and 37 of the 137 (28%) Rule-of-5 noncompliant macrocycles had average rat *F* greater than 30%. Only one of the macrocycles with human oral bioavailability (ixabepilone) was Rule-of-5 compliant.

Noteworthy examples of orally bioavailable macrocycles are discussed in more detail here. Six representative macrocycles with human oral bio-availability[2,66,67] of at least 10% are shown in Table 10.6, along with their key 2D and 3D properties. The 2D properties were computed from the structures shown, while 3D properties were computed using available X-ray crystal structures of rifampicin (CSD[54]-RIFAMP),[55] roxithromycin (CSD-FUXYOM),[56] cyclosporine A (CSD-DEKSAN),[57] and rapamycin (CSD-RAPMCN11).[58] In the case of cyclosporine A, the conformation in the crystal structure is quite similar to its NMR structure in chloroform,[44] which is believed to be a good approximation of the membrane-permeating conformation.

All examples in Table 10.6 are either immunosuppressive natural products or antibacterial semi-synthetic derivatives of rifamycin or erythromycin. Several other orally bioavailable macrocycles not shown – azithromycin, clarithromycin, and erythromycin – have human oral bioavailability above 30% and belong to the erythromycin macrolide class, exemplified in Table 10.6 by roxithromycin (15). While all six examples far exceed the MW cutoff of 500 where F_a often significantly declines,[2] their crystallographic conformations all have a radius of gyration less than 7 Å, typical for acyclic molecules with MW below 550.[6] This observation is consistent with mac-rocyclization increasing the diffusion coefficient (Equation 10.8). In add-ition, the crystallographic conformations reduce the effective surface polarity significantly (comparing 3D-PSA and TPSA). With the exception of rifampicyn, the 3D-PSAs are in the vicinity of, or below, the 140 Å^2 cutoff initially proposed by Palm *et al.*[3] Especially striking is the example of cyclosporine A, which has a far lower 3D PSA than TPSA, due to its ability to form a beta-hairpin like structure with extensive intramolecular hydrogen bonding.[25]

Examples of peptidic macrocycles, with high rat oral bioavailability, as determined in pre-clinical studies, are shown in Tables 10.7 and 10.8. The Hepatitis C Virus NS3 protease inhibitors (20, 22), ghrelin antagonist (21), and ghrelin agonist (23) shown in Table 10.7,[59,62,64,65] containing tripeptide motifs, have properties that exceed the proposed[2] threshold values for MW and TPSA for good F_a by 20–40%. Given their lower MWs and TPSA values, compared to the macrocycles in Table 10.6, one would expect their mem-brane-permeating conformations to have even lower radius of gyration and 3D-PSA. Intramolecular hydrogen bonding has been seen for 23[59] and may be a common motif for these more permeable compounds. Even the larger cyclic peptides shown in Table 10.8,[19,23,53,68] with significantly higher TPSA, may be able to shield enough of their surface polarity to make permeability through the membrane possible. (The possibility that active transport may play a role in the permeability of these peptides cannot be ruled out.) For cyclosporine A (16),[25] 24 from White *et al.*,[23] and 7 from Biron *et al.*,[19] this shielding is predominantly achieved *via* a combination of *N*-methylation and transannular IMHB's that eliminate free hydrogen bond donors. In the case of sanguinamide A (26),[53] it is a combination of transannular IMHBs and side chain shielding of the remaining H-bond donors. The crystallographic

Table 10.7 Representatives beyond Rule-of-5 macrocycles with rat oral bioavailability >20%.

Structure	Compound (Target)	Rat %F	Ref.	MW	# Ro5 Viols	ClogP	TPSA
20 Chiral	Compound 40 *Heptatitis C Virus NS3 Serine Protease*	97	64	639	3	5.5	143 Å^2
21 Chiral	Compound 1789 *Ghrelin Antagonist*	81	65	618	2	5.5	136 Å^2

42	62	789	3	8.9	181 Å^2
24	59	539	2	5.3	100 Å^2

BILN-2061
Hepatitis C Virus NS3 Protease

Ulimorelin
Ghrelin Agonist

Chiral

22

Chiral

23

Table 10.8 Representatives beyond Rule-of-5 cyclic peptides with oral bioavailability > 5%.

Structure	Name	Human (Rat) %F	Ref.	MW R-Gyr	# Ro5 Viols	ClogP	TPSA 3D-PSA
16	Cyclosporine A	28	2	1203 6.4 Å	3	14.4	279 Å² 105 Å²
24	Compound 3	(28)	23	755 5.3 Å	3	9.4	160 Å² 80 Å²
7	Peptide 8	(9.9)	19	849	4	6.1	201 A²

Peptide 1	(8.5)	68	836	3	1.2	287 A^2
Sanguinamide A	(7)	53	722	3	5.5	170 A^2

25

26

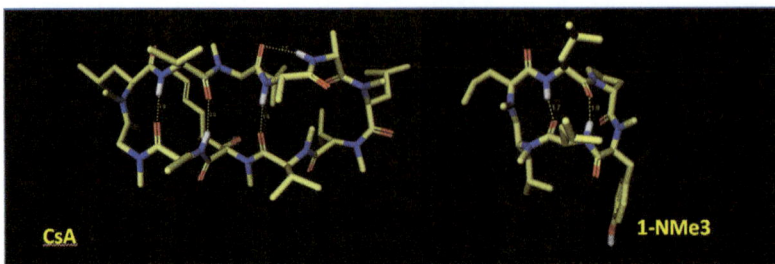

Figure 10.2   Crystallographic conformation of cyclosporine A (CsA) (CSD:DEKSAN)[57] and chloroform NMR structure of 1-NMe3 (**11**),[23] displaying the similar intramolecular hydrogen bonding and β turns of these orally bioavailable peptides.

structure of cyclosporine A[57] and the NMR structure of **24** in chloroform[23] are shown in Figure 10.2, clearly displaying the transannular IMHBs; a similar hydrogen bonding network has been seen in the NMR structure of **26**.[53]

10.5.2   Design Principles and Structure Property Relationships

Cyclosporine A (**16**) is a natural product which serves as the quintessential Beyond Rule-of-5 macrocycle, able to overcome the disadvantages of high MW (1203 Daltons) and polarity (11 amide bonds) and achieve excellent absorption ($F_a = 0.86$).[2] It appears able to do this by a combination of *N*-methylation (seven *N*-methylated amides), intramolecular hydrogen bonding (four observed in the crystal structure),[57] a compact 3D structure incorporating β turns, and a preponderance of hydrophobic sidechains. This same feature set is seen in many of the designed orally bioavailable macrocycles in Tables 10.7 and 10.8 and perhaps most closely adopted in the design of **24**.

The design of **24** and similar peptides was accomplished through the scoring of a library of virtual peptides containing the same sidechains but differing in stereochemistry and *N*-methylation.[23] Not all stereochemical combinations are consistent with optimal IMHBs, and the computational approach was able to select several peptides with the appropriate combinations of features. This work showed that a combination of IMHB and *N*-methylation is preferable for minimizing aqueous desolvation and maximizing permeability, compared to either the unmethylated analogs or permethylated analogs. Permethylation prevents IMHBs from forming and leaves backbone carbonyls exposed to solvent. Additional investigations[23,49] studied the impact of a polar sidechain replacement of leucine on permeability, clearance, and oral bioavailability. Both the location[23] and the physical properties[49] of the new polar sidechain have a significant impact on permeability, in a fashion predictable by the computational models. The measured logD of the peptides correlated well with both *in vitro* clearance (Figure 10.3) and cell-based permeability (Figure 10.4) though there were

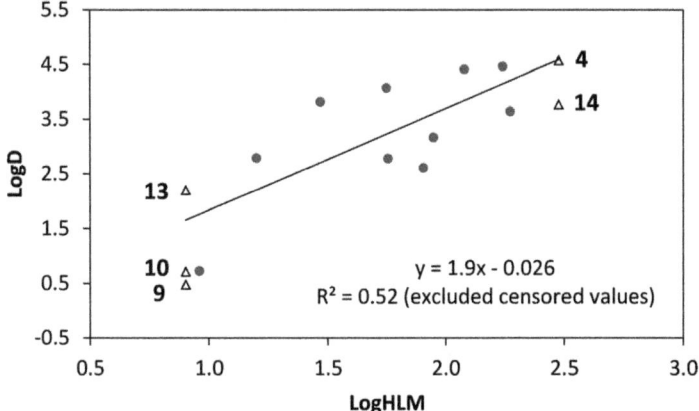

Figure 10.3 Log D[a] versus LogHLM[b] for cyclic hexapeptides[c] from ref. 49. ([a]Measured shake-flask Log D. [b]HLM = human liver microsomal intrinsic clearance, apparent in mL min^{-1} kg^{-1}. [c]Compound numbers refer to those in ref. 49.)

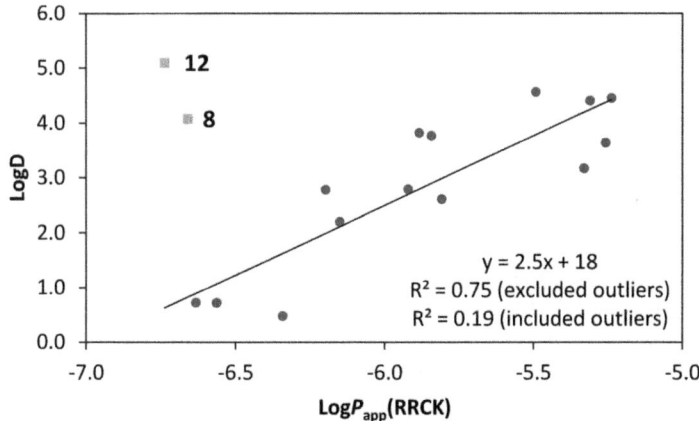

Figure 10.4 Measured LogD[a] versus cell-based permeability Log$_{Papp}$[b] for cyclic hexapeptides[c] from ref. 49. ([a]Measured shake-flask Log D. [b]P_{app} (RRCK) = cell based permeability in Ralph Russ canine kidney cell line in cm sec^{-1}. [c]Compound numbers refer to those in ref. 49.)

high logD outliers with poor measured permeability, perhaps due to the experimental challenges of measuring permeability for high logD compounds.[49] Incorporation of a threonine residue led to a peptide with only slightly reduced rat oral bioavailability ($F = 24\%$, 2.9 mg kg^{-1}, po, 0.4 mg kg^{-1}, iv), despite increased *in vivo* clearance, while incorporation of a serine, lysine, or aspartic acid caused more dramatic decreases in oral bioavailability ($F \leq 2\%$).[49]

The cyclic peptide 7[19] was designed as an *N*-methylated analog of the Veber-Hirschmann cyclic peptide *cyclo*(-PFwKTF-).[60] The goal was to obtain a peptide with both oral bioavailability and potency versus the somatostatin sst2 and sst5 receptors. Thirty of the 31 possible *N*-methylated analogs were synthesized, and seven maintained potency of 100 nM or better. Of these, the triply *N*-methylated analog 7 had the highest permeability in the Caco-2 cell monolayer assay $(4 \times 10^{-6}$ cm s$^{-1})$, good stability against proteases from serum and brush border membranes, and the highest rat oral bioavailability $(F = 10\%$, 10 mg kg^{-1}, po, 1 mg kg^{-1}, iv).[19] The unmethylated analog also had good oral exposure, despite showing lower permeability in a Caco-2 assay $(0.5 \times 10^{-6}$ cm s$^{-1})$ and lower stability versus brush border membrane proteases. Neither potency nor permeability correlates with the count of *N*-methyl groups; rather it is the specific location of *N*-methyls that is significant, most likely because of the impact on conformation and intramolecular hydrogen bonding.

The discovery of **23** came as the result of the optimization of a macrocyclic high throughput screening hit, which had promising pharmacology but poor pharmacokinetics (PK). One of the objectives of the medicinal chemistry program[59] was to reduce clearance, both by elimination of a metabolic liability (the styrenyl moiety) and reduction in flexibility through incorporation of methyl groups as steric constraints, especially adjacent to the phenoxy tether. In addition, several structure-activity features favorable for potency were also fortuitously favorable for oral bioavailability, including a preference for hydrophobic sidechains and an *N*-methyl on one of the amino acids. Crystallography and NMR both indicated the presence of an IMHB in the ring of **23**, which may reduce both aqueous desolvation and conformation flexibility, contributing to its good passive permeability $(14 \times 10^{-6}$ cm s$^{-1})$ and improved clearance. The cyclopropyl side chain of ulimorelin increases the basicity of the nearby amine, helping to stabilize the IMHB and improving solubility. Thus, both methylation and sidechain chemistry impacted ring conformation and flexibility, solubility, clearance, and permeability, enabling good oral bioavailability in a molecule that exceeded several Rule-of-5 parameters.

Macrocyclic inhibitors of Hepatitis C NS3 Protease, which have been found to be effective antivirals in humans,[61] were designed to be conformationally rigidified, cell-penetrating analogs of the acyclic protease products which were found to inhibit NS3 protease.[16] The eventual discovery of highly potent 15-membered ring macrocycles demonstrated the benefit of cyclization on receptor binding and cell penetration, leading to good cell potency. One analog had increased permeability in a Caco-2 assay (17.5% over a period of three hours[16]) and had rat oral bioavailability of 22% (25 mg kg^{-1}, po, 5 mg kg^{-1}, iv).[16] These promising leads were then further optimized, including modulation of physical properties to improve cell potency and decreased liver first-pass clearance, leading to BILN 2061 (**22**), which had rat oral bioavailability of 42% (20 mg kg^{-1}, po, 5 mg kg^{-1}, iv)[62] and was selected to become a clinical candidate. It has been shown to have excellent anti-viral efficacy in humans on oral dosing.[61] More recent publications have disclosed similar macrocycles with alternative heterocyclic substitutions, leading to compounds with Caco-2 permeability values as high as 38×10^{-6} cm sec^{-1} and rat oral bioavailability up to 73% (10 mg kg^{-1} po, 2 mg kg^{-1}, iv).[63] This class of macrocycle has aliphatic linkers not able to participate in intramolecular hydrogen bonding. Nevertheless, the 3D parameters from crystallographic structures in Tables 10.6 and 10.8 indicate that these macrocycles are often able to adopt fairly compact structures with reduced polar surface area, and this may explain the excellent permeability and bioavailability of compounds such as **22**, in spite of high MW and TPSA.

10.6   Conclusions

A growing body of literature is providing examples of Beyond Rule-of-5 macrocycles with significant oral bioavailability. Many of the earliest examples of orally bioavailable macrocycles were natural products and derivatives thereof which eventually became marketed drugs (see Table 10.6). Several of the more recent examples have arisen through medicinal chemistry optimization of Hepatitis C Virus NS3 protease inhibitors[62,64] and ghrelin antagonists[65] and agonists,[59] or through research into the impact of stereochemistry, *N*-methylation, and polarity on cyclic peptide oral bioavailability.[19,23,49] While traditional medicinal chemistry principles of oral bioavailability, such as the detrimental impact of high logD on clearance,[2] cannot be ignored (see, for example, Figure 10.3), new design principles are needed for understanding the permeability of macrocycles. These new principles are based upon an understanding of the 3D conformations of macrocycles. In order to be passively permeable, macrocycles should be designed to be compact[6] and to limit their polar surface area[6] as they permeate the hydrophobic interior of the membrane. Intramolecular hydrogen bonds[19,23,25] are especially useful for stabilizing conformations with hydrogen bond donors and acceptors shielded from the surrounding solvent; this can be supplemented by selective *N*-methylation.[19,23] Passive permeability is driven primarily by fundamental physical properties that are increasingly well understood and computationally accessible.[40] This holds out the promise of computational predictions capable of guiding the design of orally bioavailable macrocycles, a promise now beginning to be realized.[23,49]

Acknowledgments

The authors would like to thank Huijun Wang for assistance with literature searches for orally bioavailable macrocycles. MPJ is a consultant to Schrodinger LLC.

References

1. C. Lipinski, F. Lombardo, B. W. Dominy and P. J. Feeney, *Adv. Drug Delivery Rev.*, 1997, **23**, 3.

2. M. V. S. Varma, R. S. Obach, C. Rotter, H. R. Miller, G. Chang, S. J. Steyn, A. El-Kattan and M. D. Troutman, *J. Med. Chem.*, 2010, **53**, 1098.

3. K. Palm, P. Stenberg, K. Luthman and P. Artursson, *Pharm. Res.*, 1997, **14**, 568.

4. J. Kelder, P. D. J. Grootenhuis, D. M. Bayada, L. P. C. Delbressine and J.-P. Ploemen, *Pharm. Res.*, 1999, **16**, 1514.

5. P. Ertl, B. Rohde and P. Selzer, *J. Med. Chem.*, 2000, **43**, 3714.

6. C. R. W. Guimarães, A. M. Mathiowetz, M. Shalaeva, G. Goetz and S. Liras, *J. Chem. Inf. Model*, 2012, **52**, 882.

7. D. F. Veber, S. R. Johnson, H-Y. Cheng, B. R. Smith, K. W. Ward and K. D. Kopple, *J. Med. Chem.*, 2002, **45**, 2615.

8. A. L. Hopkins and C. R. Groom, *Nat. Rev. Drug Disc.*, 2002, **1**, 727.

9. Anonymous, *Nat. Med.*, 2012, **18**, 636.

10. N. Terrett, *Med. Chem. Commun.*, 2013, **4**, 474.

11. L. Ruddigkeit, R. Van Deursen, L. C. Blum and J.-L. Reymond, *J. Chem. Inf. Model.*, 2012, **52**, 2864.

12. E. M. Driggers, S. P. Hale, J. Lee and N. Terrett, *Nat. Rev. Drug Disc.*, 2008, **7**, 608.

13. J. Mallinson and I. Collins, *Future Med. Chem.*, 2012, **4**, 1409.

14. E. Marsault and M. L. Peterson, *J. Med. Chem.*, 2011, **54**, 1961.

15. J. Yang, M. Jamei, K. R. Yeo, G. T. Tucker and A. Rostami-Hodjegan, *Curr. Drug Metab.*, 2007, **8**, 676.

16. Y. S. Tsantrizos, G. Bolger, P. Bonneau, D. R. Cameron, N. Goudreau, G. Kukolj, S. R. LaPlante, M. Llinàs-Brunet, H. Nar and D. Lamarre, *Angew. Chem. Int. Ed.*, 2003, **42**, 1356.

17. C. W. Zapf, J. D. Bloom, J. L. McBean, R. G. Dushin, T. Nittoli, C. Ingalls, A. G. Sutherland, J. P. Sonye, C. N. Eid, J. Golas, H. Liu, F. Boschelli, Y. Hu, E. Vogan and J. I. Levin, *Bioorg. Med. Chem. Lett.*, 2011, **21**, 2278.

18. R. Tugyi, G. Mezö, E. Fellinger, D. Andreu and F. Hudecz, *J. Peptide Sci.*, 2005, **11**, 642.

19. E. Biron, J. Chatterjee, O. Ovadia, D. Langenegger, J. Brueggen, D. Hoyer, H. A. Schmid, R. Jelinek, C. Gilon, A. Hoffman and H. Kessler, *Angew. Chem., Int. Ed.*, 2008, **47**, 2595.

20. M. Pernot, R. Vanderesse, C. Frochot, F. Guillemin and M. Barberi-Heyob, *Exp. Opin. Drug Metab. Toxicol.*, 2011, **7**, 793.

21. M. Ishikawa and Y. Hashimoto, *J. Med. Chem.*, 2011, **54**, 1539.

22. A. R. Bogdan, N. L. Davies and K. James, *Org. Biomol. Chem.*, 2011, **9**, 7727.

23. T. R. White, C. M. Renzelman, A. C. Rand, T. Rezai, C. M. McEwen, V. M. Gelev, R. A. Turner, R. G. Linington, S. S. F. Leung, A. S. Kalgutkar, J. N. Bauman, Y. Zhang, S. Liras, D. A. Price, A. M. Mathiowetz, M. P. Jacobson and R. S. Lokey, *Nat. Chem. Biol.*, 2011, **7**, 810.

24. H. Van de Waterbeemd and B. Testa, *Drug Bioavailability: Estimation of Solubility, Permeability, Absorption and Bioavailability*, Wiley-VCH Verlag GmbH & Co. KGaA, Weinheim, 2nd edn, 2009, 71.

25. A. Alex, D. S. Millan, M. Perez, F. Wakenhut and G. A. Whitlock, *Med. Chem. Commun.*, 2011, **2**, 669.
26. M. Roth, A. Obaidat and B. Hagenbuch, *Br. J. Pharmacol.*, 2012, **165**, 1260.
27. H. van de Waterbeemd and E. Gifford, *Nat. Rev. Drug Disc.*, 2003, **2**, 192.
28. H. H. F. Refsgaard, B. F. Jensen, P. B. Brockhoff, S. B. Padkjaer, M. Guldbrandt and M. S. Christensen, *J. Med. Chem.*, 2005, **48**, 805.
29. F. Yoshida and J. G. Topliss, *J. Med. Chem.*, 2000, **43**, 4723.
30. C. Suenderhauf, F. Hammann, A. Maunz, C. Helma and J. Huwyler, *Mol. Pharmaceutics*, 2011, **8**, 213.
31. M. Fujikawa, K. Nakao, R. Shimizu and M. Akamatsu, *Bioorg. Med. Chem.*, 2007, **15**, 3756.
32. Y. H. Zhao, M. H. Abraham, A. Ibrahim, P. V. Fish, S. Cole, M. L. Lewis, M. J. de Groot and D. P. Reynolds, *J. Chem. Inf. Model.*, 2007, **47**, 170.
33. A. R. Katritzky, M. Kuanar, S. Slavov, C. D. Hall, M. Karelson, I. Kahn and D. A. Dobchev, *Chem. Rev.*, 2010, **110**, 5714.
34. T. R. Stouch, J. R. Kenyon, S. R. Johnson, X. Q. Chen, A. Doweyko and Y. Li, *J. Comput.-Aided Molec. Des.*, 2003, **17**, 83.
35. J. M. Diamond, *J. Membr. Biol.*, 1974, **17**, 121.
36. S. J. Marrink and H. J. C. Berendsen, *J. Phys. Chem.*, 1996, **100**, 16729.
37. D. Bemporad, C. Luttmann and J. W. Essex, *Biophys. J.*, 2004, **87**, 1.
38. D. Bemporad, C. Luttmann and J. W. Essex, *Biochim. Biophys. Acta-Bio-membr.*, 2005, **1718**, 1.
39. R. V. Swift and R. E. Amaro, *Chem. Bio. Drug Des.*, 2013, **81**, 61.
40. S. S. F. Leung, J. Mijalkovic, K. Borrelli and M. P. Jacobson, *J. Chem. Inf. Model.*, 2012, **52**, 1621.
41. T. X. Xiang and B. D. Anderson, *J. Membr. Biol.*, 1994, **140**, 111.
42. P. A. Shore, B. B. Brodie and C. A. M. Hogben, *J. Pharm. Exp. Therap.*, 1957, **119**, 361.
43. R. Rezai, J. E. Bock, M. V. Zhou, C. Kalyanaraman, R. S. Lokey and M. P. Jacobson, *J. Am. Chem. Soc.*, 2006, **128**, 14073.
44. J. Klages, C. Neubauer, M. Coles, H. Kessler and B. Luy, *ChemBioChem*, 2005, **6**, 1672.
45. R. V. Swift and R. E. Amaro, *J. Comput. Aided Mol. Des.*, 2011, **25**, 1007.
46. D. Remporad, J. W. Essex and C. Luttmann, *J. Phys. Chem. B.*, 2004, **108**, 4875.
47. R. V. Swift and R. E. Amaro, *Chem. Biol. Drug Des.*, 2013, **81**, 61.
48. A. Seelig, *J. Mol. Neurosci.*, 2007, **33**, 32.
49. A. C. Rand, S. S. F. Leung, H. Eng, C. J. Rotter, R. Sharma, A. S. Kalgutkar, Y. Zhang, M. V. Varma, K. A. Farley, B. Khunte, C. Limberakis, D. A. Price, S. Liras, A. M. Mathiowetz, M. P. Jacobson and R. S. Lokey, *Med. Chem. Commun.*, 2012, **3**, 1282.
50. M. P. Jacobson, D. L. Pincus, C. S. Rapp, T. J. F. Day, B. Hong, D. E. Shaw and R. A. Friesner, *Proteins: Struct., Funct., Bioinf.*, 2004, **55**, 351.
51. A. Gaulton, L. J. Bellis, A. P. Bento, J. Chambers, M. Davies, A. Hersey, Y. Light, S. McGlinchey, D. Michalovich, B. Al-Lazikani and

J. P. Overington, *Nucl. Acids Res.*, 2011, **40**, D1100. Database used: ChEMBL_14.

52. GVK BIO GOSTAR. https://gostardb.com/gostar/ Database used: January 2013.

53. D. S. Nielsen, H. N. Hoang, R.-J. Lohman, F. Diness and D. P. Fairlie, *Org. Lett.*, 2012, **14**, 5720.

54. F. H. Allen, *Acta Cryst.*, 2002, **B58**, 380.

55. M. Gadret, M. Goursolle, J. M. Leger and J. C. Colleter, *Acta Crystallogr., Sect. B: Struct. Crystallogr. Cryst. Chem.*, 1975, **31**, 1454.

56. B. Bachet, C. Brassy and J.-P. Mornon, *Acta Crystallogr., Sect. C: Cryst. Struct. Commun.*, 1988, **44**, 112.

57. H. R. Loosli, H. Kessler, H. Oschkinat, H. P. Weber, T. J. Petcher and A. Widmer, *Helv. Chim. Acta*, 1985, **68**, 682.

58. A. L. Rheingold, *Private Communication to the Cambridge Structural Database*, 2011.

59. H. R. Hoveyda, E. Marsault, R. Gagnon, A. P. Mathieu, M. Vézina, A. Landry, Z. Wang, K. Benakli, S. Beaubien, C. Saint-Louis, M. Brassard, J.-F. Pinault, L. Oullet, S. Bhat, M. Rameseshan, X. Peng, L. Foucher, S. Beauchemin, P. Bhérer, D. F. Veber, M. L. Peterson and G. L. Fraser, *J. Med. Chem.*, 2011, **54**, 8305.

60. D. F. Veber, R. M. Freidinger, D. S. Perlow, W. J. Paleveda, F. W. Holly, R. G. Strachan, R. F. Nutt, B. H. Arison, C. Homnick, W. C. Randall, M. S. Glitzer, R. Saperstein and R. Hirschmann, *Nature*, 1981, **292**, 55.

61. D. Lamarre, P. C. Anderson, M. Bailey, P. Beaulieu, G. Bolger, P. Bonneau, M. Bös, D. R. Cameron, M. Cartier, M. G. Cordingley, A.-M. Faucher, N. Goudreau, S. H. Kawai, G. Kukolj, L. Lagacé, S. R. LaPlante, H. Narjes, M.-A. Poupart, J. Rancourt, R. E. Sentjens, R. St. George, B. Simoneau, G. Steinman, D. Thibeault, Y. S. Tsantrizos, S. M. Weldon, C.-L. Yong and M. Llinàs-Brunet, *Nature*, 2003, **426**, 186.

62. M. Llinàs-Brunet, M. D. Bailey, G. Bolger, C. Brochu, A.-M. Faucher, J. M. Ferland, M. Garneau, E. Ghiro, V. Gorys, C. Grand-Maître, T. Halmos, N. Lapeyre-Paquette, F. Liard, M. Poirier, M. Rhéaume, Y. S. Tsantrizos and D. Lamarre, *J. Med. Chem.*, 2004, **47**, 1605.

63. M. Nilsson, A. K. Belfrage, S. Lindstrom, H. Wähling, C. Lindquist, S. Ayesa, P. Kahnberg, M. Pelcman, K. Benkestock, T. Agback, L. Vrang, Y. Terelius, K. Wikström, E. Hamelink, C. Rydergård, M. Edlund, A. Eneroth, P. Raboisson, T.-I. Lin, H. De Kock, P. Wigerinck, K. Simmen, B. Samuelsson and Å. Rosenquist, *Bioorg. Med. Chem. Lett.*, 2010, **20**, 4004.

64. K. X. Chen, F. G. Njoroge, A. Arasappan, S. Venkatraman, B. Vibulbhan, W. Yang, T. N. Parekh, J. Pichardo, A. Prongay, K.-C. Cheng, N. Butkiewicz, N. Yao, V. Madison and V. Girijavallabhan, *J. Med. Chem.*, 2006, **49**, 995.

65. H. Hoveyda, E. Marsault, H. Thomas, G. Fraser, B. Graeme, S. Beaubien, A. Mathieu, J. Beignet, M.-A. Bonin, S. Phoenix, D. Drutz, M. Peterson,

S. Beauchemin, M. Brassard, and M. Vezina, *Tranzyme Pharma, Inc.* USA. PCT Int. Appl. WO2011/053821, 2011.

66. R. Jain and L. H. Danziger, *Curr. Pharm. Des.*, 2004, **10**, 3045.
67. J. G. Hardman, L. E. Limbird, A. G. Gilman, *Pharmacokinetic Data, Goodman & Gilman's The Pharmacological Basis of Therapeutics*, McGraw-Hill, USA, 10th edn, 2001, 1924.
68. S. Hess, Y. Linde, O. Ovadia, E. Safrai, D. E. Shalev, A. Swed, E. Halbfinger, T. Lapidot, I. Winkler, Y. Gabinet, A. Faier, D. Yarden, Z. Xiang, F. P. Portillo, C. Haskell-Luevano, C. Gilon and A. Hoffman, *J. Med. Chem.*, 2008, **51**, 1026.

The Synthesis of Macrocycles for Drug Discovery

MARK L. PETERSON

Cyclenium Pharma Inc., 4366 Michel-Ange, Sherbrooke, Quebec J1N 1R6, Canada
Email: mpeterson@cyclenium.com

11.1 Introduction

Although macrocycles have long been known to be a pharmacologically relevant molecular class, applications in medicinal chemistry have been limited until recently due to the difficulties in their synthesis, particularly to produce libraries of such molecules in a parallel or combinatorial fashion. However, as several reviews and this volume attest, significant progress in the development of synthetic routes that provide access to these structures has resulted in a concomitant increase in their applications in the discovery of new pharmaceutical agents.[1–6] These strategies include an array of methodologies ranging from standard processes such as macrolactonization and macrolactamization, which have well-proven utility for the total synthesis of macrolides and cyclic peptides, respectively, to more complex organometallic-catalysed couplings and multi-component reactions (MCR). Some of these have even been successfully applied to the construction of libraries of macrocyclic molecules suitable for use in the high throughput screening (HTS) programs from which many current drug discovery projects originate. These synthetic approaches, both for individual compounds and libraries, are the topic of the present chapter.

RSC Drug Discovery Series No. 40
Macrocycles in Drug Discovery
Edited by Jeremy Levin
© The Royal Society of Chemistry 2015
Published by the Royal Society of Chemistry, www.rsc.org

In compiling this summary, an effort was made to be as comprehensive as possible with regard to the chemistries being utilized. Representative examples are included that illustrate the diversity of structures that can be prepared for each methodology, although this has, of necessity, been limited for the more widely employed techniques. Additionally, certain established methods that have seen application in the total synthesis realm, but which to date have seen minimal usage for the *de novo* assembly of macrocycles, are highlighted in an effort to inspire future efforts directed towards this compound class. Chemistries applicable to macrocyclic structures investigated primarily for non-pharmaceutical purposes, such as the extensive work pursued in the molecular recognition and functional materials areas, are not included.

11.2 Macrolactamization and Macrolactonization

Many of the early examples of macrocycles in drug discovery relied on these classical reaction types for the formation of the ring and they remain in regular use. This was due, in part, to the peptidomimetic nature of many of these structures, which often were targeted at protease enzyme inhibition, and thus lent themselves readily to macrolactamization for amide bond formation or macrolactonization for cyclic depsipeptide-like compounds.[7,8] Representative examples of these two general transformations are shown in Scheme 11.1 (BOP (benzotriazol-1-yloxytris(dimethylamino)-phosphonium hexafluorophosphate, Castro's reagent), EDC (1-ethyl-3-(3-dimethylamino-propyl)-carbodiimide), DMAP (4-dimethylamino-pyridine)) for the matrix metalloproteinase (MMP) inhibitor template **2**[9] and the renin inhibitor scaffold **4**.[10]

These approaches possess several advantages: (1) well-developed chemistry and procedures; (2) wide selection of readily available reagents; (3) straightforward construction of linear precursors with high diversity;

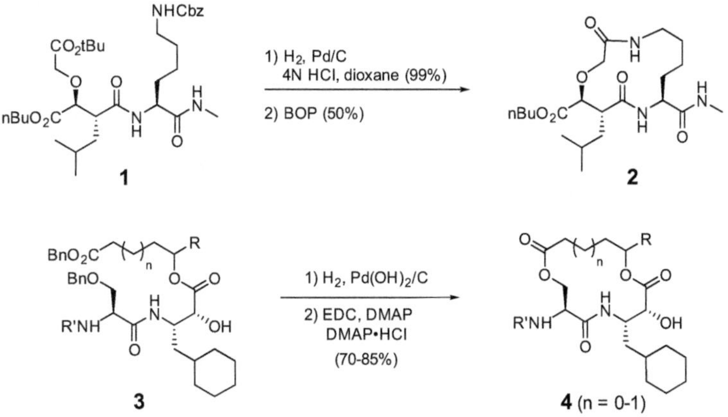

Scheme 11.1 Examples of macrolactamization and macrolactonization reactions.

(4) facile performance in either solid or solution phase; and (5) effective for a wide range of ring sizes. However, they also have a few negatives, some actually common to all macrocyclizations. Thus, they typically require high dilution conditions to prevent formation of oligomeric side-products, kinetics play a significant role in the efficiency of the cyclization, and, although amide and ester bonds are relatively ubiquitous in bioactive compounds, not all target molecules lend themselves easily to these methods.

For macrolactamization, an extensive choice of coupling agents is already available from peptide chemistry, including carbodiimides, phosphonium salts, other phosphorous derivatives, aminium/uronium salts, acylazoles, pyridinium salts, triazines and halogenating reagents, with continuing efforts constantly adding to this variety.[11–15] Some of these reagents are now available on polymer supports for ease of use in parallel synthesis and diversity investigations.[15]

Macrolactamization, not surprisingly, is often the method of choice for peptidomimetic macrocycles and has been successfully employed for a wide range of structures from the small ring inhibitors (5) of neutral endopeptidase 24.11 (NEP)[16,17] (Figure 11.1, ring closure site indicated with reagent used for cyclization (HATU (2-(1H-7-azabenzotriazol-1-yl)-1,1,3,3-tetramethyl uronium hexafluorophosphate), FDPP (pentafluorophenyl diphenylphosphinate), TCBC (2,4,6-trichlorobenzoyl chloride, Yamaguchi's reagent)) to the larger macrocycles (6) pioneered by Robinson as protein epitope mimics (PEM).[18] Two of the more advanced synthetic macrocycles in clinical trials arose from this latter methodology, POL6326, a CXCR4 antagonist currently in Phase II investigations for use in the mobilization and transplantation of stem cells,[19–21] and POL7080, an antibiotic that is in a Phase II clinical study for the treatment of life-threatening *Pseudomonas* infections.[21,22]

Intramolecular amide bond formation can be a rapid and highly efficient reaction, although it is, like every such process, subject to the ability of the linear precursor to adopt a conformation appropriate for realizing the cyclization. Also, with most reagents, care must be taken to ensure the stereocenter on the activated acid component is not compromised.

Nonetheless, this chemical approach has been used to advantage to prepare both macrocyclic peptidomimetic and non-peptidic compounds, including renin inhibitors,[23–27] thrombin inhibitors (7, Figure 11.1, ring closure site and reagent used for cyclization indicated),[28,29] human immunodeficiency (HIV) protease inhibitors,[30,31] β-secretase (BACE-1) inhibitors,[32] TNF-α converting enzyme (TACE) inhibitors,[33] selective MMP-8 inhibitors,[34] protease inhibitors,[35] calpain inhibitors,[36] cholecystokinin (CCK)-B antagonists,[37] subtype selective somatostatin analogues,[38] growth factor receptor-bound protein 2 (Grb) Src homology 2 (SH2) domain inhibitors,[39] histone deacetylase (HDAC) inhibitors,[40] heat shock protein 90 (Hsp90) inhibitors,[41] PDZ domain ligands,[42] multicyclic mimics of protein loop structures,[43,44] and a wide variety of structures that target the G-quadruplex (8).[45–47] For this latter example, it was actually simultaneous double amide bond formation that created the ring.

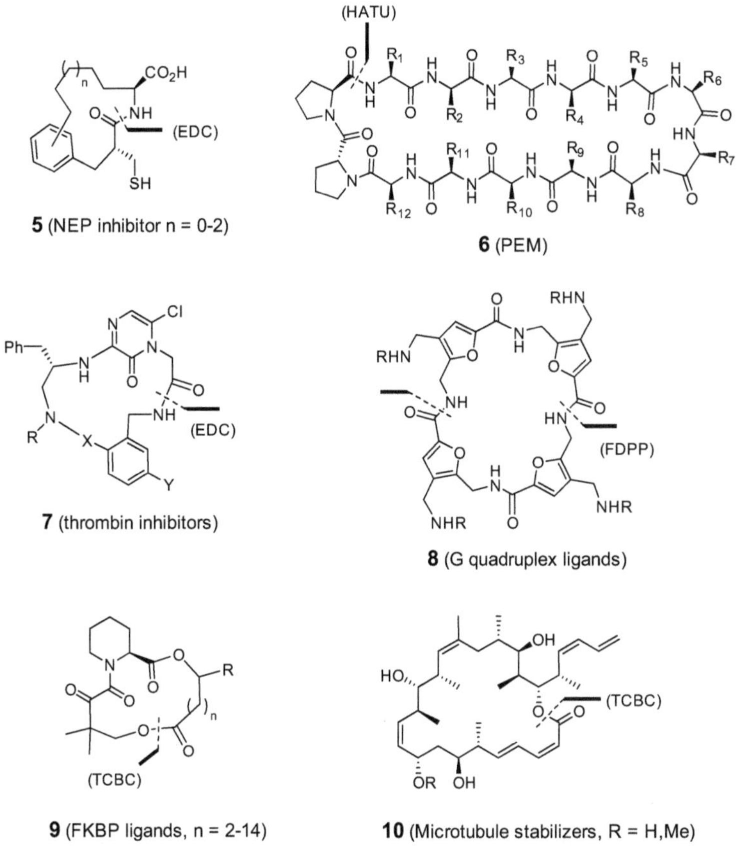

Figure 11.1 Representative macrolactamization and macrolactonization products.

In addition to employing certain of the same coupling agents as macro-lactamization, a number of alternative methods have been developed for macrolactonization, many of which originated from the myriad synthetic efforts targeted at macrolide natural products, their derivatives and analogues.[8,48] Indeed, applications for modified natural structures have been the primary use for this approach with more limited examples in the preparation of *de novo* macrocyclic molecules. The greater hydrolytic lability of the ester in the lactone compared with the lactam might play a role in this bias. However, the synthesis of a series of macrolactones as potentially immunosuppressive FK506 binding protein (FKBP) ligands has been reported (**9**, Figure 11.1),[49] as has a microtubule stabilizing agent (**10**),[50] each accessed using Yamaguchi conditions for ring closure.[51]

Returning attention to macrolactamization, a variation on the traditional amine-acid coupling was employed to access a series of finger loop inhibitors of hepatitis C virus (HCV) nonstructural protein 5B (NS5b) polymerase leading to the discovery of the clinical candidate TMC647055 (**13**, Scheme 11.2, CDI

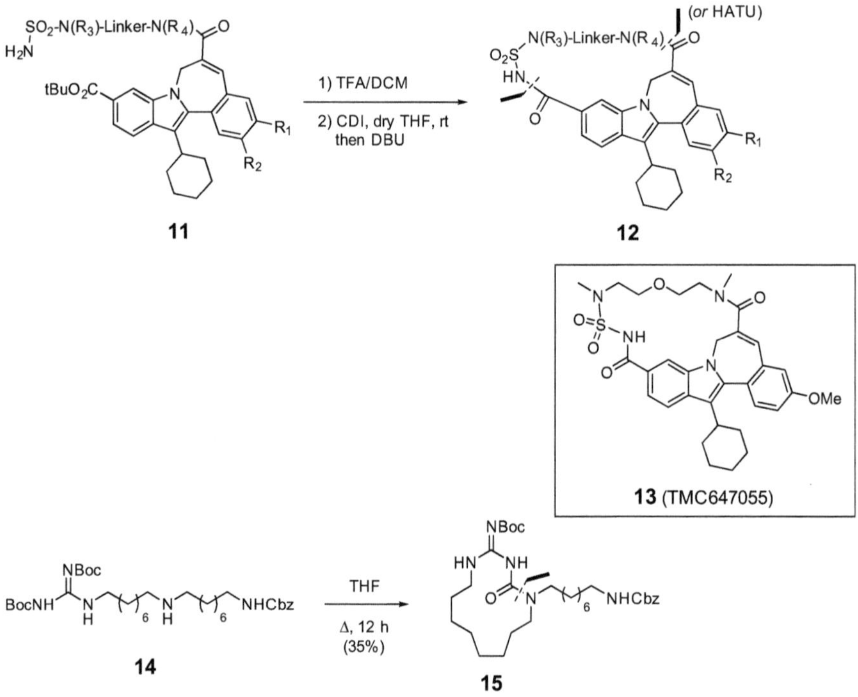

Scheme 11.2   Non-traditional macrolactamization reactions.

(carbonyl diimidazole), DBU (1,8-diazabicyclo[5.4.0]undec-7-ene)) currently in Phase II trials.[52] In addition to traditional amide bond macrocyclization (indicated as an alternative in the Scheme), ring closure of the sulphonamide moiety of **11** with the aromatic carboxylic acid was employed to further rigidify the tetracyclic system. These efforts resulted in a series of polymerase inhibitors (**12**) from which **13** displayed an acceptable pharmacokinetic profile in dogs, including high oral bioavailability ($F = 87\%$) and systemic exposure combined with moderate plasma clearance and low volume of distribution. In another variant, intramolecular reaction of a urethane (Boc group) with the secondary amine of **14** led to novel 13-membered macrocyclic amidinoureas (**15**, Scheme 11.2, ring closure site indicated), which exhibited higher antifungal activity than fluconazole against wild type and resistant clinical strains of *Candidas*.[53]

In one final strategy for macrolactamization, specifically for use on the solid phase, the cyclization can be performed such that it occurs simultaneously with release from a resin that has been appropriately functionalized with a linker that can function, or be modified to so function, as a leaving group.[54] As will be described in Section 11.14.1, this type of cyclization-release strategy can provide significant benefits for diversity investigations.

11.3 Substitution Chemistry

One of the most straightforward approaches to building a macrocyclic template is direct displacement. However, such reactions require the construction of appropriate substrates in order to be effective, encounter incompatibilities with some functional groups and require protection of other reactive moieties. They are also often plagued by side reactions, elimination in particular, and generally must be performed under high dilution conditions to reduce the formation of oligomeric side products, and they are very sensitive to the conformations of the cyclization precursor. Of course, these direct displacement strategies possess certain benefits as well: (1) availability of a myriad of reaction conditions and reagents; (2) well-established chemistries that do not require special techniques; (3) flexibility for investigation of different sites of ring closure; and (4) facile execution on resin supports as would be advantageous for diversity investigations.

11.3.1 S$_N$2 Reactions

Intramolecular application of classic S$_N$2 displacement chemistry has proven to be a versatile method for the assembly of certain macrocyclic structures, generally those that are relatively simple, even symmetrical, molecules with limited functionality. For example, this transformation has proven effective for the CXCR4-targeted immunostimulating, anti-cancer and/or antiviral cyclams AMD3100 (plerixafor, **19**, Scheme 11.3),[55,56] AMD3465[57,58] and JM2763.[59,60] Using the route to **19** as an exemplary process to construct these type of molecules, the tetraazamacrocycle (**18**) is typically synthesized from appropriate diamine or triamine precursors, for example **16**, by reaction with a bifunctional electrophile such as **17**.

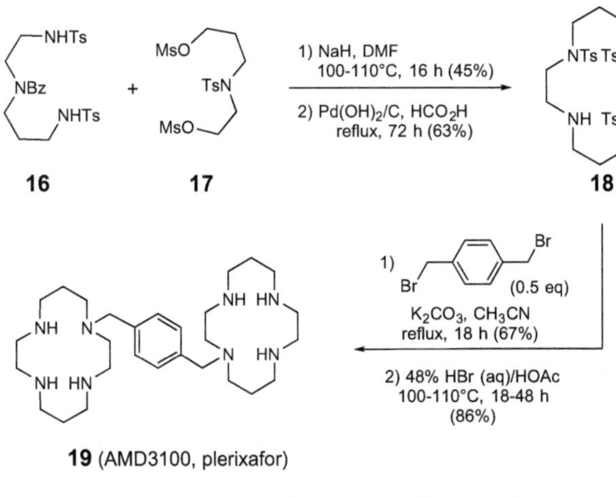

Scheme 11.3 Simultaneous S$_N$2 reaction approach towards macrocycles.

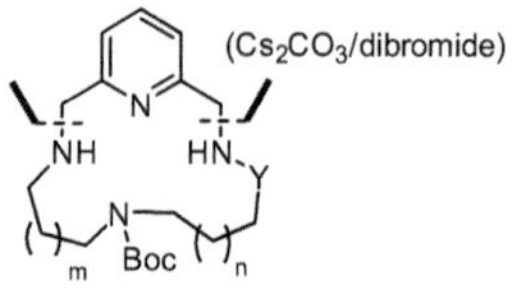

20 (m = 0,1; n = 0,1; Y = CH$_2$,O) 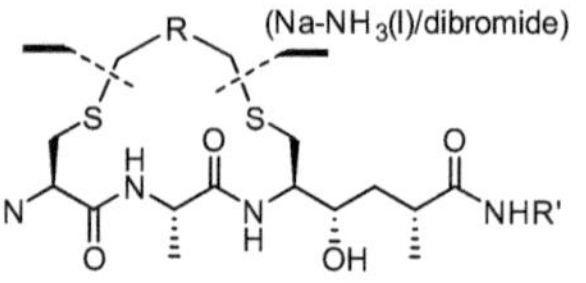   **21** (BACE-1 inhibitors)

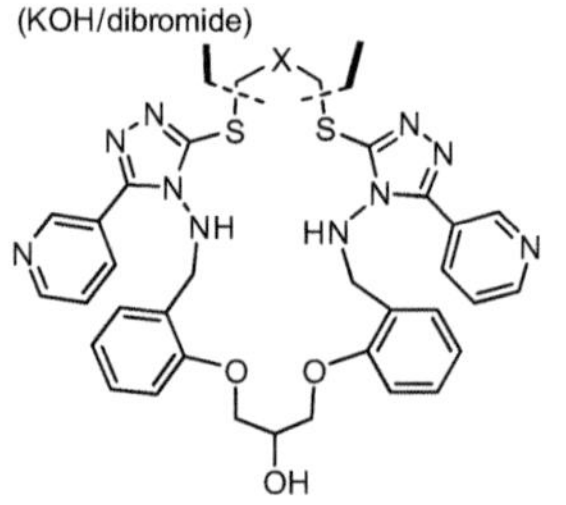

22 (antimicrobials, X = O, CH$_2$)

Figure 11.2   Representative structures from simultaneous S$_N$2 reactions.

This approach, with sequential or pseudo-simultaneous substitutions employing reactants with two nucleophilic groups in the same precursor together with two electrophilic sites in the corresponding substrate, has also been utilized to create related ring systems. For example, poly-azacyclophanes (**20**, Figure 11.2, ring closure sites, basic reagent and leaving group employed shown) were constructed in good to very good yields in this manner from differentially protected amines and 2,6-dibromomethyl-pyridine, which could then be further diversified by reaction of the free amines (Section 11.14.1).[61] In addition, double S$_N$2 displacements were used to incorporate constraints into macro-heterocyclic peptidomimetic BACE inhibitors (**21**)[62] and for the construction of macrocycles that exhibited antimicrobial activity (**22**).[63]

A nucleophilic substitution strategy has been employed for more complex structures as well. For example, an intramolecular S$_N$2 process provided the key transformation in the assembly of macrocyclic peptidomimetics designed to mimic either β-turns (**23**, Figure 11.3, ring closure site, base and leaving group indicated)[64] or β-strands (**24**).[65,66] Execution of the synthesis of the former on solid support demonstrated its applicability for library construction, whereas the latter structures were shown to be potent HIV protease inhibitors. Also on solid phase, a small collection of macro-heterocycles (**25**) was prepared utilizing an S$_N$2 process involving a halide and a malonate anion.[67]

Other bioactive macrocyclic structures have been assembled using an S$_N$2 approach including hydroxamic acid MMP and TACE inhibitors,[9,68] cyclin-dependent kinase (CDK) inhibitors (**26**, Figure 11.3, ring closure site, base and leaving group indicated),[69] MMP inhibitors (**27**),[70] thiazole-containing RGD analogues[71,72] and sodium/glucose co-transporter 2 (SGLT2) inhibitors (**28**).[73]

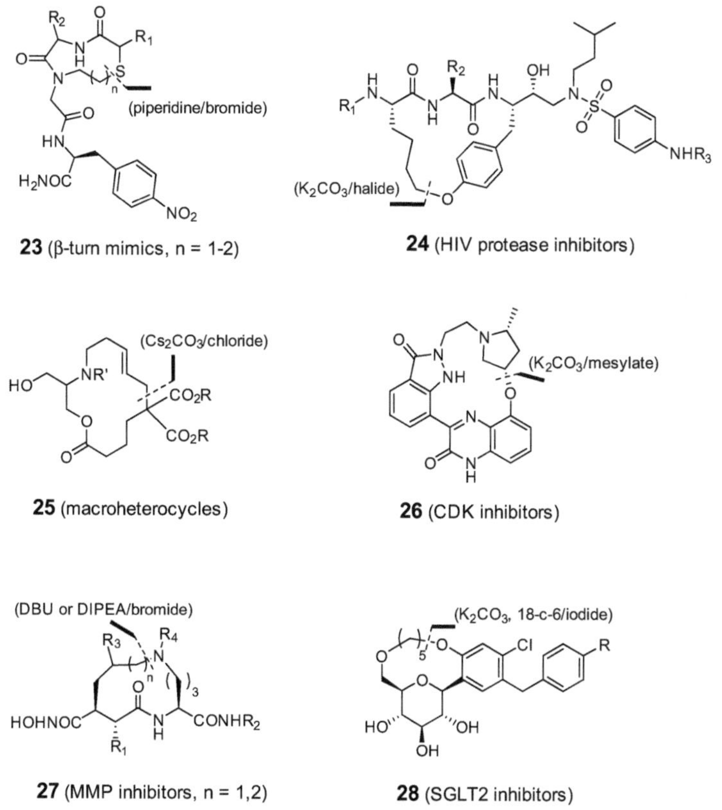

Figure 11.3 Selected macrocyclic structures from S_N2 chemistry.

In the construction of the macrocyclic amines **27**, it was found that the preferred base varied with ring size, with DBU optimal for 13-membered rings, while DIPEA (*N,N*-diisopropylethylamine) worked better for 14-membered target molecules.

11.3.2 Nucleophilic Aromatic Substitution (S_NAr)

In addition to S_N2 chemistry, substitution reactions on the aromatic ring have also been applied to the construction of macrocyclic compounds. Specifically, given the prevalence of the biaryl ether moiety as a "privileged structure" in bioactive natural products, for example vancomycin, teicoplanin, piperazinomycin and others,[74,75] it is not surprising that methods for ring closure to form this functionality have seen wide application. In particular, the ease and effectiveness of such S_NAr processes on solid support make it attractive for the synthesis of peptidomimetics containing a biaryl ether and related moieties.[76,77] This has facilitated its use for diversity investigations as well. Further, the inclusion of one or more electron-rich aromatic rings to a molecular scaffold offers the opportunity for additional target interactions with concomitant beneficial binding effects. However, such displacement reactions generally must be performed under high dilution conditions to minimize oligomeric side products, are more susceptible to cyclization difficulty due to less flexible precursors not attaining a productive conformation, and, as an anionic process, necessitate the protection of other reactive functional groups.

In a representative example, S_NAr was employed by Burgess for the solid phase synthesis of a series of β-turn mimetics (Scheme 11.4).[78–80] In this approach, a variety of nucleophiles were used to displace fluoride from the activated phenyl moiety of **29** to provide the desired ring closed products (**30**) in very good yields upon release from the resin. This versatile methodology was successfully used in the design and assembly of agonists of the Trk C neurotrophin-3 receptor (**31**) and the TrkA nerve growth factor receptor (**32**),[81–83] as well as TrkC antagonists (**33**).[84] A similar strategy was employed for the synthesis of arylthioether-containing macrocycles, where intramolecular S_NAr reactions, in addition to S_N2 processes, provided the key cyclization step in the solid phase parallel synthesis of a set of peptidomimetics.[85]

In a standard solution phase S_NAr process, extensive series of macrocyclic piperazinone, pyrrolidinone and imidazole farnesyltransferase (FTase)

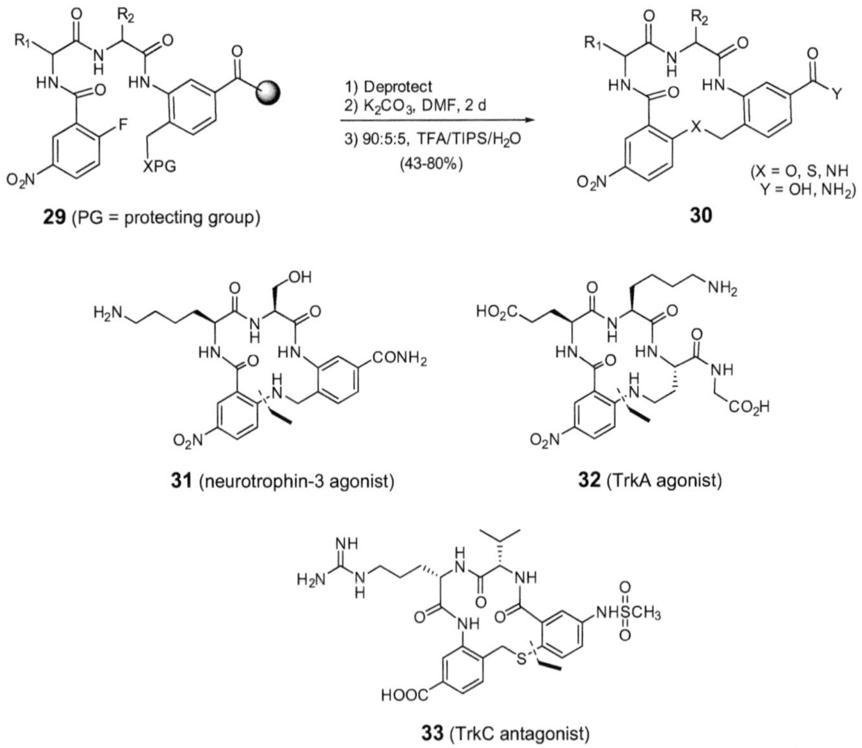

Scheme 11.4 Macrocyclic β-turn mimics *via* S_NAr.

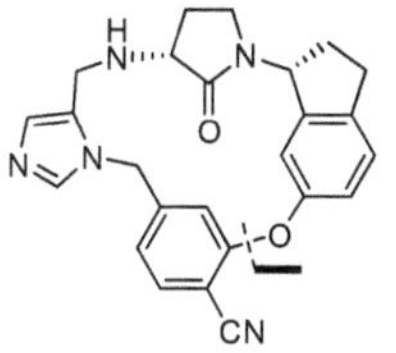

34 (FTase inhibitor)

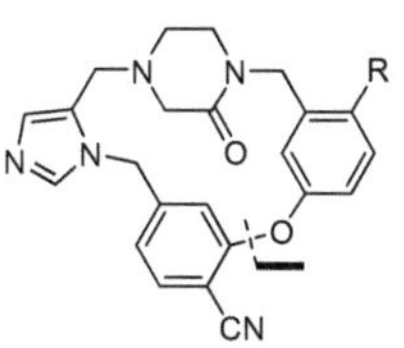

35 (dual FTase and GGTase inhibitors)

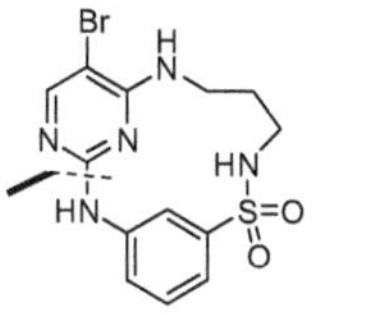

36 (dual CDK and VEGF inhibitors)

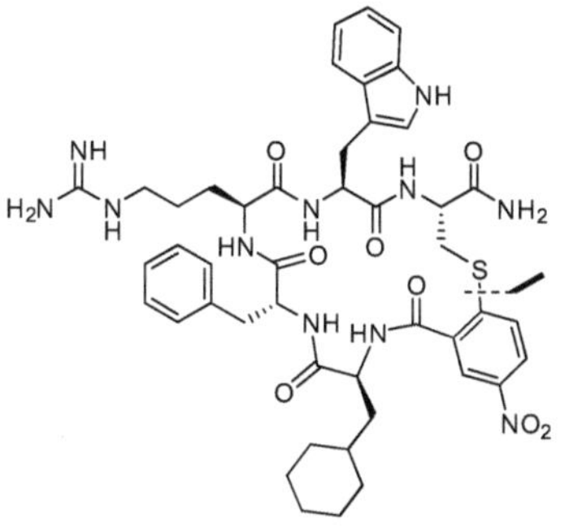

37 (selective MC5R antagonists)

Figure 11.4 Representative macrocyclic structures from S$_N$Ar chemistry.

inhibitors, with **34** as a representative example (Figure 11.4, site of ring closure indicated) were constructed,[86–88] from which were also identified dual inhibitors of FTase and geranylgeranyltransferase-1 (GGTase) (**35**).[89] Additionally, an S$_N$Ar approach proved useful for the assembly of amino-pyrimidine macrocycles (**36**) that possessed inhibitory activity against both CDK and vascular endothelial growth factor receptor-2 (VEGF-R2) and exhibited *in vivo* oral activity in a tumour xenograft model.[90] Microwaves have been shown to assist with the efficiency and speed of the S$_N$Ar process on resin,[91] which was employed by Hruby *et al.* for the preparation of potent and selective melanocortin-5 receptor (MC5R) antagonists (**37**).[92]

Another S$_N$Ar cyclization method that has benefited from the use of microwaves is the Ullmann reaction for the copper-catalysed construction of biaryl ethers, although the majority of applications for macrocycles are in the total synthesis arena. Sun and co-workers reported the initial study of the effects of microwave heating for the intramolecular and bimolecular Ullmann reaction between a diverse set of phenols and aryl bromides, which illustrated the positive effects of the process on reducing reaction time and increasing yield, even for smaller (12–14) rings.[93] However, the temperatures required for optimum results were high (220–230 °C) and, for certain substrates, dimer was the sole or predominant product. This microwave process was employed as the key step in the construction of a small library of engelhardione analogues from which antibacterial activity was garnered.[94] More recently, conditions for this transformation have been studied in detail

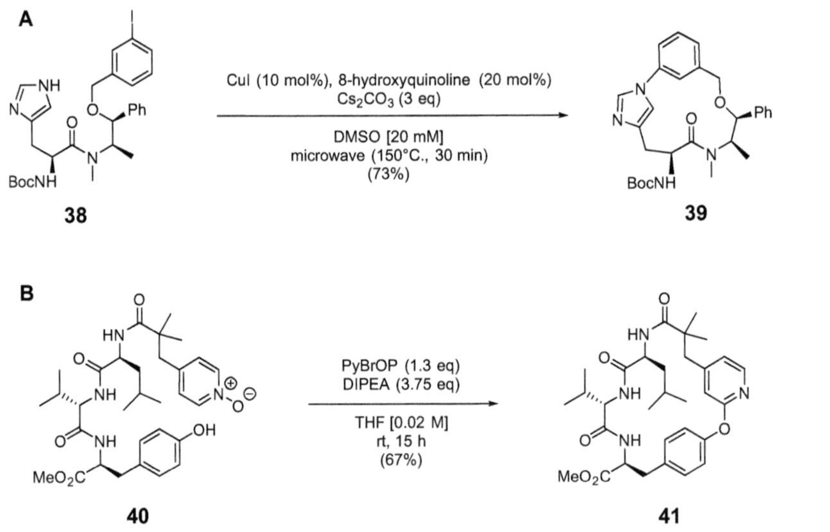

A

Cul (10 mol%), 8-hydroxyquinoline (20 mol%)
Cs₂CO₃ (3 eq)

DMSO [20 mM]
microwave (150°C., 30 min)
(73%)

38   **39**

B

PyBrOP (1.3 eq)
DIPEA (3.75 eq)

THF [0.02 M]
rt, 15 h
(67%)

40   **41**

Scheme 11.5 (A) Ullmann reaction route to macrocycles; (B) Novel macrocyclization route to peptidomimetics.

to determine a generally applicable method for coupling, with phenol and imidazole as representative nucleophiles.[95] The optimized conditions were then applied to a selection of functionalized substrates to very efficiently form 14- to 25-membered macrocycles (**39**, Scheme 11.5A for a representative example) in moderate to excellent yields (42–89%). Noteworthy are the relatively high concentration (up to 100 mM) at which these reactions were conducted, the lack of the necessity for an electron-withdrawing substituent to activate the aryl iodide, and the tolerance for a range of aryl substitution patterns. In addition, examples of organometallic-mediated S_NAr approaches whereby complexation or association of the phenyl group with a metal complex functions to activate the ring for substitution will be discussed in Sections 11.7.2 and 11.7.4.

Although not a classical substitution reaction, a recent route to macrocyclic peptidomimetics such as **41** utilizes pyridine N-oxides, activated with PyBrOP (bromotripyrrolidinophosphonium hexafluorophosphate), as substrates for an intramolecular reaction with nucleophilic groups, including phenols, amines and imidazoles, as found in certain amino acid side chains (representative example in Scheme 11.5B).[96] Adding the substrate dropwise to the other reactants was necessary to avoid polymerization. In this manner, the cyclization proceeds in fair to very good yields (22–77%) and, interestingly, does not require high dilution conditions. This could be due to the electrostatic association between the nucleophile and the presumed activated phosphonium intermediate creating a favourable conformation for macrocycle formation and minimizing the production of dimers or oligomers.

11.4 Ring-Closing Metathesis

Based upon the seminal work of Grubbs,[97] ring-closing metathesis (RCM) is an intramolecular process mediated by an organometallic catalyst in which two terminal olefins are reacted together with the formation of a cycloalkene and the concomitant loss of ethylene. Although tungsten and molybdenum catalysts have significant utility in olefin metathesis and can promote RCM, in general, their high reactivity, air and water sensitivity, and poor functional group tolerance, make ruthenium catalysts the best choice for this reaction and a number of different Ru complexes have been developed for this purpose (Figure 11.5).

The RCM methodology has proven to be one of the most versatile and widely employed reactions for the formation of macrocyclic natural products,[98,99] as well as new macrocyclic structures.[100,101] These myriad applications arise due to the many strengths of the transformation: (1) very broad scope; (2) adaptability to many ring sizes, although larger rings are often more problematic; (3) excellent tolerance for other functionality; (4) straightforward execution with gentle reaction conditions; and (5) numerous catalysts available that permit variations in reactivity and selectivity. Of course, this process is not without disadvantages. These include, for example, the alkene product is usually a mixture of geometrical isomers; the precursors often require special preparation; the amount of catalyst required for efficient conversions can be high; the reaction generally needs to be executed in high dilution to avoid forming oligomeric impurities; the ring closure can vary greatly in yield based upon the nature and size of the substrate; and catalyst removal to trace levels can be technically onerous to achieve.

Nonetheless, the benefits far outweigh the deficiencies such that RCM is very often the method of choice for the construction of macrocyclic

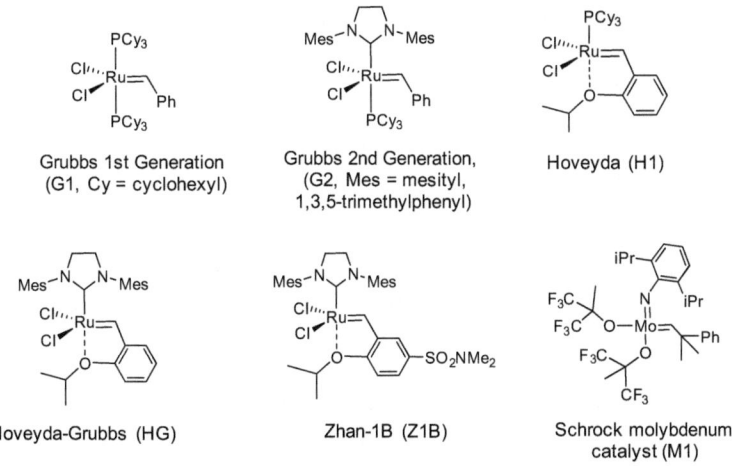

Figure 11.5 Ring-closing metathesis (RCM) catalysts.

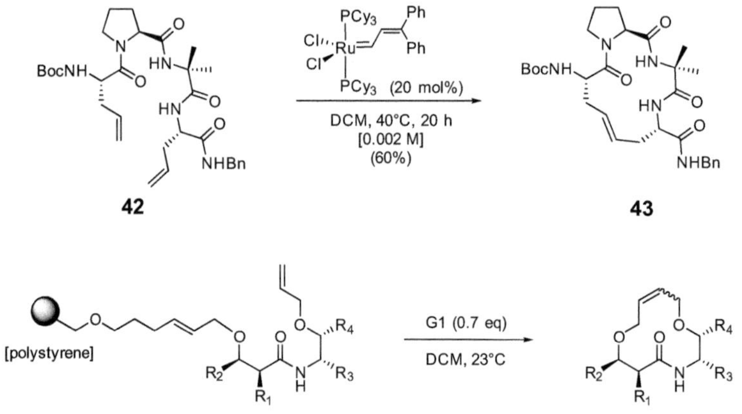

Scheme 11.6 RCM routes to macrocycles.

frameworks. Further, in many instances, the resulting double bond is subsequently reduced to yield the desired final product, so the mixture of ste-
reoisomeric RCM products is not an issue and, besides, catalysts have now
been developed that permit better control over this aspect.[102] One of the first
applications of RCM was towards the synthesis of constrained amino acids
and peptides, including β-turn mimics (**43**, Scheme 11.6) and other restricted structural mimetics.[103] This report also demonstrated that RCM
could proceed very efficiently on resin supports. Although requiring a large
percentage of catalyst, another example of RCM on the solid phase illustrates
the cyclization-release strategy mentioned in Section 11.2. The cyclic peptidomimetic products (**45**) from this process incorporate aldol-type building
blocks that provide numerous opportunities for exploring diversity
(Scheme 11.6).[104]

In an illustration of the degree of functionality and structural complexity
this reaction can accept, a number of macrocyclic taxoid derivatives (**46**,
Figure 11.6, site of cyclization indicated along with the catalyst employed
using the designations in Figure 11.5) were synthesized using RCM and
assisted in the determination of the active conformation of this class of
anticancer natural products.[105]

Indeed, the wide variety of molecular architectures that can be accessed
via RCM is illustrated by the compounds shown in Figure 11.6 (site of
cyclization indicated along with the catalyst employed using the designations
in Figure 11.5), which likewise exhibit diverse bioactivities. Specifically, this
strategy has been successfully applied to macrocyclic BACE inhibitors
(**47**),[62,106–113] calpain inhibitors (**48**),[114,115] checkpoint kinase 1 (Chk1)
inhibitors (**49**),[116–118] G-quadruplex stabilizing agents,[119] Grb2 SH2 domain
inhibitors (**50**),[39,120–122] non-natural product inspired pan-HDAC inhibitors
(**51**),[123] HIV inhibitors,[124–127] Hsp90 inhibitors (**52**),[128,129] insulin-regulated
aminopeptidase (IRAP) inhibitors,[130] neuraminidase inhibitors (**53**),[131]

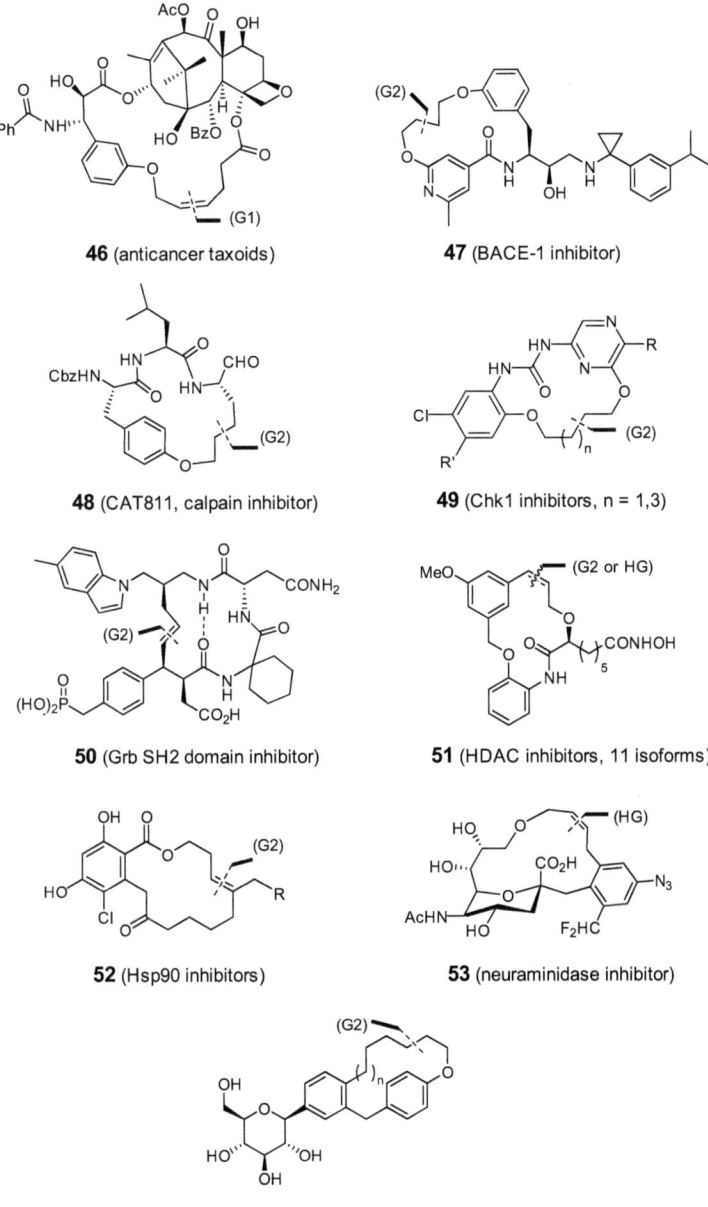

46 (anticancer taxoids)

47 (BACE-1 inhibitor)

48 (CAT811, calpain inhibitor)

49 (Chk1 inhibitors, n = 1,3)

50 (Grb SH2 domain inhibitor)

51 (HDAC inhibitors, 11 isoforms)

52 (Hsp90 inhibitors)

53 (neuraminidase inhibitor)

54 (SGLT2 inhibitors, n = 0-2)

Figure 11.6 Representative macrocyclic structures from RCM.

neuroprotective agents,[132] peptide deformylase inhibitors,[133,134] plasmepsin inhibitors,[135] RGD analogues,[136] SGLT2 inhibitors (**54**),[137] somatostatin mimetics,[138] thrombin inhibitors,[139] and human tumour susceptibility gene 101 protein (Tsg101) antagonists.[140]

However, the most significant impact of this approach has been in the discovery and development of the plethora of macrocyclic HCV NS3/4A protease inhibitors, which relied almost exclusively on RCM to assemble the macrocyclic framework.[141–143] This includes several compounds that have progressed to advanced clinical evaluation, such as ITMN-191 (danoprevir, **55**, Figure 11.7, site of cyclization indicated along with the catalyst employed using the designations in Figure 11.5),[144,145] BILN 2061 (ciluprevir, **56**),[146,147] BI 201302 (**57**),[148] MK-5172 (**58**),[149,150] MK-7009 (vaniprevir, **59**),[151] IDX320

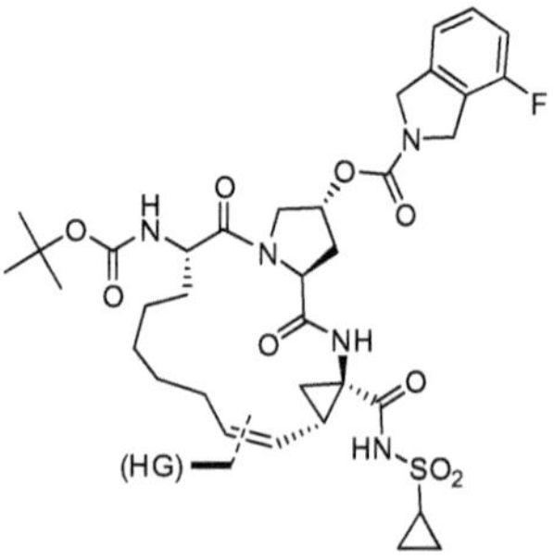

55 (ITMN-191, RG7227, danoprevir, Phase II) 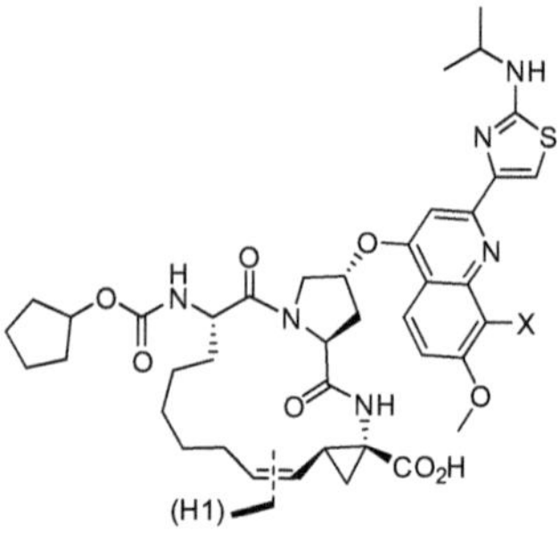 **56** (X=H, BILN2061, ciluprevir, Phase II disc.)
57 (X=Br, BI 201302)

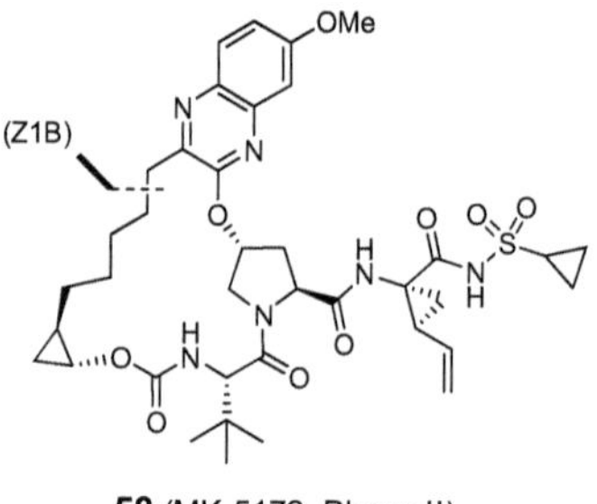

58 (MK-5172, Phase II) 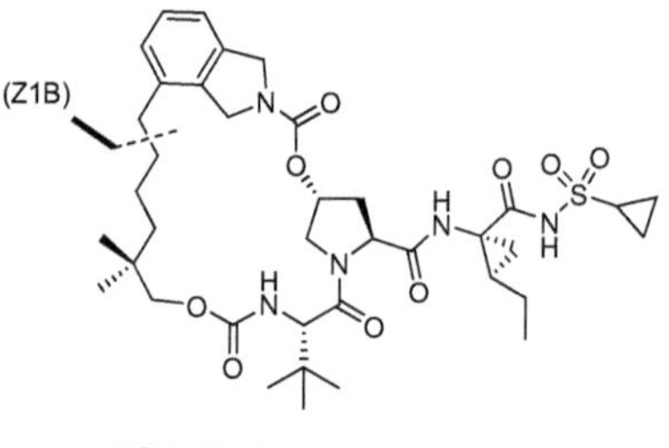 **59** (MK-7009, vaniprevir, Phase III)

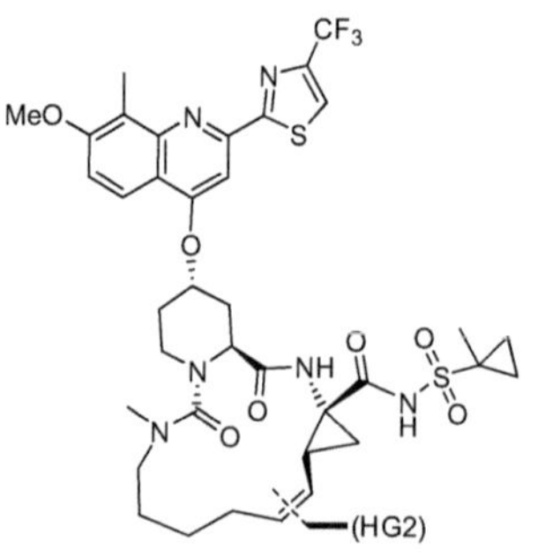

60 (IDX320, Phase IIa disc.) 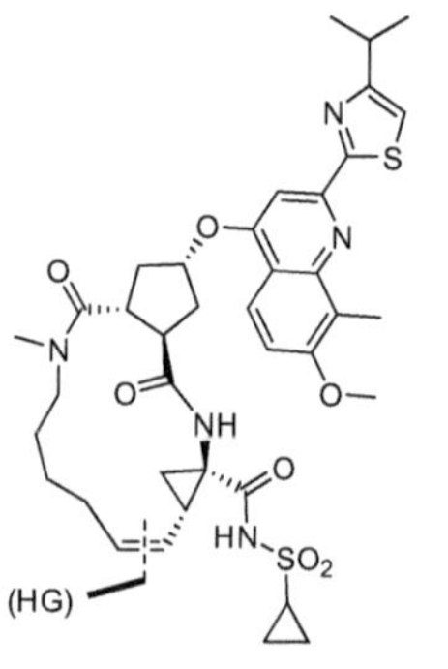 **61** (TMC-435, simeprevir, approved)

Figure 11.7 Macrocyclic HCV protease inhibitors constructed using RCM.

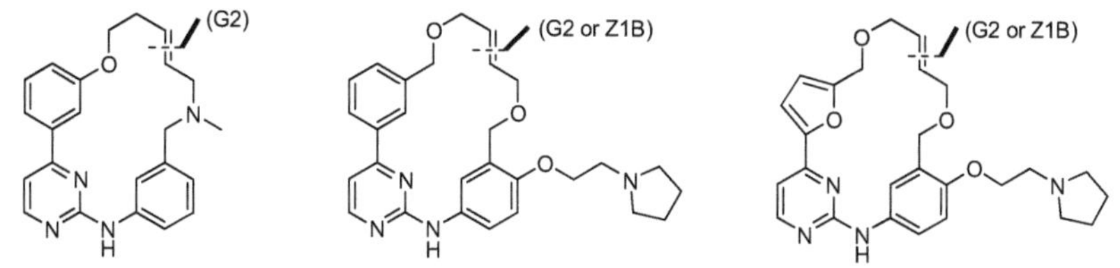

62 (SB1317, TG02)
(Phase I, leukemia)

63 (SB1518, pacritinib)
(Phase III, myelofibrosis)

64 (SB1578, CT-1578)
(Phase I, rheumatoid arthritis)

Figure 11.8 Macrocyclic kinase inhibitors *via* RCM.

(**60**),[152] and one, TMC435 (simeprevir, **61**),[153] for which marketing approval was received in 2013 for the US, Canada and Japan and in 2014 for Europe.

Another series of clinical stage compounds prepared utilizing RCM are the multi-kinase inhibitors SB1317 (TG02, **62**, Figure 11.8), an inhibitor of CDKs, Janus kinase 2 (JAK2) and Fms-like tyrosine kinase-3 (FLT3) for the treatment of cancers, including multiple myeloma and acute leukaemia,[154,155] SB1518 (pacritnib, **63**), a JAK2, FLT3 and tyrosine kinase 2 (TYK2) inhibitor for the treatment of myelofibrosis and lymphoma,[156,157] and SB1578 (**64**), an inhibitor of JAK2, FLT3 and colony stimulating factor-1 receptor kinase (c-Fms) for the treatment of rheumatoid arthritis.[158] As is evident from the structures, these all originated from the same diaminopyridine-based core template.

In the search for new pharmaceutical agents, one avenue is to create chemical structures that have little or no precedence in the scientific literature with the hope that these novel structures will produce unexpected or novel bioactivity. Given its wide applicability, ease of execution and functional group tolerance, RCM has significant potential for the assembly of novel scaffolds useful in such efforts. For example, the imidazole macrocyclic scaffold of general structure **65** (Figure 11.9) was synthesized *via* RCM and found to display a range of potentially interesting binding activities for adenosine and dopamine receptors, ion channels and transporters.[159] A series of bicyclic 1,3-bridged-2-azetidinones (**66** as a representative structure), which have been demonstrated to be inhibitors of penicillin-binding proteins, represents another novel macrocyclic structural class accessed by RCM methodology.[160–162]

Interestingly, both monomer and dimer-derived structures obtained from these latter efforts have been found to have utility. The steric and conformational constraints imposed by the bicyclic structures made RCM difficult in a number of cases. As a result, Ti(OiPr)$_4$ was utilized as an additive to suppress Ru catalyst deactivation and permit the reaction to proceed.[163] Further, in some instances, such restrictions led to the major or exclusive product being the cyclic dimer (**67**).[164,165] In contrast to the observations with some of the cyclic monomers, which often did not provide an advantage over the linear precursors, the cyclic dimers were typically more active than the acyclic molecules. Additional macrocycles of this particular type have

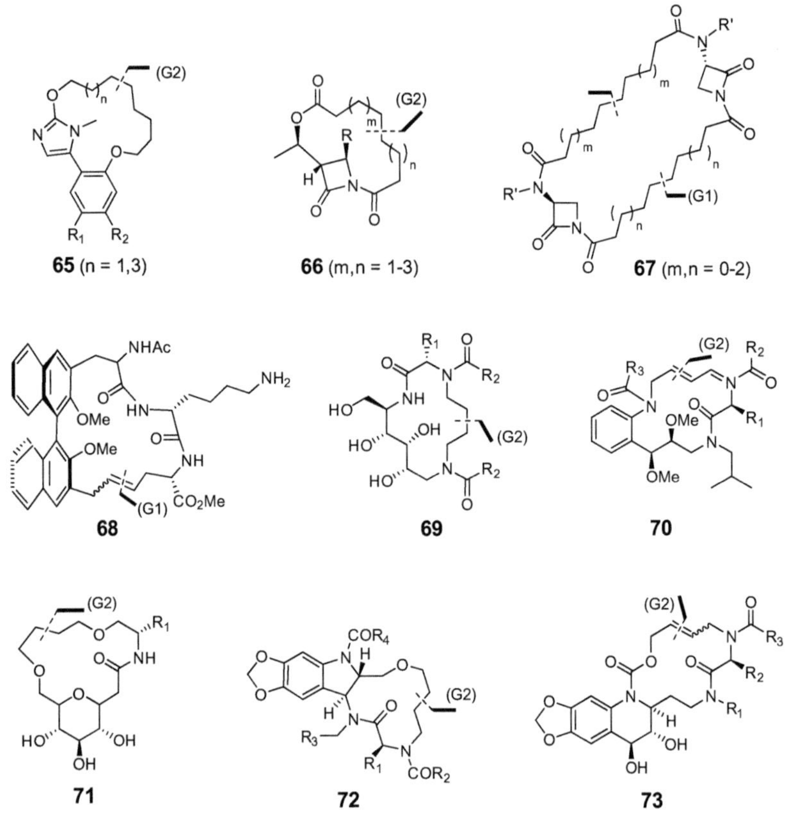

Figure 11.9 Additional macrocyclic structures accessed by RCM.

also exhibited antibacterial activity, with the consistent feature being a cationic amino acid on a hydrophobic scaffold. Hence, simple substituted benzene, carbazole, indole, benzo[b]thiophene and 1,1'-binaphthyl (**68**) macrocycles have been synthesized using RCM.[166]

Using RCM as the enabling chemistry, Arya and co-workers have reported on an impressively diverse collection of 12- to 15-membered macrocycles that exhibit activity as inhibitors of angiogenesis and early embryonic development, including glycohybrids (**69**, Figure 11.9),[167] benzo-fused analogues (**70**),[168] C-linked carbohydrate derivatives (**71**),[169] aminoindolines (**72**)[170] and tetrahydroquinolines (**73**).[171] RCM also is one of the primary methods utilized to create conformationally fixed helical peptide macrocycles, often termed "stapled peptides".[172–175] The first compound of this type, ALRN-5281 (not shown),[176] a growth hormone-releasing hormone agonist[177] for treating growth hormone deficiency and HIV lipodystrophy, has recently completed its first clinic trial.[178]

Although not nearly as widely exploited, other metathesis reactions also have potential for macrocyclization processes. For example, ring-closing alkyne metathesis (RCAM) has been explored primarily for total synthesis.[179] The use of the more difficult to handle and less stable molybdenum and tungsten catalysts, together with the synthetic inaccessibility of the precursor bis(alkynes), may explain the more limited application of this methodology to date.[180] Similarly, ring-closing enyne metathesis (RCEM) reactions have potential for wider use, but examples outside of the total synthesis field are primarily limited to small heterocycles.[181] In an example that illustrates this potential, Barrett *et al.* have reported the preparation of the macrocyclic peptidomimetic template **75** (Scheme 11.7), possessing multiple functionalities for further diversification, *via* RCEM.[182] Unfortunately, a side product apparently resulting from a cross metathesis process complicates this transformation, a reasonably common occurrence that may also contribute to the paucity of *de novo* applications of this chemistry for macrocycles as yet.

Further, Hansen and Lee have described the synthesis, both in solution and on solid support, of macrocyclic 1,3-dienes with this strategy, with the *exo*-products (**76**) predominating for 10-membered rings and the *endo* (**77**) for 12- to 15-membered rings, while 11-membered rings gave essentially equal amounts of each isomer (Figure 11.10, site of ring closure and catalyst indicated).[183]

In addition, these metathesis processes have been utilized in tandem with other reactions to create novel cyclic structures. For example, cross-enyne

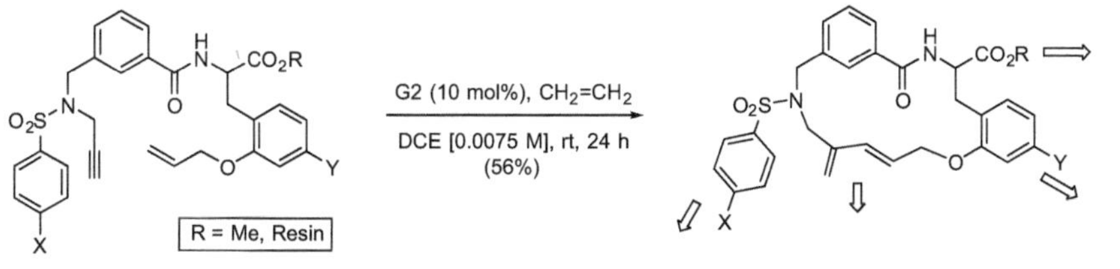

74 **75** (arrows indicate sites for further reactions)

Scheme 11.7 Macrocycles from ring-closing enyne metathesis (RCEM).

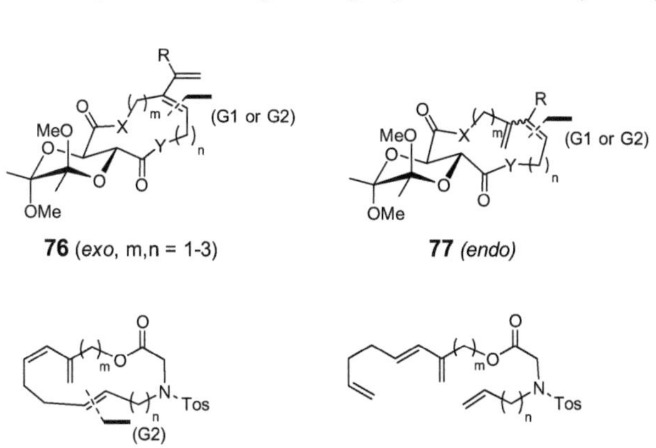

76 (*exo*, m,n = 1-3) **77** (*endo*)

78 (m = 1-2, n - 1-4) **79** (m = 1-2, n - 1-4)

Figure 11.10 Representative macrocycles from RCEM processes.

metathesis in combination with RCM can lead to 13- to 16-membered mac-roheterocycles (**78**, Figure 11.10, site of ring closure and catalyst indicated).[184] A number of variations on the substrates (chain lengths, substituents, position of the triple bond) could offer routes to generate diversity. In practice, however, this reaction is plagued by significant quantities (40–48%) of a cross-enyne product (**79**) that cannot be further converted to the cyclic material. This suggests that competing pathways with different conformations lead to each of the observed compounds, although it is noteworthy that no product from intramolecular RCEM of the enyne substrate was observed.

11.5 Wittig Chemistry

Although often exploited in the realm of total synthesis, Wittig-type reactions represent another versatile class of transformations that has surprisingly seen only limited application for the construction of macrocyclic frameworks, apart from natural products, to date. In one relatively straightforward example in the peptidomimetic area, vascular cell adhesion molecule-1 (VCAM) – very late antigen 4 (VLA-4) antagonists possessing a carbon chain in place of a disulphide linkage were constructed from the intramolecular reaction of an aldehyde with a phosphonoglycine moiety for the critical cyclization step (Scheme 11.8).[185] The precursor, **80**, was oxidized followed by treatment with DBU to effect ring closure to the macrocycle **81**. Subsequent reduction of the olefin followed by ester hydrolysis and acid deprotection gave the desired target compounds (**82**), which exhibited activity in the nanomolar range with the 13-membered rings better than the 14-membered analogues. The Wittig reaction has also been utilized in diversity investigations for macrocyclic libraries (Section 11.14.1).

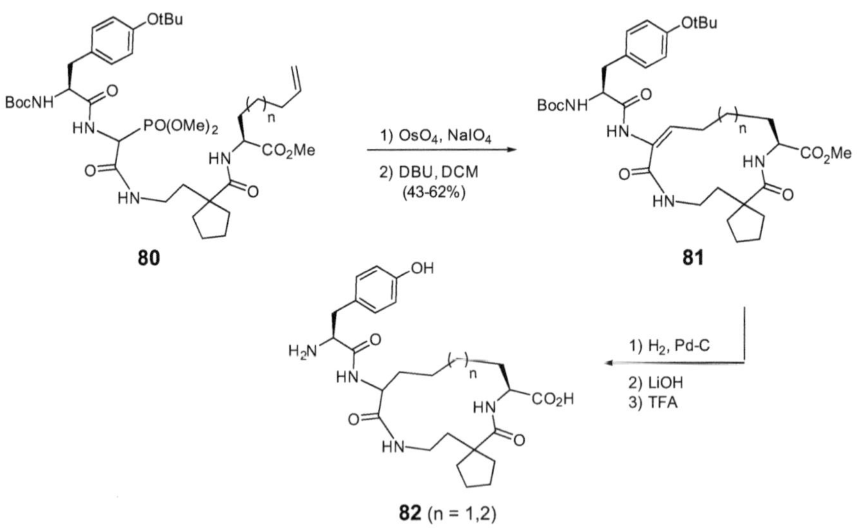

Scheme 11.8 Macrocyclic compounds from Wittig chemistry.

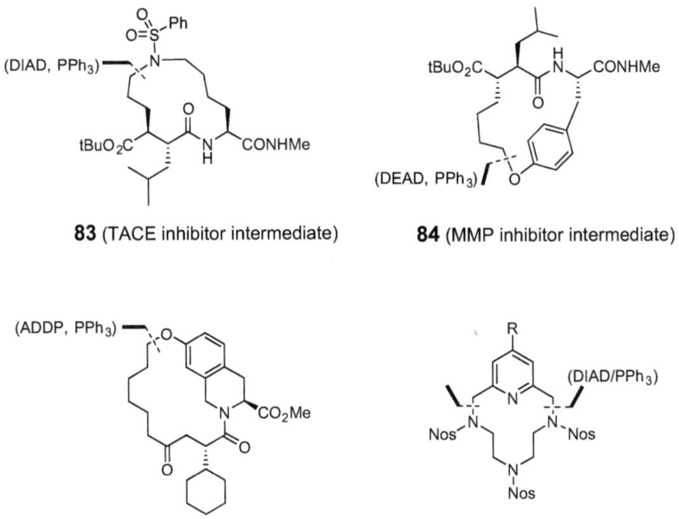

83 (TACE inhibitor intermediate)   **84** (MMP inhibitor intermediate)

85 (HCV protease inhibitor intermediate)   **86** (azamacrocycles)

Figure 11.11   Macrocycles produced using Mitsunobu-type reactions.

11.6   Mitsunobu Reactions

Similarly, despite its general utility in the synthetic arena, the Mitsunobu reaction and its variants have seen only moderate use for macrocycle ring closure.[186] The mild reaction conditions, ease of execution, known stereochemical outcome and overall versatility of the methodology led to its utilization for the synthesis of key intermediates in routes to TACE (**83**, Figure 11.11, site of ring-closure and Mitsunobu reagents indicated, ADDP (1,1'-(azodicarbonyl)piperidine), DEAD (diethylazodicarboxylate), DIAD (diisopropylazodicarboxylate)),[68] MMP (**84**)[187,188] and HCV NS3 protease inhibitors (**85**).[189–191] In the first case, the nucleophilic species was the nitrogen of a phenyl-substituted sulphonamide, while in the other two instances, a phenol served this role. As a final example, azamacrocycles such as **86** were accessed *via* double application of the Fukuyama-Mitsunobu reaction of activated (tris)sulphonamides (nosyl or p-nitrophenylsulphonyl) with diol electrophiles.[192]

11.7   Organometallic Methods

11.7.1   Palladium-mediated Reactions

Although organometallic chemistry in general has been explored to a significant extent for constructing macrocyclic systems, those involving homogeneous palladium catalysts have proven to be particularly well-suited for these structures. The myriad variations of coupling partners for such transformations have been explored to different extents, but the excellent selectivity, straightforward execution and high functional group compatibility of these processes have made them the most suitable methods for many investigations.

11.7.1.1 Suzuki

Of the Pd(0)-mediated reactions, Suzuki-type couplings of aryl or vinyl boronic esters/acids with aryl or vinyl halides/triflates are among the most widely employed for construction of complex natural structures containing an aromatic component and have found wide application for non-natural product macrocyclic compounds as well.[193] As a first illustration, an intramolecular Suzuki-Miyaura reaction provided the critical step in a route to signal peptidase inhibitors.[194] For this transformation, a detailed study of key reaction conditions, including catalyst, solvent and reaction temperature, was conducted in order to maximize yield of the strained 14-membered biaryl product **88** from linear precursor **87** (Scheme 11.9). The B-alkyl Suzuki reaction, a variant that has been widely employed in total synthesis, provided transannular access to a tricyclic system (**90**) for which an RCM strategy had previously failed.[195] The geometry of the vinyl iodide was retained in the product double bond.

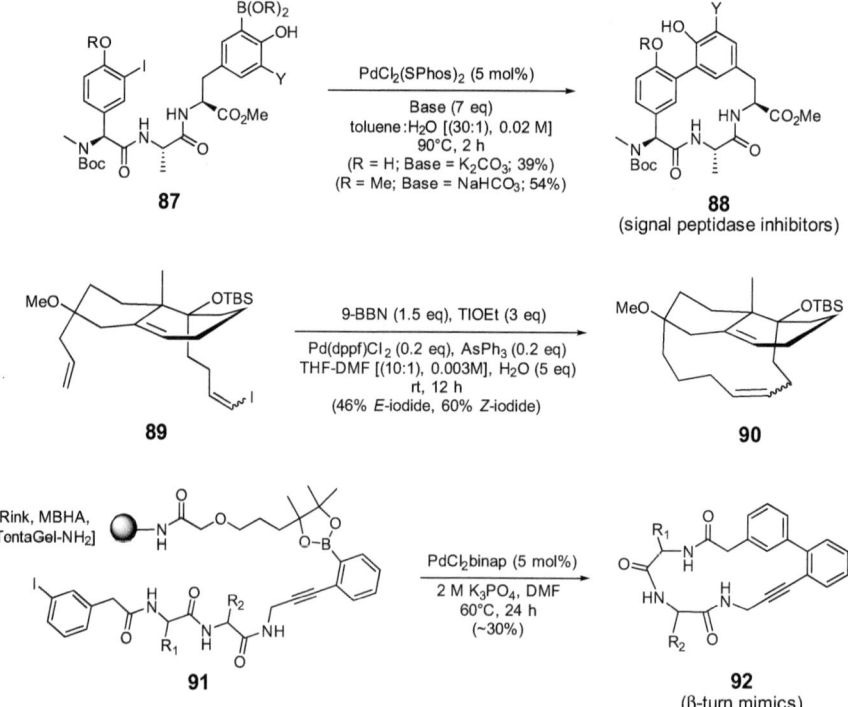

Scheme 11.9 Suzuki reactions for macrocyclic structures.

This process can also be readily performed on resin supports. For the preparation of biaryl β-turn mimetics on the solid phase, a specific linker was designed for facilitating a simultaneous Suzuki coupling, macrocyclization and resin release process (Scheme 11.9).[196] This gave only modest yields of the desired products (**92**) likely due to the strain induced by the biaryl moiety in this system. In a final example that supports this conclusion, microwave heating was used to facilitate intramolecular Suzuki–Miyaura cross-coupling of aryl iodides and boronic esters situated on amino acid side chains in order to construct biaryl cyclic peptidomimetics containing from 3–8 amino acid residues in only 23–35% purified yields.[197]

11.7.1.2 Heck

In instances where a functionalized aromatic moiety is desired in the target structure, the Heck reaction of an aryl/vinyl halide/triflate with an alkene in the presence of a palladium catalyst and base is an obvious choice and, indeed, has found application in the macrocycle arena. The first demonstration of a Pd(0) process on the solid phase actually involved Heck chemistry and was directed toward the synthesis of small libraries containing 20- to 24-membered macrocycles (**94**, Scheme 11.10).[198] Analogous procedures were employed for the assembly of macrocyclic RGD mimetics[199,200] and β-turn mimics (**97**, Figure 11.12, site of reaction and palladium species employed indicated)[201] on the solid phase. For these conversions, it was postulated that an intramolecular hydrogen bond in the precursor assisted in the formation of the cycle.

In additional applications, this methodology has been employed in solution to provide angiogenesis inhibitors (**96**, Scheme 11.10).[202] a key intermediate for the synthesis of HCV protease inhibitors (**98**, Figure 11.12,

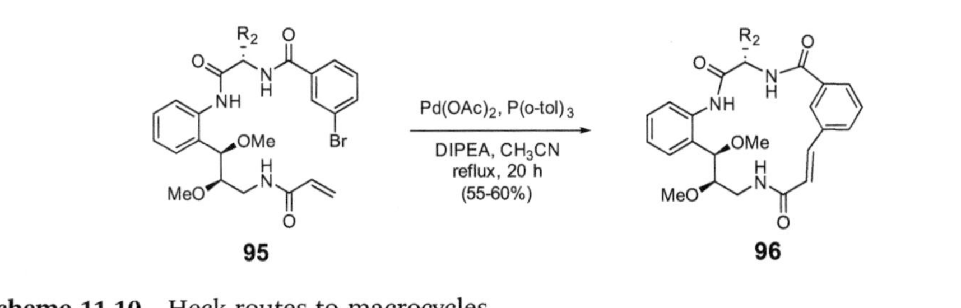

Scheme 11.10 Heck routes to macrocycles.

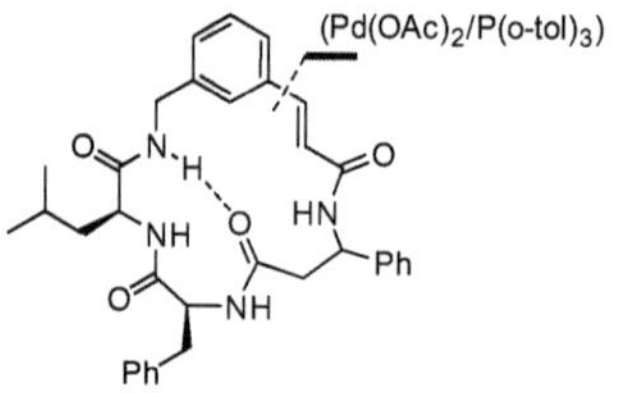

97 (β-turn mimic)

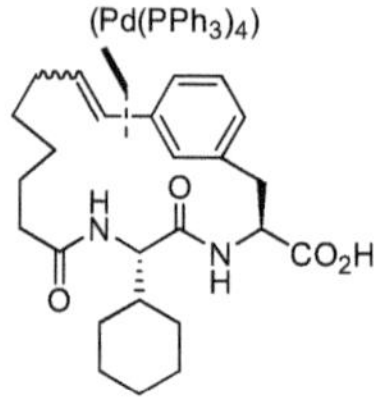

98 (HCV protease inhibitor intermediate)

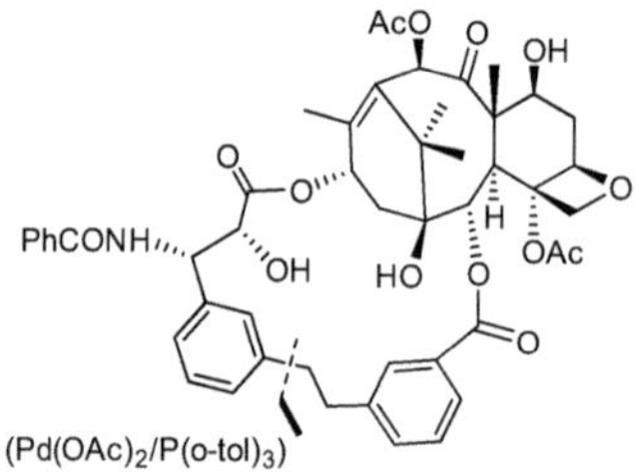

99 (macrocyclic taxoid)

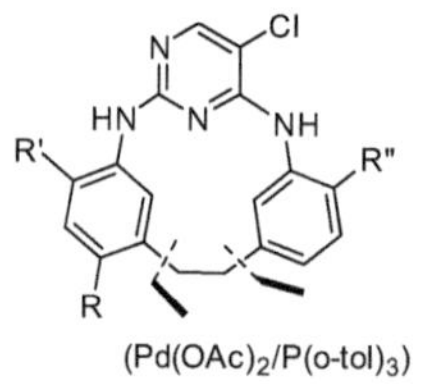

100 (ALK inhibitors)

Figure 11.12 Macrocyclic structures assembled with the Heck reaction.

site of reaction and palladium species employed indicated),[203] and several macrocyclic taxoid analogues, the latter exemplified by **99**.[204,205] In particular, these latter molecules dramatically demonstrate the complexity of substrates that the intramolecular Heck coupling can accommodate. For these taxoid structures, an alternative RCM strategy proved more sluggish.[206] Microwave heating has been reported to be useful in accelerating both solution and solid phase Heck reactions to form peptidomimetic macrocycles.[207] This procedure was also used to facilitate an intramolecular Heck reaction that was the key step in the exploration of macrocyclic inhibitors (**100**) of anaplastic lymphoma kinase (ALK).[208] The coupling proceeded equally well regardless of the ring location of the reacting vinyl and halide functionalities (indicated in the Figure by the alternative reaction sites). These molecules were designed based upon linear inhibitors, but were found to possess higher kinome selectivity while retaining the ALK inhibitory activity of their acyclic progenitors.

11.7.1.3 Stille

Another palladium-catalysed process that has proven utility for cyclic structures is the Stille coupling between organostannanes and aryl or vinyl halides/triflates.[209] Specifically for the macrocyclic framework, this chemistry was applied to the preparation of cyclic trienes (**102**) with defined geometry (Scheme 11.11) that were intermediates for transannular Diels-Alder reactions.[210] The intramolecular Stille reaction also has been efficiently conducted on solid phase to form **104**, an advanced intermediate in the synthesis of (*S*)-zearalenone, from **103** by a cyclization-release strategy.[211]

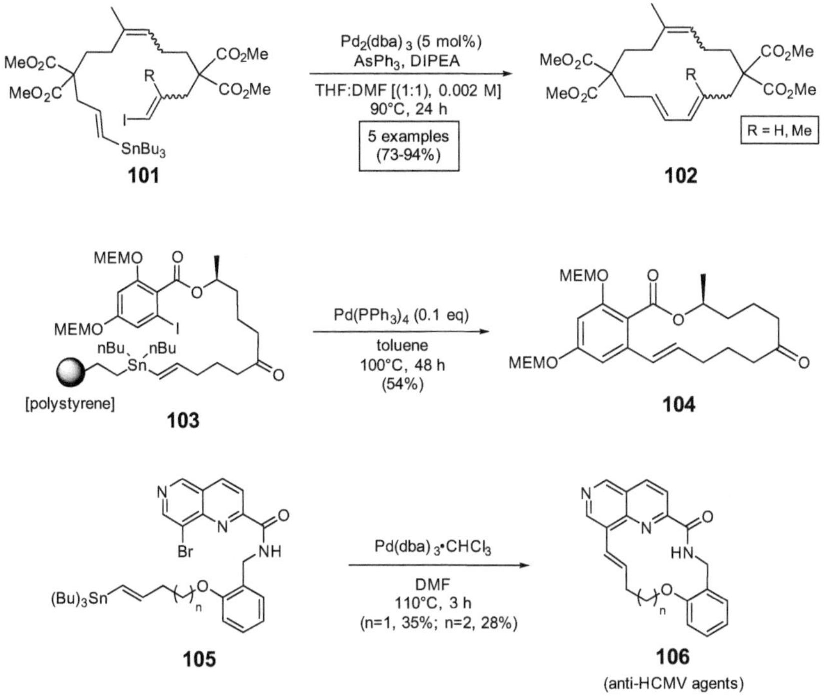

Scheme 11.11 Stille couplings for macrocyclic structures.

As another example of Stille chemistry directed towards macrocycles, 1,6-naphthyridines (**106**) were constructed from active acyclic precursors **105** (Scheme 11.11) based on the crystal structure, which revealed a proximity between substituents on the naphthyridine and phenyl rings.[212] The antiviral activity of the 14- and 15-membered cyclic compounds proved to be 25- to 150-fold higher than the linear counterpart against human cytomegalovirus (HCMV) strains with one analogue 450-fold better versus ganciclovir-resistant isolates with a selectivity index of 3000.

11.7.1.4 Sonogashira

The Sonogashira reaction of a terminal alkyne and an aryl or vinyl halide/triflate in the presence of palladium catalyst and a copper co-catalyst has become a powerful method for the formation of new carbon-carbon bonds.[213] The application of this reaction to the synthesis of macrocycles for drug discovery has to date been sparse, although its use for rigid core, shape-persistent macrocycles for supramolecular and materials chemistry, is well-established.[214] Nonetheless, some relevant pharmaceutical chemistry examples have been reported. A detailed investigation of the Sonogashira coupling for the assembly of macrocyclic peptidomimetics found that applying standard conditions for the transformation led only to dimer.[215] However,

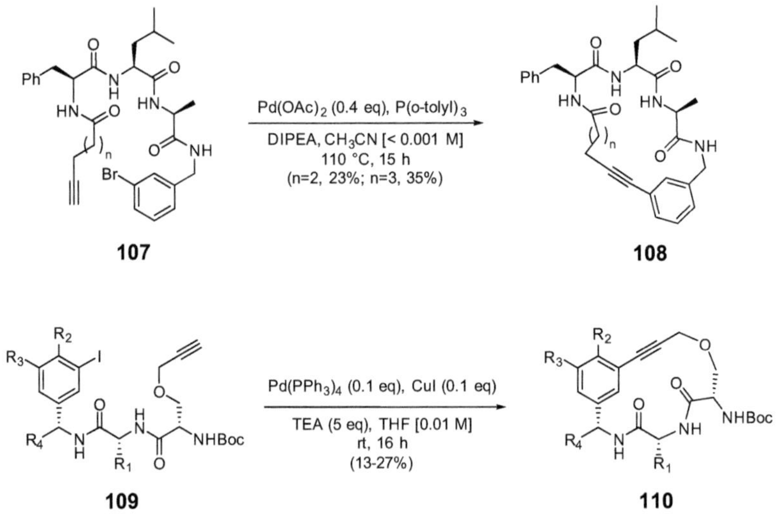

Scheme 11.12 Sonogashira chemistry for macrocyclic peptidomimetics.

utilization of a copper-free procedure did prove effective in providing the desired macrocycles (**108**) in low to moderate yields (Scheme 11.12). The process was sensitive to the number of residues, the steric demands of the amino acid side chains and the chain length attached to the alkyne.

In another study involving similar cyclic peptidomimetics, a Sonogashira approach was compared to macrolactamization, but proceeded to give the products (**110**) in lower yields (13–27% *vs.* 54–61%).[216] This route to macrocycles can also be effectively executed on the solid phase and is suitable for much larger rings, as was demonstrated in the synthesis of a constrained mimic of an immunoglobulin loop domain containing 65 atoms in the ring.[217] Lastly, simple macrolactones have been synthesized using primarily Sonogashira coupling for ring closure.[218]

11.7.1.5 Buchwald–Hartwig

Although one of the more recent additions to the armamentarium of these palladium-catalysed reactions, the Buchwald–Hartwig cross-coupling of amines with aryl halides already has found applications in macrocycle synthesis. In the first example, Iqbal *et al.* used this coupling as the cyclization step in the synthesis of constrained tri- or tetra-peptidomimetics with a biaryl linker (Scheme 11.13 illustrates a tripeptidomimetic (**112**)).[219] Fair to moderate yields were obtained for products containing 16- to 22-membered rings.

More complex aminobenzamides, **114**, designed as Hsp90 inhibitors were accessed using this transformation as the key ring-forming step in poor to excellent yields (15–93%) for 11- to 14-membered macrocycles.[220–223] The best of these molecules not only displayed good binding and functional activity, but also high solubility and an acceptable microsomal stability profile.

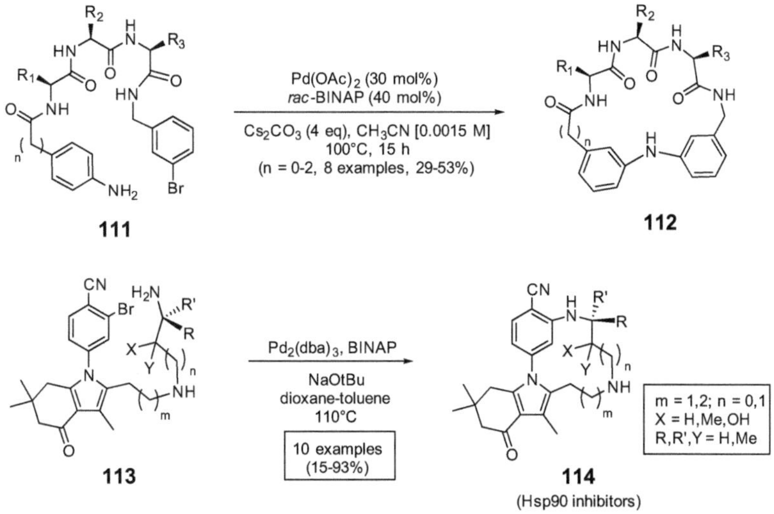

Scheme 11.13 Macrocycles from Buchwald–Hartwig reactions.

11.7.1.6 Additional Palladium-mediated Approaches

In addition to the success just described with the well-known "named" processes, a number of other macrocyclization reactions mediated by palladium complexes have been reported. The first of these approaches exploits the established chemistry of palladium π–allyl complexes for use in activation towards reaction with nucleophiles. This reaction was employed by Harran *et al.* as a critical step in the construction of a series of macrocycles such as **116** (*via* **115**) designed to significantly reduce the peptidic character of known active peptides (Scheme 11.14).[224] The approach tolerates a variety of functionality, including alcohols, amides, thioethers and selected heteroaromatics, and was also successfully conducted on solid support.

Similarly, this laboratory has recently described the synthesis of constrained peptidomimetics (**118**, Scheme 11.14) *via* intramolecular palladium-catalysed cinnamylation of a variety of amino acid side chains containing heteroatom nucleophiles (**117**, XH = amine, imidazole, phenol, carboxy).[225] This procedure is remarkable for its scope and efficiency, proceeding rapidly and in high yield independent of the nature of the residues and chain length of the peptide. Further, protection of guanidine, alcohol and amide side chains was not required. These and similar templates would appear to be quite suitable for library investigations.

As another example leading to novel conformationally restricted peptidomimetics, a Pd-catalysed enyne cycloisomerization was described as a route to macrocyclic diene structures (**119**, Figure 11.13, site of ring closure and palladium species indicated).[226] Subsequent [4+2] cycloadditions with dienophiles then gave the target molecules. An interesting application of the use of palladium catalysis in macrocyclization was reported by Barnickel and

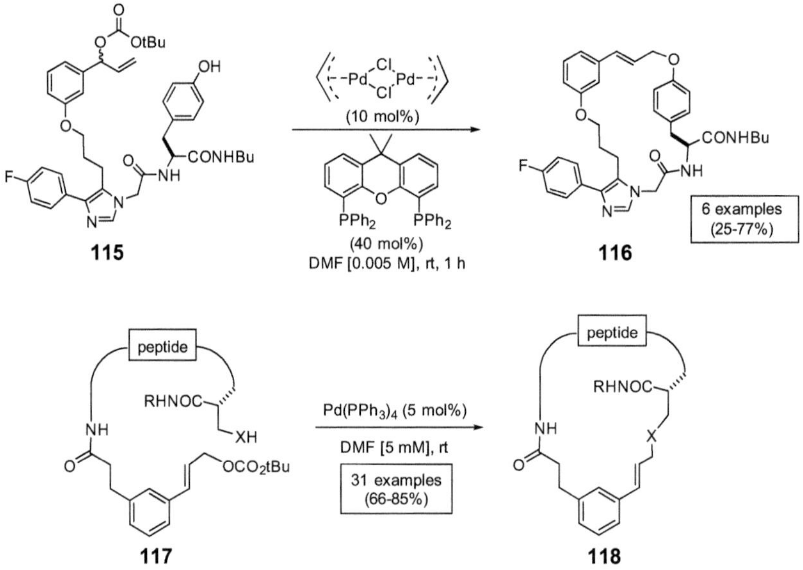

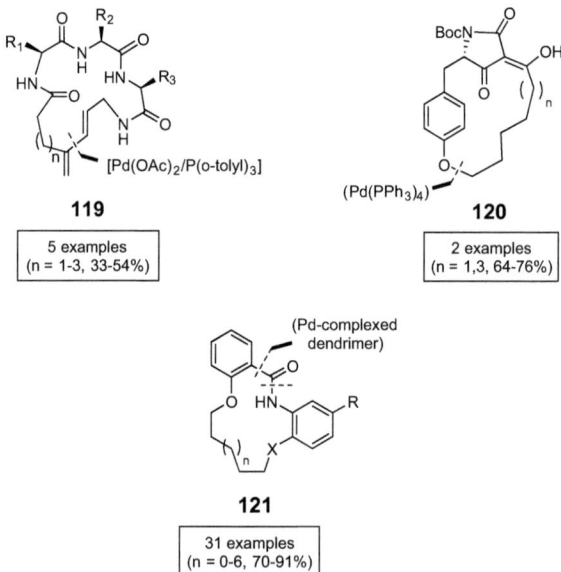

Scheme 11.14 Other palladium-mediated reactions for macrocyclic structures.

Figure 11.13 Selected macrocyclic compounds from palladium-mediated chemistry.

Schobert for a deallylation–etherification sequence.[227] Treatment of acyl tetramic acids, containing allyl protection on the phenol, with base in the presence of $Pd(Ph_3)_4$ promoted both removal of the allyl and ring closure by reaction with a primary bromide to give macrocycles **120** in good yields.

However, this process did fail for the 20-membered ring $(n = 5)$ target. Since material lacking the allyl group did not undergo cyclization with the catalyst, palladium was clearly required for ring closure, but the exact mechanism remains unclear.

Intramolecular carbonylation catalysed by palladium has been explored for the construction of macrolactams, including fused tricyclic systems (**121**, Figure 11.13, site of ring closure and palladium species indicated)[228] and rigidified RGD analogues (**123**, Scheme 11.15).[229] This latter transformation has also been effectively performed on the solid support,[230] while the former

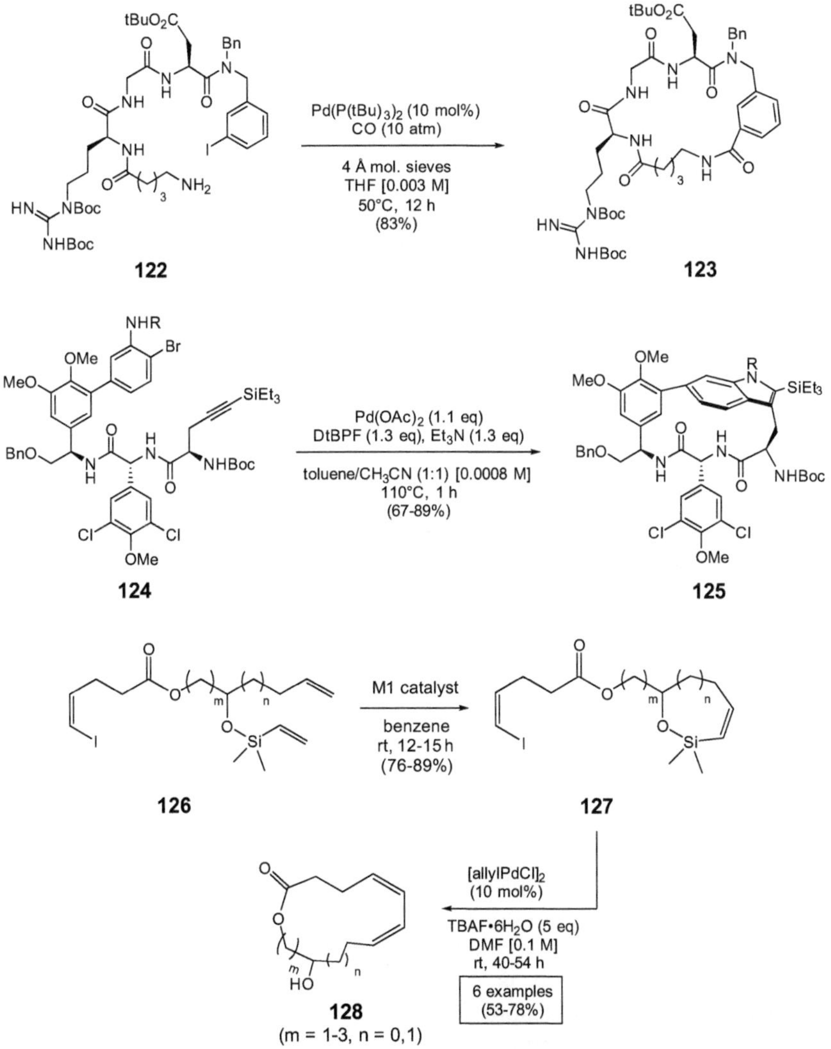

Scheme 11.15 Additional routes to macrocyclic compounds using palladium complexes.

used a supported reagent. In that study, for making **121**, palladium-complexed dendrimers on silica gel were utilized to facilitate the carbonylation and subsequent cyclization, which was found to give very good yields of 12- to 18-membered ring products. The process tolerated a variety of electron-donating and electron-withdrawing moieties on the phenyl ring, as well as the presence of sulphur, but did require higher temperatures (120 °C) for bromide substrates. The second investigation utilized homogeneous palladium catalysis and also gave high yields of the desired macrocycles (**123**) after systematic optimization of reaction conditions.

The Boger laboratory has reported on studies directed toward the total synthesis of chloropeptins, natural products which display anti-HIV activity through inhibition of gp 120-CD4 binding, that relied on the use of an intramolecular Larock indole synthesis to effect macrocyclization of **124** to give **125** (Scheme 11.15, DtBPF (1,1'-bis(di-*tert*-butylphosphino)ferrocene).[231] Subsequent detailed investigations resulted in further improvements in the optimal conditions for the transformation, which also has the potential to provide a route to complex ring systems in *de novo* macrocycles.[232]

In a final example, Denmark has described a detailed study on a tandem RCM/Si-assisted Pd cross-coupling reaction sequence that led to unsaturated macrolactones **128** (Scheme 11.15) through the intermediacy of siloxane **127**.[233] The typically difficult 11- to 14-membered ring sizes could be accessed under the optimized conditions, which included a hydrated fluoride ion activator. High dilution conditions were not required and this process was adapted to provide benzo-fused products as well.

11.7.2 Ruthenium-mediated Reactions

In addition to its critical role in RCM, ruthenium has been involved in other synthetic approaches to construct macrocyclic structures. For example, ruthenium π-arene chemistry was employed to facilitate the preparation of the biaryl ether moiety, the significance of which has been previously described in Section 11.3.2, for use as a β-turn mimic in **130**.[234,235] This was subsequently incorporated into HIV protease inhibitor **131** (Scheme 11.16).[236]

Similarly, key biphenyl intermediates **132** and **133** (Figure 11.14, site of ring closure and ruthenium species indicated) for the preparation of HCV NS3/4A protease inhibitors were accessed utilizing this particular cyclization methodology.[237–239] For these S_NAr reactions, the organometallic complex, typically prepared from $CpRu(CH_3CN)_3^+PF_6^-$, must be used in stoichiometric quantities in order to activate the ring to nucleophilic attack. In addition, the transformation needs to be conducted under high dilution conditions, while the Ru is subsequently removed by photolysis. This chemistry proceeds well despite these limitations and does provide access to a range of interesting compounds.

As another instance of a ruthenium-catalysed process, a macrocyclic taxoid, SB-T-2054 (**134**), was prepared from an unexpected diene-coupling reaction

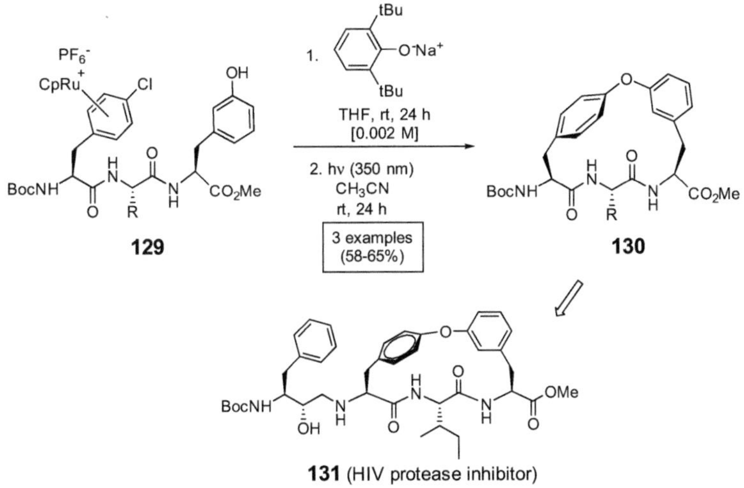

Scheme 11.16 Non-RCM ruthenium-mediated process for macrocycles.

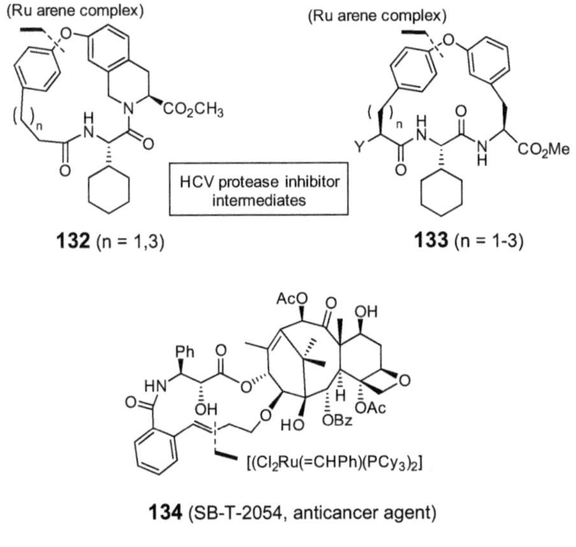

Figure 11.14 Macrocycles from Ru-mediated reactions.

that occurred instead of RCM as for analogous substrates (Figure 11.14, ring closure site and ruthenium catalyst noted).[240] This compound exhibited cytotoxic and microtubule-stabilizing activity similar to paclitaxel.

11.7.3 Nickel-mediated Reactions

Besides palladium and ruthenium, a number of other metal species have had an impact on the synthesis of macrocyclic compounds. In a first, albeit

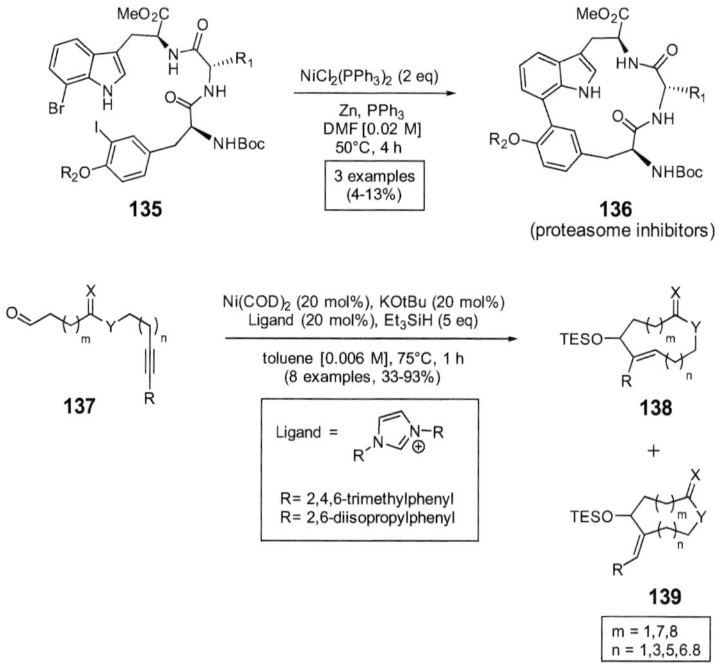

Scheme 11.17   Macrocycles from nickel-catalysed reactions.

non-scintillating due to poor yields, example, for nickel-mediated cyclization, analogues (**136**) of the proteasome inhibitor TMC-95A were constructed
from the linear bis(aromatic) dihalide **135** (Scheme 11.17).[241] This transformation could not be accomplished with multiple variations of Suzuki
coupling and, with this particular chemistry, failed with a number of substrates and gave low yields even when it succeeded.

   More successful results were obtained in the nickel-catalysed reductive
cyclization of ynals **137** to macrocyclic allylic alcohols with 14- to 22-mem-
bered rings (Scheme 11.17).[242] This reaction can provide both endocyclic
(**138**) and exocyclic (**139**) alkenes depending upon the ligand employed, the
nature of the alkyne (terminal or internal) and the reducing agent. The optimized process has been subsequently applied to the preparation of
modified macrolide structures.[243]

   In another example involving nickel, in this case as a co-catalyst, the use of
mixtures of PEG$_{400}$/MeOH as solvent enabled an intramolecular Glaser-Hay
coupling[244] of simple terminal alkynes (**140**) to form 14- to 27-membered
macrocyclic diynes (**141**, Scheme 11.18) to be conducted at comparatively
high concentrations (up to 0.1 M). This was attributed to the aggregation
properties of the PEG preferentially solubilizing the organic substrates, thus
creating a phase separation from the copper–nickel catalyst system.[245] The
approach led to a 5-fold increase in yield for the process, while use of a
PEGylated version of TMEDA as a ligand was found to exert similar effects.

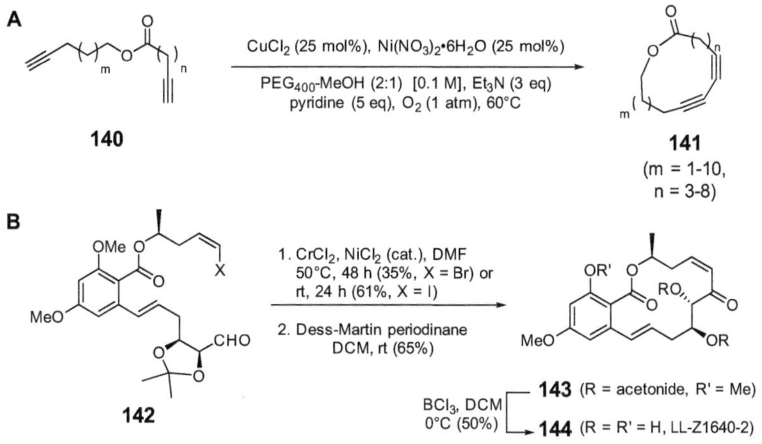

A

140

CuCl$_2$ (25 mol%), Ni(NO$_3$)$_2$•6H$_2$O (25 mol%)

PEG$_{400}$-MeOH (2:1) [0.1 M], Et$_3$N (3 eq)
pyridine (5 eq), O$_2$ (1 atm), 60°C

141
(m = 1-10,
n = 3-8)

B

142

1. CrCl$_2$, NiCl$_2$ (cat.), DMF
   50°C, 48 h (35%, X = Br) or
   rt, 24 h (61%, X = I)

2. Dess-Martin periodinane
   DCM, rt (65%)

BCl$_3$, DCM
0°C (50%)

143 (R = acetonide, R' = Me)

144 (R = R' = H, LL-Z1640-2)

Scheme 11.18 (A) Glaser–Hay and (B) Nozaki–Hiyama–Kishi routes to macrocycles.

In addition, microwave irradiation accelerated this transformation by at least 8-fold. Additives, in particular a quinolinium salt, were found to facilitate the intramolecular reaction of diynes that would not otherwise macrocyclize, apparently through an intermolecular noncovalent π-cation/arene interaction.[246] It is noteworthy that RCM also can be assisted with such additives. These studies have positioned the Glaser-Hay reaction for investigation in the preparation of macrocycles from more complex substrates.

As a final example, again with nickel as a co-catalyst, the Nozaki–Hiyama–Kishi coupling[247] between a carbonyl compound and a halide promoted by chromium (II)/nickel (II) has been widely employed in total synthesis, including for cyclic natural products.[248,249] This is illustrated by the preparation of the selective kinase inhibitor, LL-Z1640-2 (144), which used this reaction as a late step.[250] Extension to the *de novo* synthesis of macrocycles has to date been lacking. However, the mild reaction conditions, chemoselectivity and compatibility with a variety of nucleophiles provide significant advantages, so it certainly warrants investigation in that regard. However, the toxicity of chromium plus the need for high amounts of the metal are detriments.

11.7.4   Other Organometallic Reactions

In addition to the ruthenium S$_N$Ar chemistry discussed in Section 11.7.2, an analogous copper-assisted S$_N$Ar cyclization reaction of a boronic acid and a phenol has been reported to construct biaryl ethers 146 (Scheme 11.19).[251] Specifically, this functionality was then incorporated into MMP inhibitors. The mild conditions were shown to tolerate amides and esters in the substrate, although the presence of an additional phenol resulted in only trace product. Some other transformations involving copper mediation are presented in Section 11.8.

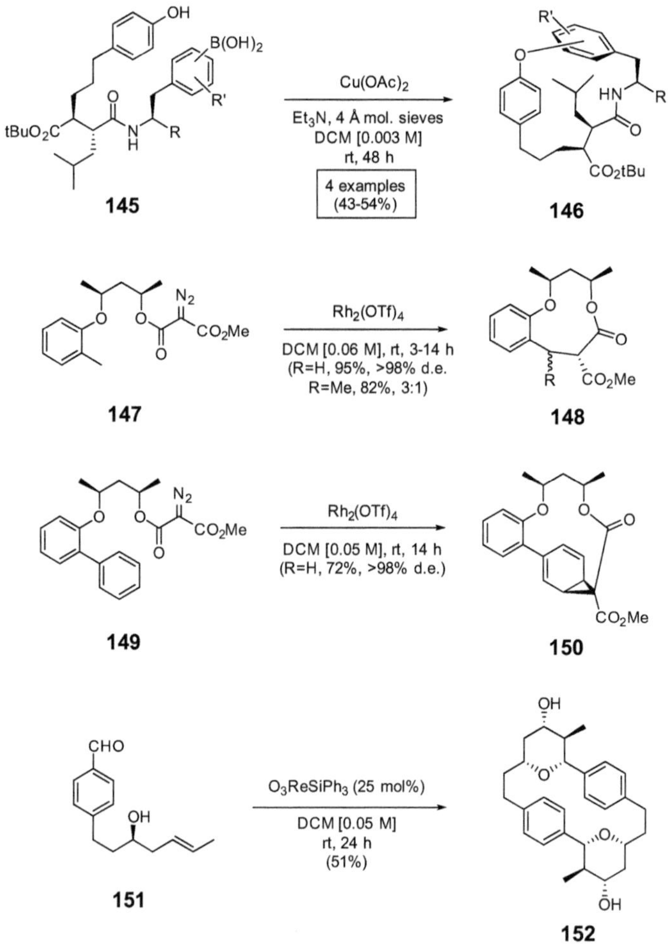

Scheme 11.19   Other metal-mediated routes to macrocyclic structures.

As another example, rhodium complexes are extremely useful for catalysing the addition of carbenes. In work on the stereocontrol of an intramolecular version of such a process, some small macrocycles with 10- and 13-member ring sizes, for example **148** and **150**, respectively, were constructed with excellent diastereoselectivity and good yields (Scheme 11.19).[252]

In a final example, again with a transition metal, rhenium (VII) catalysts were found to be effective for a tandem Prins dimerization–cyclization that provided a novel route to tetrahydropyran (THP)-containing macrocycles (**152**).[253] Intramolecular Prins reactions previously have been employed for natural product total synthesis, but this provides a route that is also amenable to *de novo* macrocycles. The difficult nature of this transformation is highlighted by the fact that the optimized conditions developed for the formation of **152** gave only a 28% yield of dimer product starting from the corresponding meta-isomer of **151** along with 13% of the trimer. Further, a related substrate, representing a model system for the natural product, clavosolide A, required reagent modification to triethylsilyl triflate-trimethylsilyl acetate in acetic acid for best results.

11.8 Cycloadditions

A methodology that has seen tremendous utility in modern medicinal chemistry is the [3+2]-cycloaddition of azides with alkynes, the Huisgen reaction, commonly referred to as "click" chemistry due to its facile nature.[254–256] The transformation is typically conducted in the presence of copper (I), although variants with other metal ions, or even no metal, have also been successfully employed. In particular, this chemistry has found application in the design and synthesis of macrocyclic peptidomimetic structures,[257,258] such as β–strand (**154**, Scheme 11.20)[259] and β-turn[260,261] mimics, although examples of non-peptidic molecules from this chemistry have also been reported (**157**, Figure 11.15, site of reaction indicated).[262,263] One drawback to the approach is its often low yields due to the strong tendency to form dimers or other oligomeric products, sometimes in preference to the monomeric products. However, this propensity also can be beneficial for the formation of novel bioactive structures, such as the Grb SH2 domain binding ligand **158** (Figure 11.15), which bound with 100-fold greater affinity than the corresponding monomer.[264]

For this cycloaddition, it has been found that monomer formation can be enhanced through the addition of a copper-chelating ligand, such as tris(benzyltriazolylmethyl)amine (TBTA).[265] Recently, detailed studies of the reaction resulted in the development of optimized conditions, including the use of TBTA as an additive, which have been successful in minimizing side

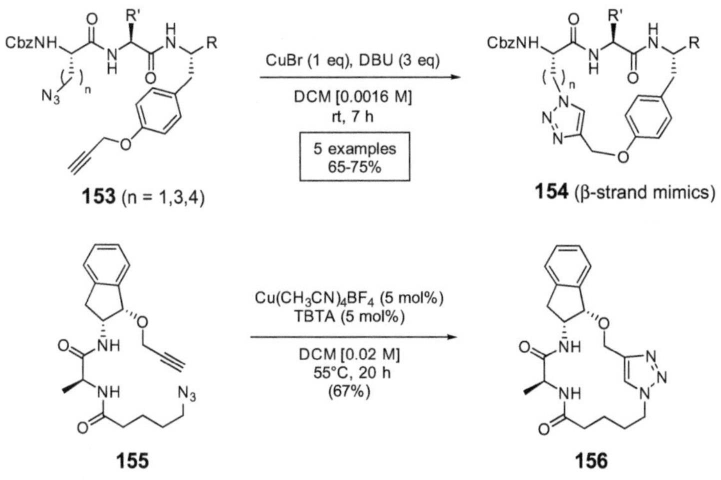

Scheme 11.20 Click chemistry for preparing macrocycles.

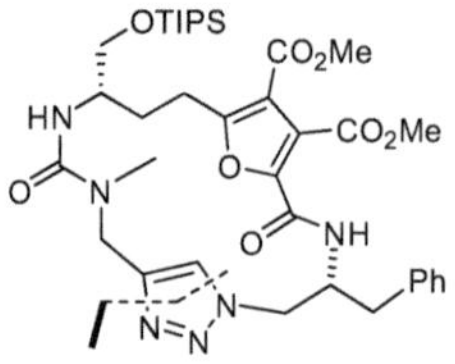

157

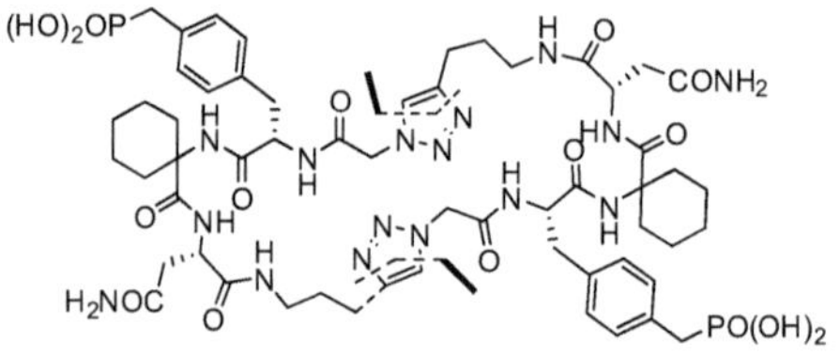

158 (Grb2 SH2 domain-binders)

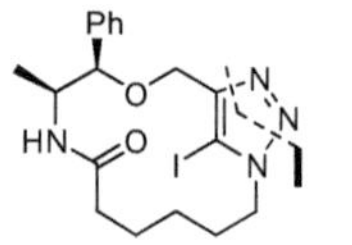

159 (library template)

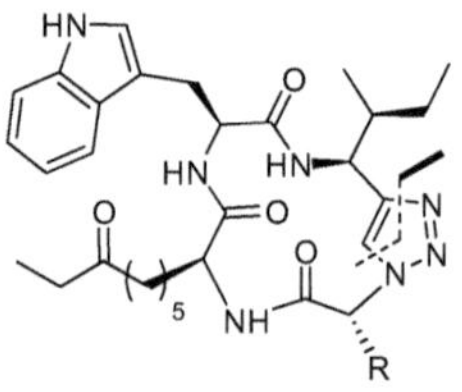

160 (HDAC inhibitors)

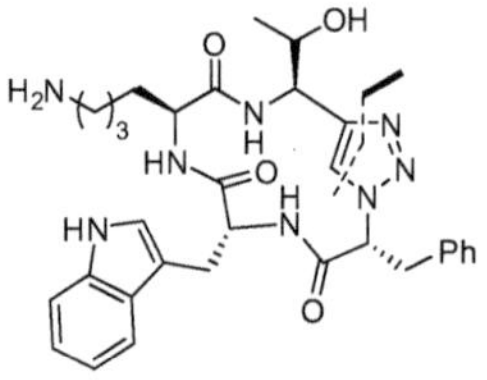

161 (sst receptor ligands)

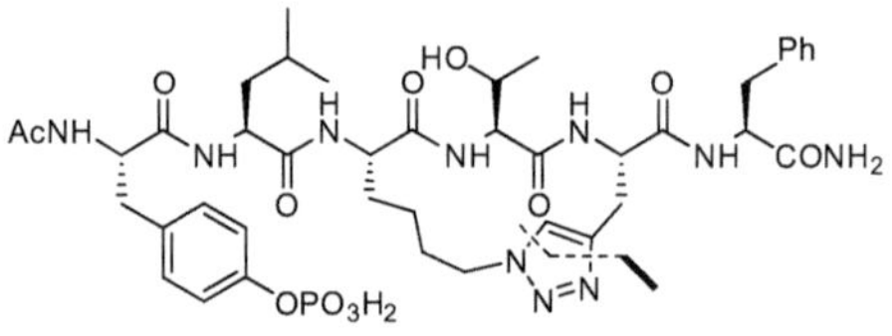

162 (STAT3 inhibitor)

Figure 11.15   Representative macrocyclic compounds from cycloaddition reactions.

products and maximizing conversions to cyclic products, **156** as an example, up to 24-membered ring size in yields of 45–95% (representative reaction shown in Scheme 11.20).[266] This procedure also has been executed on solid phase to create modified peptidic structures.[267] Further, the process can be conducted efficiently under flow conditions as was demonstrated for the formation of a series of macrocyclic 5-iodo-1,2,3-triazole-containing library templates such as **159** (Figure 11.15).[268] These 12- to 31-membered ring systems could then be further converted into a number of additional analogues using palladium-mediated cross-coupling reactions.

Most importantly, a variety of biologically active macrocycles have been constructed using this cycloaddition strategy, including HDAC inhibitors (**160**, Figure 11.15, cyclization site indicated),[269] Smac (second mitochondria-derived activator of caspase) mimetics,[270] somatostatin (sst) receptor ligands (**161**),[271] viral protease inhibitors,[272] and signal transducer and activator of transcription 3 (STAT3) inhibitors (**162**).[273]

The azide-alkyne cycloaddition can also be effected by ruthenium (II) complexes, specifically [Cp*RuCl]$_4$ (Cp* = 1,2,3,4,5-pentamethylcyclopentadiene), as has been demonstrated for monocyclic[274] and bicyclic vancomycin

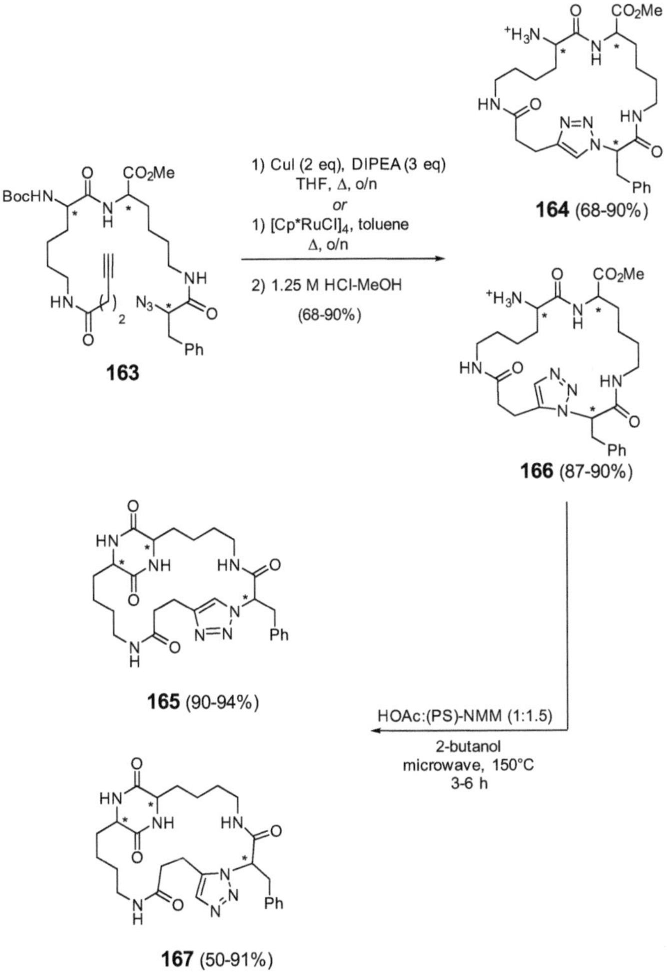

Scheme 11.21 More cycloaddition chemistry for preparing macrocycles.

mimetics.[275] The Ru(II)-mediated process resulted in 1,5-triazoles, while Cu(I) gave 1,4-triazoles from the same substrates. This reaction provided a key step in a diversity-oriented synthesis (DOS) of macrocyclic peptidomimetics reported by Spring and co-workers (Scheme 11.21).[276] In this work, a regioselective cycloaddition in the presence of either a copper (I) salt or a ruthenium (II) complex to provide the 1,4- or 1,5-triazoles **164** and **166** (* indicates all possible isomers at these stereocenters), respectively, was followed by formation of a diketopiperazine (DKP) within the resulting macrocyclic framework to give **165** and **167**. The latter reaction was found to proceed efficiently using polymer-supported N-methylmorpholine (PS-NMM) and microwave heating, which also improved the isolated yields significantly in most cases. This was successfully demonstrated on a small library of stereochemically diverse compounds, as well as on the construction of more rigid analogues with a phenyl ring replacing the methylene chain between the amide and DKP moiety as in **165** and **167**.

Another DOS approach, aimed towards multifunctional pyran-containing macrocycles represented by **169** (Scheme 11.22), relied on the tetra-butylammonium hydrogen sulphate-promoted cycloaddition of an azide onto an alkenone double bond.[277] The substrates for this transformation arise from an intermolecular azide-alkyne cycloaddition to create the initial triazole substrates (**168**). The subsequent macrocyclization provided 14- to 16-membered rings ($n = 0$–2) with the smaller sizes giving lowest yields, and with aromatic substitution having no discernible effect. Interestingly, the maximum yield of macrocycle was obtained at a relatively high (0.34 M) reaction concentration.

Relatively large cyclic RGD peptide mimics (**171**) were prepared using a different type of "click chemistry", the thiol-ene reaction,[278] which was conducted in solution or on solid support (Scheme 11.22).[279,280]

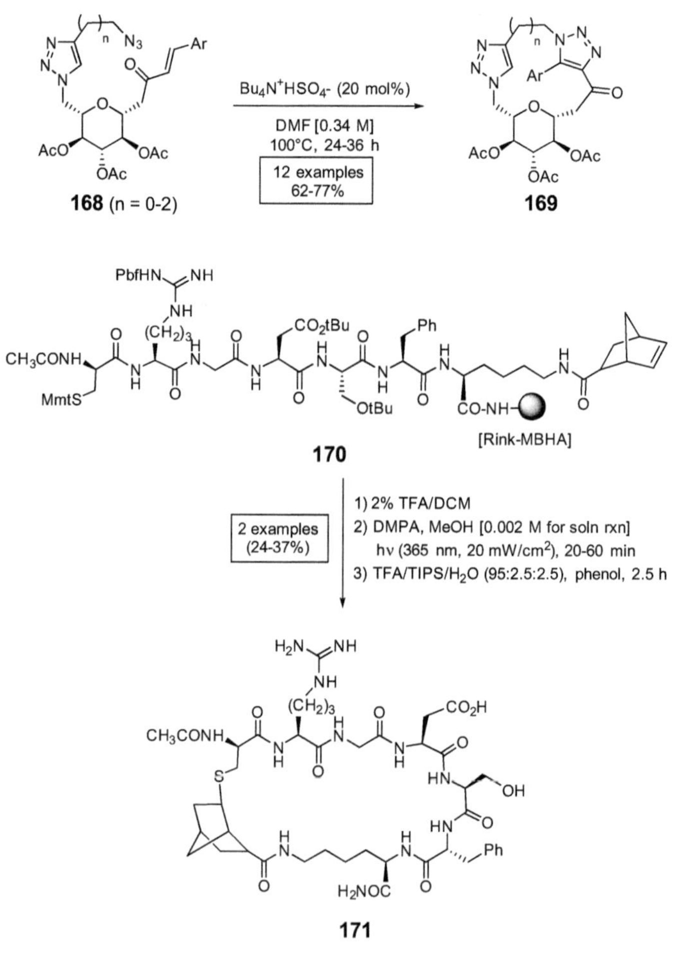

Scheme 11.22   Additional examples of cycloadditions to access macrocycles.

The cyclization itself can be promoted either photochemically (solid phase, shown) or thermally (solution). The reaction occurred rapidly and gave comparable or improved yields to other solid phase cyclization procedures. More recently, the thiol-ene cycloaddition was employed for the construction of cyclic peptides and peptoids, which could be subsequently conjugated to specific nucleosides and oligonucleotides for therapeutic or diagnostic purposes.[281] Applications relevant to drug discovery to date have been limited to these two examples, although the transformation has seen greater utility for molecular architecture investigations.[282]

Another [3+2]-cycloaddition process that has proven value in the construction of macrocyclic natural products, but has been underexplored to date for medicinal chemistry purposes, is the intramolecular addition of nitrile oxides (typically generated *in situ* from the corresponding oxime) with alkenes (Scheme 11.23). For example, this reaction has been employed for the conversion of oxime-acrylate **172** into **173**, an intermediate for the synthesis of the macrosphelide skeleton,[283] and for the construction of macrocycles useful in studies directed towards an asymmetric synthesis of brefeldin A.[284]

An alternative transformation in this class involved the generation of azomethine ylides from the decarboxylative condensation of amino acids, specifically proline, thiazolidine-4-carboxylic acid and sarcosine (not shown),

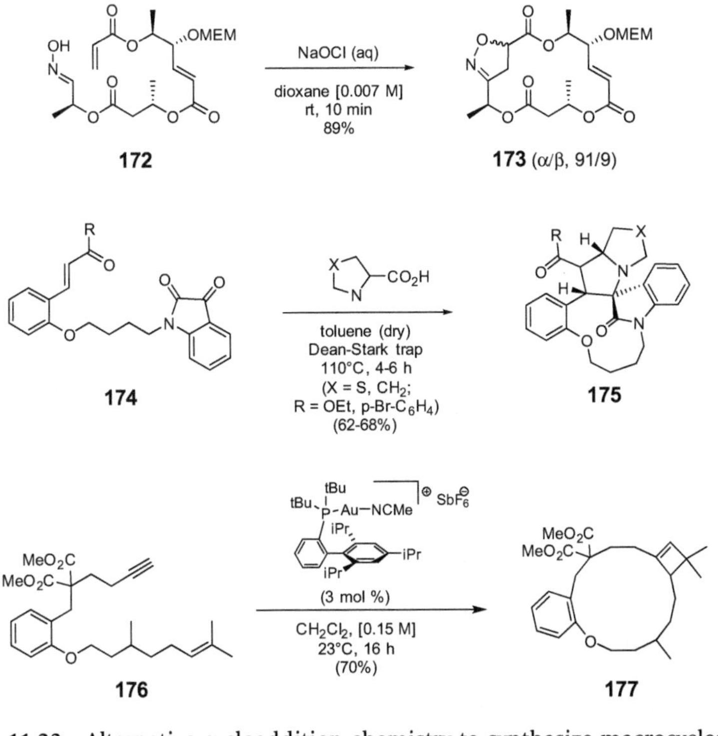

Scheme 11.23 Alternative cycloaddition chemistry to synthesize macrocycles.

with alkyl enones tethered to isatin (**174**, Scheme 11.23).[285,286] These ylides then underwent an intramolecular 1,3-dipolar cycloaddition with the enone moiety of **174** to form macrocyclic spiropyrrolidines (from sarcosine, not shown), spiropyrrolizidines or spiropyrrolothiazoles (**175**). This [3+2] process gave quite good yields particularly given the complexity of the compounds created.

In one last example of this type of reaction, a gold (I) organometallic complex has been utilized to catalyse the intramolecular [2+2]-cycloaddition of an alkene and alkyne, such as in **176**, to form 9- to 15-membered rings containing a cyclobutene moiety (for example **177**) in 20–70% yields (Scheme 11.23).[287] This reaction could be conducted at higher concentrations (as high as 0.45 M) than usual for such a process.

11.9 Multicomponent Reactions (MCR)

As methods were sought to enhance both the size and diversity of synthetic libraries, attention was directed to the general area of multicomponent reactions (MCR) due to their ability to create complex structures from simple substrates. In that regard, this chemistry, such as the Ugi, Biginelli, Passerini and Staudinger processes, has been rediscovered and applied to the search for new pharmaceutical entities.[288–290] These reactions have proven to provide very fruitful routes to libraries of compounds. However, only limited attention has been directed towards the potential of MCR for accessing the macrocyclic target class with these strategies.[291–294]

In a notable exception, Yudin has described the use of amphoteric aldehydes (**178**)[295] in an Ugi MCR with isonitriles and linear peptides (**179**) to prepare a series of modified peptidomimetic macrocycles (**180**) with ring sizes from 9 to 18 atoms (Scheme 11.24).[296] These compounds, *via* nucleophilic attack on the aziridine, also can be employed as intermediates for further reactions and, hence, provide access to additional structural diversity suitable for library production. Towards this end, the sequence was successfully transferred to an automated microfluidics platform.[297] The process did not need to be performed under high dilution conditions (0.2 M). More recently, this approach was applied successfully to the synthesis of bicyclic peptidomimetic derivatives, for example **181**, in which macrocyclization and then disulfide formation were best conducted in solution after the solid phase MCR to avoid side reactions.[298]

In another example, Kurth has reported the use of a novel three-component MCR (3CR) involving a Meldrum's acid-like substrate (**182**), an aldehyde equivalent (**183**) and a nitrile oxide (generated from the oxime **184**) in the assembly of spiromacrolactams (**185**, Scheme 11.32).[299] Similar results were observed with non-aromatic-containing counterparts of **182**. Generally, MCRs are conducted under fairly concentrated conditions to overcome entropic barriers. For this particular process, however, the use of a highly reactive, but transient, acyl ketene intermediate permitted short reaction times

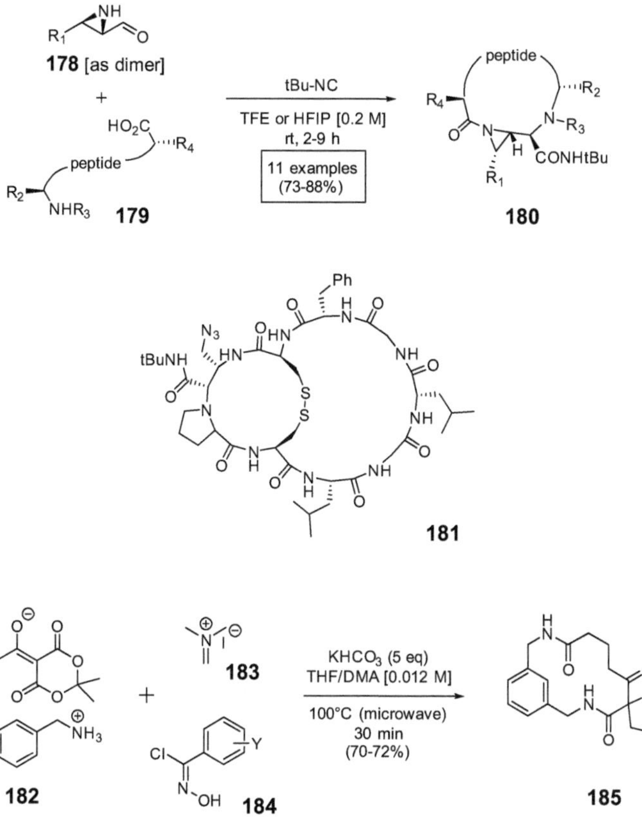

Scheme 11.24 Multicomponent reactions towards macrocycles.

even at higher dilution. Microwaves further facilitated the reaction, which proceeded in very good yields for 12- to 14-membered rings.

Although the direct use of MCR for the preparation of cyclic structures is possible as the preceding strategies amply demonstrate, such examples have been somewhat limited. However, exploiting the power of MCR in assembling complex frameworks from simpler precursors in tandem with a variety of other reactions for the construction of macrocycles has been more fruitful.[300]

In one of the initial such examples, Dömling and coworkers have reported both Ugi and Passerini-type MCR in concert with RCM.[301] The general approach is outlined in Scheme 11.25, with the linear precursor (**186**) obtained from the MCR then subjected to standard RCM to give the macrocyclic products **187** or **188**. In this manner, the representative 22-membered macrocycle (**189**) is produced from the Ugi four-component coupling reaction (4CR) of an acid, amine, isonitrile and paraformaldehyde. In a similar way, the exemplary 17-membered macrocycle (**190**) was prepared from the Passerini 3CR of an acid, aldehyde and isonitrile. Methods for the synthesis of the starting materials also needed to be developed to ensure sufficient

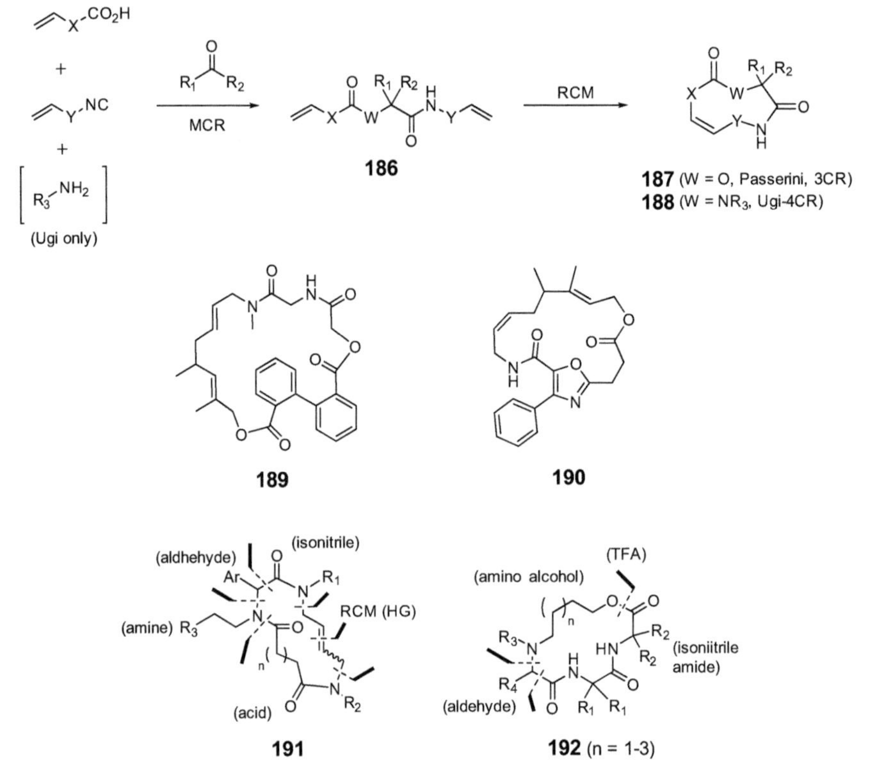

Scheme 11.25 Tandem processes for macrocycles involving MCR.

diversity could be incorporated using this process, which, particularly for the isonitrile component, can often be the case in the application of these MCR strategies.

For another application of such a tandem strategy, RCM together with Ugi 4CR was utilized in a diversity-oriented synthesis (DOS) approach suitable for small to medium ring sizes.[302] The 4CR constructs the basic framework of the structure, which, through a variety of additional transformations, can be converted to 12- to 16-membered macrocycles (for example **191**, Scheme 11.25, building block contributions to the molecule and RCM site and catalyst indicated).

In another type of tandem sequence, Zhu and co-workers have reported the synthesis of macrocyclic depsipeptides **192** that starts with the 3CR of α,α-disubstituted α-isocyanoacetamides, amino alcohols and aldehydes in the presence of ammonium chloride (Scheme 11.25, building block contributions to the molecule and cyclization site indicated).[303] The 14- to 16-membered target compounds are then formed from acid treatment of the intermediate 5-iminoisoxazolines. Evaluation of the scope indicated this sequence was quite general, and so has the potential to be applicable to the construction of macrodepsipeptide libraries.

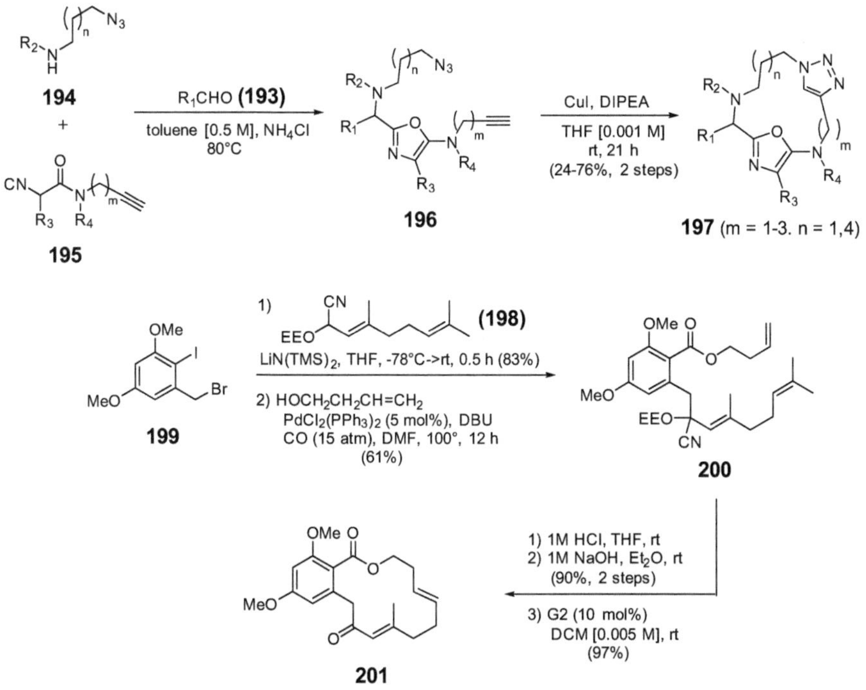

Scheme 11.26 Additional MCR tandem chemistry used to construct macrocycles.

Cycloaddition reactions also have been explored in tandem with MCR. A 3CR together with an azide-alkyne [3+2] cycloaddition has been described in an approach to functionalized macrocycles (Scheme 11.26).[304] Aldehydes (193), ω-azido-amines (194) and alkynylisocyanides (195) were used as components in the MCR to provide an intermediate 5-aminooxazole (196). This structural feature appears to rigidify and preorganize the linear molecule to the subsequent intramolecular cycloaddition. Indeed, substrates without the oxazole did not undergo cyclization, which confirmed its critical importance. The tandem process successfully gave macrocycles (197) with 14-, 15- and 16-membered rings in low to very good yield. Molecules prepared using this MCR-cycloaddition sequence have been shown to exhibit HDAC inhibitory activity.[305] This strategy and the combined MCR-RCM approaches described above would certainly appear amenable to the generation of macrocyclic libraries.

In one final tandem process, this aimed at a resorcylic acid lactone scaffold, which occurs in an established class of bioactive natural products, for example, the Hsp90 inhibitor, radicicol, and the estrogen agonist, zearalenone. The approach of Takahashi *et al.* was to employ a sequential three-component coupling strategy whereby an alkylation/carbonylation sequence was combined with RCM (Scheme 11.26).[306] Reversing the order of the initial steps was not successful. This synthetic approach can be conducted with minimal protection/deprotection sequences, although masking of the ketone as a cyanohydrin in **198** (EE = ethoxyethyl) avoided undesired iso-coumarin formation. In brief, the procedure involved alkylation of the cya-nohydrin with the benzyl bromide **199**, then the resulting product subjected to palladium-catalysed carbonylation-esterification to give **200**. After the subsequent RCM, the overall yield of the target macrolactone **201** was 44% from **199** using this protocol, which also has the potential to be applied more widely.

11.10   Ring Expansion/Opening

Although certainly not the most obvious approach to macrocyclic structures, ring expansion/ring opening chemistry provides an intriguing comple-mentary strategy to those already described.[307,308] In general for such pro-cesses, macrocycles can result from cleavage of appropriate bonds within multi-ring systems. Of course, such a strategy is often rather limited in scope as few systems can withstand the harsh reaction conditions that typically must be applied to break those bonds. Nonetheless, a Diels–Alder/ retro-Diels–Alder ring opening of steroidal precursors like **202** provided an interesting route to functionalized macrocyclic compounds **204** (Scheme 11.27). Importantly, this strategy was successful in preparing ap-proximately 500 macrocycles of general structure **205**[309,310] and also resulted in the identification of the phosphatase cdc25B inhibitor **206**.[311]

Ring expansion/opening reactions display particular success in con-structing smaller rings.[312] Indeed, it is one of the few approaches that pro-vides efficient access to such ring sizes. For example, the class of cyclic dopamine antagonists exemplified by the 10-membered ring azecine LE300 (**207**) can be synthesized using reductive opening of a quaternized multi-cyclic quinolizine precursor (Figure 11.16, site and reagents for bond breakage shown, broken bond dashed).[313] Similar procedures have been applied to generate a wide range of potent dopamine antagonists.[314–317]

Ring expansion likewise has proven applicable for some macrocycles, but is also restricted in scope. For example, construction of the scaffold for the

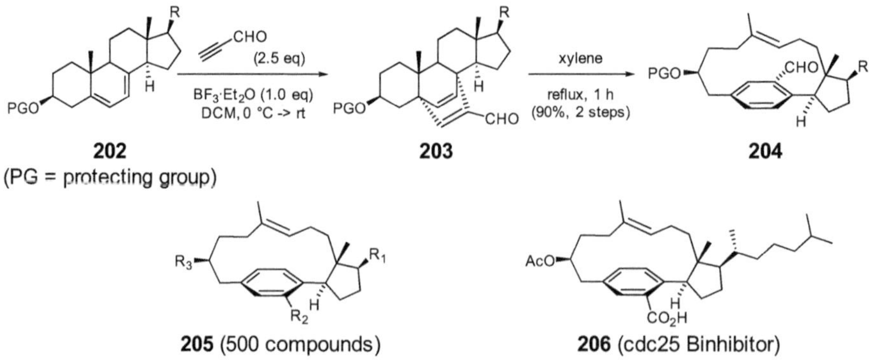

Scheme 11.27   Ring opening chemistry yielding macrocyclic products.

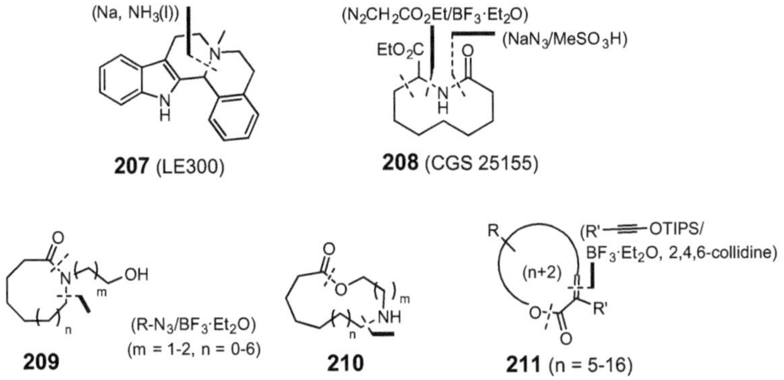

Figure 11.16 Selected macrocycles from ring expansion/ring opening.

neutral endopeptidase 24.11 inhibitor CGS 25155 (**208**) and related analogues was achieved utilizing two successive one atom ring expansions from cyclooctanone.[318] Subsequent transformations then resulted in the 10-membered ring target molecules (Figure 11.16, reagents for ring expansion noted). In another such process, nitrogen insertion/ring expansion of cyclic ketones provided either macrolactams (**209**) or macrolactones (**210**), with the relative proportions dependent on the ring size of the precursor and the pH of the reaction medium (Figure 11.16, reagents common for both products indicated).[319] The relative simplicity of these structures speaks clearly to the limitations of such approaches.

Similarly non-complex ring-expanded macrolactones **211** can be accessed from the reaction of acetals and electron-rich siloxyalkynes in the presence of a Lewis acid and an additive (Figure 11.16, reagents for reaction indicated).[320] This transformation, which is postulated to proceed *via* an initial intermediate oxetene formed by a [2+2] cycloaddition, is then followed by ring opening. This results in lactones possessing a ring two atoms larger than the precursor. It is noteworthy that this procedure works for a range of small to large ring sizes and that high dilution is not required, with the reaction occurring efficiently at 0.1 M. Indeed, most ring expansion and ring opening processes are insensitive to concentration, certainly much less so than many other macrocycle-forming reactions.

In a method aimed towards more complex molecules, which utilizes natural product macrocycles as substrates, the potential anti-parasitic compounds **213** were constructed from the precursor tetrapeptides **212** by reductive carbon–nitrogen bond cleavage of the pyrrolidine ring of proline with samarium iodide (Scheme 11.28).[321] The resulting structures are three atoms larger than the original macrocycle and provide an interesting avenue to create skeletal diversity. This process seems to be favoured by the strain caused by the fused 5-membered ring system in conjunction with the quaternary carbon on the larger ring. Such a hypothesis was confirmed in that molecules with a piperidine ring, or lacking the quaternary carbon, fail to undergo the transformation. Unfortunately, this same less flexible system

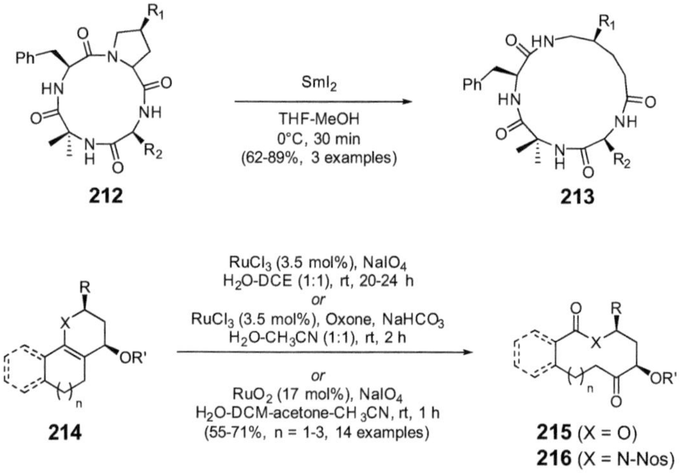

Scheme 11.28   Additional ring opening reactions for macrocycles.

appeared to be important for bioactivity as the ring-expanded compounds (**213**) displayed reduced or no desired anti-parasitic action.

Oxidative ring expansion has been utilized in a diversity-oriented synthesis approach to smaller ring macrocyclic compounds from polycyclic precursors such as **214** (Scheme 11.28).[322] These product structures are not able to be accessed through conventional macrolactamization/macrolactonization chemistry. A variety of oxidants can be used to break the internal double bond in **214** and prepare 10- to 12-membered macrolactones (**215**, X = O) or macrolactams (**216**, X = N-Nos), including analogues with a fused benzene ring. Not surprisingly, the optimal conditions were found to be dependent on the electronic nature of the substrate. This oxidative process, in contrast to alternative ring closure reactions, was not sensitive to the stereochemistry of the substrate and was shown to be efficient on gram scale. The conditions are mild enough that the reaction proceeds in the presence of latent functionalities, including protected alcohols, benzyl ethers and aryl iodides. Hence, the ring-opened products serve as effective scaffolds for access to diversity since they can be further converted through a variety of chemistries to additional macrocyclic compounds.

In another example suitable for smaller cycle sizes, 9- to 12-membered rings can be generated from vinylogous acyl triflates **217** through a reductive cyclization followed by ring expanding fragmentation (Scheme 11.29).[323] This is initiated by halogen–metal exchange to first provide intermediate **218**, which then undergoes carbon–carbon bond cleavage. The optimized conditions developed for the transformation produced the macrocycles in 39–95% yields. Either aryl or vinyl iodides are viable substrates for the reaction, although competing dehydroiodination can lower the yield with the latter. The ring-expanded products (**219**) contain several functionalities that offer opportunities for further structural diversification.

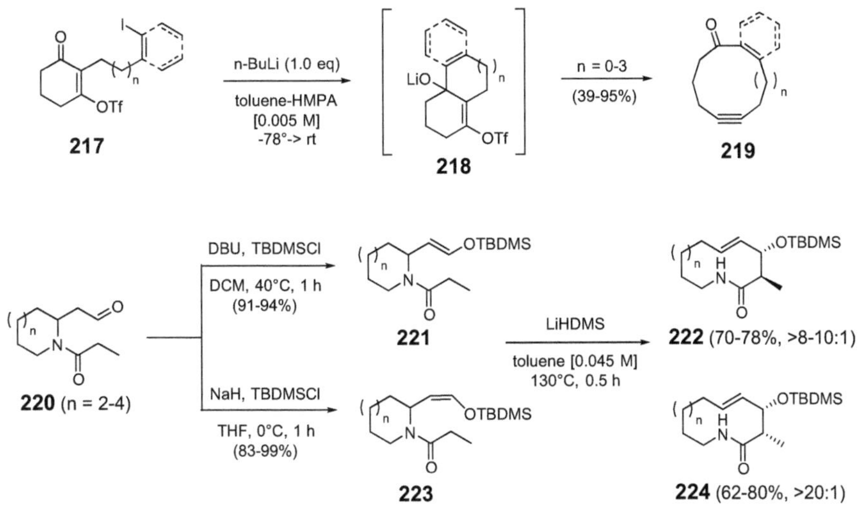

Scheme 11.29 Macrocyclic compounds from ring expansion chemistry.

In a final example of this type of process, functionalized macrolactams like **222** and **224** can be prepared through the ring expansion of smaller cyclic lactams *via* an aza-Claisen rearrangement (Scheme 11.29).[324] Highly stereoselective preparation of either the (*E*)- or (*Z*)-enol ether precursors from the aldehydes **220** was dictated by the choice of reactants with DBU at 40 °C. providing (*E*) and NaH at 0 °C. leading to (*Z*). Treatment with strong base facilitated the aza-Claisen and resulted in ring expansion, with the (*E*)-substrate leading to the *syn* stereoisomer (**222**, > 8–10 : 1), while the (*Z*)-isomer gave the *anti*-product (**224**, >20 : 1). In this manner, 7–10 membered starting lactams were efficiently converted to 11–14 atom macrolactams in very good yields (62–80%).

11.11   Reductive Amination

Reductive amination is another standard transformation that has been applied, although not yet widely, to macrocycle synthesis. For example, the synthesis of the series of BACE inhibitors represented by **227** was effected utilizing this reaction for cyclization of amino-aldehyde **225**. This was then followed by formation of the 2-amino-3,4-dihydroquinazoline ring from intermediate **226** (Scheme 11.30).[325] These products exhibited low nM potency with **227** found to reduce plasma levels of β-amyloid after oral dosing.

Analogously, the aspartic protease inhibitor **228** (Figure 11.17, site of reaction and reducing reagent indicated) was constructed *via* an intramolecular reductive amination.[326] In addition, multiple reductive aminations can be applied to assemble molecules such as the symmetrical G-quadruplex macrocyclic ligand BOQ1 (**229**)[327] and antiprotozoal polyazamacrocycles such as **230**.[328,329] For the latter, an iron (II) complex was employed as an intermediate to assist with the ring closure.

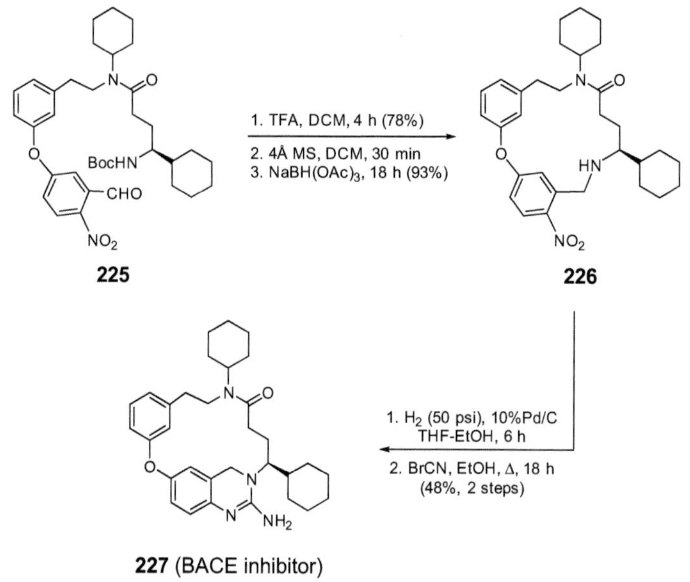
BocHN
CHO
NO2
225
1. TFA, DCM, 4 h (78%)
2. 4Å MS, DCM, 30 min
3. NaBH(OAc)3, 18 h (93%)
HN
NO2
226
1. H2 (50 psi), 10%Pd/C
THF-EtOH, 6 h
2. BrCN, EtOH, Δ, 18 h
(48%, 2 steps)
NH2
227 (BACE inhibitor)

Scheme 11.30 Reductive amination route to macrocycles.

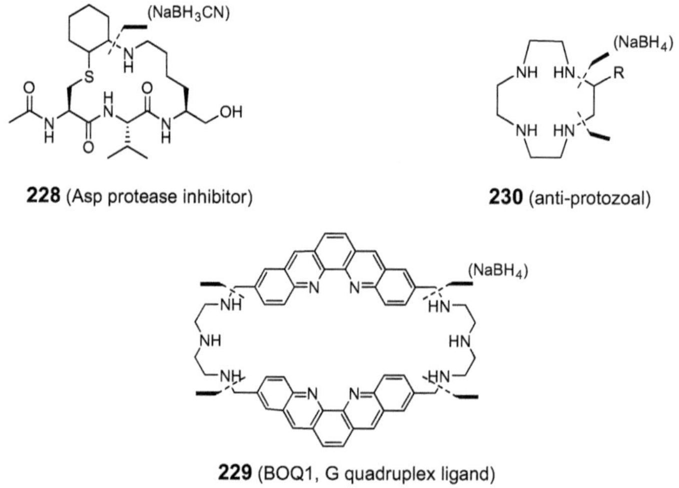
(NaBH3CN)
OH
228 (Asp protease inhibitor)
(NaBH4)
R
230 (anti-protozoal)
(NaBH4)
229 (BOQ1, G quadruplex ligand)

Figure 11.17 Macrocyclic compounds *via* reductive amination.

A double reductive amination was one of several approaches used to build macrocycles from diol precursors or their electrophilic derivatives (aldehydes, halides) described by Clausen (Figure 11.18, sites of reaction indicated).[330,331] Specifically, reaction of the bis-functionalized substrates with appropriate diactivated reagents were utilized to form cyclic carbonates (**231**), sulphites (**232**), phosphates (**233**), sulphides (**234**), amines (**235, 236**) and malonates (**237**) with ring sizes of 15–19 members. Although yields were

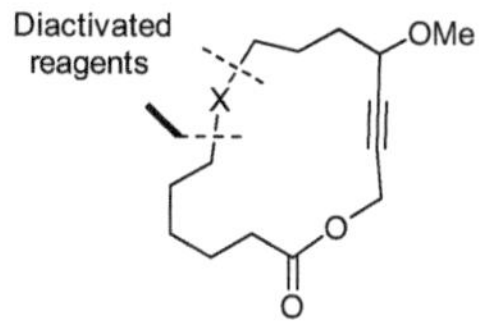

231 X= -OC(=O)O- (45%)
232 X= -OS(=O)O- (55%)
233 X= -OP(=O)(OPNP)O- (60%)
234 X= -S- (56%)
235 X= -NBn- (48%)

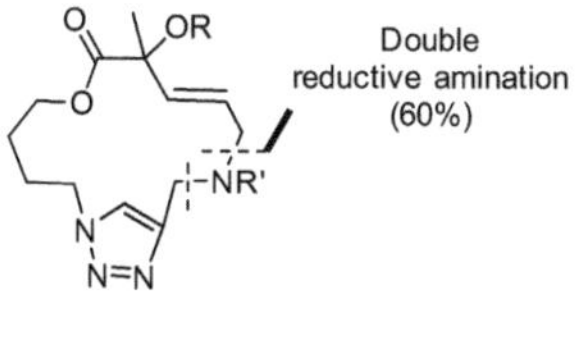

236 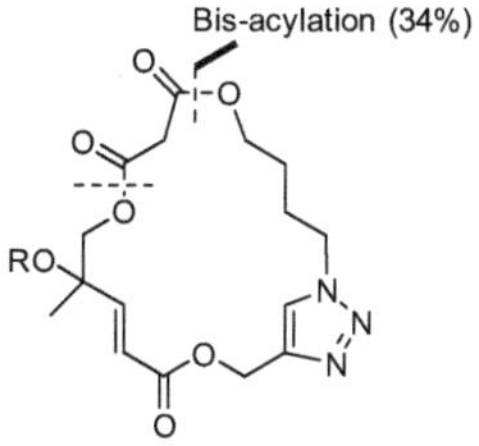 **237**

Figure 11.18 Macrocycles from bis-functionalized substrates.

generally modest, these sequences do provide a route to impart significant diversification to a single functionalized precursor.

11.12 Miscellaneous Methods

A number of other reaction methodologies have seen at least limited application to macrocyclic structures, although they have not yet been explored widely, so their overall utility remains to be determined. For example, in addition to the aza-Claisen ring expansion method described earlier in Section 11.10, another sigmatropic process, a novel oxy-oxonia Cope rearrangement, has been employed in a route to a series of simple macrocyclic compounds potentially useful as musks.[332] Treatment of dialdehyde substrates **238** with boron trifluoride etherate prompted the rearrangement to form the 14- to 18-membered macrocyclic products **239** ($n = 8$–12, Scheme 11.31), favouring the (Z)-stereoisomer by a ratio of $4:1$ to $99:1$. Smaller ring sizes failed to provide the desired macrocycle, as did alternative Lewis acids, while addition by syringe pump to maintain high dilution was necessary to minimize dimer formation.

As a route to more highly functionalized molecules, MCR of a sugar amino acid or alcohol, an aldehyde, and an isocyanoacetamide was used to prepare the acyclic precursor (**240**) for an acid-promoted cyclization that produced interesting macrodepsipeptides **241** (Scheme 11.31).[333] In this approach, the 5-aminooxazole in **240** acts as an internal activator of the terminal carboxylic acid to facilitate the macrolactonization.[334] Subsequent saponification followed by treatment with excess trifluoroacetic acid led to the cyclic target molecules.

In studies directed at the synthesis of the furanocembranoids, marine diterpenoid natural products, investigation on the use of an intramolecular oxidative coupling strategy for ring closure led to an interesting result whereby the desired macrocyclic product or its dimer could be obtained

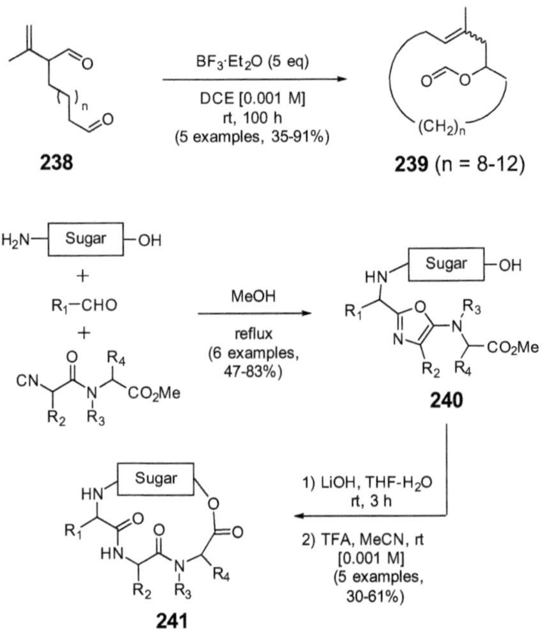

Scheme 11.31 Miscellaneous methods for preparing macrocycles.

depending on the reaction conditions employed.[335] Slow addition of substrate **242** to the oxidant (CAN, ceric ammonium nitrate) along with high dilution was required to provide fair to good yields of monomeric product **243** (Scheme 11.32). The desired reaction succeeded on ring sizes from 10–20 atoms and tolerated alkene, alkyne, ester, triazole and butenolide functionalities. In contrast, at higher reactant concentrations and with addition of CAN all at once to the substrate, only dimer was observed.

Macrocycles have also been synthesized using free radical chemistry. In a representative transformation, the cyclic tripeptidomimetic **245** (Scheme 11.32) was prepared from acryloyl bromide **244** using standard conditions for radical generation.[336] The reaction gave similar results for dipeptidomimetics and substrates with additional steric constraints, such as a proline residue. This is postulated to be assisted by the presence of an intramolecular hydrogen bond that preorganizes the structure to cyclization.

In another macrocyclization method, Katritzky and coworkers have reported a Staudinger-type ring closure procedure for cyclic peptides that was successfully applied to the more difficult smaller ring sizes (7–10 atoms).[337] Rapid reaction of azido-thioester substrate **246** with tributylphosphine under the influence of microwaves rapidly gave acceptable yields (48–75%) of the macrocyclic product **247** (Scheme 11.33). Although not examined in this work, the process also could have applications to larger ring sizes.

Although the result from a complex reaction, a Friedel–Crafts (F–C) alkylation of tryptophan was observed in the construction of a series of

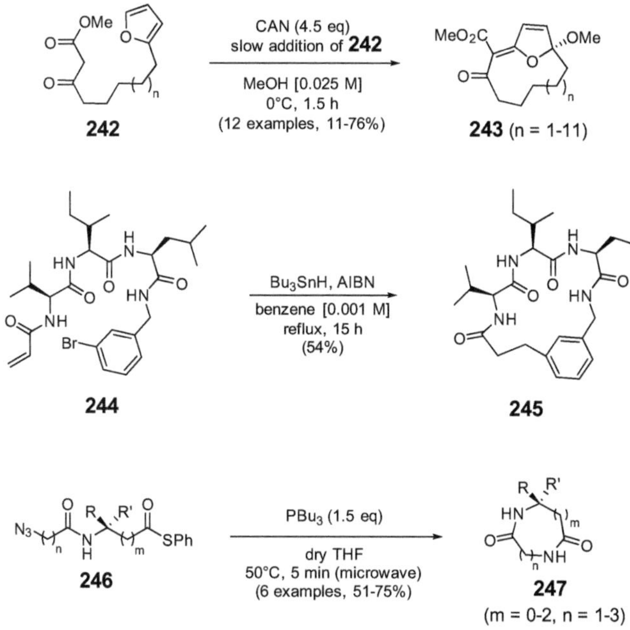

Scheme 11.32 Additional routes to synthesize macrocycles.

macrocyclic peptidomimetics containing 15- to 21-membered rings *via* acid-catalysed rearrangements of linear precursors containing an allyl carbonate moiety.[338] Reaction conditions, including the use of $Sc(OTf)_3$ as Lewis acid, could be modified such that a single F–C product predominated, but appreciable levels of other compounds were still present. At least in its current state, this transformation is not feasible for preparative use.

Another reaction that has seen only minimal use to date for macrocyclization outside the total synthesis area is the intramolecular Julia–Kocienski methylenation of carbonyl groups. For example, a series of simple macrocyclic lactones (**251**) has been synthesized utilizing this procedure, although a competing intermolecular process that produces macrodiolides (**252**) complicates this reaction (Scheme 11.33).[339] For both products, the (*Z*)-olefin configuration ((*ZZ*) in the case of the diolide) is favored. Smaller to medium cycles tend to favor the latter due to strain in the transition state for olefination, while larger ring sizes produce modest yields of the desired intramolecular product. It is possible to tune the reaction conditions by varying mode of addition and temperature to change the predominant product. The synthetic potential of this reaction is perhaps better illustrated by its use with a more complex substrate (**253**) in the construction of intermediate **254**, which was used in the total synthesis of spirohexenolide B, an anti-tumor natural product targeting human macrophage inhibitory factor (MIF). In this instance, only one diastereomer of **253** successfully cyclized.[340]

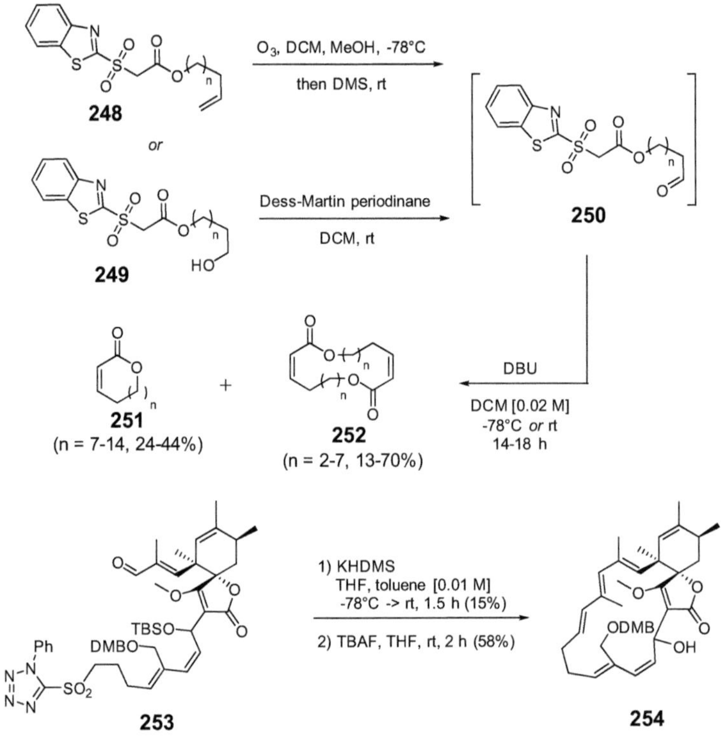

Scheme 11.33 Macrocycles from a Julia–Kocienski olefination process.

11.13 Synthesis at Scale

One of the issues that often has been raised regarding macrocyclic molecules is the difficulty in accessing these compounds at the scale necessary for advanced preclinical and clinical investigations. However, the steady progression of an increasing number of such entities in the pipelines of pharmaceutical and biotechnology companies would seem to indicate that this challenge is beginning to be addressed. Given the advanced nature of the clinical trials for many of the macrocyclic HCV protease inhibitors (see Chapter 7 in this volume), it is not surprising that these compounds represent those on which the greatest amount of information on the large scale synthesis of macrocyclic structures is currently known.

As a first example, the HCV NS3/4A protease inhibitor ciluprevir (BILN 2061, **56**) relied on RCM for the key cyclization step during its original preparation and it remained so upon scale-up. After a detailed investigation of the discovery route, with significant attention directed at the cyclization, the optimal conditions developed were those illustrated in Scheme 11.34A.[341,342] This streamlined convergent process was used to successfully prepare 400 kg of **256**, which led to more than 100 kg of **56**. Nonetheless, certain aspects of the RCM reaction were identified that were

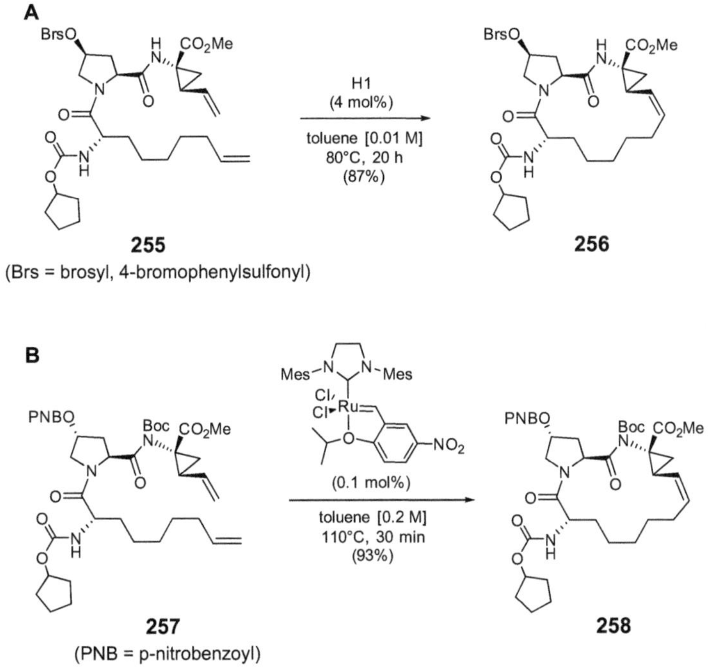

Scheme 11.34 Process improvements for ciluprevir (BILN 2061, **56**).

expected to benefit from additional study, including catalyst load, reaction rate and concentration. The second generation process (Scheme 11.34B), which included a change to a modified ruthenium catalyst and a different protection strategy on the cyclization substrate **257**, was indeed even further improved, resulting in a 10-fold increase in reaction efficiency and a 20-fold reduction in solvent consumption.[343] The process of a related clinical candidate from Boehringer-Ingelheim, the 15-membered macrocycle BI 201302 (**57**), which also relied on RCM, was investigated with similar results obtained for the optimal conditions required in this critical step.[148]

For scale-up of another advanced HCV NS3/4A protease inhibitor candidate, vaniprevir (MK-7009, **59**), different methods were evaluated for the cyclization step, including RCM, which was employed in the medicinal chemistry route, palladium-mediated couplings and macrolactamization (Scheme 11.35, site of cyclization and reaction chemistry indicated in the structure of **59**).[344] RCM, targeting the RCM1 position indicated in the Scheme, required high catalyst loading and reaction concentrations of less than 0.003 M. Efforts at modification only led to lower yields of cyclized product. A variety of palladium-mediated techniques also were investigated at the site on the structure so highlighted. A Heck process for ring closure was successful, but with only modest yield (47%) and numerous side products. Multiple conditions for the Suzuki reaction failed to produce meaningful amounts of the macrocycle, while a Sonogashira approach was

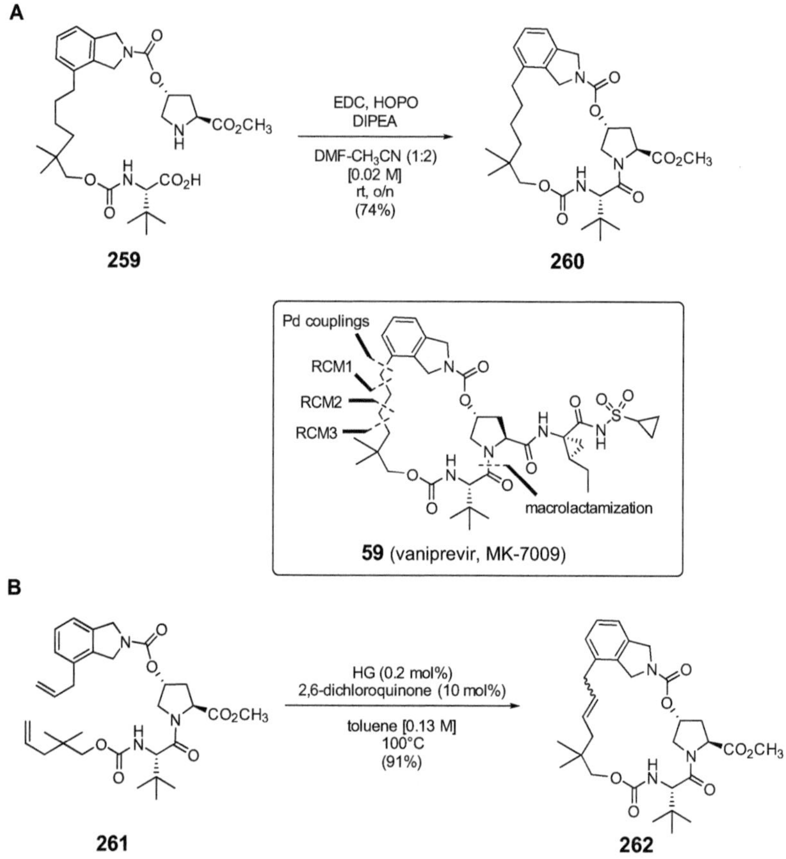

A

259 → **260**

EDC, HOPO
DIPEA

DMF-CH₃CN (1:2)
[0.02 M]
rt, o/n
(74%)

59 (vaniprevir, MK-7009)

Pd couplings
RCM1
RCM2
RCM3
macrolactamization

B

261 → **262**

HG (0.2 mol%)
2,6-dichloroquinone (10 mol%)

toluene [0.13 M]
100°C
(91%)

Scheme 11.35 Vaniprevir (MK-7009, **59**) scale-up investigations.

plagued by dimer formation. Systematic studies of various reagents for macrolactamization resulted in selection of HATU and EDC/HOPO (hydroxyl pyridine N-oxide)[345] as viable alternatives for this transformation. Although the former resulted in a more rapid reaction and could be conducted at higher substrate concentrations, the yields of **260** with both methods were comparable and the significant cost advantages of the latter reagents became the driving factor for proceeding further with this combination. The overall yield of **59** from the optimized process, which also included improved preparations for the precursor compounds, was ~20% (Scheme 11.35A).

Much as for **56**, a re-examination of the RCM strategy for **59**, investigating three different disconnection points (RCM1, RCM2, RCM3 on the structure of **59** in Scheme 11.35), led to substantial yield enhancement as compared to the first generation macrolactamization process.[346] In particular, this optimized procedure, which targeted the RCM2 disconnection site, resulted in lower catalyst loading and relatively high reaction concentration. Further, simultaneous slow introduction of catalyst and diene **261** over 1 h, along with a 2,6-dichloroquinone additive, were also necessary for best results in the cyclization to afford **262** (Scheme 11.35B). The additive was required to suppress the formation of a 19-membered impurity identified during these studies that apparently results from catalyst decomposition. Overall, the improved synthesis was accomplished in nine linear steps and provided a 55% yield of **59**.

For another Merck HCV inhibitor, MK-5172 (**58**), RCM was again utilized in the original route to the structure, but macrolactamization was chosen for the scale-up chemistry (Scheme 11.36A).[347] The protected linear substrate **263** was assembled through a Sonogashira reaction (reaction site indicated

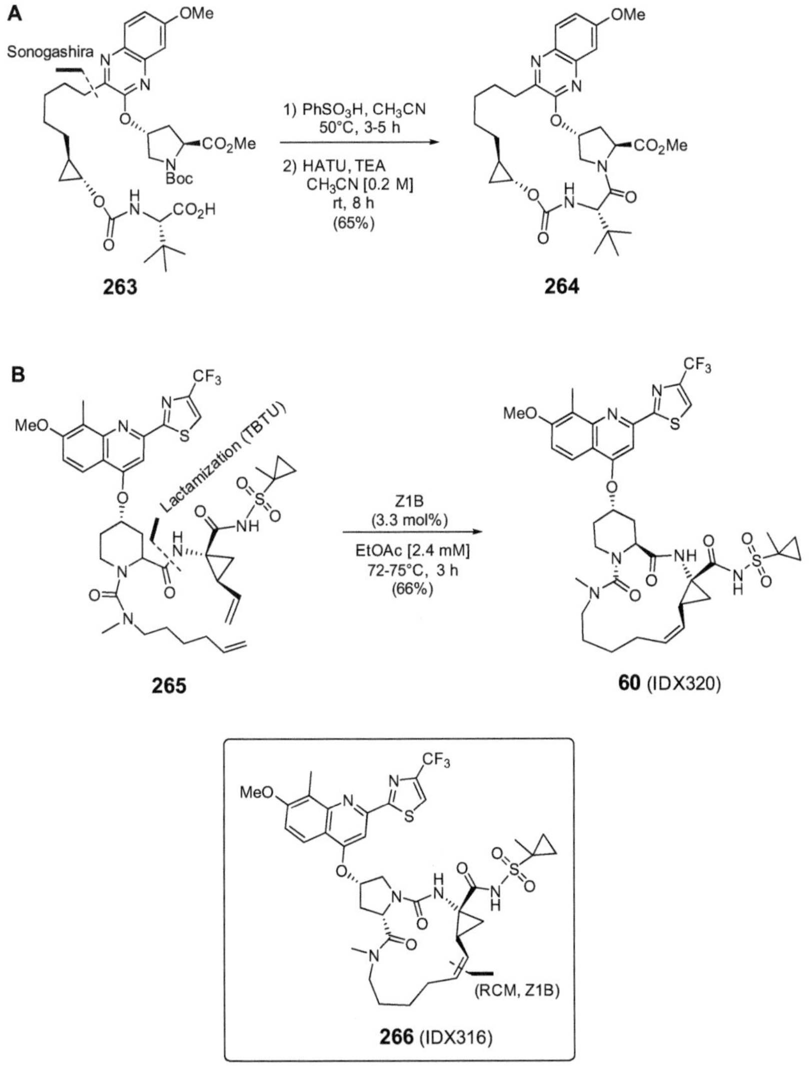

Scheme 11.36 Large scale synthetic routes for (A) MK-5172 (**58**) and (B) IDX320 (**60**).

on structure) followed by reduction of the alkyne. The cyclization was conducted, after Boc deprotection, using HATU without the need for high dilution. Macrocycle **264** was obtained as a crystalline material after concentration of the reaction mixture. Subsequent transformations then yielded the target macrocyclic product **58**. This sequence was successful at providing kilogram quantities of **58** with no chromatographic purification in 42% overall yield and 99.7% purity with less than 0.2% epimerization.

In yet one final example from the HCV protease area, process development efforts have been reported for two closely-related 14-membered ring macrocycles, IDX316 (**266**) and IDX320 (**60**).[348] Again, RCM was the cyclization method of choice. Due to numerous deficiencies within the original medicinal chemistry method, two alternative routes were investigated with the strategy ultimately modified such that the RCM became the final step, in contrast to the initial approach in which the RCM was executed much earlier in the synthetic scheme. The remainder of the structure of the cyclization substrate **265** was assembled using lactamization (site of coupling indicated in the structure). Optimized conditions for the RCM as shown led to the desired product **60** in 66% yield from **265** at 1 kg scale (Scheme 11.36B). Similar results were also obtained with **266**, although clinical development of that compound was discontinued in favour of **60** after the proof of concept studies. Crystallization of **60** achieved a ruthenium content in the isolated product of less than 10 ppm with overall yields from all four starting materials ranging from 10% to 35%. However, this inhibitor was halted in development as well due to the appearance of drug–drug interactions with other pharmaceutical agents used in the treatment of HCV.

As an example outside the realm of HCV protease inhibitors, the multi-kilo scale process for the clinical ghrelin agonist ulimorelin (TZP-101, **268**)[349] relied on a convergent assembly strategy with a macrolactamization to form the ring (Scheme 11.37).[350] The initial synthesis of this molecule was performed on solid phase, so for scale-up, an alternative approach was necessary. Hence, the dipeptide portion was coupled to the alkylated amino acid component under standard conditions to provide the protected linear precursor **267** (bond formation site indicated), containing all the necessary structural features and functionality of the target molecule. Simultaneous deprotection of the two terminal groups was followed by cyclization, for

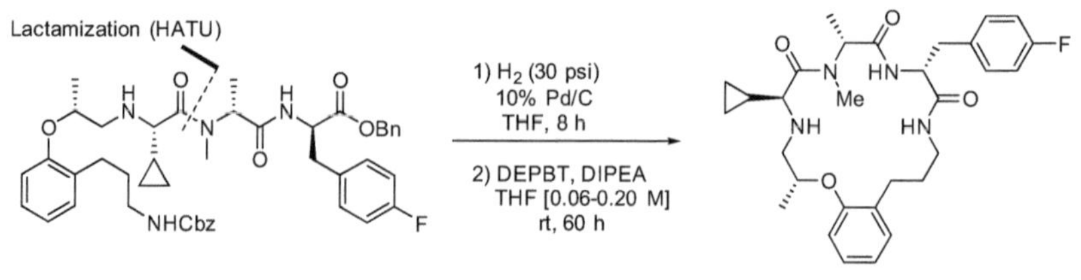

Scheme 11.37   Ulimorelin (TZP-101, **268**) process chemistry.

which the DEPBT (3-(diethoxyphosphoryloxy)-3H-benzo[d][1,2,3]triazin-4-one) reagent of Goodman[351] gave the best results. A crystallization sequence led to ulimorelin (**268**) as the monohydrochloride monohydrate salt in very good overall yield and 99.7% purity. It is noteworthy that high dilution conditions were not required as the macrolactamization could be executed at a concentration as high as 0.2 M, similar to that employed for **58**, albeit with different reagents and reaction conditions.

Beyond these few examples, the reports of larger scale syntheses of macrocyclic molecules remain relatively sparse. Nonetheless, as more macrocyclic drug candidates advance through the clinic, additional successful scale-up processes for their preparation are expected to appear, which should eventually remove one of the barriers to wider utilization and acceptance of these structures.

11.14   Macrocyclic Library Synthesis

11.14.1   Standard Chemistry Methods

As has already been indicated, the utility of macrocyclic structures for pharmaceutical purposes has lagged at least in part due to the challenges of accessing screening libraries of these molecules. With many discovery programs relying on HTS for generation of initial lead structures, macrocycles typically have entered the discussion during the optimization phase of a program as a method for adding conformational constraints to an active molecule rather than as *de novo* actives themselves. Fortunately, several innovative technologies have now proven successful at generating libraries of macrocyclic compounds and represent significant steps in remedying this situation. Some commonalities are evident in these various approaches, however. Many take advantage of the wide diversity of commercially available amino acid building blocks and are performed on solid support, which lends itself better to handling larger numbers of compounds and provides a pseudo-dilution effect to minimize formation of oligomeric side products as well.

In a pioneering attempt at generating macrocyclic libraries, technology focused on the generation of tripeptidomimetic macrocycles designed to incorporate a non-peptidic topological control element, termed the tether, embodies both these features.[352,353] Noteworthy aspects of the solid phase process, which yielded a screening library of over 40,000 diverse compounds (general structure **269**, Figure 11.19, site of cyclization and reagent employed indicated), were (a) the use of a thioester linker that enabled cyclization to form the macrolactam to occur simultaneous with cleavage from the resin ("cyclization-release" as described in Section 11.2),[54] (b) the formation of the C-N sp^3 bond between the amino acid chain and the tether utilized an N-benzothiazole-2-sulphonyl (Bts)[354] moiety for dual roles, first as protection of the amine and then for activation towards use in a Fukuyama–Mitsunobu reaction, and (c) the optional addition of silver to assist with difficult

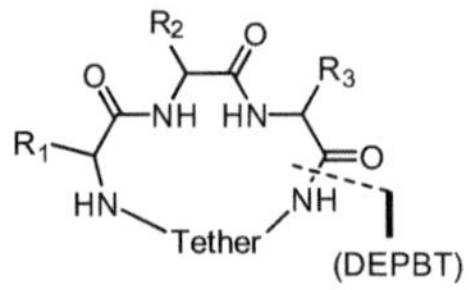

269

40,000+ member library

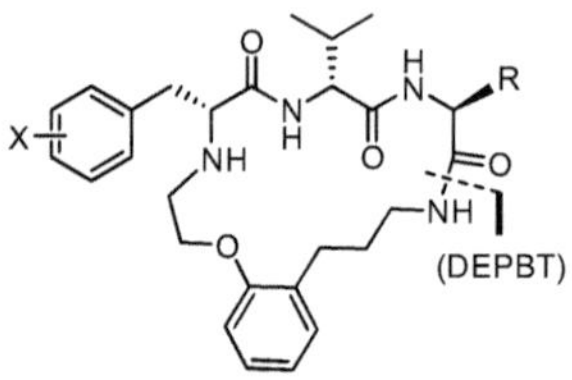

270 (motilin antagonists)

R = basic, heteroaryl moieties
X = 3-CF$_3$, 3-F, 3-Cl

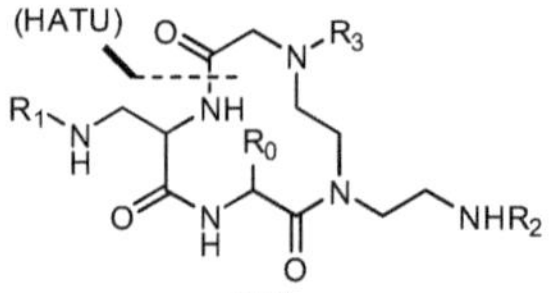

271

16 templates (R$_0$)
7 x R$_1$, R$_2$, R$_3$
3987 analogues

Figure 11.19 Macrocyclic libraries from lactamization routes.

cyclizations.[355] Compounds of this type were also accessed using RCM.[356] Screening of these libraries led to the discovery of highly active and selective ghrelin agonists (ulimorelin, **268**)[349] and motilin antagonists (**270**, Figure 11.19).[357,358]

For solution phase approaches as well, macrolactamization has often been the method of choice for the key step in the synthesis of macrocyclic libraries, in part because of its high efficiency and wide reagent selection. For example, research on construction of a library of smaller cyclic peptidomimetics led to optimized conditions for an intramolecular lactamization (HATU, DMF-CH$_3$CN, slow addition) to create the triply orthogonal protected template **271** (Figure 11.19, site of cyclization and reagent employed indicated),[359] which could then be further diversified using a variety of standard transformations. This procedure proved effective in constructing a series of 12-membered ring scaffolds with four diversity sites that were expanded into a collection of almost 4000 members.

To accomplish this, the initial cyclic compounds thus obtained were serially transformed through selective deprotection of one of the amines followed by amide coupling, sulphonamide formation, reductive amination or even S$_N$Ar with appropriate heteroaryls. For these structures, the formation of the ring was facilitated through the use of (2-nitrophenyl)sulphonyl (Nos) protection for one of the amine nitrogens, which essentially acts as a hinge on the linear peptide backbone as had been utilized previously for apicidin analogues.[360,361] Such preorganization also permitted the reaction to be conducted at relatively high concentration, although careful control of reaction parameters was required to minimize dimer formation.

Interestingly, the concentration actually could be increased at gram scale, as the slow addition of substrate becomes more effective at avoiding dimer formation. An interesting finding was that the cellular permeability of these analogues varied based upon stereochemistry, which also directly correlated with the degree of intramolecular hydrogen-bonding.[362,363]

In work that led to one of the first macrocycle libraries, the poly-azacyclophane **20** (Section 11.3.1, Scheme 11.3) was reacted with appropriate halides to prepare a small mixture library (14×100 compounds each).[61] Essentially the same strategy, using an S_N2 process to prepare the macrocycle followed by reaction of the amine with various electrophilic species, was employed to construct a variety of piperidinyl polyazacyclophane libraries (**272**, Figure 11.20, site of ring closure, base and leaving group employed indicated) containing four diversity sites.[364]

Similarly, a series of 19- to 26-membered polyazadipyridinocyclophane scaffolds (**273**) was assembled as a screening collection of almost 25,000 compounds.[365] Perhaps not surprisingly, the yields in the macrocyclization decreased as the ring size increased, from 95% for the 19-membered ring (m = 2, n = 1) to 40% for the 26-ring size (m = 6, n = 4). These libraries proved to be sources of antibacterial activity and inhibitors of HIV-1 tat (trans-activator of transcription)/TAR (trans-activation responsive region) protein–RNA interactions.

The seminal work of Liu and co-workers on the uses of DNA-templated synthesis included a strategy applicable to very large macrocycle libraries.[366,367] Complementary DNA strands function both to pre-organize substrates for the cyclization reaction and track the individual reactants. Although this technique is compatible with a variety of chemistries, including macrolactamization, cycloaddition and RCM, it was initially demonstrated for macrocycles utilizing a Wittig reaction for ring closure in the construction of a small 65-member library.[368] This approach was then expanded and utilized for a much larger 13,824 compound library (**274** as a representative scaffold, Figure 11.21),[369] from which selective kinase inhibitors and activators were developed (**275**, **276**).[370,371] The strategy has also

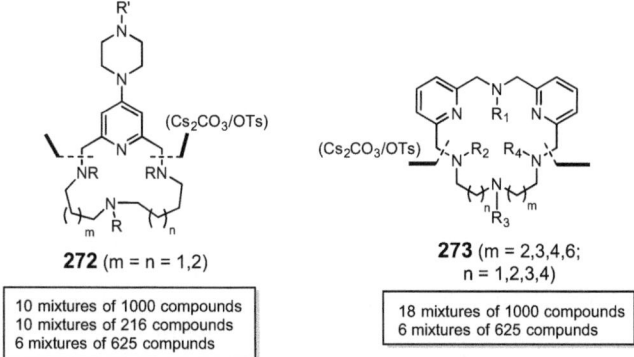

272 (m = n = 1,2)

10 mixtures of 1000 compounds
10 mixtures of 216 compounds
6 mixtures of 625 compunds

273 (m = 2,3,4,6; n = 1,2,3,4)

18 mixtures of 1000 compounds
6 mixtures of 625 compunds

Figure 11.20 Polyazacyclophane libraries from S_N2 chemistry.

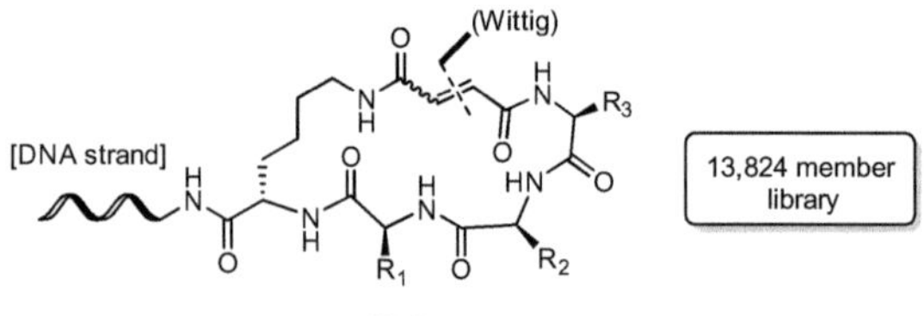

274

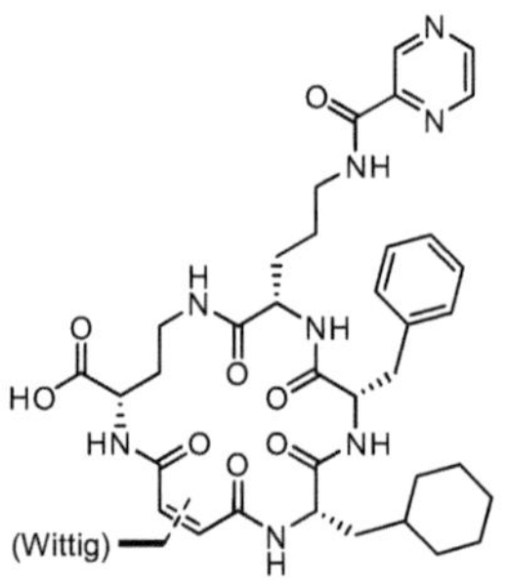

275 (Src kinase inhibitor)

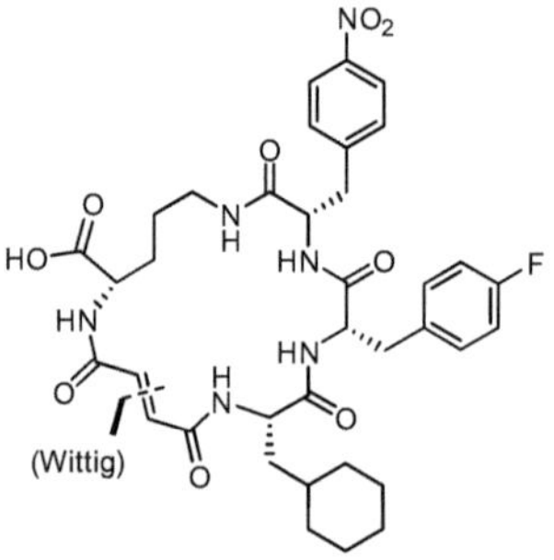

276 (Src kinase inhibitor)

Figure 11.21 Libraries created using DNA-templates.

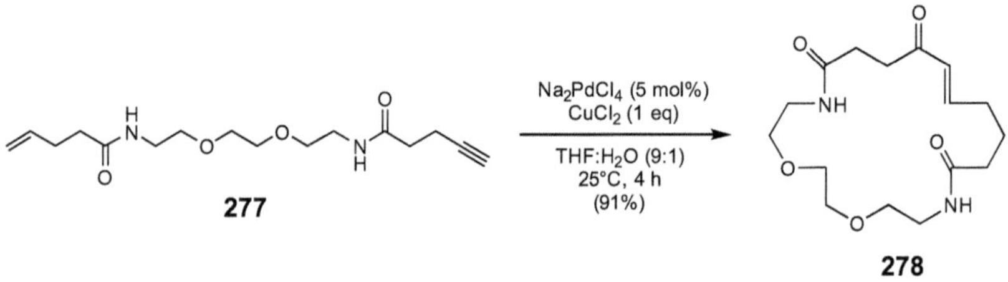

Scheme 11.38 Novel reaction discovery from DNA-template technology.

been applied to the identification of TNF-α inhibitors[372] and IL-17 antagonists.[373,374]

In an alternative application of this DNA-based technology, a novel palladium-catalysed alkyne-alkene macrocyclization reaction was identified (Scheme 11.38).[375] Optimization of this reaction for metal catalyst system, solvent, temperature and time was also enabled by using the DNA-template methodology, which led to a highly efficient ring closure of **277** to **278** in excellent yield.

MCR has also been found to be a methodology suitable for libraries of macrocycles. In particular, the multiple multicomponent macrocyclizations including bifunctional building blocks (MiB) technique has been used for a number of potentially interesting structures (Figure 11.22).[376] Although the Ugi MCR has proven to be the most versatile in this approach, Staudinger and Passerini approaches have also been employed. The MiB strategy has

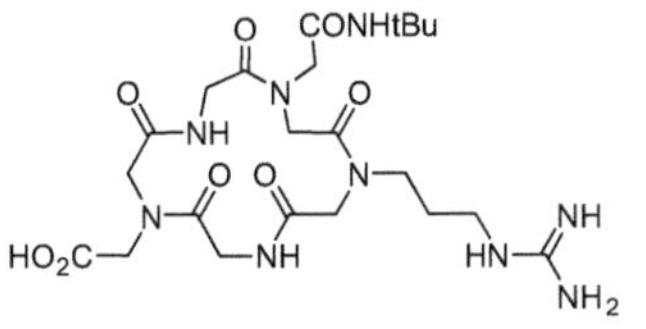

Figure 11.22 Macrocyclic libraries constructed using MCR.

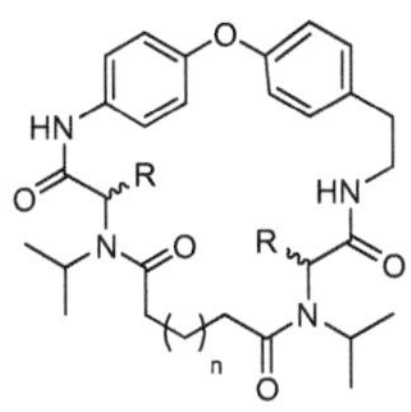

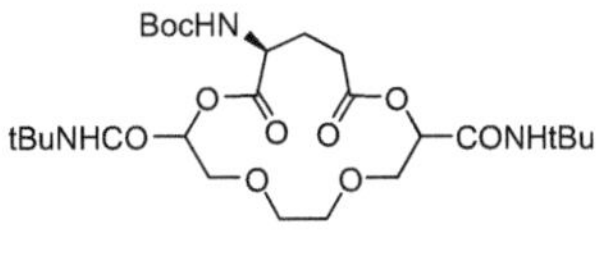

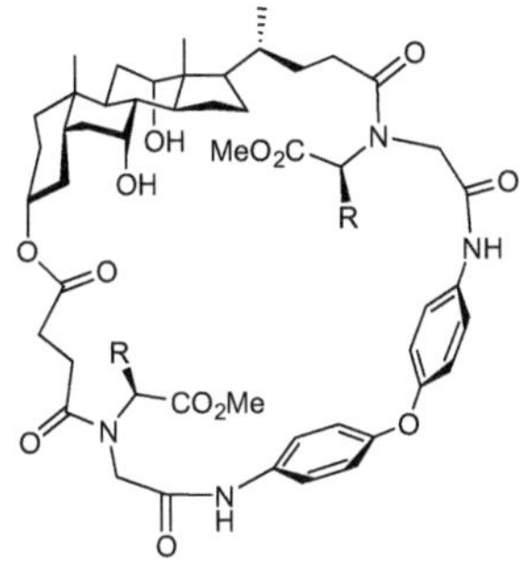

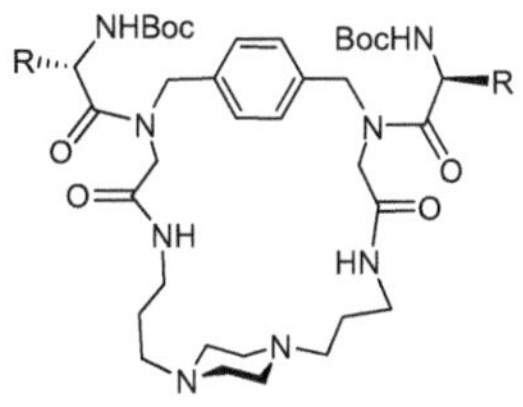

yielded a variety of biologically relevant structures, including peptoids (**279**), biaryl ether macrocycles (**280**), macrolactones (**281**), β-lactam-containing macrocycles, steroid-peptoid macrocycles (**282**), macroheterocycles (**283**) and large macrobicycles. However, specific applications for these libraries in pharmaceutical discovery have not been reported.

Not surprisingly, the excellent utility of the S_NAr in intramolecular ring closure and ease of execution on solid phase has been explored for library preparation as well. For example, a combinatorial library of 12,000 macrocycles was synthesized on solid phase capitalizing on this approach for the cyclization step (**284**, Figure 11.23, site of ring closure indicated).[377] Compounds that inhibited bacterial protein synthesis were identified from this collection. Similarly, antibacterial lead compounds were identified from a library of 1,350 compounds possessing a quinolone pharmacophore (**285**)[378] and a DOS approach gave a variety of macro-heterocycles,[379] such as shown in general structures **286** and **287**, each of which relied on an intramolecular S_NAr process for cyclization.

In another example, this one conducted in solution phase, a library of pyran-containing macrocycles exemplified by **288** and **289** was constructed

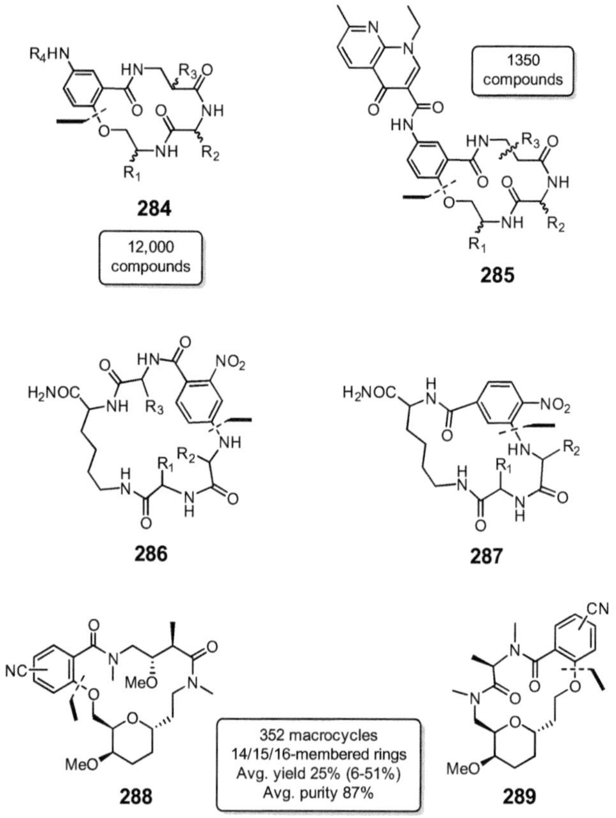

Figure 11.23 S$_N$Ar chemistry for macrocyclic libraries.

utilizing S$_N$Ar for the critical transformation. The reaction featured a nitrile-substituted aromatic as the electrophilic species (Figure 11.23) rather than the more commonly used fluoroaryl moiety.[380] The ring closure proceeded well with a range of amino acid components, substrate stereochemistries, aromatic substitution patterns and cycle sizes. Of particular note, the physicochemical properties of this library were found to be in the acceptable "drug-like" range and the degree of three-dimensional diversity, including rod-, disc- and sphere-like topologies, obtained from this small number of structures was impressive.

The pervasive use of an RCM strategy for macrocycle construction prompted a detailed investigation to optimize this chemistry, including reactions conducted on resin supports, for diversity generation with a stereochemically complex 12-membered ring (**290**) as a representative objective (Figure 11.24, site of ring closure and RCM catalyst employed shown).[381] Generally, the transformation proceeded quite well, although the appearance of dimers and stereoisomers were occasionally confounding factors. The product could be chemically manipulated post-cyclization to incorporate additional diversity. A small library of 122 fused macrocyclic sugar

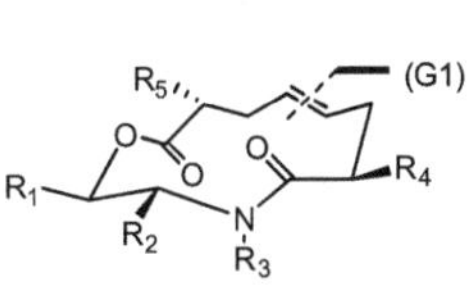

290

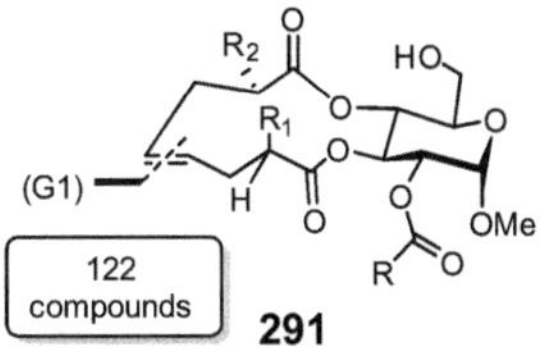

291

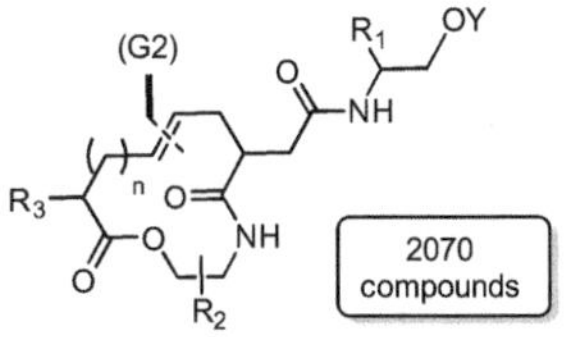

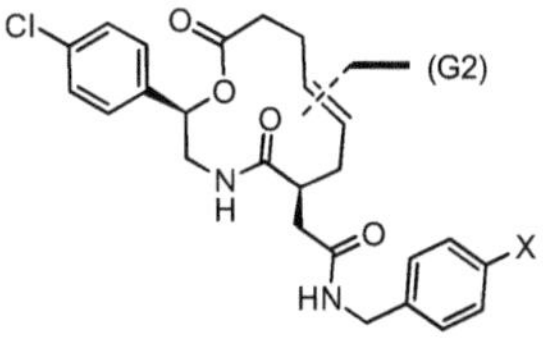

292 (n = 1-3, Y = protecting group, polystyrene resin)

293 (X=H, robotnikinin, Shh inhibitor)
294 (X=Cl, BRD-6851, Smo antagonist)

Figure 11.24 Libraries of macrocycles made *via* RCM.

molecules (**291**) was prepared *via* an RCM process based upon these studies.[382]

Not surprisingly, RCM also has been instrumental for accessing a variety of other libraries, including a 2070 member collection of 12-, 13- and 14-membered macrocycles (**292**, Figure 11.24). This library was primarily assembled on solid phase, although was also conducted in solution phase, and yielded robotnikin (**293**), a novel inhibitor of the hedgehog (Shh) pathway.[383,384] RCM also was utilized to synthesize analogues of **293** with improved cellular activity that were found to specifically act as antagonists of the smoothened (Smo) receptor, with BRD-6851 (**294**) being the most potent.[385]

In a demonstration of methodology amenable to larger library construction, a fluorous tagging strategy[386,387] that included RCM for cyclization enabled the synthesis of a small stereoisomer library of macrolactones **295** (Figure 11.25, site of ring closure and chemistry utilized indicated, along with catalyst for RCM).[388] A fluorous strategy was also utilized by Nelson in studies employing an extensive series of reactions, including metathesis cascades, that created over 80 different natural product-like scaffolds that included macrocycles among the novel structural types prepared.[389]

The Schreiber research group, which had performed the exploratory studies on the RCM mentioned earlier in this section, also conducted a systematic investigation of the cyclization step in a DOS approach to macrolactones, exemplified by the representative compound **296** (Figure 11.25, site of ring closure, chemistry used and reagent for macrolactonization indicated).[390] The optimized reaction conditions (TCBC, DIPEA, toluene, rt, 20 h) thus developed on solid phase were used to construct a small 36 compound pilot library. Interestingly, the chirality of the linear precursors was not found to dramatically affect the macrolactonization, which stood in contrast to the results with RCM substrates where a significant stereochemical bias had been observed.

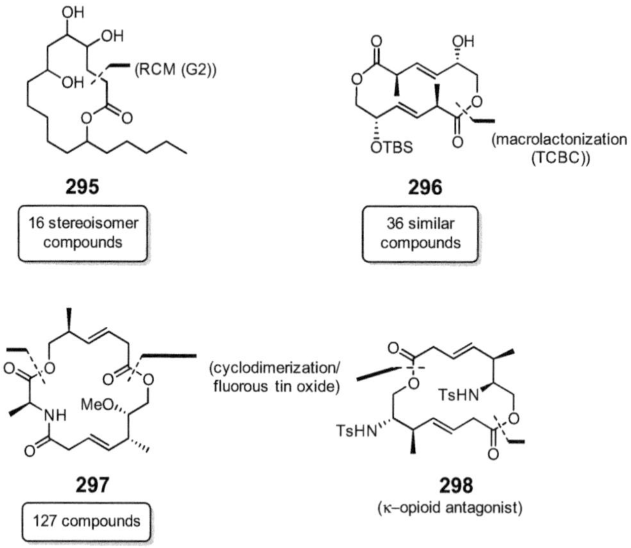

Figure 11.25   Macrolactone libraries.

The synthesis of a modest library of macrocyclic dilactones (or macro-diolides), a known class of active natural products, also capitalized on fluorous chemistry.[391] These compounds were accessed from the homo- or hetero-dimerization of chiral hydroxy ester substrates catalysed by a fluorous tin oxide using microwave irradiation to facilitate the transesterification ring closure. This resulted in a variety of macrocycle sizes (11–23 members) with **297** as a representative example (Figure 11.25, site of ring closure, chemistry used and reagents indicated), although larger rings (>19 atoms) were dis-favored. A novel κ-opioid receptor antagonist (**298**) was identified from this work.

As described in Section 11.7.1, palladium (0) chemistry has been found particularly well-suited for constructing macrocyclic structures and, hence, applications for libraries have also been pursued. Indeed, as already noted, one of the first macrocyclic library efforts actually used the Heck reaction for solid phase construction of small collections of 20- to 24-membered semi-peptidic macrocycles (**299**, Figure 11.26, site of ring closure and chemistry indicated).[198] In addition, modest-sized libraries of RGD mimic macrocycles (**300**)[230] and macrosphelide analogues (**301**)[392] were prepared using palladium-catalysed cyclocarbonylation on resin. This particular method proved to be tolerant of a variety of functional groups, including halides, ethers, ketones and esters.

With most corporate compound collections notably lacking in macrocyclic structures, continued work in this area is expected to develop additional methodologies robust enough for preparation of libraries possessing suf-ficient diversity for generating HTS hits for the initiation of medicinal chemistry programs. Of particular note in this regard is the recent

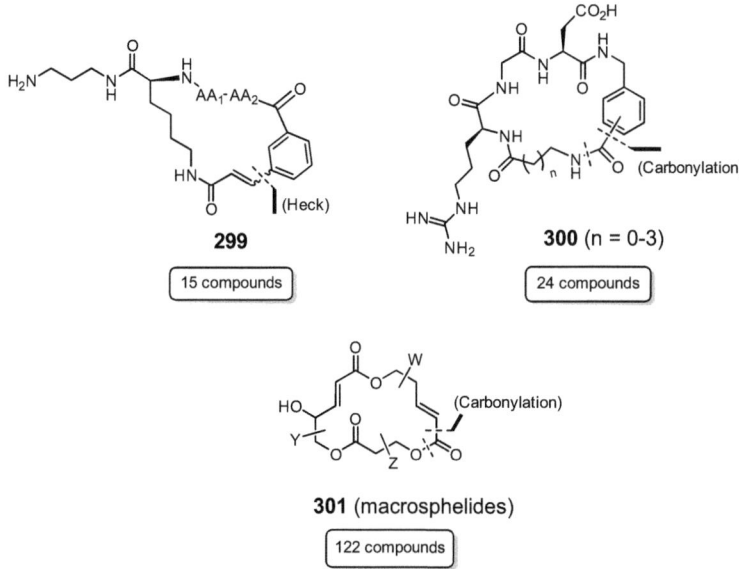

Figure 11.26 Macrocyclic libraries from palladium-catalysed processes.

appearance of the hybrid strategies outlined in the next section, which can generate enormous numbers of macrocycles.

11.14.2   Biological-Chemical Hybrid Approaches

A number of innovative methods for macrocycle synthesis have attempted to harness the power and selectivity of biological methods in conjunction with one or more chemical transformations. These hybrid processes have by necessity focused on peptidic structures, often relatively large in ring size, but also have proven very capable of the rapid synthesis of extremely high numbers of macrocyclic compounds. Several recent reviews have detailed these strategies, some of the most useful of which will be outlined here.[393–397]

Recent advances in protein engineering and molecular biology have enabled the biosynthesis of large libraries of cyclic peptides using standard expression systems.[398] Techniques such as expressed protein ligation,[399] intein-mediated trans-splicing reactions,[400,401] protease-catalysed trans-peptidation[402,403] and sortase-mediated ligation[404,405] produce backbone cyclized peptides, but are not yet directly applicable for non-peptidic structures and generally generate larger macrocyclic structures.

In addition, directed evolution can be used to re-engineer non-ribosomal peptide synthetases (NRPS) that in turn may be applied to the biosynthesis of novel macrocyclic products.[406] Formation of the ring relies on application of an appropriate chemical step, often utilizing specific residues incorporated into each sequence. For many of these approaches, cysteine (Cys) is employed to cyclize the linear precursor molecules through the formation of disulphide bonds, chemoselective ligation with a thioester, or the nucleophilic attack of the thiol with an appropriate electrophilic species. Lantipeptide-like structures, resulting from the Michael addition of the Cys thiol to an α,β-unsaturated amino acid, have also been generated in this manner.[407]

In contrast, split-intein circular ligation of peptides and proteins (SICLOPPS),[408] first reported by Benkovic, utilizes split-intein chemistry to cyclize randomized peptide sequences. However, the size of the resulting cyclopeptide is limited by the transformation efficiency of *E. coli*, specific amino acids are required in order to obtain efficient splicing, and random residues are generally limited to five, although additional amino acids, including unnatural ones, can be incorporated into the backbone, thus varying the structure and ring size of the cyclic peptide.

As another hybrid method, Suga has pioneered genetic code reprogramming to permit the *in vitro* production of ribosomally expressed peptides that contain non-natural amino acid residues.[409] This technology relies on the use of an engineered ribozyme that permits the transfer of essentially any amino acid into tRNA. Ligation chemistry and attack by the thiol of a Cys residue on an N-chloroacetyl tyrosine or tryptophan provide the ring closure routes as part of the associated discovery strategy that creates compounds such as **302** (Figure 11.27, ring closure site indicated). Selective kinase[410] and ligase[409] inhibitors, as well as VEGF-R2 antagonists and multidrug and toxic compound extrusion (MATE) family transporter inhibitors,[411,412] have been

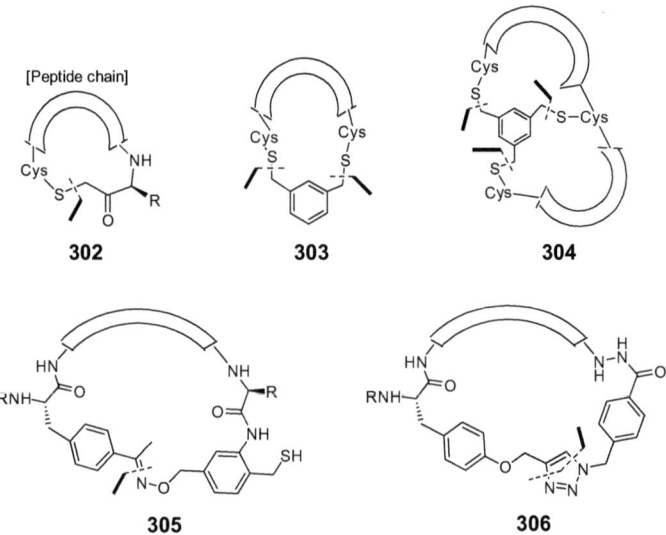

Figure 11.27 Biological–chemical hybrid methods for very large macrocyclic libraries.

found from macrocycle libraries produced by these methods and illustrate the versatility of this strategy.

The Szostak laboratory has utilized mRNA display to produce a library of macrocyclic peptides in which a number of unusual amino acids were successfully incorporated.[413] The cyclization in this case was done through the use of dibromoxylene cross-linking agents that reacted with two cysteine residues in the precursor. The resulting cyclic library, represented by **303** (Figure 11.27, sites of ring closure indicated) yielded a new thrombin inhibitor. In a variation on this approach, Heinis *et al.* have utilized a trifunctional cross-linking agent to create bicyclic peptides such as **304** (Figure 11.27, cyclization sites indicated) on phage.[414] Potent inhibitors of plasma kallikrein were identified *via* this effort. More recently, a series of alternative cross-linking agents have been reported by this group, which were shown to significantly diversify the conformations displayed by the bicyclic peptide products.[415]

Fasan and co-workers have developed multiple methods for constructing macrocyclic organo-peptide hybrids (MOrPHs).[416,417] This technology utilizes a variety of synthetic linker units to cyclize ribosomally-generated precursor polypeptides. Cyclization can be achieved through hydrazide/ thioester ligation, oxime formation (**305**, Figure 11.27, cyclization site indicated), or azide–alkyne cycloaddition (**306**).

As another example, from the Schmidt and Schultz laboratories, in a route amenable to smaller macrocyclic molecules with less peptidic character, the ribosomal peptide natural product pathway for cyanobactins was manipulated in a manner that permitted the incorporation of multiple non-proteinogenic amino acids.[418] This produced structures, **307** (Figure 11.28) as a representative example, with rings as small as 18-membered and possessing more "drug-like" features.

In addition to these more elegant methodologies, the straightforward application of enzymes for macrocycle synthesis has also been explored. In particular, thioesterases catalyse the intramolecular reaction of linear acyl chains and are involved in the construction of cyclic natural products such

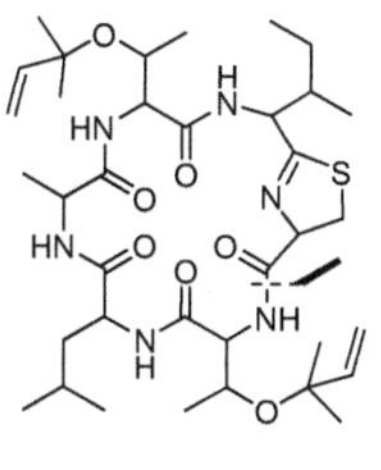

307 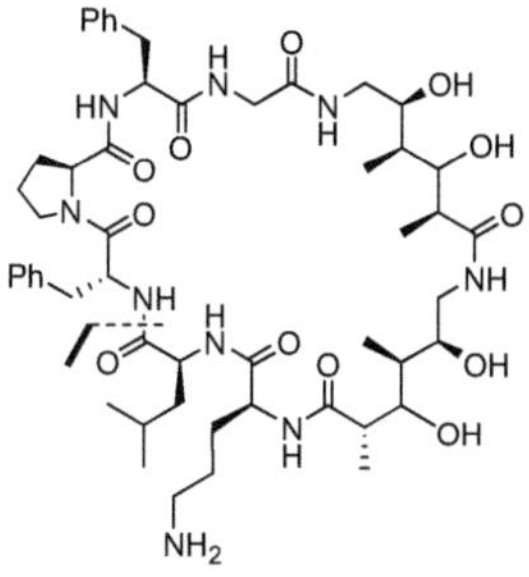   **308**

Figure 11.28 Additional biological–chemical hybrid methods for macrocycle libraries.

as polyketides and peptides.[419,420] These enzymes tolerate significant diversity in substrates and, hence, it is not surprising that they, or "reprogrammed" versions thereof, have been studied as efficient catalysts for the stereoselective assembly of synthetic macrocyclic molecules as well.[406,421] In many cases these efforts have been directed at modified cyclopeptides or macrolides, although Walsh has reported macrocyclic molecules containing both peptide and polyketide elements, such as **308** (Figure 11.28, ring closure site indicated), that were accessed by cyclization with TycC thioesterase.[422] This process was also demonstrated to perform well on solid phase. Other enzymes can also be employed for cyclization, including proteases,[423] transglutamases,[424] and leucyl/phenylalanyl tRNA-protein transferase,[425] although investigations have been confined to cyclic peptides and modified peptides to date.

11.15   Cyclization Studies

Due to the critical nature of the cyclization step for the synthesis of macrocyclic structures, a number of efforts have been devoted to attempting to better understand and define this process. Initial studies focused on the factors involved in the formation of cyclic peptides.[426] These investigations revealed the positive effects of preorganization of cyclization precursors on the reaction rate and yield.[427] They also showed the benefits of mixed absolute configurations,[428,429] *N*-methylation[430,431] and other conformational constraints on cyclization.

More recently, a systematic study on efficiency of peptide cyclization was conducted using libraries of 4–12 amino acids with some fixed and some random sites.[432] Over 2 million peptide sequences were surveyed using standard Fmoc chemistry on TentaGel® and on resin cyclization. Use of the differential swelling properties of the PEG (polyethylene glycol) support permitted different sequences to be constructed on the interior and surface sites ("one bead, two compounds"). The results demonstrated that cyclization was very efficient (≥ 96% success, monomer only) for sequences greater than six amino acids, but that significant amounts of dimer were obtained with 4–5 residues. Other key observations were (a) poor yields with Lys and Arg rich sequences; (b) bulky side chains at N-terminus slow cyclization; and (c) the positive effect of additives [LiCl, KSCN, "Magic Mixture" (1 : 1 : 1 DMF/DCM/NMP plus 1% Triton X-100)] that break up hydrogen-bonding networks in improving efficiency. It was noted by the researchers that certain parameters were not evaluated that also may have had an impact on the results, such as the nature and loading of the resin.

In a comprehensive analysis, a literature survey of macrocyclization reactions reported from 2009 to 2011, 896 total reactions, revealed an average concentration of 3.7 mM with only 3% conducted ≥ 100 mM, not surprising given the known beneficial effects of high dilution for these transformations.[433] Perhaps somewhat unexpectedly, however, a reasonably high average yield in the 60–80% range was obtained, which was attributed to the attention directed at this critical step during synthesis optimization. This work also included an attempt to define a measure of the efficiency of the macrocyclization reaction, Emac. Across a range of reaction types and ring sizes, a mean Emac of 5.80 was calculated, with a value of 2–5 indicating poor and 8–9 optimized, which would suggest that overall further improvements would be possible and should be pursued.

These recent efforts to gain an in-depth understanding of this fundamental process are not only another demonstration of the growing importance of the macrocyclic compound class, but also an indication of just how much remains to be learned in this area.

11.16 Conclusions

Despite the significant increase in reports on the use of macrocyclic compounds in drug discovery, they remain alien and unfamiliar to many medicinal chemists. Such structures do not display the typical characteristics or obey the rules usually associated with traditional small molecule pharmaceutical agents.[434] One of the primary initial barriers to wider exploration of these compounds had been the difficulty in their efficient synthesis. As the preceding compilation has amply demonstrated, however, a myriad of synthetic methods are now available for the reliable and efficient construction of a diverse range of macrocyclic structures, including libraries. These methods were initially focused on peptidomimetic type compounds, but have now progressed towards creating molecules with little or no peptidic character. This is expected to open the way to more thorough examination of the chemical space of this compound class and a concomitant increase in their applications for the discovery of new pharmaceutical entities.

Acknowledgements

The author wishes to thank Professor Eric Marsault, Dr Eileen Larkin and the anonymous reviewers for their constructive input and helpful comments on this chapter.

References

1. E. M. Driggers, S. P. Hale, J. Lee and N. K. Terrett, *Nat. Rev. Drug Discovery*, 2008, 7, 608.
2. N. K. Terrett, *Drug Discovery Today: Technol.*, 2010, 7, e97.
3. E. Marsault and M. L. Peterson, *J. Med. Chem.*, 2011, 54, 1961.
4. X. Yu and D. Sun, *Molecules*, 2013, **18**, 6230.
5. J. Mallinson and I. Collins, *Future Med. Chem.*, 2012, 4, 1409.
6. C. M. Madsen and M. H. Clausen, *Eur. J. Org. Chem.*, 2011, **2011**, 3107.
7. J. S. Davies, *J. Pept. Sci.*, 2003, **9**, 471.

8. A. Parenty, X. Moreau, G. Niel and J. M. Campagne, *Chem. Rev.*, 2012, **113**, PR1.

9. C. B. Xue, X. He, J. Roderick, W. F. DeGrado, R. J. Cherney, K. D. Hardman, D. J. Nelson, R. A. Copeland, B. D. Jaffee and C. P. Decicco, *J. Med. Chem.*, 1998, **41**, 1745.

10. A. E. Weber, M. G. Steiner, P. A. Krieter, A. E. Colletti, J. R. Tata, T. A. Halgren, R. G. Ball, J. J. Doyle, T. W. Schorn, R. A. Stearns and et al., *J. Med. Chem.*, 1992, **35**, 3755.

11. F. Albericio and L. A. Carpino, *Methods Enzymol.*, 1997, **289**, 104.

12. F. Albericio, R. Chinchilla, D. J. Dodsworth and C. Najera, *Org. Prep. Proced. Int.*, 2001, **33**, 203.

13. F. Albericio, *Curr. Opin. Chem. Biol.*, 2004, **8**, 211.

14. S.-Y. Han and Y.-A. Kim, *Tetrahedron*, 2004, **60**, 2447.

15. A. El-Faham and F. Albericio, *Chem. Rev.*, 2011, **111**, 6557.

16. G. M. Ksander, R. de Jesus, A. Yuan, R. D. Ghai, A. Trapani, C. McMartin and R. Bohacek, *J. Med. Chem.*, 1997, **40**, 495.

17. G. M. Ksander, R. de Jesus, A. Yuan, R. D. Ghai, C. McMartin and R. Bohacek, *J. Med. Chem.*, 1997, **40**, 506.

18. J. A. Robinson, *J. Pept. Sci.*, 2013, **19**, 127.

19. S. J. DeMarco, H. Henze, A. Lederer, K. Moehle, R. Mukherjee, B. Romagnoli, J. A. Robinson, F. Brianza, F. O. Gombert, S. Lociuro, C. Ludin, J. W. Vrijbloed, J. Zumbrunn, J. P. Obrecht, D. Obrecht, V. Brondani, F. Hamy and T. Klimkait, *Bioorg. Med. Chem.*, 2006, **14**, 8396.

20. F. de Nigris, C. Schiano, T. Infante and C. Napoli, *Recent Pat. Anti-Cancer Drug Discovery*, 2012, 7, 251.

21. N. Srinivas, P. Jetter, B. J. Ueberbacher, M. Werneburg, K. Zerbe, J. Steinmann, B. Van der Meijden, F. Bernardini, A. Lederer, R. L. Dias, P. E. Misson, H. Henze, J. Zumbrunn, F. O. Gombert, D. Obrecht, P. Hunziker, S. Schauer, U. Ziegler, A. Kach, L. Eberl, K. Riedel, S. J. DeMarco and J. A. Robinson, *Science*, 2010, **327**, 1010.

22. The specific structures of these molecules have not been publicly disclosed, although their origin from the PEM technology has been acknowledged.

23. H. L. Sham, G. Bolis, H. H. Stein, S. W. Fesik, P. A. Marcotte, J. J. Plattner, C. A. Rempel and J. Greer, *J. Med. Chem.*, 1988, **31**, 284.

24. A. E. Weber, T. A. Halgren, J. J. Doyle, R. J. Lynch, P. K. Siegl, W. H. Parsons, W. J. Greenlee and A. A. Patchett, *J. Med. Chem.*, 1991, **34**, 2692.

25. D. S. Dhanoa, W. H. Parsons, W. J. Greenlee and A. A. Patchett, *Tetrahedron Lett.*, 1992, **33**, 1725.

26. M. D. Reily, V. Thanabal, E. A. Lunney, J. T. Repine, C. C. Humblet and G. Wagner, *FEBS Lett.*, 1992, **302**, 97.

27. C. Sund, O. Belda, D. Wiktelius, C. Sahlberg, L. Vrang, S. Sedig, E. Hamelink, I. Henderson, T. Agback, K. Jansson, N. Borkakoti, D. Derbyshire, A. Eneroth and B. Samuelsson, *Bioorg. Med. Chem. Lett.*, 2011, **21**, 358.

28. M. N. Greco, E. T. Powell, L. R. Hecker, P. Andrade-Gordon, J. A. Kauffman, J. M. Lewis, V. Ganesh, A. Tulinsky and B. E. Maryanoff, *Bioorg. Med. Chem. Lett.*, 1996, **6**, 2947.

29. P. G. Nantermet, J. C. Barrow, C. L. Newton, J. M. Pellicore, M. Young, S. D. Lewis, B. J. Lucas, J. A. Krueger, D. R. McMasters, Y. Yan, L. C. Kuo, J. P. Vacca and H. G. Selnick, *Bioorg. Med. Chem. Lett.*, 2003, **13**, 2781.

30. B. L. Podlogar, R. A. Farr, D. Friedrich, C. Tarnus, E. W. Huber, R. J. Cregge and D. Schirlin, *J. Med. Chem.*, 1994, **37**, 3684.

31. G. Abbenante, D. A. Bergman, R. I. Brinkworth, D. R. March, R. C. Reid, P. A. Hunt, I. W. James, R. J. Dancer, B. Garnham, M. L. Stoermer and D. P. Fairlie, *Bioorg. Med. Chem. Lett.*, 1996, **6**, 2531.

32. S. J. Stachel, C. A. Coburn, S. Sankaranarayanan, E. A. Price, G. Wu, M. Crouthamel, B. L. Pietrak, Q. Huang, J. Lineberger, A. S. Espeseth, L. Jin, J. Ellis, M. K. Holloway, S. Munshi, T. Allison, D. Hazuda, A. J. Simon, S. L. Graham and J. P. Vacca, *J. Med. Chem.*, 2006, **49**, 6147.

33. C. B. Xue, X. He, R. L. Corbett, J. Roderick, Z. R. Wasserman, R. Q. Liu, B. D. Jaffee, M. B. Covington, M. Qian, J. M. Trzaskos, R. C. Newton, R. L. Magolda, R. R. Wexler and C. P. Decicco, *J. Med. Chem.*, 2001, **44**, 3351.

34. R. J. Cherney, L. Wang, D. T. Meyer, C. B. Xue, Z. R. Wasserman, K. D. Hardman, P. K. Welch, M. B. Covington, R. A. Copeland, E. C. Arner, W. F. DeGrado and C. P. Decicco, *J. Med. Chem.*, 1998, **41**, 1749.

35. E. Dumez, J. S. Snaith, R. F. Jackson, A. B. McElroy, J. Overington, M. J. Wythes, J. M. Withka and T. J. McLellan, *J. Org. Chem.*, 2002, **67**, 4882.

36. H. Chen, W. Jiao, M. A. Jones, J. M. Coxon, J. D. Morton, R. Bickerstaffe, A. D. Pehere, O. Zvarec and A. D. Abell, *Chem. Biodiversity*, 2012, **9**, 2473.

37. G. L. Bolton, B. D. Roth and B. K. Trivedi, *Tetrahedron*, 1993, **49**, 525.

38. D. J. Suich, S. A. Mousa, G. Singh, G. Liapakis, T. Reisine and W. F. DeGrado, *Bioorg. Med. Chem.*, 2000, **8**, 2229.

39. K. Lee, M. Zhang, H. Liu, D. Yang and T. R. Burke, Jr, *J. Med. Chem.*, 2003, **46**, 2621.

40. S. C. Mwakwari, V. Patil, W. Guerrant and A. K. Oyelere, *Curr. Top. Med. Chem.*, 2010, **10**, 1423.

41. A. Suda, H. Koyano, T. Hayase, K. Hada, K.-i. Kawasaki, S. Komiyama, K. Hasegawa, T. A. Fukami, S. Sato, T. Miura, N. Ono, T. Yamazaki, R. Saitoh, N. Shimma, Y. Shiratori and T. Tsukuda, *Bioorg. Med. Chem. Lett.*, 2012, **22**, 1136.

42. G. Udugamasooriya, D. Saro and M. R. Spaller, *Org. Lett.*, 2005, 7, 1203.

43. Y. Singh, M. J. Stoermer, A. J. Lucke, M. P. Glenn and D. P. Fairlie, *Org. Lett.*, 2002, **4**, 3367.

44. Y. Singh, M. J. Stoermer, A. J. Lucke, T. Guthrie and D. P. Fairlie, *J. Am. Chem. Soc.*, 2005, **127**, 6563.

45. M. C. Nielsen and T. Ulven, *Curr. Med. Chem.*, 2010, **17**, 3438.

46. D. Monchaud, A. Granzhan, N. Saettel, A. Guedin, J. L. Mergny and M. P. Teulade-Fichou, *J. Nucleic Acids*, 2010, **2010**, DOI: 10.4061/2010/525862 and DOI: 10.4061/2010/460561.

47. A. Granzhan, D. Monchaud, N. Saettel, A. Guedin, J. L. Mergny and M. P. Teulade-Fichou, *J. Nucleic Acids*, 2010, **2010**, DOI: 10.4061/2010/460561.

48. E. Gonthier and R. Breinbauer, *Mol. Diversity*, 2005, **9**, 51.

49. J. I. Luengo, A. Konialian-Beck, M. A. Levy, M. Brandt, D. S. Eggleston and D. A. Holt, *Bioorg. Med. Chem. Lett.*, 1994, **4**, 321.

50. I. Paterson, G. J. Naylor, N. M. Gardner, E. Guzman and A. E. Wright, *Chem. - Asian J.*, 2011, **6**, 459.

51. J. Inanaga, K. Hirata, H. Saeki, T. Katsuki and M. Yamaguchi, *Bull. Chem. Soc. Jpn.*, 1979, **52**, 1989.

52. S. Vendeville, T.-I. Lin, L. Hu, A. Tahri, D. McGowan, M. D. Cummings, K. Amssoms, M. Canard, S. Last, I. Van den Steen, B. Devogelaere, M.-C. Rouan, L. Vijgen, J. M. Berke, P. Dehertogh, E. Fransen, E. Cleiren, L. van der Helm, G. Fanning, K. Van Emelen, O. Nyanguile, K. Simmen and P. Raboisson, *Bioorg. Med. Chem. Lett.*, 2012, **22**, 4437.

53. M. Sanguinetti, S. Sanfilippo, D. Castagnolo, D. Sanglard, B. Posteraro, G. Donzellini and M. Botta, *ACS Med. Chem. Lett.*, 2013, **4**, 852.

54. J. H. van Maarseveen, *Comb. Chem. High Throughput Screening*, 1998, **1**, 185.

55. G. J. Bridger, R. T. Skerlj, D. Thornton, S. Padmanabhan, S. A. Martellucci, G. W. Henson, M. J. Abrams, N. Yamamoto and K. D. Vreese, *J. Med. Chem.*, 1995, **38**, 366.

56. S. P. Fricker, *Expert Opin. Invest. Drugs*, 2008, **17**, 1749.

57. G. J. Bridger, R. T. Skerlj, P. E. Hernandez-Abad, D. E. Bogucki, Z. Wang, Y. Zhou, S. Nan, E. M. Boehringer, T. Wilson, J. Crawford, M. Metz, S. Hatse, K. Princen, E. De Clercq and D. Schols, *J. Med. Chem.*, 2010, **53**, 1250.

58. X. Ling, E. Spaeth, Y. Chen, Y. Shi, W. Zhang, W. Schober, N. Hail, Jr, M. Konopleva and M. Andreeff, *PLoS One*, 2013, **8**, e58426.

59. M. Ciampolini, L. Fabbrizzi, A. Perotti, A. Poggi, B. Seghi and F. Zanobini, *Inorg. Chem.*, 1987, **26**, 3527.

60. E. De Clercq, N. Yamamoto, R. Pauwels, M. Baba, D. Schols, H. Nakashima, J. Balzarini, Z. Debyser, B. A. Murrer and D. Schwartz, *Proc. Natl. Acad. Sci., U. S. A.*, 1992, **89**, 5286.

61. H. An and P. D. Cook, *Tetrahedron Lett.*, 1996, **37**, 7233.

62. S. Hanessian, G. Yang, J. M. Rondeau, U. Neumann, C. Betschart and M. Tintelnot-Blomley, *J. Med. Chem.*, 2006, **49**, 4544.

63. N. S. A. M. Khalil, *Eur. J. Med. Chem.*, 2010, **45**, 5265.

64. A. A. Virgilio and J. A. Ellman, *J. Am. Chem. Soc.*, 1994, **116**, 11580.

65. J. D. Tyndall, R. C. Reid, D. P. Tyssen, D. K. Jardine, B. Todd, M. Passmore, D. R. March, L. K. Pattenden, D. A. Bergman, D. Alewood, S. H. Hu, P. F. Alewood, C. J. Birch, J. L. Martin and D. P. Fairlie, *J. Med. Chem.*, 2000, **43**, 3495.

66. M. P. Glenn, L. K. Pattenden, R. C. Reid, D. P. Tyssen, J. D. Tyndall, C. J. Birch and D. P. Fairlie, *J. Med. Chem.*, 2002, **45**, 371.
67. M. Ramaseshan, Y. L. Dory and P. Deslongchamps, *J. Comb. Chem.*, 2000, **2**, 615.
68. C. B. Xue, M. E. Voss, D. J. Nelson, J. J. Duan, R. J. Cherney, I. C. Jacobson, X. He, J. Roderick, L. Chen, R. L. Corbett, L. Wang, D. T. Meyer, K. Kennedy, W. F. DeGradodagger, K. D. Hardman, C. A. Teleha, B. D. Jaffee, R. Q. Liu, R. A. Copeland, M. B. Covington, D. D. Christ, J. M. Trzaskos, R. C. Newton, R. L. Magolda, R. R. Wexler and C. P. Decicco, *J. Med. Chem.*, 2001, **44**, 2636.
69. N. Kawanishi, T. Sugimoto, J. Shibata, K. Nakamura, K. Masutani, M. Ikuta and H. Hirai, *Bioorg. Med. Chem. Lett.*, 2006, **16**, 5122.
70. J. J. Duan, L. Chen, C. B. Xue, Z. R. Wasserman, K. D. Hardman, M. B. Covington, R. R. Copeland, E. C. Arner and C. P. Decicco, *Bioorg. Med. Chem. Lett.*, 1999, **9**, 1453.
71. A. Nefzi, S. Arutyunyan and J. E. Fenwick, *J. Org. Chem.*, 2010, **75**, 7939.
72. A. Nefzi and J. E. Fenwick, *Tetrahedron Lett.*, 2011, **52**, 817.
73. M. J. Kim, S. H. Lee, S. O. Park, H. Kang, J. S. Lee, K. N. Lee, M. E. Jung, J. Kim and J. Lee, *Bioorg. Med. Chem.*, 2011, **19**, 5468.
74. J. Zhu, *Synlett*, 1997, **1997**, 133.
75. E. N. Pitsinos, V. P. Vidali and E. A. Couladouros, *Eur. J. Org. Chem.*, 2011, **2011**, 1207.
76. K. Burgess, D. Lim, M. Bois-Choussy and J. Zhu, *Tetrahedron Lett.*, 1997, **38**, 3345.
77. C. Fotsch, G. Kumaravel, S. K. Sharma, A. D. Wu, J. S. Gounarides, N. R. Nirmala and R. C. Petter, *Bioorg. Med. Chem. Lett.*, 1999, **9**, 2125.
78. Y. Feng, Z. Wang, S. Jin and K. Burgess, *J. Am. Chem. Soc.*, 1998, **120**, 10768.
79. L. Jiang and K. Burgess, *Tetrahedron*, 2002, **58**, 8743.
80. H. B. Lee, M. C. Zaccaro, M. Pattarawarapan, S. Roy, H. U. Saragovi and K. Burgess, *J. Org. Chem.*, 2004, **69**, 701.
81. S. Maliartchouk, Y. Feng, L. Ivanisevic, T. Debeir, A. C. Cuello, K. Burgess and H. U. Saragovi, *Mol. Pharmacol.*, 2000, **57**, 385.
82. M. Pattarawarapan, M. C. Zaccaro, U. H. Saragovi and K. Burgess, *J. Med. Chem.*, 2002, **45**, 4387.
83. M. C. Zaccaro, H. B. Lee, M. Pattarawarapan, Z. Xia, A. Caron, P. J. L'Heureux, Y. Bengio, K. Burgess and H. U. Saragovi, *Chem. Biol.*, 2005, **12**, 1015.
84. F. Brahimi, A. Malakhov, H. B. Lee, M. Pattarawarapan, L. Ivanisevic, K. Burgess and H. U. Saragovi, *Peptides*, 2009, **30**, 1833.
85. S. Derbel, K. Ghedira and A. Nefzi, *Tetrahedron Lett.*, 2010, **51**, 3607.
86. C. J. Dinsmore, M. J. Bogusky, J. C. Culberson, J. M. Bergman, C. F. Homnick, C. B. Zartman, S. D. Mosser, M. D. Schaber, R. G. Robinson, K. S. Koblan, H. E. Huber, S. L. Graham, G. D. Hartman, J. R. Huff and T. M. Williams, *J. Am. Chem. Soc.*, 2001, **123**, 2107.

87. D. C. Beshore, I. M. Bell, C. J. Dinsmore, C. F. Homnick, J. C. Culberson, R. G. Robinson, C. Fernandes, E. S. Walsh, M. T. Abrams, H. G. Bhimnathwala, J. P. Davide, M. S. Ellis-Hutchings, H. A. Huber, K. S. Koblan, C. A. Buser, N. E. Kohl, R. B. Lobell, I. W. Chen, D. A. McLoughlin, T. V. Olah, S. L. Graham, G. D. Hartman and T. M. Williams, *Bioorg. Med. Chem. Lett.*, 2001, **11**, 1817.

88. I. M. Bell, S. N. Gallicchio, M. Abrams, L. S. Beese, D. C. Beshore, H. Bhimnathwala, M. J. Bogusky, C. A. Buser, J. C. Culberson, J. Davide, M. Ellis-Hutchings, C. Fernandes, J. B. Gibbs, S. L. Graham, K. A. Hamilton, G. D. Hartman, D. C. Heimbrook, C. F. Homnick, H. E. Huber, J. R. Huff, K. Kassahun, K. S. Koblan, N. E. Kohl, R. B. Lobell, J. J. Lynch, Jr, R. Robinson, A. D. Rodrigues, J. S. Taylor, E. S. Walsh, T. M. Williams and C. B. Zartman, *J. Med. Chem.*, 2002, **45**, 2388.

89. C. J. Dinsmore, C. B. Zartman, J. M. Bergman, M. T. Abrams, C. A. Buser, J. C. Culberson, J. P. Davide, M. Ellis-Hutchings, C. Fernandes, S. L. Graham, G. D. Hartman, H. E. Huber, R. B. Lobell, S. D. Mosser, R. G. Robinson and T. M. Williams, *Bioorg. Med. Chem. Lett.*, 2004, **14**, 639.

90. U. Lucking, G. Siemeister, M. Schafer, H. Briem, M. Kruger, P. Lienau and R. Jautelat, *ChemMedChem*, 2007, **2**, 63.

91. P. Grieco, P. Campiglia, I. Gomez-Monterrey, T. Lama and E. Novellino, *Synlett*, 2003, **2003**, 2216.

92. P. Grieco, M. Cai, L. Liu, A. Mayorov, K. Chandler, D. Trivedi, G. Lin, P. Campiglia, E. Novellino and V. J. Hruby, *J. Med. Chem.*, 2008, **51**, 2701.

93. L. Shen, C. J. Simmons and D. Sun, *Tetrahedron Lett.*, 2012, **53**, 4173.

94. L. Shen, M. M. Maddox, S. Adhikari, D. F. Bruhn, M. Kumar, R. E. Lee, J. G. Hurdle, R. E. Lee and D. Sun, *J. Antibiot.*, 2013, **66**, 319.

95. J. C. Collins, K. A. Farley, C. Limberakis, S. Liras, D. Price and K. James, *J. Org. Chem.*, 2012, **77**, 11079.

96. A. T. Londregan, K. A. Farley, C. Limberakis, P. B. Mullins and D. W. Piotrowski, *Org. Lett.*, 2012, **14**, 2890.

97. R. H. Grubbs, S. J. Miller and G. C. Fu, *Acc. Chem. Res.*, 1995, **28**, 446.

98. T. Gaich and J. Mulzer, *Curr. Top. Med. Chem.*, 2005, **5**, 1473.

99. A. Gradillas and J. Perez-Castells, *Angew. Chem., Int. Ed.*, 2006, **45**, 6086.

100. P. Van de Weghe and J. Eustache, *Curr. Top. Med. Chem.*, 2005, **5**, 1495.

101. W. H. Martin and S. Blechert, *Curr. Top. Med. Chem.*, 2005, **5**, 1521.

102. V. M. Marx, M. B. Herbert, B. K. Keitz and R. H. Grubbs, *J. Am. Chem. Soc.*, 2013, **135**, 94.

103. S. J. Miller, H. E. Blackwell and R. H. Grubbs, *J. Am. Chem. Soc.*, 1996, **118**, 9606.

104. S. Sasmal, A. Geyer and M. E. Maier, *J. Org. Chem.*, 2002, **67**, 6260.

105. I. Ojima and M. Das, *J. Nat. Prod.*, 2009, **72**, 554.

106. A. K. Ghosh, T. Devasamudram, L. Hong, C. DeZutter, X. Xu, V. Weerasena, G. Koelsch, G. Bilcer and J. Tang, *Bioorg. Med. Chem. Lett.*, 2005, **15**, 15.

107. I. Rojo, J. A. Martin, H. Broughton, D. Timm, J. Erickson, H. C. Yang and J. R. McCarthy, *Bioorg. Med. Chem. Lett.*, 2006, **16**, 191.
108. R. Machauer, S. Veenstra, J. M. Rondeau, M. Tintelnot-Blomley, C. Betschart, U. Neumann and P. Paganetti, *Bioorg. Med. Chem. Lett.*, 2009, **19**, 1361.
109. R. Machauer, K. Laumen, S. Veenstra, J. M. Rondeau, M. Tintelnot-Blomley, C. Betschart, A. L. Jaton, S. Desrayaud, M. Staufenbiel, S. Rabe, P. Paganetti and U. Neumann, *Bioorg. Med. Chem. Lett.*, 2009, **19**, 1366.
110. A. Lerchner, R. Machauer, C. Betschart, S. Veenstra, H. Rueeger, C. McCarthy, M. Tintelnot-Blomley, A. L. Jaton, S. Rabe, S. Desrayaud, A. Enz, M. Staufenbiel, P. Paganetti, J. M. Rondeau and U. Neumann, *Bioorg. Med. Chem. Lett.*, 2010, **20**, 603.
111. T. Huber, F. Manzenrieder, C. A. Kuttruff, C. Dorner-Ciossek and H. Kessler, *Bioorg. Med. Chem. Lett.*, 2009, **19**, 4427.
112. V. Sandgren, T. Agback, P. O. Johansson, J. Lindberg, I. Kvarnstrom, B. Samuelsson, O. Belda and A. Dahlgren, *Bioorg. Med. Chem.*, 2012, **20**, 4377.
113. L. D. Pennington, D. A. Whittington, M. D. Bartberger, S. R. Jordan, H. Monenschein, T. T. Nguyen, B. H. Yang, Q. M. Xue, F. Vounatsos, R. C. Wahl, K. Chen, S. Wood, M. Citron, V. F. Patel, S. A. Hitchcock and W. Zhong, *Bioorg. Med. Chem. Lett.*, 2013, **23**, 4459.
114. A. D. Abell, M. A. Jones, J. M. Coxon, J. D. Morton, S. G. Aitken, S. B. McNabb, H. Y. Lee, J. M. Mehrtens, N. A. Alexander, B. G. Stuart, A. T. Neffe and R. Bickerstaffe, *Angew. Chem., Int. Ed.*, 2009, **48**, 1455.
115. B. G. Stuart, J. M. Coxon, J. D. Morton, A. D. Abell, D. Q. McDonald, S. G. Aitken, M. A. Jones and R. Bickerstaffe, *J. Med. Chem.*, 2011, **54**, 7503.
116. Z. F. Tao, L. Wang, K. D. Stewart, Z. Chen, W. Gu, M. H. Bui, P. Merta, H. Zhang, P. Kovar, E. Johnson, C. Park, R. Judge, S. Rosenberg, T. Sowin and N. H. Lin, *J. Med. Chem.*, 2007, **50**, 1514.
117. G. Li, Z. F. Tao, Y. Tong, M. K. Przytulinska, P. Kovar, P. Merta, Z. Chen, H. Zhang, T. Sowin, S. H. Rosenberg and N. H. Lin, *Bioorg. Med. Chem. Lett.*, 2007, **17**, 6499.
118. Z. F. Tao, Z. Chen, M. H. Bui, P. Kovar, E. Johnson, J. Bouska, H. Zhang, S. Rosenberg, T. Sowin and N. H. Lin, *Bioorg. Med. Chem. Lett.*, 2007, **17**, 6593.
119. M. Satyanarayana, S. G. Rzuczek, E. J. Lavoie, D. S. Pilch, A. Liu, L. F. Liu and J. E. Rice, *Bioorg. Med. Chem. Lett.*, 2008, **18**, 3802.
120. C. Q. Wei, Y. Gao, K. Lee, R. Guo, B. Li, M. Zhang, D. Yang and T. R. Burke, Jr, *J. Med. Chem.*, 2003, **46**, 244.
121. S. U. Kang, Z. D. Shi, K. M. Worthy, L. K. Bindu, P. G. Dharmawardana, S. J. Choyke, D. P. Bottaro, R. J. Fisher and T. R. Burke, Jr, *J. Med. Chem.*, 2005, **48**, 3945.
122. F. Liu, K. M. Worthy, L. K. Bindu, R. J. Fisher and T. R. Burke, Jr, *J. Org. Chem.*, 2007, **72**, 9635.

123. L. Auzzas, A. Larsson, R. Matera, A. Baraldi, B. Deschenes-Simard, G. Giannini, W. Cabri, G. Battistuzzi, G. Gallo, A. Ciacci, L. Vesci, C. Pisano and S. Hanessian, *J. Med. Chem.*, 2010, **53**, 8387.

124. A. K. Ghosh, L. M. Swanson, C. Liu, K. A. Hussain, H. Cho, D. E. Walters, L. Holland and J. Buthod, *Bioorg. Med. Chem. Lett.*, 2002, **12**, 1993.

125. A. K. Ghosh, L. M. Swanson, H. Cho, S. Leshchenko, K. A. Hussain, S. Kay, D. E. Walters, Y. Koh and H. Mitsuya, *J. Med. Chem.*, 2005, **48**, 3576.

126. A. K. Ghosh, S. Kulkarni, D. D. Anderson, L. Hong, A. Baldridge, Y. F. Wang, A. A. Chumanevich, A. Y. Kovalevsky, Y. Tojo, M. Amano, Y. Koh, J. Tang, I. T. Weber and H. Mitsuya, *J. Med. Chem.*, 2009, **52**, 7689.

127. E. N. Prabhakaran, V. Rajesh, S. Dubey and J. Iqbal, *Tetrahedron Lett.*, 2001, **42**, 339.

128. J. E. Day, S. Y. Sharp, M. G. Rowlands, W. Aherne, P. Workman and C. J. Moody, *Chem. - Eur. J.*, 2010, **16**, 2758.

129. J. E. Day, S. Y. Sharp, M. G. Rowlands, W. Aherne, A. Hayes, F. I. Raynaud, W. Lewis, S. M. Roe, C. Prodromou, L. H. Pearl, P. Workman and C. J. Moody, *ACS Chem. Biol.*, 2011, **6**, 1339.

130. H. Andersson, H. Demaegdt, A. Johnsson, G. Vauquelin, G. Lindeberg, M. Hallberg, M. Erdelyi, A. Karlen and A. Hallberg, *J. Med. Chem.*, 2011, **54**, 3779.

131. H. Kai, H. Hinou, K. Naruchi, T. Matsushita and S. Nishimura, *Chem. - Eur. J.*, 2013, **19**, 1364.

132. P. W. Harris and M. A. Brimble, *Org. Biomol. Chem.*, 2006, **4**, 2696.

133. X. Hu, K. T. Nguyen, V. C. Jiang, D. Lofland, H. E. Moser and D. Pei, *J. Med. Chem.*, 2004, **47**, 4941.

134. G. Shen, J. Zhu, A. M. Simpson and D. Pei, *Bioorg. Med. Chem. Lett.*, 2008, **18**, 3060.

135. K. Ersmark, M. Nervall, H. Gutierrez-de-Teran, E. Hamelink, L. K. Janka, J. C. Clemente, B. M. Dunn, A. Gogoll, B. Samuelsson, J. Qvist and A. Hallberg, *Bioorg. Med. Chem.*, 2006, **14**, 2197.

136. D. S. Maxwell, D. Sun, Z. Peng, D. V. Martin, B. A. Bhanu Prasad and W. G. Bornmann, *Tetrahedron Lett.*, 2013, **54**, 5799.

137. S. Y. Kang, M. J. Kim, J. S. Lee and J. Lee, *Bioorg. Med. Chem. Lett.*, 2011, **21**, 3759.

138. J. Zhou, M.-C. Matos and P. V. Murphy, *Org. Lett.*, 2011, **13**, 5716.

139. S. Hanessian, A. Larsson, T. Fex, W. Knecht and N. Blomberg, *Bioorg. Med. Chem. Lett.*, 2010, **20**, 6925.

140. F. Liu, A. G. Stephen, A. A. Waheed, E. O. Freed, R. J. Fisher and T. R. Burke, Jr, *Bioorg. Med. Chem. Lett.*, 2010, **20**, 318.

141. S. Venkatraman and F. G. Njoroge, *Curr. Top. Med. Chem.*, 2007, 7, 1290.

142. S. Venkatraman and F. G. Njoroge, *Expert Opin. Ther. Pat.*, 2009, **19**, 1277.

143. S. Avolio and V. Summa, *Curr. Top. Med. Chem.*, 2010, **10**, 1403.

144. M. Deutsch and G. V. Papatheodoridis, *Curr. Opin. Invest. Drugs*, 2010, **11**, 951.

145. Y. Jiang, S. W. Andrews, K. R. Condroski, B. Buckman, V. Serebryany, S. Wenglowsky, A. L. Kennedy, M. R. Madduru, B. Wang, M. Lyon, G. A. Doherty, B. T. Woodard, C. Lemieux, M. G. Do, H. Zhang, J. Ballard, G. Vigers, B. J. Brandhuber, P. Stengel, J. A. Josey, L. Beigelman, L. Blatt and S. D. Seiwert, *J. Med. Chem.*, 2014, **57**, 1753.

146. D. Lamarre, P. C. Anderson, M. Bailey, P. Beaulieu, G. Bolger, P. Bonneau, M. Bos, D. R. Cameron, M. Cartier, M. G. Cordingley, A. M. Faucher, N. Goudreau, S. H. Kawai, G. Kukolj, L. Lagace, S. R. LaPlante, H. Narjes, M. A. Poupart, J. Rancourt, R. E. Sentjens, R. St George, B. Simoneau, G. Steinmann, D. Thibeault, Y. S. Tsantrizos, S. M. Weldon, C. L. Yong and M. Llinas-Brunet, *Nature*, 2003, **426**, 186.

147. M. Llinas-Brunet, M. D. Bailey, G. Bolger, C. Brochu, A. M. Faucher, J. M. Ferland, M. Garneau, E. Ghiro, V. Gorys, C. Grand-Maitre, T. Halmos, N. Lapeyre-Paquette, F. Liard, M. Poirier, M. Rheaume, Y. S. Tsantrizos and D. Lamarre, *J. Med. Chem.*, 2004, **47**, 1605.

148. X. Wei, C. Shu, N. Haddad, X. Zeng, N. D. Patel, Z. Tan, J. Liu, H. Lee, S. Shen, S. Campbell, R. J. Varsolona, C. A. Busacca, A. Hossain, N. K. Yee and C. H. Senanayake, *Org. Lett.*, 2013, **15**, 1016.

149. S. Harper, J. A. McCauley, M. T. Rudd, M. Ferrara, M. DiFilippo, B. Crescenzi, U. Koch, A. Petrocchi, M. K. Holloway, J. W. Butcher, J. J. Romano, K. J. Bush, K. F. Gilbert, C. J. McIntyre, K. T. Nguyen, E. Nizi, S. S. Carroll, S. W. Ludmerer, C. Burlein, J. M. DiMuzio, D. J. Graham, C. M. McHale, M. W. Stahlhut, D. B. Olsen, E. Monteagudo, S. Cianetti, C. Giuliano, V. Pucci, N. Trainor, C. M. Fandozzi, M. Rowley, P. J. Coleman, J. P. Vacca, V. Summa and N. J. Liverton, *ACS Med. Chem. Lett.*, 2012, **3**, 332.

150. V. Summa, S. W. Ludmerer, J. A. McCauley, C. Fandozzi, C. Burlein, G. Claudio, P. J. Coleman, J. M. Dimuzio, M. Ferrara, M. Di Filippo, A. T. Gates, D. J. Graham, S. Harper, D. J. Hazuda, C. McHale, E. Monteagudo, V. Pucci, M. Rowley, M. T. Rudd, A. Soriano, M. W. Stahlhut, J. P. Vacca, D. B. Olsen, N. J. Liverton and S. S. Carroll, *Antimicrob. Agents Chemother.*, 2012, **56**, 4161.

151. J. A. McCauley, C. J. McIntyre, M. T. Rudd, K. T. Nguyen, J. J. Romano, J. W. Butcher, K. F. Gilbert, K. J. Bush, M. K. Holloway, J. Swestock, B. L. Wan, S. S. Carroll, J. M. DiMuzio, D. J. Graham, S. W. Ludmerer, S. S. Mao, M. W. Stahlhut, C. M. Fandozzi, N. Trainor, D. B. Olsen, J. P. Vacca and N. J. Liverton, *J. Med. Chem.*, 2010, **53**, 2443.

152. J. de Bruijne, A. van Vliet, C. J. Weegink, W. Mazur, A. Wiercinska-Drapalo, K. Simon, G. Cholewinska-Szymanska, J. Kapocsi, I. Varkonyi, X. J. Zhou, M. F. Temam, J. Molles, J. Chen, K. Pietropaolo, J. F. McCarville, J. Z. Sullivan-Bolyai, D. Mayers and H. Reesink, *Antiviral Ther.*, 2012, **17**, 633.

153. Y. S. Tsantrizos, *Curr.Opin. Invest. Drugs*, 2009, **10**, 871.
154. A. D. William, A. C. Lee, K. C. Goh, S. Blanchard, A. Poulsen, E. L. Teo, H. Nagaraj, C. P. Lee, H. Wang, M. Williams, E. T. Sun, C. Hu, R. Jayaraman, M. K. Pasha, K. Ethirajulu, J. M. Wood and B. W. Dymock, *J. Med. Chem.*, 2012, **55**, 169.
155. A. Poulsen, A. William, S. Blanchard, H. Nagaraj, M. Williams, H. Wang, A. Lee, E. Sun, E. L. Teo, E. Tan, K. C. Goh and B. Dymock, *J. Mol. Model.*, 2013, **19**, 119.
156. A. D. William, A. C. Lee, S. Blanchard, A. Poulsen, E. L. Teo, H. Nagaraj, E. Tan, D. Chen, M. Williams, E. T. Sun, K. C. Goh, W. C. Ong, S. K. Goh, S. Hart, R. Jayaraman, M. K. Pasha, K. Ethirajulu, J. M. Wood and B. W. Dymock, *J. Med. Chem.*, 2011, **54**, 4638.
157. A. Poulsen, A. William, S. Blanchard, A. Lee, H. Nagaraj, H. Wang, E. Teo, E. Tan, K. C. Goh and B. Dymock, *J. Comput.-Aided Mol. Des.*, 2012, **26**, 437.
158. A. D. William, A. C. Lee, A. Poulsen, K. C. Goh, B. Madan, S. Hart, E. Tan, H. Wang, H. Nagaraj, D. Chen, C. P. Lee, E. T. Sun, R. Jayaraman, M. K. Pasha, K. Ethirajulu, J. M. Wood and B. W. Dymock, *J. Med. Chem.*, 2012, **55**, 2623.
159. P. Nshimyumukiza, E. Van Den Berge, B. Delest, T. Mijatovic, R. Kiss, J. Marchand-Brynaert and R. Robiette, *Tetrahedron*, 2010, **66**, 4515.
160. A. Urbach, G. Dive and J. Marchand-Brynaert, *Eur. J. Org. Chem.*, 2009, **2009**, 1757.
161. A. Urbach, G. Dive, B. Tinant, V. Duval and J. Marchand-Brynaert, *Eur. J. Med. Chem.*, 2009, **44**, 2071.
162. A. Sliwa, G. Dive and J. Marchand-Brynaert, *Chem. - Asian J.*, 2012, 7, 425.
163. A. Fürstner and K. Langemann, *J. Am. Chem. Soc.*, 1997, **119**, 9130.
164. A. Sliwa, G. Dive, J.-L. Habib Jiwan and J. Marchand-Brynaert, *Tetrahedron*, 2010, **66**, 9519.
165. G. Dive, C. Bouillon, A. Sliwa, B. Valet, O. Verlaine, E. Sauvage and J. Marchand-Brynaert, *Eur. J. Med. Chem.*, 2013, **64**, 365.
166. D. R. Coghlan, J. B. Bremner, P. A. Keller, S. G. Pyne, D. M. David, K. Somphol, D. Baylis, J. Coates, J. Deadman, D. I. Rhodes and A. D. Robertson, *Bioorg. Med. Chem.*, 2011, **19**, 3549.
167. B. Dasari, S. Jogula, R. Borhade, S. Balasubramanian, G. Chandrasekar, S. S. Kitambi and P. Arya, *Org. Lett.*, 2013, **15**, 432.
168. M. Aeluri, C. Pramanik, L. Chetia, N. K. Mallurwar, S. Balasubramanian, G. Chandrasekar, S. S. Kitambi and P. Arya, *Org. Lett.*, 2013, **15**, 436.
169. S. Jogula, B. Dasari, M. Khatravath, G. Chandrasekar, S. S. Kitambi and P. Arya, *Eur. J. Org. Chem.*, 2013, **2013**, 5036.
170. S. Chamakuri, S. K. R. Guduru, S. Pamu, G. Chandrasekar, S. S. Kitambi and P. Arya, *Eur. J. Org. Chem.*, 2013, **2013**, 3959.
171. S. K. Reddy Guduru, S. Chamakuri, G. Chandrasekar, S. S. Kitambi and P. Arya, *ACS Med. Chem. Lett.*, 2013, **4**, 666.

172. K. Estieu-Gionnet and G. Guichard, *Expert Opin. Drug Discovery*, 2011, **6**, 937.
173. G. L. Verdine and G. J. Hilinski, *Drug Discovery Today: Technol.*, 2012, **9**, e41.
174. G. L. Verdine and G. J. Hilinski, *Methods Enzymol.*, 2012, **503**, 3.
175. L. D. Walensky and G. H. Bird, *J. Med. Chem.*, 2014, **57**, DOI: 10.1021/jm4011675.
176. The structure of this 29-amino acid compound has not been publicly released.
177. K. Olson, H. Cai, S. J. DeMarco, N. Kawahata, A. Mukherjee, E. Shi, A. M. Manning, A. Annis and H. C. Chen, *The Endocrine Socety's 95th National Meeting and Exposition*, 2013. https://endo.confex.com/endo/2013endo/webprogram/Paper5438.html.
178. Aileron Therapeutics, Inc. Press Release, 7 May 2013. http://www.businesswire.com/news/home/20130507005467/en/Aileron-Therapeutics-Successfully-Completes-First-Ever-Stapled-Peptide.
179. A. Furstner and P. W. Davies, *Chem. Commun.*, 2005, 2307.
180. X. Wu and M. Tamm, *Beilstein J. Org. Chem.*, 2011, **7**, 82.
181. H. Villar, M. Frings and C. Bolm, *Chem. Soc. Rev.*, 2007, **36**, 55.
182. A. G. M. Barrett, A. J. Hennessy, R. L. Vézouët, P. A. Procopiou, P. W. Seale, S. Stefaniak, R. J. Upton, A. J. P. White and D. J. Williams, *J. Org. Chem.*, 2004, **69**, 1028.
183. E. C. Hansen and D. Lee, *J. Am. Chem. Soc.*, 2003, **125**, 9582.
184. S. Kotha and K. Singh, *Eur. J. Org. Chem.*, 2007, **2007**, 5909.
185. J. Tilley, G. Kaplan, N. Fotouhi, B. Wolitzky and K. Rowan, *Bioorg. Med. Chem. Lett.*, 2000, **10**, 1163.
186. K. C. K. Swamy, N. N. B. Kumar, E. Balaraman and K. V. P. P. Kumar, *Chem. Rev.*, 2009, **109**, 2551.
187. D. H. Steinman, M. L. Curtin, R. B. Garland, S. K. Davidsen, H. R. Heyman, J. H. Holms, D. H. Albert, T. J. Magoc, I. B. Nagy, P. A. Marcotte, J. Li, D. W. Morgan, C. Hutchins and J. B. Summers, *Bioorg. Med. Chem. Lett.*, 1998, **8**, 2087.
188. R. J. Cherney, L. Wang, D. T. Meyer, C. B. Xue, E. C. Arner, R. A. Copeland, M. B. Covington, K. D. Hardman, Z. R. Wasserman, B. D. Jaffee and C. P. Decicco, *Bioorg. Med. Chem. Lett.*, 1999, **9**, 1279.
189. A. Arasappan, K. X. Chen, F. G. Njoroge, T. N. Parekh and V. Girijavallabhan, *J. Org. Chem.*, 2002, **67**, 3923.
190. A. Arasappan, F. G. Njoroge, K. X. Chen, S. Venkatraman, T. N. Parekh, H. Gu, J. Pichardo, N. Butkiewicz, A. Prongay, V. Madison and V. Girijavallabhan, *Bioorg. Med. Chem. Lett.*, 2006, **16**, 3960.
191. K. X. Chen, F. G. Njoroge, J. Pichardo, A. Prongay, N. Butkiewicz, N. Yao, V. Madison and V. Girijavallabhan, *J. Med. Chem.*, 2006, **49**, 567.
192. J. Hovinen and R. Sillanpää, *Tetrahedron Lett.*, 2005, **46**, 4387.
193. Q. Wang and J. Zhu, *Chimia*, 2011, **65**, 168.
194. J. Dufour, L. Neuville and J. Zhu, *Chem. - Eur. J.*, 2010, **16**, 10523.
195. S. R. Chemler and S. J. Danishefsky, *Org. Lett.*, 2000, **2**, 2695.

196. W. Li and K. Burgess, *Tetrahedron Lett.*, 1999, **40**, 6527.
197. A. Afonso, L. Feliu and M. Planas, *Tetrahedron*, 2011, **67**, 2238.
198. M. Hiroshige, J. R. Hauske and P. Zhou, *J. Am. Chem. Soc.*, 1995, **117**, 11590.
199. K. Akaji and Y. Kiso, *Tetrahedron Lett.*, 1997, **38**, 5185.
200. K. Akaji, K. Teruya, M. Akaji and S. Aimoto, *Tetrahedron*, 2001, **57**, 2293.
201. P. Rajamohan Reddy, V. Balraju, G. R. Madhavan, B. Banerji and J. Iqbal, *Tetrahedron Lett.*, 2003, **44**, 353.
202. M. Aeluri, J. Gaddam, D. V. K. S. Trinath, G. Chandrasekar, S. S. Kitambi and P. Arya, *Eur. J. Org. Chem.*, 2013, **2013**, 3955.
203. K. X. Chen, F. G. Njoroge, A. Prongay, J. Pichardo, V. Madison and V. Girijavallabhan, *Bioorg. Med. Chem. Lett.*, 2005, **15**, 4475.
204. T. C. Boge, Z. J. Wu, R. H. Himes, D. G. Vander Velde and G. I. Georg, *Bioorg. Med. Chem. Lett.*, 1999, **9**, 3047.
205. X. Geng, M. L. Miller, S. Lin and I. Ojima, *Org. Lett.*, 2003, **5**, 3733.
206. I. Ojima, X. Geng, S. Lin, P. Pera and R. J. Bernacki, *Bioorg. Med. Chem. Lett.*, 2002, **12**, 349.
207. G. Byk, M. Cohen-Ohana and D. Raichman, *Biopolymers*, 2006, **84**, 274.
208. H. J. Breslin, B. M. Lane, G. R. Ott, A. K. Ghose, T. S. Angeles, M. S. Albom, M. Cheng, W. Wan, R. C. Haltiwanger, K. J. Wells-Knecht and B. D. Dorsey, *J. Med. Chem.*, 2012, **55**, 449.
209. M. A. J. Duncton and G. Pattenden, *J. Chem. Soc., Perkin Trans. 1*, 1999, 1235.
210. E. Marsault and P. Deslongchamps, *Org. Lett.*, 2000, **2**, 3317.
211. K. C. Nicolaou, N. Winssinger, J. Pastor and F. Murphy, *Angew. Chem., Int. Ed.*, 1998, **37**, 2534.
212. G. Falardeau, H. Lachance, A. St-Pierre, C. G. Yannopoulos, M. Drouin, J. Bedard and L. Chan, *Bioorg. Med. Chem. Lett.*, 2005, **15**, 1693.
213. R. Chinchilla and C. Nájera, *Chem. Rev.*, 2007, **107**, 874.
214. W. Zhang and J. S. Moore, *Angew. Chem., Int. Ed.*, 2006, **45**, 4416.
215. V. Balraju, D. S. Reddy, M. Periasamy and J. Iqbal, *J. Org. Chem.*, 2005, **70**, 9626.
216. H. T. ten Brink, D. T. S. Rijkers and R. M. J. Liskamp, *J. Org. Chem.*, 2006, **71**, 1817.
217. A. C. Spivey, J. McKendrick, R. Srikaran and B. A. Helm, *J. Org. Chem.*, 2003, **68**, 1843.
218. J. Krauss, D. Unterreitmeier, C. Neudert and F. Bracher, *Arch. Pharm.*, 2005, **338**, 605.
219. V. Balraju and J. Iqbal, *J. Org. Chem.*, 2006, **71**, 8954.
220. C. W. Zapf, J. D. Bloom, J. L. McBean, R. G. Dushin, T. Nittoli, C. Ingalls, A. G. Sutherland, J. P. Sonye, C. N. Eid, J. Golas, H. Liu, F. Boschelli, Y. Hu, E. Vogan and J. I. Levin, *Bioorg. Med. Chem. Lett.*, 2011, **21**, 2278.
221. C. W. Zapf, J. D. Bloom, J. L. McBean, R. G. Dushin, T. Nittoli, M. Otteng, C. Ingalls, J. M. Golas, H. Liu, J. Lucas, F. Boschelli, Y. Hu, E. Vogan and J. I. Levin, *Bioorg. Med. Chem. Lett.*, 2011, **21**, 3411.

222. C. W. Zapf, J. D. Bloom, J. L. McBean, R. G. Dushin, J. M. Golas, H. Liu, J. Lucas, F. Boschelli, E. Vogan and J. I. Levin, *Bioorg. Med. Chem. Lett.*, 2011, **21**, 3627.

223. C. W. Zapf, J. D. Bloom, Z. Li, R. G. Dushin, T. Nittoli, M. Otteng, A. Nikitenko, J. M. Golas, H. Liu, J. Lucas, F. Boschelli, E. Vogan, A. Olland, M. Johnson and J. I. Levin, *Bioorg. Med. Chem. Lett.*, 2011, **21**, 4602.

224. Q. Wei, S. Harran and P. G. Harran, *Tetrahedron*, 2003, **59**, 8947.

225. K. V. Lawson, T. E. Rose and P. G. Harran, *Proc. Natl. Acad. Sci. U.S.A.*, 2013, **110**, 3753.

226. V. Balraju, R. V. Dev, D. S. Reddy and J. Iqbal, *Tetrahedron Lett.*, 2006, **47**, 3569.

227. B. Barnickel and R. Schobert, *J. Org. Chem.*, 2010, **75**, 6716.

228. S. M. Lu and H. Alper, *Chem. - Eur. J.*, 2007, **13**, 5908.

229. T. Doi, S. Kamioka, S. Shimazu and T. Takahashi, *Org. Lett.*, 2008, **10**, 817.

230. S. Kamioka, S. Shimazu, T. Doi and T. Takahashi, *J. Comb. Chem.*, 2008, **10**, 681.

231. H. Shimamura, S. P. Breazzano, J. Garfunkle, F. S. Kimball, J. D. Trzupek and D. L. Boger, *J. Am. Chem. Soc.*, 2010, **132**, 7776.

232. S. P. Breazzano, Y. B. Poudel and D. L. Boger, *J. Am. Chem. Soc.*, 2013, **135**, 1600.

233. S. E. Denmark and J. M. Muhuhi, *J. Am. Chem. Soc.*, 2010, **132**, 11768.

234. J. W. Janetka and D. H. Rich, *J. Am. Chem. Soc.*, 1995, **117**, 10585.

235. C. W. West and D. H. Rich, *Org. Lett.*, 1999, **1**, 1819.

236. J. W. Janetka, P. Raman, K. Satyshur, G. R. Flentke and D. H. Rich, *J. Am. Chem. Soc.*, 1997, **119**, 441.

237. S. Venkatraman, F. George Njoroge and V. Girijavallabhan, *Tetrahedron*, 2002, **58**, 5453.

238. S. Venkatraman, F. G. Njoroge, V. M. Girijavallabhan, V. S. Madison, N. H. Yao, A. J. Prongay, N. Butkiewicz and J. Pichardo, *J. Med. Chem.*, 2005, **48**, 5088.

239. A. Marchetti, J. M. Ontoria and V. G. Matassa, *Synlett*, 1999, **1999**, 1000.

240. L. Sun, X. Geng, R. l. Geney, Y. Li, C. Simmerling, Z. Li, J. W. Lauher, S. Xia, S. B. Horwitz, J. M. Veith, P. Pera, R. J. Bernacki and I. Ojima, *J. Org. Chem.*, 2008, **73**, 9584.

241. A. Berthelot, S. Piguel, G. Le Dour and J. Vidal, *J. Org. Chem.*, 2003, **68**, 9835.

242. B. Knapp-Reed, G. M. Mahandru and J. Montgomery, *J. Am. Chem. Soc.*, 2005, **127**, 13156.

243. A. R. Shareef, D. H. Sherman and J. Montgomery, *Chem. Sci.*, 2012, **3**, 892.

244. M. H. Vilhelmsen, J. Jensen, C. G. Tortzen and M. B. Nielsen, *Eur. J. Org. Chem.*, 2013, **2013**, 701.

245. A. C. Bedard and S. K. Collins, *Chem. - Eur. J.*, 2013, **19**, 2108.

246. P. Bolduc, A. Jacques and S. K. Collins, *J. Am. Chem. Soc.*, 2010, **132**, 12790.

247. Z. Wang, in *Comprehensive Organic Name Reactions*, John Wiley & Sons, Hoboken, NJ, 2009, vol. 2, p. 2076.

248. A. Furstner, *Chem. Rev.*, 1999, **99**, 991.

249. L. A. Wessjohann and G. Scheid, *Synthesis*, 1999, 1.

250. C. A. LeClair, M. B. Boxer, C. J. Thomas and D. J. Maloney, *Tetrahedron Lett.*, 2010, **51**, 6852.

251. C. P. Decicco, Y. Song and D. A. Evans, *Org. Lett.*, 2001, **3**, 1029.

252. C. Y. Im and T. Sugimura, *Tetrahedron*, 2012, **68**, 3744.

253. M. R. Gesinski, K. Tadpetch and S. D. Rychnovsky, *Org. Lett.*, 2009, **11**, 5342.

254. G. C. Tron, T. Pirali, R. A. Billington, P. L. Canonico, G. Sorba and A. A. Genazzani, *Med. Res. Rev.*, 2008, **28**, 278.

255. C. Hein, X.-M. Liu and D. Wang, *Pharm. Res.*, 2008, **25**, 2216.

256. P. Thirumurugan, D. Matosiuk and K. Jozwiak, *Chem. Rev.*, 2013, **113**, 4905.

257. Y. L. Angell and K. Burgess, *Chem. Soc. Rev.*, 2007, **36**, 1674.

258. J. M. Holub and K. Kirshenbaum, *Chem. Soc. Rev.*, 2010, **39**, 1325.

259. A. D. Pehere and A. D. Abell, *Org. Lett.*, 2012, **14**, 1330.

260. G. Chouhan and K. James, *Org. Lett.*, 2013, **15**, 1206.

261. Y. Angell and K. Burgess, *J. Org. Chem.*, 2005, **70**, 9595.

262. R. E. Looper, D. Pizzirani and S. L. Schreiber, *Org. Lett.*, 2006, **8**, 2063.

263. D. Pasini, *Molecules*, 2013, **18**, 9512.

264. W. J. Choi, Z. D. Shi, K. M. Worthy, L. Bindu, R. G. Karki, M. C. Nicklaus, R. J. Fisher and T. R. Burke, Jr, *Bioorg. Med. Chem. Lett.*, 2006, **16**, 5265.

265. T. R. Chan, R. Hilgraf, K. B. Sharpless and V. V. Fokin, *Org. Lett.*, 2004, **6**, 2853.

266. G. Chouhan and K. James, *Org. Lett.*, 2011, **13**, 2754.

267. R. A. Turner, A. G. Oliver and R. S. Lokey, *Org. Lett.*, 2007, **9**, 5011.

268. A. R. Bogdan and K. James, *Org. Lett.*, 2011, **13**, 4060.

269. W. S. Horne, C. A. Olsen, J. M. Beierle, A. Montero and M. R. Ghadiri, *Angew. Chem., Int. Ed.*, 2009, **48**, 4718.

270. H. Sun, L. Liu, J. Lu, S. Qiu, C.-Y. Yang, H. Yi and S. Wang, *Bioorg. Med. Chem. Lett.*, 2010, **20**, 3043.

271. J. M. Beierle, W. S. Horne, J. H. van Maarseveen, B. Waser, J. C. Reubi and M. R. Ghadiri, *Angew. Chem., Int. Ed.*, 2009, **48**, 4725.

272. S. R. Mandadapu, P. M. Weerawarna, A. M. Prior, R. A. Uy, S. Aravapalli, K. R. Alliston, G. H. Lushington, Y. Kim, D. H. Hua, K. O. Chang and W. C. Groutas, *Bioorg. Med. Chem. Lett.*, 2013, **23**, 3709.

273. J. Chen, Z. Nikolovska-Coleska, C. Y. Yang, C. Gomez, W. Gao, K. Krajewski, S. Jiang, P. Roller and S. Wang, *Bioorg. Med. Chem. Lett.*, 2007, **17**, 3939.

274. J. Zhang, J. Kemmink, D. T. Rijkers and R. M. Liskamp, *Org. Lett.*, 2011, **13**, 3438.

275. J. Zhang, J. Kemmink, D. T. Rijkers and R. M. Liskamp, *Chem. Commun.*, 2013, **49**, 4498.

276. A. Isidro-Llobet, T. Murillo, P. Bello, A. Cilibrizzi, J. T. Hodgkinson, W. R. Galloway, A. Bender, M. Welch and D. R. Spring, *Proc. Natl. Acad. Sci. U.S.A.*, 2011, **108**, 6793.

277. A. Ajay, S. Sharma, M. P. Gupt, V. Bajpai, Hamidullah, B. Kumar, M. P. Kaushik, R. Konwar, R. S. Ampapathi and R. P. Tripathi, *Org. Lett.*, 2012, **14**, 4306.

278. C. E. Hoyle and C. N. Bowman, *Angew. Chem., Int. Ed.*, 2010, **49**, 1540.

279. A. A. Aimetti, R. K. Shoemaker, C. C. Lin and K. S. Anseth, *Chem. Commun.*, 2010, **46**, 4061.

280. A. A. Aimetti, K. R. Feaver and K. S. Anseth, *Chem. Commun.*, 2010, **46**, 5781.

281. X. Elduque, E. Pedroso and A. Grandas, *J. Org. Chem.*, 2014, **79**, 2843.

282. A. C. Fahrenbach and J. F. Stoddart, *Chem. - Asian J.*, 2011, **6**, 2660.

283. S.-M. Paek, H. Yun, N.-J. Kim, J.-W. Jung, D.-J. Chang, S. Lee, J. Yoo, H.-J. Park and Y.-G. Suh, *J. Org. Chem.*, 2008, **74**, 554.

284. D. Kim, J. Lee, P. J. Shim, J. I. Lim, T. Doi and S. Kim, *J. Org. Chem.*, 2002, **67**, 772.

285. S. Purushothaman, R. Prasanna, S. Lavanya and R. Raghunathan, *Tetrahedron Lett.*, 2013, **54**, 5744.

286. S. Purushothaman, R. Prasanna and R. Raghunathan, *Tetrahedron*, 2013, **69**, 9742.

287. C. Obradors, D. Leboeuf, J. Aydin and A. M. Echavarren, *Org. Lett.*, 2013, **15**, 1576.

288. L. Weber, *Curr. Med. Chem.*, 2002, **9**, 2085.

289. C. Hulme and V. Gore, *Curr. Med. Chem.*, 2003, **10**, 51.

290. I. Akritopoulou-Zanze, *Curr. Opin. Chem. Biol.*, 2008, **12**, 324.

291. L. Weber, *Drug Discovery Today*, 2002, 7, 143.

292. A. Domling, *Curr. Opin. Chem. Biol.*, 2002, **6**, 306.

293. A. Ulaczyk-Lesanko and D. G. Hall, *Curr. Opin. Chem. Biol.*, 2005, **9**, 266.

294. J. E. Biggs-Houck, A. Younai and J. T. Shaw, *Curr. Opin. Chem. Biol.*, 2010, **14**, 371.

295. A. K. Yudin and R. Hili, *Chem. - Eur. J.*, 2007, **13**, 6538.

296. R. Hili, V. Rai and A. K. Yudin, *J. Am. Chem. Soc.*, 2010, **132**, 2889.

297. M. J. Jebrail, A. H. Ng, V. Rai, R. Hili, A. K. Yudin and A. R. Wheeler, *Angew. Chem., Int. Ed.*, 2010, **49**, 8625.

298. B. K. W. Chung, J. L. Hickey, C. C. G. Scully, S. Zaretsky and A. K. Yudin, *MedChemComm*, 2013, **4**, 1124.

299. J. M. Knapp, J. C. Fettinger and M. J. Kurth, *Org. Lett.*, 2011, **13**, 4732.

300. G. Koopmanschap, E. Ruijter and R. Orru, *Beilstein J. Org. Chem.*, 2014, **10**, 544.

301. B. Beck, G. Larbig, B. Mejat, M. Magnin-Lachaux, A. Picard, E. Herdtweck and A. Dömling, *Org. Lett.*, 2003, **5**, 1047.

302. M. Oikawa, S. Naito and M. Sasaki, *Heterocycles*, 2007, **73**, 377.

303. T. Pirali, G. C. Tron, G. Masson and J. Zhu, *Org. Lett.*, 2007, **9**, 5275.

304. T. Pirali, G. C. Tron and J. Zhu, *Org. Lett.*, 2006, **8**, 4145.
305. T. Pirali, V. Faccio, R. Mossetti, A. A. Grolla, S. Di Micco, G. Bifulco, A. A. Genazzani and G. C. Tron, *Mol. Diversity*, 2010, **14**, 109.
306. S. Sugiyama, S. Fuse and T. Takahashi, *Tetrahedron*, 2011, **67**, 6654.
307. C. J. Roxburgh, *Tetrahedron*, 1995, **51**, 9767.
308. C. J. Roxburgh, *Tetrahedron*, 1993, **49**, 10749.
309. S. Baurle, T. Blume, A. Mengel, C. Parchmann, W. Skuballa, S. Basler, M. Schafer, D. Sulzle and H. P. Wrona-Metzinger, *Angew. Chem., Int. Ed.*, 2003, **42**, 3961.
310. S. Bäurle, T. Blume, E. Leroy, A. Mengel, C. Parchmann, K. Schmidt and W. Skuballa, *Tetrahedron Lett.*, 2004, **45**, 9569.
311. S. Baurle, T. Blume, J. Gunther, D. Henschel, R. C. Hillig, M. Husemann, A. Mengel, C. Parchmann, E. Schmid and W. Skuballa, *Bioorg. Med. Chem. Lett.*, 2004, **14**, 1673.
312. H. Stach and M. Hesse, *Tetrahedron*, 1988, **44**, 1573.
313. T. Witt, F. J. Hock and J. Lehmann, *J. Med. Chem.*, 2000, **43**, 2079.
314. B. Hoefgen, M. Decker, P. Mohr, A. M. Schramm, S. A. Rostom, H. El-Subbagh, P. M. Schweikert, D. R. Rudolf, M. U. Kassack and J. Lehmann, *J. Med. Chem.*, 2006, **49**, 760.
315. C. Enzensperger, S. Kilian, M. Ackermann, A. Koch, K. Kelch and J. Lehmann, *Bioorg. Med. Chem. Lett.*, 2007, **17**, 1399.
316. D. Robaa, C. Enzensperger, D. Abul Azm Sel, S. El Khawass el, O. El Sayed and J. Lehmann, *J. Med. Chem.*, 2010, **53**, 2646.
317. D. Robaa, R. Kretschmer, O. Siol, S. E. Abulazm, E. Elkhawass, J. Lehmann and C. Enzensperger, *Arch. Pharm.*, 2011, **344**, 28.
318. L. J. MacPherson, E. K. Bayburt, M. P. Capparelli, R. S. Bohacek, F. H. Clarke, R. D. Ghai, Y. Sakane, C. J. Berry, J. V. Peppard and A. J. Trapani, *J. Med. Chem.*, 1993, **36**, 3821.
319. J. E. Forsee and J. Aubé, *J. Org. Chem.*, 1999, **64**, 4381.
320. W. Zhao, Z. Li and J. Sun, *J. Am. Chem. Soc.*, 2013, **135**, 4680.
321. M. Traoré, F. Mietton, D. Maubon, M. Peuchmaur, F. Francisco Hilário, R. Pereira de Freitas, A. Bougdour, A. Curt, M. Maynadier, H. Vial, H. Pelloux, M.-A. Hakimi and Y.-S. Wong, *J. Org. Chem.*, 2013, **78**, 3655.
322. F. Kopp, C. F. Stratton, L. B. Akella and D. S. Tan, *Nat. Chem. Biol.*, 2012, **8**, 358.
323. J. Tummatorn and G. B. Dudley, *Org. Lett.*, 2011, **13**, 1572.
324. Y. G. Suh, Y. S. Lee, S. H. Kim, J. K. Jung, H. Yun, J. Jang, N. J. Kim and J. W. Jung, *Org. Biomol. Chem.*, 2012, **10**, 561.
325. Y. Huang, E. D. Strobel, C. Y. Ho, C. H. Reynolds, K. A. Conway, J. A. Piesvaux, D. E. Brenneman, G. J. Yohrling, H. Moore Arnold, D. Rosenthal, R. S. Alexander, B. A. Tounge, M. Mercken, M. Vandermeeren, M. H. Parker, A. B. Reitz and E. W. Baxter, *Bioorg. Med. Chem. Lett.*, 2010, **20**, 3158.
326. A. S. Ripka, K. A. Satyshur, R. S. Bohacek and D. H. Rich, *Org. Lett.*, 2001, **3**, 2309.

327. O. Baudoin, M.-P. Teulade-Fichou, J.-P. Vigneron and J.-M. Lehn, *J. Org. Chem.*, 1997, **62**, 5458.

328. C. M. Reid, C. Ebikeme, M. P. Barrett, E. M. Patzewitz, S. Muller, D. J. Robins and A. Sutherland, *Bioorg. Med. Chem. Lett.*, 2008, **18**, 2455.

329. C. M. Reid, C. Ebikeme, M. P. Barrett, E. M. Patzewitz, S. Muller, D. J. Robins and A. Sutherland, *Bioorg. Med. Chem. Lett.*, 2008, **18**, 5399.

330. M. J. Wingstrand, C. M. Madsen and M. H. Clausen, *Tetrahedron Lett.*, 2009, **50**, 693.

331. C. M. Madsen, M. Hansen, M. V. Thrane and M. H. Clausen, *Tetrahedron*, 2010, **66**, 9849.

332. Y. Zou, H. Mouhib, W. Stahl, A. Goeke, Q. Wang and P. Kraft, *Chem. - Eur. J.*, 2012, **18**, 7010.

333. C. Bughin, G. Masson and J. Zhu, *J. Org. Chem.*, 2007, **72**, 1826.

334. G. Zhao, X. Sun, H. Bienayme and J. Zhu, *J. Am. Chem. Soc.*, 2001, **123**, 6700.

335. K. C. Nicolaou, C. R. Hale, C. Ebner, C. Nilewski, C. F. Ahles and D. Rhoades, *Angew. Chem., Int. Ed.*, 2012, **51**, 4726.

336. V. Balraju, D. Srinivasa Reddy, M. Periasamy and J. Iqbal, *Tetrahedron Lett.*, 2005, **46**, 5207.

337. K. Ha, J. C. Monbaliu, B. C. Williams, G. G. Pillai, C. E. Ocampo, M. Zeller, C. V. Stevens and A. R. Katritzky, *Org. Biomol. Chem.*, 2012, **10**, 8055.

338. K. V. Lawson, T. E. Rose and P. G. Harran, *Tetrahedron*, 2013, **69**, 7683.

339. H. E. Giesbrecht, B. J. Knight, N. R. Tanguileg, C. R. Emerson and P. R. Blakemore, *Synlett*, 2010, **2010**, 374.

340. B. D. Jones, J. J. La Clair, C. E. Moore, A. L. Rheingold and M. D. Burkart, *Org. Lett.*, 2010, **12**, 4516.

341. N. K. Yee, V. Farina, I. N. Houpis, N. Haddad, R. P. Frutos, F. Gallou, X. J. Wang, X. Wei, R. D. Simpson, X. Feng, V. Fuchs, Y. Xu, J. Tan, L. Zhang, J. Xu, L. L. Smith-Keenan, J. Vitous, M. D. Ridges, E. M. Spinelli, M. Johnson, K. Donsbach, T. Nicola, M. Brenner, E. Winter, P. Kreye and W. Samstag, *J. Org. Chem.*, 2006, **71**, 7133.

342. C. Shu, X. Zeng, M. H. Hao, X. Wei, N. K. Yee, C. A. Busacca, Z. Han, V. Farina and C. H. Senanayake, *Org. Lett.*, 2008, **10**, 1303.

343. V. Farina, C. Shu, X. Zeng, X. Wei, Z. Han, N. K. Yee and C. H. Senanayake, *Org. Process Res. Dev.*, 2009, **13**, 250.

344. Z. J. Song, D. M. Tellers, M. Journet, J. T. Kuethe, D. Lieberman, G. Humphrey, F. Zhang, Z. Peng, M. S. Waters, D. Zewge, A. Nolting, D. Zhao, R. A. Reamer, P. G. Dormer, K. M. Belyk, I. W. Davies, P. N. Devine and D. M. Tschaen, *J. Org. Chem.*, 2011, **76**, 7804.

345. G.-J. Ho, K. M. Emerson, D. J. Mathre, R. F. Shuman and E. J. J. Grabowski, *J. Org. Chem.*, 1995, **60**, 3569.

346. J. Kong, C. Y. Chen, J. Balsells-Padros, Y. Cao, R. F. Dunn, S. J. Dolman, J. Janey, H. Li and M. J. Zacuto, *J. Org. Chem.*, 2012, **77**, 3820.

347. J. Kuethe, Y. L. Zhong, N. Yasuda, G. Beutner, K. Linn, M. Kim, B. Marcune, S. D. Dreher, G. Humphrey and T. Pei, *Org. Lett.*, 2013, **15**, 4174.

348. J. Arumugasamy, K. Arunachalam, D. Bauer, A. Becker, C. A. Caillet, R. Glynn, G. M. Latham, J. Lim, J. Liu, B. A. Mayes, A. Moussa, E. Rosinovsky, A. E. Salanson, A. F. Soret, A. Stewart, J. Wang and X. Wu, *Org. Process Res. Dev.*, 2013, **17**, 811.

349. H. R. Hoveyda, E. Marsault, R. Gagnon, A. P. Mathieu, M. Vezina, A. Landry, Z. Wang, K. Benakli, S. Beaubien, C. Saint-Louis, M. Brassard, J. F. Pinault, L. Ouellet, S. Bhat, M. Ramaseshan, X. Peng, L. Foucher, S. Beauchemin, P. Bherer, D. F. Veber, M. L. Peterson and G. L. Fraser, *J. Med. Chem.*, 2011, **54**, 8305.

350. E. Marsault, L. Ouellet, C. St-Louis, S. Beaubien, K. Benakli, H. R. Hoveyda, M. L. Peterson, S. Bhat, *Tranzyme Pharma Inc.*, Canada. *U.S. Pat. Appl.*, US 2009/0198050, 2009.

351. H. Li, X. Jiang, Y. H. Ye, C. Fan, T. Romoff and M. Goodman, *Org. Lett.*, 1999, **1**, 91.

352. E. Marsault, H. R. Hoveyda, R. Gagnon, M. L. Peterson, M. Vezina, C. Saint-Louis, A. Landry, J. F. Pinault, L. Ouellet, S. Beauchemin, S. Beaubien, A. Mathieu, K. Benakli, Z. Wang, M. Brassard, D. Lonergan, F. Bilodeau, M. Ramaseshan, N. Fortin, R. Lan, S. Li, F. Galaud, V. Plourde, M. Champagne, A. Doucet, P. Bherer, M. Gauthier, G. Olsen, G. Villeneuve, S. Bhat, L. Foucher, D. Fortin, X. Peng, S. Bernard, A. Drouin, R. Deziel, G. Berthiaume, Y. L. Dory, G. L. Fraser and P. Deslongchamps, *Bioorg. Med. Chem. Lett.*, 2008, **18**, 4731.

353. E. Marsault, H. R. Hoveyda, M. L. Peterson, R. Gagnon, M. Vezina, J. F. Pinault, A. Landry, C. Saint-Louis, L. G. Ouellet, S. Beauchemin, K. Benakli, S. Beaubien, M. Brassard, Z. Wang, M. Champagne, F. Galaud, N. Fortin, D. Fortin, V. Plourde, M. Ramaseshan, S. Bhat, F. Bilodeau, D. Lonergan, R. Lan, S. Li, G. Berthiaume, L. Foucher, X. Peng, Y. Dory and P. Deslongchamps, *Adv. Exp. Med. Biol.*, 2009, **611**, 15.

354. E. Vedejs, S. Lin, A. Klapars and J. Wang, *J. Am. Chem. Soc.*, 1996, **118**, 9796.

355. L. Zhang and J. P. Tam, *J. Am. Chem. Soc.*, 1999, **121**, 3311.

356. S. Beaubien, H. R. Hoveyda, M. Vezina, E. Marsault, H. Tremblay, L. Foucher and K. Benakli, *Adv. Exp. Med. Biol.*, 2009, **611**, 13.

357. E. Marsault, H. R. Hoveyda, M. L. Peterson, C. Saint-Louis, A. Landry, M. Vezina, L. Ouellet, Z. Wang, M. Ramaseshan, S. Beaubien, K. Benakli, S. Beauchemin, R. Deziel, T. Peeters and G. L. Fraser, *J. Med. Chem.*, 2006, **49**, 7190.

358. E. Marsault, K. Benakli, S. Beaubien, C. Saint-Louis, R. Deziel and G. Fraser, *Bioorg. Med. Chem. Lett.*, 2007, **17**, 4187.

359. J. Chen, F. Rong, B. Shan, Y. Chen, Y. Li, H. Yu, L. Chen, T. Kuang, S. Li, Y. Chen, J. Du, C. Ai, J. Li, X. Li, C. Shi, Z. Jiang, Y. Long, Q. Gao, Z. Wang, K. Xu, X. Ran, H. Yi, D. Zhao, H. Qiao, J. Shen, B. Liu, C. Liu, K. Wu, X. Geng, J. Tan, D. McLeod, H. Frost, G. Bai, G. Goetz, J. Federico Iii, C. Whitney-Pickett, M. Troutman, M. C. Noe, C. Guimaraes, D. W. Piotrowski and T. V. Magee, *Tetrahedron Lett.*, 2013, **54**, 3298.

360. P. J. Murray, M. Kranz, M. Ladlow, S. Taylor, F. Berst, A. B. Holmes, K. N. Keavey, A. Jaxa-Chamiec, P. W. Seale, P. Stead, R. J. Upton, S. L. Croft, W. Clegg and M. R. Elsegood, *Bioorg. Med. Chem. Lett.*, 2001, **11**, 773.
361. F. Berst, M. Ladlow and A. B. Holmes, *Chem. Commun.*, 2002, 508.
362. A. Alex, D. S. Millan, M. Perez, F. Wakenhut and G. A. Whitlock, *MedChemComm*, 2011, **2**, 669.
363. B. Over, P. McCarren, P. Artursson, M. Foley, F. Giordanetto, G. Gronberg, C. Hilgendorf, M. D. t. Lee, P. Matsson, G. Muncipinto, M. Pellisson, M. W. Perry, R. Svensson, J. R. Duvall and J. Kihlberg, *J. Med. Chem.*, 2014, **57**, 2746.
364. H. An, B. D. Haly and P. D. Cook, *Bioorg. Med. Chem. Lett.*, 1998, **8**, 2345.
365. T. Wang, H. An, T. A. Vickers, R. Bharadwaj and P. D. Cook, *Tetrahedron*, 1998, **54**, 7955.
366. X. Li and D. R. Liu, *Angew. Chem., Int. Ed.*, 2004, **43**, 4848.
367. C. T. Calderone and D. R. Liu, *Curr. Opin. Chem. Biol.*, 2004, **8**, 645.
368. Z. J. Gartner, B. N. Tse, R. Grubina, J. B. Doyon, T. M. Snyder and D. R. Liu, *Science*, 2004, **305**, 1601.
369. B. N. Tse, T. M. Snyder, Y. Shen and D. R. Liu, *J. Am. Chem. Soc.*, 2008, **130**, 15611.
370. R. E. Kleiner, C. E. Dumelin, G. C. Tiu, K. Sakurai and D. R. Liu, *J. Am. Chem. Soc.*, 2010, **132**, 11779.
371. G. Georghiou, R. E. Kleiner, M. Pulkoski-Gross, D. R. Liu and M. A. Seeliger, *Nat. Chem. Biol.*, 2012, **8**, 366.
372. J. Lee, J. F. Bond, N. Terrett, F. G. Favaloro, D. Wang, T. F. Briggs, B. A. Seigal, W.-C. Sun and S. F. Hale, Ensemble Discovery Corp., USA. *PCT Int. Appl.*, WO 2010/022249, 2010.
373. M. Taylor, N. K. Terrett, W. H. Connors, K. C. Shortsleeves, B. A. Seigal, C. Snedeker, S. P. Hale, T. F. Briggs, F. G. Favaloro, T. J. Cipriani, D. Yan, S. L. Alexander, A. Thorarensen and L. Xing, Ensemble Therapeutics Corp. USA, *PCT Int. Appl.*, WO 2013/116682, 2013.
374. D. Livingston, American College of Rheumatology (ACR) Annual Meeting, 2012, Abstract #1810. http://www.ensemblediscovery.com/news/pdfs/ACR%20Poster%20DJL-v1-1%20(2).pdf.
375. M. W. Kanan, M. M. Rozenman, K. Sakurai, T. M. Snyder and D. R. Liu, *Nature*, 2004, **431**, 545.
376. L. A. Wessjohann, D. G. Rivera and O. E. Vercillo, *Chem. Rev.*, 2009, **109**, 796.
377. E. A. Jefferson, S. Arakawa, L. B. Blyn, A. Miyaji, S. A. Osgood, R. Ranken, L. M. Risen and E. E. Swayze, *J. Med. Chem.*, 2002, **45**, 3430.
378. E. A. Jefferson, E. E. Swayze, S. A. Osgood, A. Miyaji, L. M. Risen and L. B. Blyn, *Bioorg. Med. Chem. Lett.*, 2003, **13**, 1635.
379. M. Giulianotti and A. Nefzi, *Tetrahedron Lett.*, 2003, **44**, 5307.
380. E. Comer, H. Liu, A. Joliton, A. Clabaut, C. Johnson, L. B. Akella and L. A. Marcaurelle, *Proc. Natl. Acad. Sci., U.S.A.*, 2011, **108**, 6751.

381. D. Lee, J. K. Sello and S. L. Schreiber, *J. Am. Chem. Soc.*, 1999, **121**, 10648.
382. Y. K. Kim, M. A. Arai, T. Arai, J. O. Lamenzo, E. F. Dean, 3rd, N. Patterson, P. A. Clemons and S. L. Schreiber, *J. Am. Chem. Soc.*, 2004, **126**, 14740.
383. B. Z. Stanton, L. F. Peng, N. Maloof, K. Nakai, X. Wang, J. L. Duffner, K. M. Taveras, J. M. Hyman, S. W. Lee, A. N. Koehler, J. K. Chen, J. L. Fox, A. Mandinova and S. L. Schreiber, *Nat. Chem. Biol.*, 2009, **5**, 154.
384. L. F. Peng, B. Z. Stanton, N. Maloof, X. Wang and S. L. Schreiber, *Bioorg. Med. Chem. Lett.*, 2009, **19**, 6319.
385. C. Dockendorff, M. M. Nagiec, M. Weiwer, S. Buhrlage, A. Ting, P. P. Nag, A. Germain, H. J. Kim, W. Youngsaye, C. Scherer, M. Bennion, L. Xue, B. Z. Stanton, T. A. Lewis, L. Macpherson, M. Palmer, M. A. Foley, J. R. Perez and S. L. Schreiber, *ACS Med. Chem. Lett.*, 2012, **3**, 808.
386. D. P. Curran, *Med. Res. Rev.*, 1999, **19**, 432.
387. W. Zhang, *Curr. Opin. Drug Discovery Dev.*, 2004, 7, 784.
388. J. D. Moretti, X. Wang and D. P. Curran, *J. Am. Chem. Soc.*, 2012, **134**, 7963.
389. D. Morton, S. Leach, C. Cordier, S. Warriner and A. Nelson, *Angew. Chem., Int. Ed.*, 2009, **48**, 104.
390. D. R. Schmidt, O. Kwon and S. L. Schreiber, *J. Comb. Chem.*, 2004, **6**, 286.
391. A. B. Beeler, D. E. Acquilano, Q. Su, F. Yan, B. L. Roth, J. S. Panek and J. A. Porco, *J. Comb. Chem.*, 2005, 7, 673.
392. T. Takahashi, S. Kusaka, T. Doi, T. Sunazuka and S. Omura, *Angew. Chem., Int. Ed.*, 2003, **42**, 5230.
393. T. Katoh, Y. Goto, M. S. Reza and H. Suga, *Chem. Commun.*, 2011, 47, 9946.
394. T. L. Aboye and J. A. Camarero, *J. Biol. Chem.*, 2012, **287**, 27026.
395. A. A. Bowers, *MedChemComm*, 2012, **3**, 905.
396. J. M. Smith, J. R. Frost and R. Fasan, *J. Org. Chem.*, 2013, **78**, 3525.
397. J. R. Frost, J. M. Smith and R. Fasan, *Curr. Opin. Struct. Biol.*, 2013, **23**, 571.
398. H. Sancheti and J. A. Camarero, *Adv. Drug Delivery Rev.*, 2009, **61**, 908.
399. R. Kimura and J. A. Camarero, *Protein Peptide Lett.*, 2005, **12**, 789.
400. J. A. Camarero and T. W. Muir, *J. Am. Chem. Soc.*, 1999, **121**, 5597.
401. R. H. Kimura, A. T. Tran and J. A. Camarero, *Angew. Chem., Int. Ed.*, 2006, **45**, 973.
402. B. F. Conlan, A. D. Gillon, D. J. Craik and M. A. Anderson, *Biopolymers*, 2010, **94**, 573.
403. B. F. Conlan and M. A. Anderson, *Curr. Pharm. Des.*, 2011, **17**, 4318.
404. S. Tsukiji and T. Nagamune, *ChemBioChem*, 2009, **10**, 787.
405. R. Parthasarathy, S. Subramanian and E. T. Boder, *Bioconjugate Chem.*, 2007, **18**, 469.

406. J. Grunewald and M. A. Marahiel, *Microbiol. Mol. Biol. Rev.*, 2006, **70**, 121.
407. T. Bosma, A. Kuipers, E. Bulten, L. de Vries, R. Rink and G. N. Moll, *Appl. Environ. Microbiol.*, 2011, 77, 6794.
408. A. Tavassoli and S. J. Benkovic, *Nat. Protoc.*, 2007, **2**, 1126.
409. Y. Yamagishi, I. Shoji, S. Miyagawa, T. Kawakami, T. Katoh, Y. Goto and H. Suga, *Chem. Biol.*, 2011, **18**, 1562.
410. Y. Hayashi, J. Morimoto and H. Suga, *ACS Chem. Biol.*, 2012, 7, 607.
411. Y. Tanaka, C. J. Hipolito, A. D. Maturana, K. Ito, T. Kuroda, T. Higuchi, T. Katoh, H. E. Kato, M. Hattori, K. Kumazaki, T. Tsukazaki, R. Ishitani, H. Suga and O. Nureki, *Nature*, 2013, **496**, 247.
412. C. J. Hipolito, Y. Tanaka, T. Katoh, O. Nureki and H. Suga, *Molecules*, 2013, **18**, 10514.
413. Y. V. Schlippe, M. C. Hartman, K. Josephson and J. W. Szostak, *J. Am. Chem. Soc.*, 2012, **134**, 10469.
414. C. Heinis, T. Rutherford, S. Freund and G. Winter, *Nat. Chem. Biol.*, 2009, **5**, 502.
415. S. Chen, J. Morales-Sanfrutos, A. Angelini, B. Cutting and C. Heinis, *ChemBioChem*, 2012, **13**, 1032.
416. J. M. Smith, F. Vitali, S. A. Archer and R. Fasan, *Angew. Chem., Int. Ed.*, 2011, **50**, 5075.
417. M. Satyanarayana, F. Vitali, J. R. Frost and R. Fasan, *Chem. Commun.*, 2012, **48**, 1461.
418. M. D. Tianero, M. S. Donia, T. S. Young, P. G. Schultz and E. W. Schmidt, *J. Am. Chem. Soc.*, 2012, **134**, 418.
419. R. M. Kohli and C. T. Walsh, *Chem. Commun.*, 2003, 297.
420. F. Kopp and M. A. Marahiel, *Nat. Prod. Rep.*, 2007, **24**, 735.
421. C. T. Walsh, *Acc. Chem. Res.*, 2008, **41**, 4.
422. R. M. Kohli, M. D. Burke, J. Tao and C. T. Walsh, *J. Am. Chem. Soc.*, 2003, **125**, 7160.
423. J. A. McIntosh, C. R. Robertson, V. Agarwal, S. K. Nair, G. W. Bulaj and E. W. Schmidt, *J. Am. Chem. Soc.*, 2010, **132**, 15499.
424. J. Touati, A. Angelini, M. J. Hinner and C. Heinis, *ChemBioChem*, 2011, **12**, 38.
425. T. Hamamoto, M. Sisido, T. Ohtsuki and M. Taki, *Chem. Commun.*, 2011, **47**, 9116.
426. C. J. White and A. K. Yudin, *Nat. Chem.*, 2011, 3, 509.
427. J. Blankenstein and J. Zhu, *Eur. J. Org. Chem.*, 2005, **2005**, 1949.
428. S. F. Brady, S. L. Varga, R. M. Freidinger, D. A. Schwenk, M. Mendlowski, F. W. Holly and D. F. Veber, *J. Org. Chem.*, 1979, **44**, 3101.
429. A. B. Yongye, Y. Li, M. A. Giulianotti, Y. Yu, R. A. Houghten and K. Martinez-Mayorga, *J. Comput.-Aided Mol. Des.*, 2009, **23**, 677.
430. T. R. White, C. M. Renzelman, A. C. Rand, T. Rezai, C. M. McEwen, V. M. Gelev, R. A. Turner, R. G. Linington, S. S. Leung, A. S. Kalgutkar,

J. N. Bauman, Y. Zhang, S. Liras, D. A. Price, A. M. Mathiowetz, M. P. Jacobson and R. S. Lokey, *Nat. Chem. Biol.*, 2011, 7, 810.

431. A. C. Rand, S. S. F. Leung, H. Eng, C. J. Rotter, R. Sharma, A. S. Kalgutkar, Y. Zhang, M. V. Varma, K. A. Farley, B. Khunte, C. Limberakis, D. A. Price, S. Liras, A. M. Mathiowetz, M. P. Jacobson and R. S. Lokey, *MedChemComm*, 2012, **3**, 1282.

432. A. Thakkar, T. B. Trinh and D. Pei, *ACS Comb. Sci.*, 2013, **15**, 120.

433. J. C. Collins and K. James, *MedChemComm*, 2012, **3**, 1489.

434. For a recent review on the PK-ADME characteristics of macrocyclic drugs on the market and in development see: F. Giordanetto and J. Kihlberg, *J. Med. Chem.*, 2014, **57**, 278.

Subject Index